Handbuch der Urologie
Encyclopedia of Urology · Encyclopédie d'Urologie

Gesamtdisposition · Outline · Disposition générale

HANDBUCH DER UROLOGIE

ENCYCLOPEDIA OF UROLOGY

ENCYCLOPÉDIE D'UROLOGIE

HERAUSGEGEBEN VON · EDITED BY
PUBLIÉE SOUS LA DIRECTION DE

C. E. ALKEN   V. W. DIX   H. M. WEYRAUCH
HOMBURG (SAAR) LONDON   SAN FRANCISCO

E. WILDBOLZ
BERN

V/1

SPRINGER-VERLAG BERLIN HEIDELBERG GMBH 1962

DIAGNOSTIC RADIOLOGY

BY

RUBIN H. FLOCKS
IOWA CITY

GÖSTA JÖNSSON
LUND

KNUT LINDBLOM
STOCKHOLM

OLLE OLSSON
LUND

RAGNAR ROMANUS
GÖTEBORG

CHESTER C. WINTER
COLUMBUS

WITH 402 FIGURES

SPRINGER-VERLAG BERLIN HEIDELBERG GMBH 1962

ISBN 978-3-642-45989-4   ISBN 978-3-642-45987-0 (eBook)
DOI 10.1007/978-3-642-45987-0

© Springer-Verlag Berlin Heidelberg 1962
Ursprünglich erschienen bei Springer-Verlag OHG/Berlin · Göttingen · Heidelberg 1962
Softcover reprint of the hardcover 1st edition 1962

Contents

Contributors to volume V/1

RUBIN H. FLOCKS, M. D., Professor, Department of Urology, University of Iowa, Iowa City, Iowa (USA).

GÖSTA JÖNSSON, M. D., Ass. Professor of Urology, University of Lund, Head of Urologic Unit at Surgical Department, University Hospital, Lund (Sweden).

KNUT LINDBLOM, M. D., Professor, Karolinska Sjukhuset, Roentgendiagnostic Department, Stockholm (Sweden).

OLLE OLSSON, M. D., Professor of Diagnostic Radiology, University of Lund, Director of Roentgendiagnostic Department of University Hospital, Lund (Sweden).

RAGNAR ROMANUS, M. D., Professor of Surgery, University of Göteborg, Sahlgrenska Sjukhuset, Göteborg (Sweden).

CHESTER C. WINTER, M. D., Professor and Head of the Department of Urology, Ohio State University Medical School, Columbus, Ohio (USA).

Roentgen examination of the kidney and the ureter

By

OLLE OLSSON

In collaboration with

GÖSTA JÖNSSON

With 258 figures

Preface

This volume is based on the accumulated experience gained in daily routine work in a large roentgen-diagnostic centre and on continuous research by members of the staff. The centre serves *all* departments of the University Hospital, Lund, Sweden, which also includes a highly specialized department of urology (Director: Ass. Professor GÖSTA JÖNSSON, M. D.) and a corresponding medical department for renal diseases (Director: Professor NILS ALWALL, M. D.).

It is a pleasure for me to have this opportunity of expressing the gratitude of all members of the roentgen-diagnostic centre to the directors and staffs of the above-mentioned departments for close and fruitful co-operation.

Roentgen-diagnostic Department,
University Hospital, Lund, Sweden

OLLE OLSSON

A. Introduction

The previous edition of the Encyclopedia of Urology, Handbuch der Urologie, did not include a special volume on roentgen-diagnostics. The decision of the editors to include urologic roentgenology in the series of monographs may have been dictated by the importance they attach to diagnostic radiology in general and special examinations of patients with urologic diseases. Another reason may be that the range of methods has been widened and that the need of a comprehensive discussion of the methods including new techniques in a separate volume therefore appears obvious. Technical advances have also made it necessary to revise our opinions of various fundamental examination methods, and cumulative experience concerning the roentgenology of some diseases and new achievements in others have modified our conceptions.

This volume deals exclusively with roentgen-diagnostics of the kidney and ureter. Other aspects are dealt with comprehensively in other volumes. The differential-diagnostic problems have therefore received little space in this volume. The diagnostic criteria are, however, described in detail in the various chapters and the roentgenologic differential-diagnosis is stressed when considered important.

The bladder and the urethra are dealt with in a special volume. For details on the lower urinary tract in diseases involving the entire urinary system the reader is therefore referred to that volume.

Perusal of the urologic literature and current journals will convince any critical reader of the need of a comprehensive presentation of urologic diagnostic radiology in which the examination techniques and evaluation of the findings are based on fundamental roentgen-diagnostic principles. It is apparent from the literature that diagnostic radiology is widely practised without sufficient fundamental knowledge of physics, of the different examination methods, of radiation protection, pharmacology of the contrast media, physiologic principles of dynamics, etc., all factors to be considered in the planning and performance of the examinations and in the interpretation of the findings.

Diagnostic radiology requires special training. Such training should first span the entire field before specialization is attempted in any particular branch of it. It is not possible to master any sector of diagnostic radiology without wide knowledge of the subject as a whole. Diagnostic radiology of the urinary tract occupies a central position in general diagnostic radiology: therefore it is not desirable to separate it off as a special branch. On the contrary, roentgen-diagnostics of the urinary tract places high demands on the examiner's knowledge of diagnostic radiology in general because the original urologic disease may manifest itself outside the urinary tract, e.g. in the skeleton, lungs, vascular system, etc. just as the urologic disease may be only one component of a more or less generalized disease.

Several fundamental technical details such as film, processing units, roentgen machines, high voltage technique, automatization, radiation protection, pharmacology and side effects of contrast media etc. must be studied and tested in various branches of diagnostic radiology and evaluated on the basis of experience as wide as possible. Technical skill in the performance of certain details such as arterial puncture and catheterization can only be acquired and maintained if the daily work includes a number of angiographic examinations. All technical variations as well as measures to avoid complications require cumulative experience.

The technical equipment, particularly for angiography, is specialized and expensive and thus cannot be procured for occasional examinations.

Technical advances and clinical research have given diagnostic radiology a value of its own: therefore it is wrong to regard it or use it simply as a gratuitous supplement to the clinical investigation of any disease. Diagnostic radiology yields information on anatomic, pathologic and to no small extent also on physiologic conditions. The method is based on a refined technique permitting wide variation and on detailed roentgen anatomy, which is ordinary normal anatomy with special attention to the many normal variants and presented in detailed densograms known as roentgen pictures.

Normal and pathologic conditions should be studied as closely as possible with all necessary variations of the examination technique, and the results of the examination should be described in anatomic and pathologic nomenclature and not in photographic terms.

Only findings made in complete examinations should be considered, but then in full detail.

If a roentgen examination is performed only half-heartedly or if it is interrupted simply because preliminary findings happen to fit in with a preconceived opinion, or if technically poor examinations are accepted, the result may be a serious misdiagnosis.

Roentgen examination must be properly performed, and definite conclusions must only be drawn against the background of the clinical picture. The best results are obtained if the examination is carried out with close co-operation between the roentgenologist and the urologist.

Principles of examination. The indications for the examination should be well founded, problems to be solved well defined, and the examination planned accordingly.

The doctor requesting the examination must know what knowledge might be gained from it, and he should be able to assess the strain the examination implies to his patient.

The examiner should be competent and be able to perform the examination in the most rational manner. The examination should therefore always be performed by, or under the supervision of, the roentgenologist. Amateurish examinations are condemnable.

The equipment should be of good quality. The roentgen machines must give the necessary output. The tubes, film, cassette material etc. must be of good quality.

The patient should be properly prepared for the examination.

Every examination should be performed in such a way as to yield as much information as possible. This implies that the examination should include all necessary technical variations.

No examination should be performed in a standardized way but varied according to the information desired and problems arising in the course of the examination.

During an examination planned in a certain way new problems may arise. The subsequent procedure should then be modified in a manner providing the best possibilities of solving such new problems.

Utilization of all possible modifications of a method are necessary to obtain the information desired. The roentgenologist must therefore perform or supervise the examination and study the films continuously while the patient is still available for further study, if necessary.

The films should document the results of a competent examination. Diagnostic radiology consisting of examination of films produced under standardized conditions is liable to lead to much guesswork and is therefore condemnable.

B. Equipment

The following presentation is limited to a few points of general interest concerning the equipment necessary for urologic roentgen-diagnosis.

The roentgen apparatus should have a high output to permit performance of examinations with high voltage technique. The apparatus should satisfy the highest requirements of routine work, *i.e.* renal angiography. This examination thus dictates the capacity of the apparatus. The frequency of exposures necessary for routine work, 5—10 representing the various phases of the renal circulation, can be secured with a 6-valve machine, which is also preferable to a large 4-valve machine from the point of view of radiation dose.

All types of roentgen examinations require strict consideration of the radiation dose. This holds especially for urologic roentgen examinations.

The radiation quantity needed to produce a roentgen picture is represented by the product of current and time, MaS. The tube potential controls the passage of roentgen quanta produced in the roentgen tube through the object to the intensifying screens in the cassette, which transform the roentgen quanta into light quanta producing the picture in the film. High voltage, so to say, forces more radiation through the object to the film, whereas at low voltage more radiation is absorbed in the object. Therefore the MaS product is influenced by the potential in that the higher the voltage that can be used, the lower the MaS product need be. The ratio is most favourable for voltages up to about 150 kV.

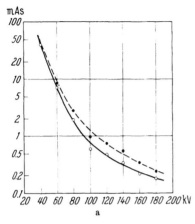

a

The higher the voltage below this limit the smaller the radiation quantity delivered (Fig. 1 a– c).

High voltage, however, implies increased secondary radiation. When working with high voltage, secondary radiation must be controlled as far as possible. This can be achieved by means of careful primary coning and, if possible, compression of the object, and the use of good secondary screening. If the examiner is used to working with low voltages, he will have to familiarize himself with the type of pictures obtained when high voltage is used. In his daily routine work the radiologist should regularly use maximal voltages compatible with an optimal yield of diagnostic data.

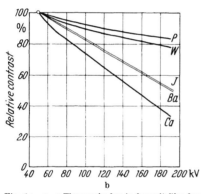

b

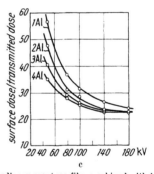

c

Fig. 1a—c. a The required mAs for unit film density with an ordinary roentgen film combined with barium lead sulphate screens ("high-voltage screens"). The dotted line, which is introduced for comparison, represents the values of the calcium tungstate screens. (Film: Cea Vicor X. Screens: Kodak Type 80. 16 cm wax phantom.) b Relative contrast of some different substances recorded with a screen-film combination. 50 kV = 100 %. c Surface dose in relation to transmitted dose at different voltages with 1, 2, 3 and 4 mm Al total filtration. (After MATTSSON)

High voltage results in loss of contrast because of increasing secondary radiation and because of specific absorption. Calcifications in necrotic tissue, for example, and calcareous stones will lose in contrast. Particularly in the detection of small or less opaque calculi the voltage plays an important rôle. The contrast element most commonly used in contrast media for urologic diagnostic roentgenology is iodine. With high voltage this, too, approaches the risk zone. For these reasons one must make a compromise between intensity of contrast and choice of voltage.

High voltage produces well exposed pictures showing structure rather than outline. In principle, a roentgenogram should be judged by the information it yields and not by its appearance from an aesthetic point of view. This is certainly a truism but experience has nevertheless taught that it is well worth pointing out.

High voltage implies low MaS. The MaS-product can be represented in high current and short time. This permits a shortening of the exposure time and thereby a better possibility of securing sharp pictures. It cannot be emphasized sufficiently that good quality films are necessary for all diagnostic work.

Pyelography must be done under fluoroscopic control. Any examination table for pyelography not permitting fluoroscopy is unsatisfactory. It must offer the possibility of taking films under fluoroscopy and with a Potter-Bucky grid. Fluoroscopy should be done under optimal conditions: The examiner should be well dark adapted. Current should be low (1—3 Ma), voltage high (about 90 kV), tube filter corresponding to at least 3 mm Al, tube-object-distance reasonable, and fluoroscopy time the shortest possible. For fluoroscopy in connexion with an operation of any kind an image amplifier should preferably be used in order to permit illumination. As pointed out by KOCKUM, LIDÉN & NORMAN (1958), work with image intensifiers requires the same precautions as work with conventional fluoroscopes.

Angiography requires satisfactory equipment. To perform this type of examination with make-shift apparatus is no longer defensible. A film changer for film sheets or rolls should be available, though only one-plane films are necessary. The changer should be equipped with a program selector and preferably with a timing accessory in order to be able to keep the dose of contrast medium low and to take a series of films at a rate dictated by the pulse frequency and the circulation rate. It is better not to do renal angiography at all than to do it incompletely or in a *laissez-faire* manner.

For cineradiography some sort of image amplifying technique should be used, with an image amplifier with or without television technique. Other methods give far too large a radiation dose.

The films should be examined under optimal conditions. This implies, among other things, that the viewing box space should be large enough to permit simultaneous examination of all the films taken during a urographic examination and permit comparison with one or more previous examinations. To examine single films from a urographic series without the possibility of comparing them with films taken on previous occasions is not satisfactory.

All work should be done with the right tool. Special work may require special tools. If such tools are not available, the work should not be done.

C. Radiation protection

Radiologists have always endeavoured to reduce the radiation dose received by patients and personnel. Investigations, particularly of genetic hazards of ionizing radiation, have increased the interest in such endeavours. Many conclusions on the proportion between radiation for diagnostic purposes and the total radiation of the population and on genetic effect as well as general effect of roentgen radiation are based on loose grounds. Reliable research, however, has shown that there is every reason to secure maximum protection against radiation, particularly of the gonads. A fair proportion of the radiation received by the reproductive organs is due to urologic diagnostic radiology. A reduction of the dose in this field is thus highly desirable.

In highly civilized countries the cumulative dose received in association with roentgen examinations is said to be less than 25 per cent of the background radiation. Of artificial radiation sources, roentgen examination is the most important. In Sweden urography including plain roentgenograms represents about 20 % of the genetically significant dose produced by roentgen examinations

(LARSSON 1958). A marked reduction in the radiation dose during urography thus markedly influences the dose received by the entire population.

For radiation protection the first point to be borne in mind is that examinations, particularly of patients in fertile age, should be performed only for proper indications. The range of indication should be kept extremely narrow for pregnant women. The reasons for which the examination is requested must be properly defined.

The second point to be stressed is that every examination should be performed with proper skill and the technique selected should be such as to give the best possible information.

The third point is to keep the radiation dose as low as possible. This can be achieved by using fluoroscopy—in spite of well trimmed technique—as seldom and for as short a time as possible, and by the use of a minimal number of exposures with the smallest possible field and highest possible voltage. Such a small increase in voltage as from 60 to 90 kV can bring down the MaS-product from 250 to 30 with a corresponding reduction of the radiation dose.

Reduction of the radiation dose to which the patient is exposed during urologic roentgen examination can also be secured by covering the gonads of the patient with lead rubber. This is simple as far as males are concerned, but can also be secured to a fair degree in females. It is important that this precaution be strictly observed. We have found that during urography without protection of the gonads the testes will receive an average dose of 1,900 mr as against only 140 mr with lead protection and 20 mr with all proper radiation protection measures. On plain radiography including a film of the bladder the dose could be reduced to 5 mr. In females proper protection will reduce the gonadal dose received in association with roentgenography of the kidneys by 30—40%. In examinations in which the films must include the bladder, such as in complete urography, the reduction in the dose of females is small because some of the films must include the ovaries. The number of such films should therefore be kept as low as possible.

As to the personnel, regulations for radiation protection should be meticulously observed. During the exposure no member of the staff should be in the examination room but in the well protected control room. The examination table for fluoroscopy should be equipped with well designed protective arrangements and the examiner should wear a lead rubber apron and gloves. Should it be necessary for the roentgenologist to be in the examination room during the exposure, e.g. during pyelography, effective screening must be possible. This is best secured by hanging up a suitably designed rubber curtain. The curtain may be placed and shaped according to specific requirements.

Continuous control of the personnel by the film method, for example, is to be recommended. For this purpose all members of our staff wear a film readily visible on their lapel or blouse. Half of the film is completely protected. The film is developed after it has been worn for a week. If the wearer is found to have been exposed to radiation, he is kept under special observation and given necessary instructions.

Continous control and instruction of radiation protection is always necessary and should be part and parcel of daily routine work.

D. Preparation of the patient for roentgen examination

For a roentgen examination to yield a maximum amount of information, the patient must be properly prepared.

A self-evident but unfortunately often neglected part of the preparation is to inform the patient about what is to be done and why. This is all the more important if the examination is liable to cause discomfort or pain or imply a strain on the patient. Such information promotes co-operation with the patient and thereby facilitates the examination.

In addition special preparation is sometimes necessary. Since the kidneys and the urinary tract are situated in the retroperitoneal space behind the peritoneal organs, the contents of the digestive tract can be projected onto the urinary tract. The digestive tract should therefore be as empty as possible at examination of the kidneys and ureters. This can be secured by ordering the patient not to eat on the morning of the examination and by cleansing the tract. We generally give the patient a purgative the day before the examination and two enemas, one the evening before, and one on the morning of the examination. As a purgative we usually use castor oil, which is given early on the day before the examination. If it is given late in the day, it will disturb the patient's sleep. If the patient cannot tolerate such a strong purgative as castor oil, a milder laxative may be used, but then preferably on two days in succession. Occasionally drastic purgatives are necessary, such as neodrast (dioxophenyl-isatin and sacch. lactis) or Clysodrast® (diacetoxidifenyl-pyridyl-uretan and tannic acid). These purgatives exert their effect mainly on the large intestine. Sometimes, on the other hand, simpler preparation is sufficient if intestinal function is normal.

The most important factor in all preparation is to get rid of intestinal gas, particulary in the colon. The gas is often abundant owing to air swallowed or to impaired absorption of gas. The major part of intestinal gas is swallowed air, which can pass rapidly into the colon. It has thus been shown (MAGNUSSON 1931) that air introduced into the stomach by means of a stomach tube passes to the caecum within 6—15 minutes. Swallowed air is usually removed by eructation. In bedridden patients, however, swallowed air passes through the pylorus, particularly if they lie on the left side, *i.e.* when the pylorus is the highest part of the stomach. This is one of the reasons why patients confined to bed generally have more intestinal gas than others. Before the examination the patient should therefore, if possible, be up and about or sitting up or lying on the right side, but not on the left. Certain factors decrease the production of gas, such as suitable composition of the diet. The diet should not contain foodstuffs rich in cellulose such as cabbage.

According to LILJA & WAHREN (1934), in pyelography meteorism is to a large extent due to impaired absorption of gas as a consequence of cystoscopy and trauma of catheterization, which causes a reflexogenic circulatory disturbance in the splenic area. They claim that meteorism is less pronounced if cystoscopy is performed under good anesthesia.

Various drugs have been used to diminish the intestinal gas, such as absorbents, atropine, pitressin, etc. The simplest and most important procedure is, however, to cleanse the intestine of gas and fecal matter by purgation and enema in the way described above. In addition the examination should be performed early in the morning and without undue delay after the last enema, besides which the patient should, if possible, be up and about before the examination. If disturbing meteorism or fecal contents persists, the patient may be prepared again the following day or he may be given a tannic acid enema, which empties and contracts the intestine. Such an enema should be prepared very carefully and contain $7^1/_2$ g tannic acid in $1^1/_2$ litres of water. It should not be given to old or very ill patients. The intestine may, of course, be cleansed in various ways modified according to the patient's condition, age etc. and sensitivity to inconvenience experienced by purgation. The only important thing is that the intestine is really properly cleansed.

Opinions differ on the use of enema, particularly in the preparation of the patient for urography. It is claimed that the fluid infused can be absorbed from the bowel and cause diuresis with consequent dilution of the contrast excreted and decrease in density. It has, however, been shown (STEINERT 1952) that absorption of the water is so slow as to be negligible provided urography is performed soon after the enema. Our experience definitely endorses this opinion.

In children meteorism is more common than in adults. WYATT (1941) recommends the same measures to control meteorism in children as in adults, *i.e.* before the examination the child should be erect, prone with the head slightly raised or lying on the right side, but never on the left. A detailed rationale for managing meteorism has been devised by GYLLENSVÄRD, LODIN & MYKLAND (1953). They recommend sedatives, the postures described above, and that the child be given a milk meal with addition of a viscosing agent.

The most important thing is to remove gas liable to be projected over the kidneys. An simple measure for this purpose has been suggested by KOSENOW (1955). He gives children 100—250 cm³ fluid in the form of milk beverage or tea or juice before urography. The stomach thus filled with gas and fluid pushes aside intestinal gas so that with the patient supine the kidneys will be projected over the homogenous stomach. One can, however, also fill the stomach with gas and thus secure a large homogenous gas bubble over the kidneys. This can be performed with the use of a carbonated fruit salt or carbonated beverage (BERG & ALLEN 1952, BERG & DUFRESNE 1956).

Examination of a patient during an acute attack of a disease requires no preparation. More specific preparations are discussed in connection with specific examination methods.

E. Examination methods

The commonest basic roentgen diagnostic methods routinely used in urologic diseases will be discussed with due attention to the prerequisites of the methods and to their technique. In addition a description will be given of the normal roentgen anatomy constituting the basis on which any discussion of pathologic conditions must be founded. Plain roentgenography will be dealt with first, this method being a fundamental prerequisite of all other roentgen examinations; and then the supplementary examinations such as tomography, retroperitoneal pneumography and examination of the mobility of the kidney during respiration. The next section will be concerned with the methods where contrast media are used for examination of the kidneys, the renal pelves and the ureters, *i.e.* above all urography and pyelography. Here *urography* means excretion urography or intravenous urography. *Pyelography* means retrograde, antegrade, and instrumental pyelography. Accordingly *urogram* means a picture obtained by urography, and *pyelogram* a picture obtained by pyelography.

The angiographic methods including examination of the entire vascular system or of the venous system only will be dealt with last under the common name of renal angiography.

Methods concerning examination of the bladder, the urethra and the genital organs such as urethro-cystography, vesiculography etc. are not dealt with here. Regarding these methods and organs and the problems they give rise to, the reader is referred to Part II of this volume.

I. Plain radiography

Plain radiography of the urinary tract constitutes the basis of all other roentgen examinations of the kidney and the urinary tract.

The kidneys are of the same density as the surrounding tissue. The kidney can, however, as a rule be delimited because of its fatty capsule. It is also often possible to demonstrate the hilum and part of the sinus because of their content of fat. The medial outline of the kidney pelvis can sometimes be recognized, particularly if it is dilated. Normal ureters will, on the other hand, not be visible in plain roentgenograms. The upper part of the urinary bladder is well outlined because of the surrounding layer of fat, and in women a clear border is usually seen between the bladder and the uterus. It is difficult to distinguish the outline of normal kidneys if the fatty capsule is thin. In early infancy and in old age the capsule is normally thin. Turning the patient about 45⁰ to the right on examination of the right kidney, or to the left on examination of the left kidney (so-called oblique views), will enhance definition because then a much larger area of the fatty capsule will coincide with the direction of the roentgen rays.

Since the difference in density permitting distinction between the kidneys and the surrounding tissue is small, the patient must be well prepared for the examination and the examination technique be satisfactory.

Plain radiography of the urinary tract of adults should preferably include two exposures: one of the kidneys and the major part of the ureters with the region of the suprarenals in the upper margin of the film (with a film 30 × 40 cm, 12 × 17 inches), and one (usually 18 × 24 cm, 8 × 10 inches) of the lower part of the ureters and the bladder. The two films should, of course, overlap one another in order to be sure that the films cover the entire urinary tract. The focus-film distance should preferably be 1 m. The exposure of a separate film of the lower urinary tract and bladder has the advantage that the beam can then be directed roughly in line with the longitudinal axis of the pelvic canal. In such a film the contents of the small pelvis are projected free from the skeleton. Moreover, in the examination of patients above fertile age the method also permits suitable adjustment of the voltage and exposure time. The kidneys are influenced by the respiration and by the heart beat. Therefore the exposure time must be fairly short and the voltage high with consequent loss of contrast. The urinary bladder, which is not influenced by respiration and heart beat, tolerates a longer exposure time, so that films may be taken with lower voltage and consequently better contrast. This is of importance in the evaluation of the thickness of the wall of the bladder, for example, and for demonstrating small, less opaque ureteric or vesical concrements.

1. Position of kidneys

The position of the kidneys varies within a fairly wide range. The right kidney is usually somewhat lower than the left. In one third of all persons both kidneys are situated at the same level, and the left is seldom higher than the right. In children the kidneys are relatively lower than in adults and it is claimed (PETRÉN 1934) on the basis of anatomic studies that the right kidney assumes its definitive position at the age of 5—7 years, the left at 8—10 years.

The posterior surface of the kidney is usually situated 5—9 cm ventral to the surface of the skin of the back. The kidneys are usually related to the twelfth rib. As a rule, the level is such that the middle of the kidney is projected at the level of the upper half of the second lumbar vertebra. Sometimes, however, the poles of the kidneys may be situated the height of a vertebral body above or below the ordinary level (Fig. 2a, b). The most medial part of the kidney is usually projected onto or close to the tip of a transverse process, usually that of the first lumbar vertebra (Fig. 3a, b). The longitudinal axis of the kidneys forms an angle

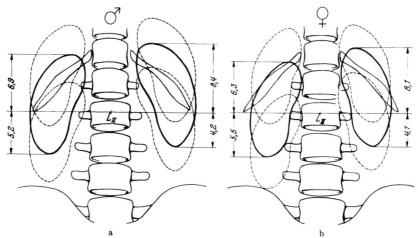

Fig. 2 a and b. Distances in cm, cranially and caudally from the middle of vertebra LII, of the poles of normal adult kidneys in plain roentgenograms. Dotted lines indicate ±2 s. (After MoËLL)

of up to about 20⁰ with the midline of the body (Fig. 4a, b). The medial outline of the kidney usually runs parallel to, and at a distance from, the psoas muscle varying with the thickness of the fatty capsule. The positions of the kidneys in

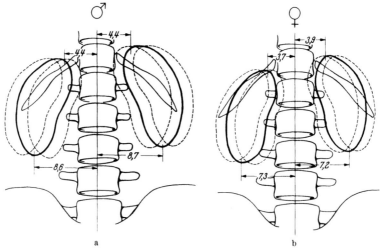

Fig. 3 a and b. Distances in cm of the cranial and caudal poles of normal adult kidneys from the midline in plain roentgenograms. Dotted lines indicate ± 2 s. (After MoËLL)

relation to the midline (distance and angle) and to the middle of the second lumbar vertebra was determined in 100 normal men and 100 women, aged 20 to 49 years, with apparently healthy kidneys. Statistical analysis showed that in males both kidneys are situated more laterally and that the angle between the longitudinal axis of the kidney and the midline is greater than in females. In both sexes the right kidney was lower than the left. The results are "given graphically" in the diagrams (MoËLL).

The mobility of the kidneys in cranio-caudal direction is not insignificant. Respiratory excursions, which are well known from anatomic and roentgenologic

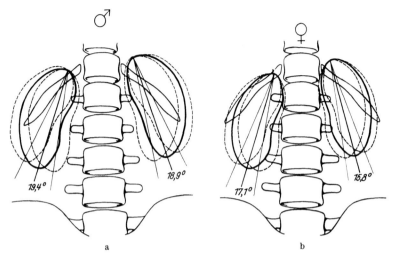

a b

Fig. 4a and b. The angle between the longitudinal axis of the kidneys and the midline. a Males, b Females. Dotted lines indicate ± 2 s. (After MOÉLL)

studies, are made possible by the fact that the renal fascia encloses a space, closed cranially up to the diaphragm and laterally but open caudally (Fig. 5). The posterior leaf of the renal fascia is the muscle fascia of the psoas muscle. This posterior leaf is more or less fixed while the anterior leaf is fairly slack. Since this cranially closed sac is attached to the diaphragm, the upper part of the sac and the kidney follow the excursions of respiration. Since the perirenal fascia is a direct extension from the diaphragm, the movable diaphragm is a *sine qua non* for normal renal mobility. The range of mobility is limited by the vascular pedicle, by the attachment of the kidney to the suprarenal and by the fact that connective tissue runs from the renal fascia through the fatty capsule to unite with the fibrous capsule of the kidney. But even then the kidney is still fairly movable. Normally the range of movement is about 3 cm, somewhat less on the right side than on the left and somewhat larger for women than for men. On deep respiration, however, excursions of up to 10 cm may be recorded. These respiratory excursions of the kidneys have long been utilized for diagnostic purposes and have been systematically charted to form the basis of a supplementary examination method (HILGENFELDT 1936, HESS 1939, BACON 1940). It may be useful for locating calculi and metal fragments, for example, within or outside the kidney. It can also be used in the dia-

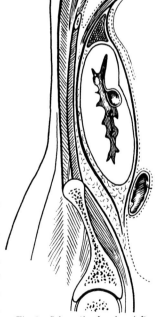

Fig. 5. Schematic drawing (after GEROTA) demonstrating relation of renal fascia to kidney and adrenal and to diaphragm

gnosis of processes preventing excursions, *e. g.* edema, perinephritis etc. It is, however, of value only as a supplement to other examination methods.

Extrarenal processes can displace the kidney. Enlargement of the liver, for example, can displace the right kidney distally, while shrinkage of the liver, as in cirrhosis, may be accompanied by cranial displacement of the right kidney. An enlarged spleen may displace the left kidney caudally and medially and flatten it, and so on.

A certain range of movement of the kidney in ventrodorsal direction is demonstrable, the position of the kidney in supine position is sometimes different from that in prone position. In the supine position the upper pole can fall ventrally and sometimes laterally (see Fig. 20).

The range of movement of the kidney in mediolateral direction is very small. Definitely pathologic are cases where the kidney can be shifted manually across the midline, which is due to a defect in the fascial attachment medially (SANDERS 1957). A moderate range of movement towards the midline is sometimes demonstrable on examination of the patient in the lateral position and with the beam horizontal (PRATHER 1948).

In ptosis approaching a pathologic condition the kidney is displaced, usually the right, in caudal direction. As the kidney is also displaced forwards along the psoas muscle, it rotates with the lower pole directed ventrally. Therefore in plain roentgenograms in supine position the caudally displaced kidney will appear shorter than usual, and the increase in object-film distance will result in geometric enlargement of the lower renal pole, which will then appear plump. The ptotic kidney is also situated more laterally than normally.

It is clear from the remarks set forth above that it is sometimes difficult to decide whether the position and mobility of the kidney in a given case is normal or pathologic.

2. Shape of kidneys

The normal range of variation of the shape of the kidneys is wide. Sometimes the kidneys are long and narrow, sometimes short and thick. The upper pole of the left kidney is often very narrow owing to modelling of the kidney by the spleen. The lower pole on that side then appears plump, or its lateral outline will be bulgent. The relationship between the kidney and the liver produces a corresponding shape on the right side. The kidneys are most frequently bean-shaped, though long kidneys with hardly any rolling of the hilum are sometimes seen. Occasionally, however, the kidney is markedly rolled and angular and then its lateral outline will be bulgent. The distance between the surface of the kidney and the pelvis may be large, sometimes so large that it is not possible to exclude the presence of a space occupying lesion in the kidney.

The outline of the kidney is, as a rule, smooth with the exception of the medial portion, where it may be interrupted or a recess may be seen owing to the renal hilum. The width of the hilum varies and it is often only possible to delimit the cranial or caudal border distinctly. In double renal pelvis an unusually wide hilum or two hili may be seen. Below the hilum the medial outline of the kidney is more bulgent than cranially to the hilum. This medial outline usually runs parallel to the edge of the psoas muscle, alongside it or, if the fatty capsule is thick, some distance from it. The surface of the kidney may be uneven owing to persistent fetal lobation. Such lobation corresponds to the pyramids and occurs regularly before 4 years of age, but then sometimes persists. Usually only the deep furrows persist, namely those bordering the pars cranialis, pars intermedia and pars caudalis of the kidney (LÖFGREN 1949). Otherwise the outline of the kidney is smooth.

3. Size of kidneys

The size of the kidneys is important *per se* and for estimating the amount of kidney parenchyma, especially in cases of generalized parenchymal diseases (see chapter U). The kidneys vary widely in length and breadth. In roentgenograms taken at a focus-film distance of 1 metre and without correction for ordinary variation in the object-film distance the length and breadth of the kidneys has been measured by MOËLL (1956). His investigation is the most thorough on record in this field. Pertinent references are given in his paper of 1961.

The determinations were made on plain roentgenograms of the abdomen of 100 males and 100 females 20—49 years of age with apparently healthy kidneys. The total area (sum of products of length × width of right and left kidney) and kidney weights found *post mortem* were also correlated to form an opinion of the mass of the renal parenchyma. In males both the right and the left kidney were significantly larger than in females, and then also the total area. The left kidney

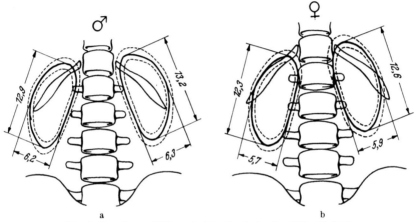

Fig. 6. Size of normal kidneys in (a) males (b) females. (After MOËLL)

was also significantly larger than the right in males and females. The results are given in the figures (Fig. 6a, b).

The sizes of normal kidneys in adults are as follows with the standard deviation within brackets:

males $\begin{cases} \text{right } 12.9 \ (0.80) \times 6.3 \ (0.45) \\ \text{left } \quad 13.2 \ (0.49) \times 6.3 \ (0.49) \end{cases}$ females $\begin{cases} \text{right } 12.3 \ (0.79) \times 5.7 \ (0.46) \\ \text{left } \quad 12.6 \ (0.77) \times 5.9 \ (0.42) \end{cases}$

The kidney-weight can be predicted from the diagram (Fig. 7) representing a material of over one hundred pairs of kidneys. The figures are treated logarithmically. The thin lines indicate a range of 2 s.

The size of the kidneys was not found to vary appreciably with body-build (stature, body-weight, m^2 body surface, and area of vertebra L_{II}, as measured in the roentgenogram).

4. Calcifications projected onto the urinary tract

Plain roentgenography of the urinary tract often shows calcifications. They may be situated within or outside the urinary tract. Calcifications in the kidneys may be of many types and will be discussed in association with various diseases. Calcifications projected onto the urinary tract but situated outside the urinary pathways are, for instance, calcified lymph nodes, gallstones, extra-renal vascular calcifications, or fecal matter etc. It has, of course, to be decided whether they are intra- or extra-renal. This may be readily determined by changing the projection and taking oblique views in the way described above. Calcifications situated within the kidney, thus in the renal parenchyma or renal pelvis, are then projected onto the kidney regardless of the angle of projection. Calcifications lying outside the kidney will, on suitable projection, be projected outside the kidney. The more distant a calcification is from the anterior or posterior surface of the kidney the less the angle of projection need be changed to project it outside the kidney. The closer an extrarenal calcification is situated to the kidney the more the angle of projection must be changed to show that it really lies outside the kidney. Judging from certain urologic hand-books various elaborate and unnecessary procedures are sometimes used for ascertaining whether calcifications are situated within or outside the kidney. Such procedures can be replaced by the simple measures described above.

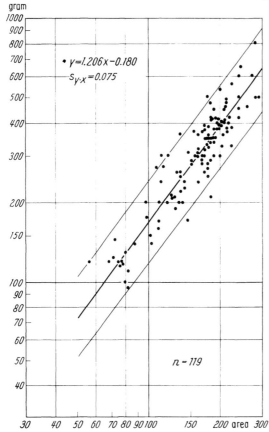

Fig. 7. Diagram for estimation of kidney weight from area of kidney in roentgenogram. Thin borderlines represent 2 s.
(After MOËLL)

Also in the examination of calcifications in or beneath the ureter, change in projection is of importance.

In this connection it might be convenient to mention a source of error which, though less common, is very embarrassing if it leads to erroneous interpretation. A fibroma or atheroma in the skin of the back and raised above the surface of the skin may cause a local increase in density which may be projected onto the kidney and simulate a stone (Fig. 8). The source of error is well known from chest examinations but should be borne in mind even in the examination of kidneys. Oblique views will show that it is a question of something dorsal to the kidney and a glance at the patient's back will explain the finding.

Calcifications in the veins, phlebolites, are very common. They may be unilateral or bilateral, solitary or multiple and of various size and shape. They are often very dense and laminated. Sometimes they occur exclusively on one side. They are of importance in differentiation from ureteric stones. It may be difficult in some cases to decide whether a calcification or one of many calcifications is a phlebolite or a ureteric stone. Urography or pyelography will solve the problem (see chapter G).

Prostatic calcifications are often seen. They vary widely in size, number and distribution. They are usually symmetric, but sometimes they occur almost exclusively on one side.

The suprarenals are fairly often seen as triangular soft tissue densities surrounded by fat and situated cranial to the kidneys. In plain roentgenograms a rounded soft tissue formation is often seen above the left kidney. This has been misinterpreted as a suprarenal tumour. In reality, however, it is the contracted fornix part of the stomach which because of its backward tilt lies with its axis in line with the beam, with the result that the organ is prone to appear as a density in the roentgenogram.

Plain roentgenography is important *per se* and as a guide to planning of subsequent examination with contrast medium. *It is wrong to undertake roentgen examination of the urinary tract with contrast medium without previous, careful plain roentgenography.*

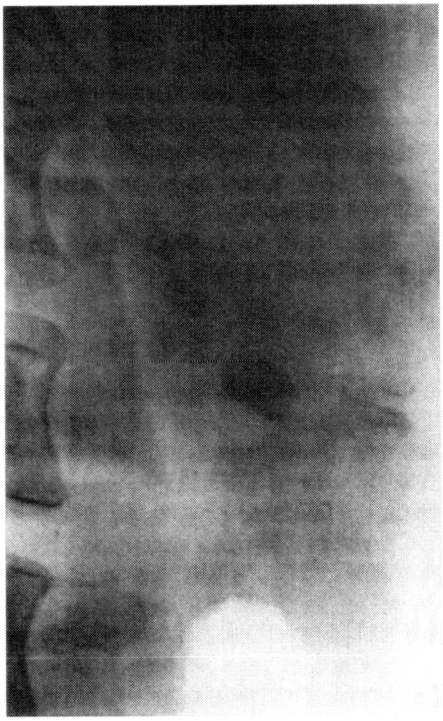

II. Additional methods

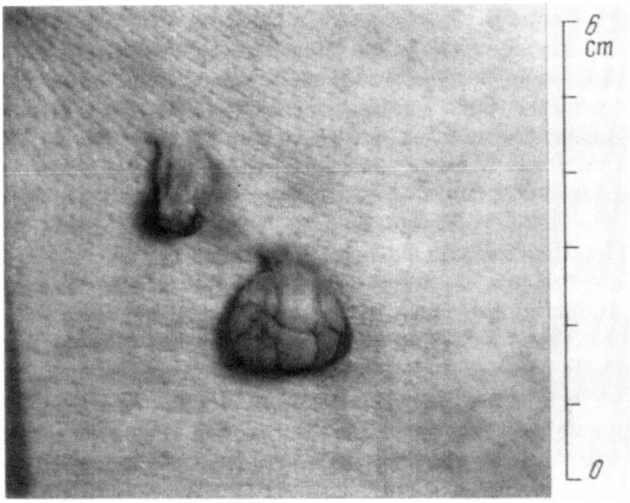

1. Tomography

If it is difficult to delimit the kidneys because of lack of perirenal fat, tomography may be resorted to. Tomography can, by enhancing the contrast, facilitate recognition of the outline of the kidney. If for some reason, the intestine cannot be cleansed satisfactorily, it may be difficult to study the kidney. In such cases tomography is valuable. But the method should not be used routinely as a substitute for plain roentgenography. Neither should it be used simply to avoid proper preparation of the patient.

In order to reduce the radiation dose and

Fig. 8a and b. a Plain roentgenography. Two stone-like densities within contour of kidney. Oblique view showed them to be situated outside and far behind kidney. b Densities produced by two pedunculated fibromas in skin on back. Roentgenogram reversed to facilitate comparison

to facilitate tomography the examination should be performed as simultaneous multiplane tomography with the use of several films in one package at a distance of 0.5—1 cm and with continually calibrated intensifying screens (BACKLUND

1956). An 18 × 24 cm casette will as a rule cover kidneys and 7 films 0.5—1 cm apart and adjusted to a depth beginning with 4 cm from the back of the patient, will cover the entire thickness of the kidneys in a single exposure.

Another indication for tomography is to delimit kidneys in association with retroperitoneal pneumography. Occasionally it might be used with advantage in connection with nephrography, for example. But it should not be resorted to as HAJÓS (1959) seems to recommend for purposes served equally well by simpler, ordinary methods.

Transversal tomography may on occasion be of value in association with retroperitoneal pneumography.

2. Retroperitoneal pneumography

If it is difficult to demonstrate the kidneys and suprarenals by plain roentgenography, gas may be injected into the retroperitoneal space to increase the contrast between these organs and the surrounding tissue. The gas may be injected directly around the kidney, and the examination is usually known as perirenal gas insufflation or pneumoren (ROSENSTEIN 1921, CARELLI 1921). This method has been used to some extent and has also lately been discussed in the literature (SINNER 1955). It has, however, been more or less superseded by the method described by RUIZ RIVAS 1947 in a preliminary report and in further detail in 1950. This method is more reliable and simpler. It has been described under various names such as retropneumoperitoneum, pneumoretroperitoneum, retroperitoneal emphysema, retroperitoneal gas insufflation, perirenal gas contrast, extraperitoneal pneumography. It will be referred to here as retroperitoneal pneumography. This method has received much space in the literature (see COCCHI 1957).

Anatomy. The method is based on the fact that retroperitoneal organs, in this case the kidneys and suprarenals, are embedded in more or less fatty connective tissue continuous with connective tissue in other regions. The pelvic connective tissue thus continues directly upwards *inter alia* into the retroperitoneum and further upwards through and above the diaphragm. The retroperitoneal connective tissue is voluminous in those spaces situated on either side of the lumbar spine and containing the kidneys and suprarenals enclosed in the renal fascia. This fascia is described as surrounding the kidneys and suprarenals like a veil closed laterally and cranially but more or less wide open caudally (Fig. 9). Gas injected into the connective tissue space retrorectally can pass up into this retroperitoneal space and, via the caudal opening, enter the renal fascia and surround the kidney and suprarenal and find its way into the interstices in the connective tissue between these two organs. The fatter the connective tissue the quicker the gas will enter the loose tissue, while denser connective tissue will offer more resistance to the passage of the gas. Sometimes the connection between the kidney and the suprarenal may be so dense as not to permit the passage of gas between the two organs.

Technique. The patient is prepared for the examination in the same way as for urography, thus with purgatives and enema. Some authors recommend premedication of one sort or another, mainly sedatives, but this is, as a rule, unnecessary.

Contrast media: Various types of gas such as nitrogen, carbon dioxide, nitrous oxide, and helium have been used. Attempts have been made to use pentane, whose boiling point is lower than normal body temperature and which thus volatilizes in the tissues. Oxygen is most commonly used because it is rapidly absorbed, usually within 24 hours, and secondly because it involves hardly any risk of embolism. This gas may, if it enters the vascular system be bound by the blood pigments (but see Hazards below). The gas most readily soluble in the blood is, however, carbon dioxide whereas air is absorbed only slowly. The use of helium has been suggested by LEVINE (1952) and SENGER, HORTON, BOTTONE, CHIN & WILSON (1953). This gas, however, should *not* be used because it is the least soluble and therefore the most dangerous. Statements that helium "casts a somewhat darker shadow than the air", and that it gives a "slightly sharper contrast than air" only reveal astonishing lack of knowledge of the fundaments of diagnostic radiology.

The amount of gas used varies between $^1/_2$—$1^1/_2$ litres. In children the dose may be reduced down to 100 ml.

Many authors have expressed the view that tomography is necessary in association with retroperitoneal pneumography (GANDINI and GIBBA 1954, GIRAUD,

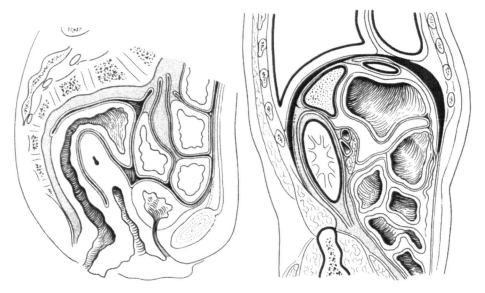

Fig. 9. Schematic drawing (after RUIZ RIVAS) illustrating relation between retrorectal-retroperitoneal connective tissue space and renal fascia

BETOULIERES, LATOUR and PELISSIER 1956 and others). It is not necessary but may sometimes be helpful. When used, simultaneous multisection tomography should be done. Transverse section tomography may also be used. Abdominal angiography has been done in association with the examination method (GOODWIN, MOORE, PEIRCE 1955 and others) and, judging from illustrations in the literature, the method is used in connection with many other methods, mostly unjustified.

The use of high voltage technique, about 200 kV, rational in methods where gas is used as contrast agent, is advocated by ENGELKAMP (1960).

Puncture technique. The coccyx is identified and puncture is done with an ordinary lumbar needle immediately adjacent this bone. The tip of the needle is directed medially and cranially and directed towards the sacrum. Penetration of the rectal mucosa can be avoided by the palpation with a finger in the rectum. A modification with the introduction of the needle through one of the coccygeal intervertebral spaces has been suggested (PALUBINSKAS & HODSON 1958). The advantage of this procedure is that the needle is held more firmly in position.

Another modification is presented by LANDES & RANSOM (1959). They place two thin vinyl catheters in the retro-rectal space.

To be sure that the tip of the needle is not situated within a blood vessel, aspiration is tried and, to secure a free injection space, a small amount of physiologic saline can be injected. Via a sterile pipette with a layer of cotton wool for sterilising the gas, the needle is then connected with a gas container of the type used for therapeutic pneumothorax or gas myelography, for example. During puncture and injection of the gas the patient may be in the knee-elbow position or lying on his side, preferably with the side of greater diagnostic interest uppermost. The gas is injected fairly slowly. Some authors check the position of the gas under fluoroscopy after a few hundred millilitres have been injected. This is, as a rule, not necessary. After the gas has been injected films are exposed, usually plain films and possibly with the patient in different positions, including the erect position to secure passage of the gas to those areas of greatest diagnostic interest. During and after the injection of gas the patient has a feeling of fullness or abdominal tension and occasionally slight pain in the diaphragm, sometimes radiating up to the shoulders.

The equipment necessary for the procedure is simple. The items are listed by BLAND (1958).

Hazards. Deaths, mostly from gas embolism, have been known to occur in association with pneumoren. This is not surprising since the gas is injected quite close to the kidney and might therefore be accidentally injected directly into the kidney. The lesion caused by the actual puncture may also result in bleeding with the formation of a perirenal haematoma (COPE & SCHATZKI 1939). RUIZ RIVAS' method, on the other hand, has been described by many authors as involving no risks. In his original publication RUIZ RIVAS stated that the risk of gas emboli was small because the most vascular tissue encountered during puncture is the actual skin, while the retrorectal tissue is very poor in vessels. STEINBACH & SMITH (1955) performed the examination on 1,995 patients without any fatalities or serious complications. In a collection of 1,500 cases, of which some were probably included in the above collection, MOSCA (1951) found no serious reactions. STEINBACH & SMITH, however, described 4 cases in which gas had been injected into the presacral tissue with very serious complications, 2 fatal, one resulting in hemiplegia and one in severe shock which, however, disappeared without sequelae. In the two fatal cases air had been used as contrast medium. One of the patients in whom oxygen had been used was placed on the left side as soon as the reaction occurred and the symptoms disappeared. DURANT, LONG & OPPENHEIMER (1947) observed in animal experiments that in this posture no air trap arose in the right ventricular outflow tract.

RANSOM, LANDES and McLELLAND (1956) made a survey including over 9,000 retroperitoneal pneumographies by the presacral route. In 24 of these cases the examination had been fatal and in 33 it had caused severe non-fatal reactions (over 2,000 examinations of the type pneumoren had caused 34 deaths and 31 severe non-fatal reactions). The investigation showed that the frequency of fatalities was equal whether air or oxygen was used, and they concluded that oxygen is not safer than air to any significant degree and recommend the use of carbon dioxide which is 20 times more soluble in blood than oxygen is. (STAUFFER, OPPENHEIMER, Soloff & Stewart 1957, like GROSSE-BROCKHOFF, LÖHR, LOOGEN & VIETEN 1959, used this gas as a contrast medium for angiocardiography and thus injected large amounts directly into the vascular system without undesired reactions.)

Since then further cases of general reactions have been described without, however, contributing to our knowledge of the risks involved by the method.

A strange case of gas embolism in association with the use of oxygen, 600 ml, described by SCHULTE (1959) must, however, be mentioned. The examination was accompanied not only by shock, but also by the simultaneous appearance of cherry-sized livid spots on the skin of the back at the level of the low ribs. The general reactions disappeared as soon as the patient was placed on the left side.

It is obvious that all precautions must be taken. It must be checked, for example, that the tip of the needle is not situated within the lumen of a vessel and this must be repeated on observation of any change in the position of the needle during the examination. The gas must be injected slowly, and gas soluble in blood should be used.

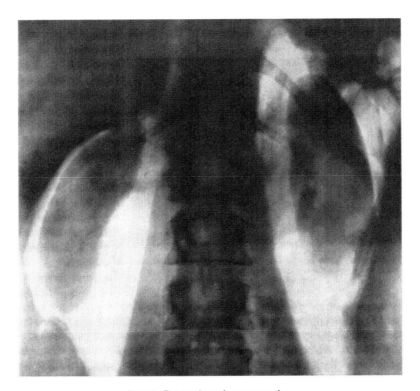

Fig. 10. Retroperitoneal pneumography

Other complications are emphysema of the scrotum, of the mediastinum and of the neck. In addition, cases of pneumothorax and pneumoperitoneum have been described. Poor asepsis will, of course, favour infection.

In the evaluation of the risks it might be convenient first to consider the indications. Retroperitoneal pneumography should not be used unless other roentgen methods have first been tried without success. The large series of retroperitoneal pneumography reported by some authors only show that the method is undoubtedly often used for very loose indications or quite unnecessarily.

The method is contraindicated by any local inflammatory process at the intended site of injection and by poor general condition, particularly when due to cardiac insufficiency.

Normal anatomy. Normally it is not difficult for the gas to enter the renal fascia and surround the kidneys (Fig. 10). Since the gas may flow into the renal fascia and partly accumulate outside the latter, the fascia is sometimes seen as a

2*

thin membrane along part of the lateral outline of the kidney (Fig. 11). As previously mentioned, the kidney is held in position by a large number of connective tissue bands running from the fascia to the surface of the kidney, and they can be loosened by the gas when it forces its way into the connective tissue. The kidney may then be mobilized, and COONEY, AMELAR & ORRON (1955) described a case of complete tilting of the kidney, which rotated 90° without, however, causing any symptoms whatsoever. As a rule, the mobility of the kidney in this type of examination appears to be small, as judged by a comparative examination of 7 cases by POLVAR and BRAGGION (1952). The fat forming the capsule of the kidney, a thick layer on the posterior surface of the kidney and thinner ventrally, often has a reticular or areolar appearance owing to the division of the connective tissue which can vary from one individual to another and with the examination technique, such as with varying thickness of the layers on tomography and with

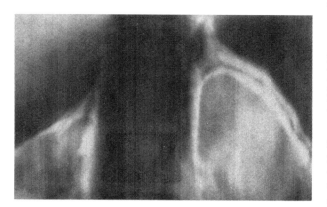

the amount of gas (VESPIGNANI & ZENNARO 1951). It will sometimes give the outline of the kidney an irregular appearance which must not be interpreted as pathologic.

On occasion, only a small amount of gas or no gas at all will enter the interstices between the kidney and the suprarenal if the connective tissue is dense, and then the upper pole of the kidney cannot be defined.

Fig. 11. Retroperitoneal pneumography. Tomogram (film from simultaneous serial multisection tomography) showing renal fascia on left side and adrenals

The suprarenals vary in size, position and shape (see Fig. 11). Judging from the literature, demonstration of suprarenals by this method appears to be both simple and reliable. But this is by no means always the case. The right suprarenal is usually situated adjacent the upper pole of the kidney like a cap and is more or less triangular with an elongated cranial tip. The depths in sagittal direction may vary widely, for which reason many advocate not only frontal tomography, but also lateral tomography. The shape of the left suprarenal is more irregular and has been described as semilunar. It is situated more medially and lower in relation to the renal pole. It may sometimes be difficult to define the outline of the suprarenals exactly because they vary in consistency with the amount of fat in the parenchyma or because of the thickness and reticulation of the fatty capsule. They also vary in size. Thus on the basis of frontal films, STEINBACH & SMITH (1955) gave the following planimetric values: for the right suprarenal 2—7.8 cm with a mean of 4.2 cm² and for the left suprarenal: 2—8.7 cm² with an average of 4.3 cm². This wide range, which does not take into account the above mentioned wide variation in sagittal diameter, makes it difficult to diagnose hyper- and hypoplasia. In the evaluation of the appearance of the suprarenal the examiner must rely largely on his experience.

3. Roentgen examination of the surgically exposed kidney

Roentgen examination of the kidney during operation has been used particularly for locating calculi and for checking that no stones have been left at operation.

On examination of the kidney during operation a cassette is placed over the operative field (SUTHERLAND 1935, ASTRALDI & URIBURU 1937) or a film is placed in the actual wound. The latter method is the more important. The procedure is briefly as follows. The kidney is exposed, a film is inserted and placed against the kidney, the roentgen tube is adjusted and the beam coned to cover the kidney. As a rule a suitably sized film is wrapped in black paper and then packed in a sheet of rubber, a sterilized operation sleeve or the like. Special cases have, however, also been designed for this purpose. ÅKERLUND (1937) had ready-packed films made similar to those employed in dentistry. A ready-packed film of this type is placed in a sterilized rubber glove. In order to prevent infection when the packed film is being introduced into the glove, use is made of a loading guide, consisting of a metal sleeve. The whole package is held against the exposed kidney

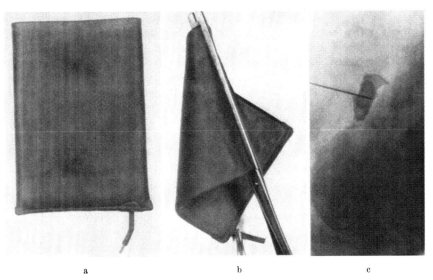

a   b   c

Fig. 12 a—c. Flexible, easily sterilizable rubber cassette (with flexible intensifying screens) for roentgen examination of operatively exposed kidney. Film obtained with cassette

by means of elastic ribbons. The disadvantage of a package of this type is the lack of intensifying screens which reduces contrast and makes a longer exposure time necessary, which may cause poor definition, and then small stone fragments may not be demonstrable.

In an attempt to eliminate these disadvantages ordinary cassettes have been used (JACHES; FRANCOIS 1932) or thin cassettes made particularly for the purpose (BENJAMIN 1931, PUIGVERT GORRO 1943). Such stiff cassettes are, however, difficult to insert into the operative wound.

In order to secure a flexible, small, suitably packed film with intensifying screens, OLLE OLSSON (1948) designed a rubber cassette similar to that employed in industry for the roentgen inspection of material (Fig. 12). The cassette consists simply of a flat rubber bag 10 × 15 cm. The film and two intensifying screens are dropped into the bag. The mouth of the bag is closed by means of a clamp. The bottom of the bag is provided with a spout through which the air content of the closed bag may be withdrawn by means of a syringe. This decreases the thickness of the cassette and at the same time presses the screens tight against the film, which is important for obtaining sharp pictures.

The screens are of the type used for industrial purposes. They are supplied in standard sizes such as 9×12 cm. In these screens the fluorescent coating has been applied to a flexible material.

Thanks both to the material of which the cassette is made and the construction of the screens the loaded cassette is very flexible. In other words: it is an easily sterilizable, convenient and flexible cassette with intensifying screens. The cassette has been dimensioned to suit a standard-sized film 9×12 cm, 4×5 inches. As mentioned, standard screens, coarse and fine-grained, are available for this size of film.

The rubber cassette is sterilized in the same manner as the rest of the rubber articles used at operation. An assistant with sterilized gloves holds up the sterilized cassette in the dark room of the operation department, where it is loaded with the aid of a guide consisting of a metal sleeve. The mouth of the cassette is closed by the assistant with a single pair of resection tongs or with two, one on each side. The mouth may also be closed in any other suitable manner. If tongs are used, such types should be chosen as may be used as handles when the cassette is being introduced into the operative wound. When loaded the cassette is placed on the assistant's table and the air is withdrawn. Every time the syringe is removed from the spout, the latter is closed by means of a clip. As a rule, about 60 cc air can be sucked out of the cassette. When the air has been withdrawn the spout is sealed by means of a small stopper. The cassette is then ready for use. It is immaterial which of the two screens is placed next to the organ to be examined. To render the double-sided use of this cassette possible the practice of making one of the sides of the cassette of lead rubber, for example, to prevent secondary radiation from the underlayer, has been discarded.

Roentgen examination for stones in the surgically exposed kidney has been used mainly for locating concrements in the renal pelvis (see chapter on Renal Calculi). Pyelography (FRANCOIS 1932, HEUSSER 1937) and renal angiography (ALKEN 1951, GRAVES 1956) have also been performed during operation. Fluoroscopy with a specially modified apparatus has also been described (BASKIN, HARVARD & JANZEN 1957). Apart from the difficulty in securing sterile conditions such fluoroscopic examinations, like all other fluoroscopic examinations during operation, are not to be recommended because of the difficulty in securing satisfactory radiation protection and acceptable conditions for fluoroscopy. If fluoroscopy is nevertheless considered indicated, it should be done with the use of an image amplifier. This has been used in combination with television (LINDBLOM 1960) the image of the screen of the amplifier being taken up by a television tube (Vidikon or Orthikon) and transferred to an ordinary television monitor. With the use of two tubes and covering of the right and left eye alternately and synchronously with the indirect current the image can be viewed stereoscopically.

III. Pyelography and urography

1. Pyelography

In pyelography contrast medium is injected directly into the renal pelvis or via the ureter, as a rule through a catheter with the tip in the renal pelvis or at any desired level of the ureter. The contrast medium may also be deposited in the ureteric orifice or the urinary bladder and the ureter then filled by gravity or by reflux by high pressure in the bladder (see Fig. 47). Particularly in children with an incompetent ureteric orifice it is usually easy to obtain a filling of the renal pelvis by lowering the head and allowing the contrast medium to flow from the bladder into the ureter and further into the renal pelvis. A filling can also be obtained by percutaneous puncture of the renal pelvis or the ureter and injection via a needle or cannula, or via an opening after pyelostomy or via a fistula, so-called antegrade pyelography.

a) Contrast media

Formerly silver was used as a contrast element in the form of Collargol (Ag has the atomic number 47 atomic weight 107,88 the corresponding figures for iodine are 53 and 126,92 for barium 56 and 137,37 and for thorium 90 and 232,15). Collargol, however, was often attended by serious side reactions. It was soon superseded by halogen salts such as sodium and potassium bromide or iodide respectively lithium iodide. These contrast media are also sometimes attended by clinical reactions and experimentally they have been proved to damage the epithelium of the renal pelvis and the ureter with desquamation, edema, hyperemia and hemorrhage.

Later a colloidal thorium dioxide was used as a contrast medium. It was believed to be ideal because it was almost non-irritable. It was soon realized, however, that if this insoluble and non-absorbable contrast medium escaped into the tissues in association with reflux, for example, it would remain there and give rise to granuloma. That the radioactive effect of thorium can lead to malignant metaplasia, is well known. Therefore thorium should be completely abandoned as a contrast agent. Judging from the literature, it is still in use in some quarters for special purposes, but even then it is not acceptable. Thorotrast is still of clinical interest because rests of the medium persistent after pyelography performed many years ago with thorotrast and with the medium lodged in the tissues, possibly in granulomatous masses, are still occasionally observed.

Later the contrast media which we now use for urography became available, and they are the only media that should be used for pyelography.

Judging from illustrations in papers and textbooks, there seems to be a tendency to use contrast media of too high a density. High concentration of the contrast media will produce sharp outlines of the hollow organs examined, but too high a density is liable to mask changes within the renal pelvis, even fairly marked ones, such as polyps or stones. Therefore one should use the contrast medium in a concentration that can give well detailed pyelograms.

Possibly as a reaction against too high a density of contrast medium with its above mentioned disadvantages, gas, particularly oxygen, has been used as a contrast medium. Gas can undoubtedly be indicated in certain investigations, e.g. in so-called double contrast examinations. A mixture of hydrogen superoxide solution with ordinary contrast medium has been suggested (KLAMI 1954) to induce the formation of gas bubbles in pathologic processes in the renal pelvis, which liberate oxygen from hydrogen peroxide. The advantage, if any, of this method appears to be very small.

b) Method

Pyelography can be performed in two essentially different ways, namely with and without fluoroscopic control.

Usually it is performed without such control. Contrast medium warmed to body temperature is injected via the indwelling catheter, and films are taken after a certain amount of contrast medium has been injected or when the patient complains of a feeling of tension or pain. Attempts have been made to calculate the amount of contrast medium that should preferably be injected by measuring the volume of the contents of the normal renal pelvis. This volume varies normally, namely from 4 to 12 cc. In addition some of the contrast medium may flow back, or on malposition of the catheter it may be deposited in a single calyx. This method is therefore not reliable. Injection of contrast medium until the patient reports discomfort in the region of the kidneys has also been taken as a sign that the renal pelvis is filled. This method has severe inherent sources of error, particularly regarding the difficulty in obtaining a suitable degree of filling of the renal pelvis, but also because reflux (see chapter O) often occurs which *inter alia* may make interpretation of the films difficult.

The other, and in my opinion better, procedure is to carry out the examination under fluoroscopic control. It can be improved by the use of an image amplifier. This variation of the method of pyelography has been called pyeloscopy, which name is obviously not correct. A better and more correct designation is pyeloradioscopy or pyelofluoroscopy.

On performance of fluoroscopy the examiner must of course be well dark adapted, the field must be well coned, the voltage relatively high, and the current as low as possible. The time of radioscopy should be reduced to a minimum. This holds for every type of fluoroscopy, thus also when an image amplifier is used. Manufacturers' advertisments and less conscientious roentgenologists seem to neglect the fact that fluoroscopy with the use of image amplifiers calls for the same restrictions as all fluoroscopic work regarding radiation safety. The output from an image amplifier working with 3 mA gives the same output as an ordinary fluoroscope working with the same current, other data being equal. In an investigation on radiation hazards attending the use of transportable image intensifiers KOCKUM, LIDÉN & NORMAN (1958) conclude that roentgen units of this type, especially when placed in the hands of radiologically unskilled workers, require additional radiation safety standards. This, of course, also holds when a TV-system is used.

During fluoroscopy well coned films can be obtained in suitable projection and with a suitable degree of compression.

In pyelography, the position of the catheter must be checked. The tip of the catheter should be situated in the confluence of the renal pelvis or in the upper part of the ureter. If it is too high *e.g.* in a calyx, a filling may be obtained of that calyx only, which may then be inflated and incur the risk of misinterpretation. Occasionally, though rarely, the tip of the catheter might be inadvertently pushed into the renal parenchyma and the contrast medium deposited there, or inserted through the renal parenchyma with deposition of the contrast medium subcapsularly.

If the ureter is to be examined, the catheter is withdrawn a suitable distance. The entire ureter can be examined by using a so-called Chevassu catheter with an olive-shaped tip or a Braasch acorn bulb, Woodruff or Ravich metal bulb or Foley cone tip catheter. These catheters block the ureteric orifice. Films may also be taken during the actual injection of the contrast medium, during which protective measures against radiation hazards should, of course, be strictly observed.

If the renal pelvis is dilated and its drainage is obstructed, attempts may be made to aspirate the contrast medium after the examination, or the catheter may be left *in situ* for some hours to facilitate drainage.

Some authors have recommended a modified pyelographic technique: the movements of the kidney are studied on application of manual pressure or during the respiratory cycle (SCHEELE 1930, ALFERMANN 1950).

Particularly during pyelography, but also during urography (JUNKER 1936, PREVÔT 1939), fluoroscopy, and spot-film radiography is valuable not only for reasons given above but also to study the motility of the renal pelvis and the ureter. For this purpose kymography has also been used and recently also cineradiography with or without the use of an intensifier. The latter method permits exposure of films with a small radiation dose.

It is possible clearly to distinguish systole and diastole in the renal pelvis (NARATH) and to study the course of certain contractions. The two renal pelves contract independently of one another with regard to rhythm and frequency with pressure fluctuations of 3—4 mm/Hg (KIIL 1957).

The literature on the motility of the renal pelvis is considerable. It must, however, be stressed that it is to a large extent of at most limited value. Examination with the use of a catheter partly obstructing the flow and influencing the motility, and retrograde injection of a contrast medium, which is in addition not quite inert, interferes with physiology. An experimental situation in which pyelography is used does not provide a sound basis for investigation of true physiologic conditions in the urinary pathways. It may be assumed that a refined

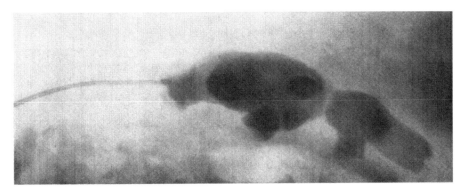

Fig. 13. Position of calyces, confluence and ureter when patient is examined in supine position. Cranial calyces lowest, confluence highest

technique with the use of *inter alia* image amplifier and urography would imply a great advance in this field. In this conjunction reference might be made to PREVÔT & BERNING, DAVIS (1950), NARATH (1951), and KIIL (1957), for example, who have given extensive surveys of pertinent literature.

As mentioned, the kidney is tilted so that the cranial pole of the kidney is situated more dorsally than the caudal, and the medial part is higher *i.e.* more ventral than the lateral (Fig. 13). The confluence is therefore situated further ventrally than the rest of the renal pelvis. This is of importance in the performance of urography and pyelography.

The specific gravity of ordinary contrast media is higher than that of body fluids such as urine, blood etc. This gives rise to a *layer formation* between contrast medium and the rest of the contents of a cavity (the phenomenon is sometimes incorrectly called sedimentation). Ignorance of this phenomenon has often resulted in misinterpretation and erroneous evaluation of the actual findings in examinations of different kinds with contrast media particularly in urologic radiology. The phenomenon was first described by LAURELL (1924) and has since been studied in further detail by RIBBING (1933) in retrograde pyelography and by ETTINGER (1943) in urography. Formerly it was believed that only Thorotrast was capable of causing this phenomenon, owing to its poor miscibility with urine, but it has since been shown that water soluble contrast media infused into the renal pelvis via the catheter for retrograde pyelography or contrast urine coming from the papillae during urography can produce the same phenomenon, which is also confirmed by daily experience. This is why the dorsal and cranial calyces are filled first and most completely, which, because of the position of the kidney, are situated lowest when the patient is in the supine position.

Layer formation is of importance in the evaluation of the pelviureteric junction. A narrow junction in the film or a band-like transverse filling defect at the site of the junction may be caused only by incomplete filling of this most ventrally located anatomic part. What looks like narrowing of the junction may thus mean just incomplete filling of a lumen of ordinary diameter. This also holds for "narrowing" of the ureter, which may be caused by a bend of the ureter in the ventral-dorsal plane and incomplete filling of the bend. Suitable and complete filling of all parts of the renal pelvis and the ureter therefore requires examination of the patient in different positions.

This is necessary for free projection and suitable filling of single calyces and for obtaining a three-dimensional impression of the renal pelvis, and therefore provides further support for the view that the examination should be carried out under fluoroscopic control. In certain conditions the layer formation plays a special rôle and dictates several steps in the method (see chapter N).

In association with pyelography contractions of the renal pelvis are sometimes seen, especially on less gentle catheterization. Cases have been described (HEN-DRIOCK 1934) in which marked contractions of the entire renal pelvis have been observed during catheterization. The examination should therefore be performed as carefully as possible.

c) Roentgen anatomy

The discussion of the anatomy of the renal pelvis requires an acceptable nomenclature. The nomenclature used by anatomists differs from that used by clinicians. In addition the nomenclature in the clinical literature is by no means uniform. Thus, some authors use the term renal pelvis to designate the entire renal pelvis, while others mean only that part of it formed after the confluence of the individual calyces. Some authors call this part the saccus or ampulla, which is sometimes a very inappropriate name. The term calyx is used with the epithet minor to describe a single calyx, but is also used with the epithet major to designate a group of calyces. Important parts, as far as nomenclature is concerned, are the stems of the calyces minores and majores. We use a nomenclature presented in 1946 by JOHNSSON of our department. According to this, that part of the renal pelvis where the different calyces conflow is called the confluence; the calyces majores, the branches; after which come the stems of the calyces and the calyces (see Fig. 14).

Wide variations occur in the shape, width and branching of the renal pelvis, in the number of calyces, in size and length of the stems and in the important region of the pelviureteric junction (Fig. 14, 15, 16). The kidney is built up of 14 papillae with 6 in a cranial part, 4 in an intermediate part and 4 in a caudal part. These papillae are arranged in a ventral and a dorsal row. Often several papillae fuse, always in the tips of the papillae, so that the number found in a normal kidney is usually 8 or 9 (LÖFGREN 1949). This fusion of the papillae has a strong moulding effect on the calyces with the result that calyces of widely different shapes occur. The shape also varies with degree of filling. On urography and pyelography it is necessary to take films at suitable angles, usually by turning the patient, so as to obtain true lateral projections of the individual calyces of particular interest in a given case.

The renal pelvis is often divided into two parts, the division coinciding with the primary bifurcation angle. The upper branch is then of the same shape as the

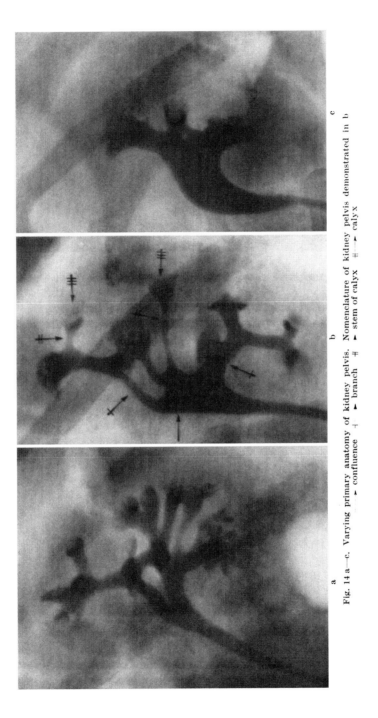

Fig. 14 a—c. Varying primary anatomy of kidney pelvis. Nomenclature of kidney pelvis demonstrated in b ⊸ confluence ⊣ ▸ branch ╫ ▸ stem of calyx ╫—▸ calyx

upper part of a double kidney (see Chapter Anomalies) and the upper pole may be large and the lower pole smaller than ordinarily.

A not uncommon variant of the renal pelvis is a small sprout usually from the base of the upper branch (Fig. 17). It has the appearance of a calyx that has been blocked and is probably due to some slight disorder during embryologic develop-

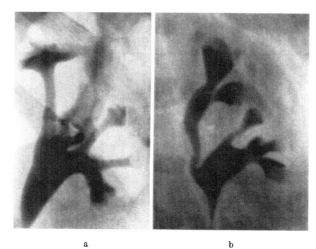

a   b
Fig. 15 a and b. Other examples of infinite variation in morphology of kidney pelvis

ment. A microcalyx or otherwise unusually shaped calyx is sometimes seen at this site, which corresponds to the primary bifurcation angle in embryonal life (Fig. 18).

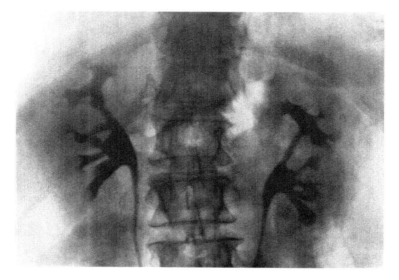

Fig. 16. Both upper kidney poles dominant with large upper branches

The calyces vary widely in shape, even when they are completely filled with contrast medium. The stem may be very long or short, wide or very narrow. Several calyces may lie close together with a common stem. The actual calyx can vary widely in diameter and deviate from its normally round shape. The edge of the calyx may be angular or rounded and vary in different parts of the circumference of one and the same calyx and may be of different height. Detailed

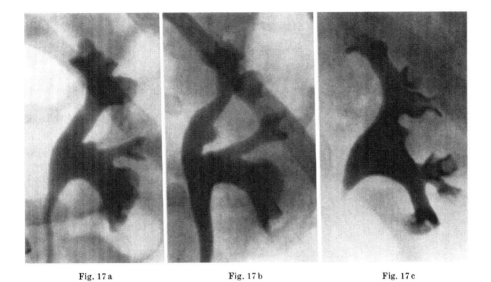

Fig. 17 a   Fig. 17 b   Fig. 17 c

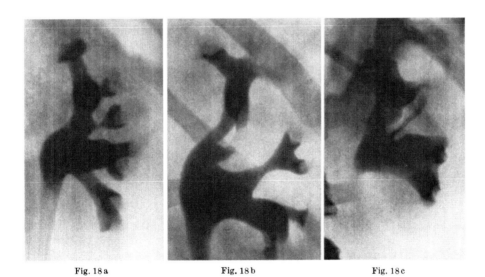

Fig. 18 a   Fig. 18 b   Fig. 18 c

Fig. 17 a—c. Small sprout from
caudal branch, cranial branch and
confluence without a calyx. This
anatomic variant is not
uncommon

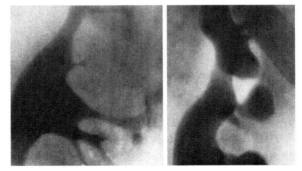

Fig. 18 a—e. Different types of
calyces at the same site as of sprout
formation illustrated in fig. 17

Fig. 18 d   Fig. 18 e

examination of the anatomy may require several well coned films in different projections secured by turning the patient or angulating the beam. Sometimes very small calyces with long or short stems, so-called micro-calyces, are seen (Fig. 19).

Not only the size and shape of the papillae influence the form of the calyces, but also the form of the sinus and the amount of sinus fat. The branches and stems may form different-sized angles with one another, usually acute. If the sinus fat is abundant, however, the branches may be pushed apart and one or more of the angles between them may then be rounded to such an extent as to simulate a space-occupying lesion.

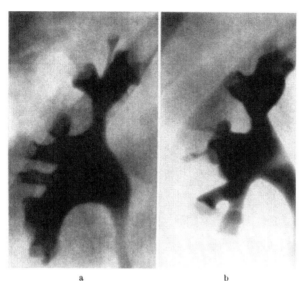

a   b

Fig. 19a and b. Microcalyces in cranial (a) and middle (b) part of kidney pelvis

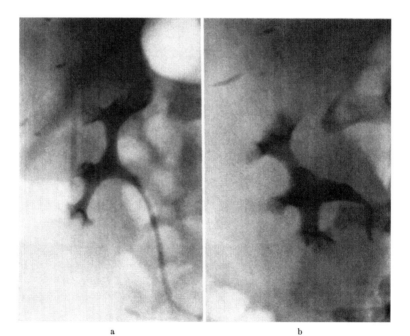

a   b

Fig. 20a and b. Roentgen anatomy: Position of kidney in (a) supine position and (b) prone position of patient with mobile kidney

A certain similarity is often, though not always, seen between the shapes of the renal pelves on either side. To my knowledge, no investigation has been published on the possible heredity of the shape of the renal pelvis.

In a renal pelvis with many and long branches pathologic changes are easier to recognize than in renal pelves in which the calyces are, so to say,

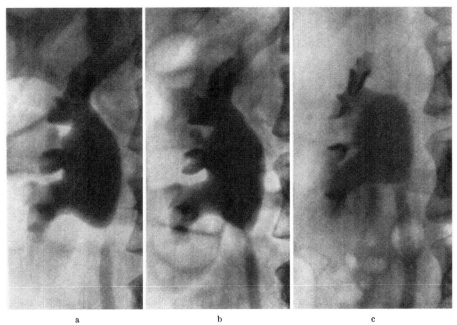

a   b   c

Fig. 21a—c. Pelviureteric junction. Urography (a) diastole, pelviureteric junction not filled (b) systole, junction filled and of ordinary width (c) ureteric compression released. Slight ptosis of kidney causes fold at junction

situated directly on the confluence.

The confluence may have the shape of a sac or ampulla, but it may also be very narrow. If the confluence is wide, it may, of course, be difficult to draw a line of distinction between normal width and pathologic widening.

Change of position of the patient may cause an apparent change of the shape of the kidney pelvis (Fig. 20).

The pelviureteric junction varies widely from a confluence gradually tapering and merging with the ureter to a distinctly outlined confluence merging abruptly with the ureter. The actual pelviureteric junction in such cases varies considerably in width. The level of the pelviureteric

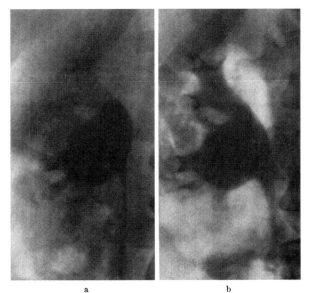

a   b

Fig. 22a and b. Pelviureteric junction. Urography (a) frontal (b) oblique projection. The junction is flat and therefore of narrow appearance in (a) but of ordinary width in (b)

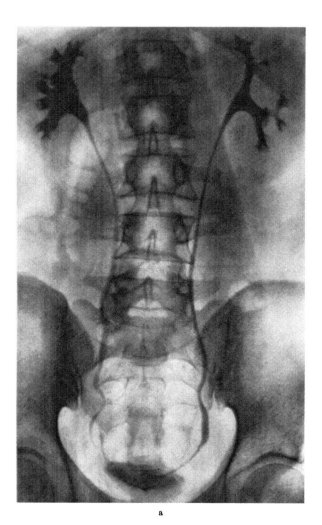

a

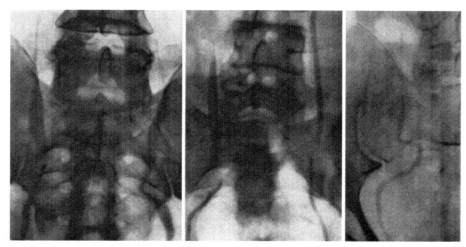

b

Fig. 23a and b. Course of ureters (a). b Variation in roentgen anatomy of ureters at point of intersection between
ureter—iliac artery

junction also varies and the ureter may be referred to as being of high or low departure from the renal pelvis. In the evaluation of the width, films must be taken in different planes, and then it is important that the region under examination be completely filled with contrast medium (Fig. 21, 22).

Pyelography provides good possibilities of studying the ureter in the way described under b) Method (page 23), urography, in films taken immediately after release of ureteric compression. Normally, the filling obtained of the ureter during urography is never continuous. If it is, it is due to the examination technique or to some pathologic condition, usually a more or less pronounced stasis in the ureteric orifice or distal thereto.

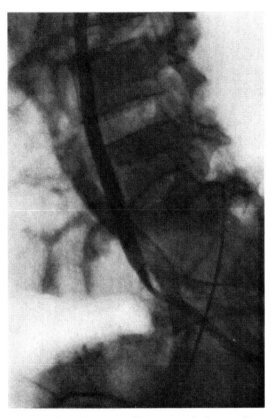

The ureters run from the kidneys medially, often in a slight curve up along the psoas muscle and then more or less parallel and fairly close to the spine to the lower part of the ileosacral joints. There they bend, sometimes markedly, sometimes less markedly, laterally, make an extra bend over the iliac artery, and then again run medially to the ureteric orifice in the bladder. This last mentioned section extends in a fairly sharp angle medially and ventrally (Fig. 23, 24). This part can be shown best with the patient sitting and leaning forward and the beam directed obliquely downwards from behind. The ureteric orifice is often distinct when a small amount of contrast medium is in the bladder and the inter-ureteric ridge can be seen (as a result of layer formation). If a

Fig. 24. Relationship ureter—iliac artery. Contrast medium injected into right femoral artery backwards and into right ureter, oblique view. Narrowing by impression of ureter at level crossed by artery

normal sized uterus is not situated in the midline, it can dislocate the ureter. If the floor of the bladder is high, the lowest segment or the distal part of the ureters may be lifted.

The spina ischiadica is often used as a landmark in the description of stones in the distal part of the ureter, for example. It should, however, be observed that the ureter is situated about one and one half inches away from the spina ischiadica both cranially and ventrally, and that the ureter comes nowhere in its course near the spina (WADSWORTH & UHLENHUTH 1956). Sometimes the ureter may be very tortuous during ureteric compression, which need not imply disease. Often the ureter is slightly widened, particularly on the right side immediately above the level where the ureter crosses the iliac artery. In fact the ureter is nearly always somewhat wider above this level than below.

Ureteric peristalsis can be studied cinematographically or kymographically. Ureteric contractions always travel to the end of the ureter without any relationship between pressure amplitude and travel rate. Retrograde contractions

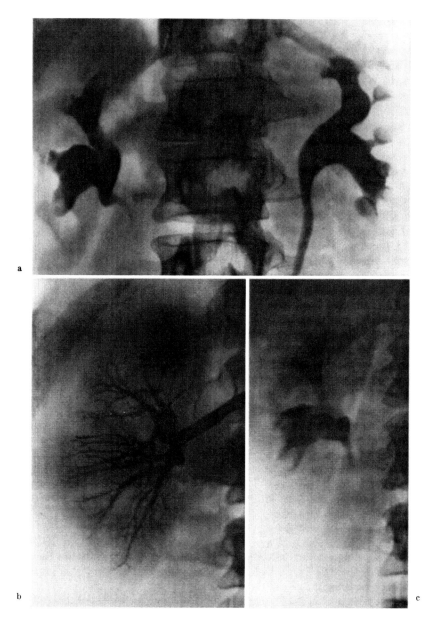

a

b

c

Fig. 25a—c. Filling defect in right kidney pelvis, caused by artery. Comparison with arteriogram shows complete agreement between defect in urogram shown in end-phase of angiography and ventral branch, which impresses kidney pelvis. a Urography, b renal angiography, c urography in end-phase of angiography

occasionally occur (KIIL 1957). JULIANI & GIBBA (1957) state that the average speed of the peristaltic wave varies between 2 and 6 cm per sec. and that the renal excretory rate determines the frequency of the contractile waves, usually three or four per minute.

The renal pelvis often shows filling defects in the form of indentations in various parts of the edge of the renal pelvis or band shaped defects across a branch, the stem of a calyx or across the confluence. The changes responsible for some of these defects have long been known. Thus WOLKE (1936) showed that a rigid artery may cause such a defect. These phenomena have, however, also been the subject of much discussion in which spastic conditions have been supposed, but not proved. Such spastic conditions have also been supposed to occur locally in sphincters, the existence of which has not always been proved either. BORGARD (1944, 1948) compared pyelograms with the vascular anatomy as seen at operation, and in some cases he believed to have observed that normal vessels can produce stasis in the calyces with pyelitis as a consequence. GÜNTHER (1950) tried to explain the defects as spasms due to pyelitis and described the cause (1952) as "Unruhe, Spasmophilie" etc. but presented no evidence in support of his claim.

Since the cause of the filling defects was not properly understood and since they had sometimes given rise to misinterpretations BOIJSEN (1958) in our department studied the problem on the basis of roentgen diagnostic materiel yielding much more reliable evidence than formerly, namely a series in which each patient had been examined by urography and complete angiography (arterial, venous and nephrographic phases).

The anatomy of the hilum can usually be studied completely in the nephrogram. Large anatomic variations can be seen, and the nephrogram will also show distinctly that certain defects in the renal pelvis, especially in its edges, correspond to and are thus due to, the edge of the parenchyma. Certain other marginal filling defects are caused by vessels, particularly if they are tortuous. The linear filling defects can be explained by vessels, usually arteries, sometimes veins, sometimes a combination of the edge of the parenchyma and vessels. Common to most of these changes is that they can be observed when the renal pelvis is not completely filled, *i.e.* before application of ureteric compression, and that they disappear as soon as the renal pelvis has been filled during compression. They can also appear distinctly during diastole, while they will disappear on increase in tonus during systole. Decrease in tonus of the renal pelvis favours demonstration. BOIJSEN has thus provided a simple and interesting explanation for many of the obscure filling defects and at the same time been able to dismiss from the discussion many unconfirmed claims and much speculation (Fig. 25).

The distance between the renal pelvis and the outer border of the parenchyma is of diagnostic interest because it decreases on scar formation in the parenchyma and increases in the presence of a space-occupying lesion. In normal kidneys the measurement at a focus-film distance of 100 cm was found to be 2—2.7 cm and in only one instance did it reach 3 cm (BILLING 1954). The distance between the renal pelvis and the outer margin of the parenchyma in the poles of the kidney may, however, exceed 3 cm.

d) Antegrade pyelography

In certain cases in which the renal pelvis is dilated and in which no excretion is obtained on urography and in which retrograde pyelography cannot be resorted to because it is not possible to pass the catheter, for example, and in which angiography does not yield sufficient information, the renal pelvis may be punctured percutaneously and contrast medium be deposited directly into it (WEENS & FLORENCE 1947, WICKBOM 1954, FLOYD & GUY 1956). The method has been called antegrade pyelography. A special type of antegrade pyelography is that in which the contrast medium is deposited directly into the renal pelvis via a catheter inserted for pyelostomy or via a fistula out to the skin.

e) Contraindications

As a rule pyelography should not be performed if urography will yield the desired information. Broadly speaking, in these cases pyelography is a supplementary method to urography. The more the examiner is familiar with urography the less will he resort to pyelography. The most inportant risk of pyelography is infection, and rise in temperature is not uncommon after pyelography. Attempts have been made to control or eliminate this risk by incorporation of an antibacterial agent in the contrast medium (BLOOM & RICHARDSON 1959). The problem is, however, complicated and made still more difficult by the nosocomial infections with resistant bacteria regularly occurring in large hospitals, especially in departments of thoracic surgery and neurosurgery, but also in departments of urology.

According to many experienced urologists, retrograde pyelography should, as a rule, not be used in the investigation of patients with tuberculosis and co-existent cystitis or in patients with obstructed drainage of the renal pelvis, thus in many cases of hydronephrosis. In such cases in which the renal pelvis contains stagnant urine, the risk of infection is great. Other risks are instrumental lesions (see chapter H) and perforation (see chapter P).

If retrograde pyelography is done instead of urography because of renal insufficiency, measures should be taken to avoid reflux. In such cases one may in fact give an intravenous injection via the backflow (see chapter O). Retrograde pyelography is sometimes performed instead of urography, because of hypersensitivity to the contrast medium. Especially in such cases of course, the risk of reflux should be observed, as mentioned. Symptoms of hypersensitivity may occur also in association with retrograde pyelography without backflow. One case was described by BURROS, BORROMEO & SELIGSON (1958) in which bilateral retrograde pyelography was followed by anuria, probably because of oedema of the ureteric mucosa due to hypersensitivity to the contrast medium.

For cases in which catheterization is nevertheless considered indicated and the risk of infection regarded as slight, pyelography is, of course, preferred by many urologists. The tendency is, however, to start the investigation with urography and continue with pyelography only if really necessary. The better the urographic examination is performed and the more the examiner is familiar with the diagnostic possibilities of the method and the more he is able to use suitable modifications for all aspects of problems presenting themselves during the examination, the less often will pyelography be necessary.

As to the question whether pyelography can be done on both sides in one session, experienced urologists and roentgenologists can, from their personal experience, produce evidence both for and against either alternative. Suffice it here to say that limitation of the procedure to one side at a time is naturally the safer procedure and this is the technique we use.

2. Urography

Since the end of the nineteen-twenties urography has an established place as a diagnostic adjunct in the management of urologic problems. The method is based on the capacity of the kidneys to clear the blood of certain crystalline substances in which for the purpose of urography two or three iodine atoms have been incorporated in the molecule, and which are concentrated in the kidneys because of their reabsorption of water.

a) Contrast media

Most contrast media for urography contain two or three iodine atoms per molecule bound to a pyridine or benzene ring. All of the media contain a carboxyl group to make them water-soluble. As a rule, the carboxyl group is attached directly to the ring, but a CH_2-group may be inserted between the ring and the carboxyl group. If a larger hydrocarbon group radical is inserted, less will be excreted in the urine and more in the bile. If the amino-groups are acylated with lower fatty acid radicals (acetyl-respectively propionyl) it will make the salts more soluble and less toxic. If higher fatty acids are used for acylation, less will be excreted in the urine and more in the bile. A keto-group or an amino-group facilitates the introduction of iodine in the pyridine benzene ring respectively. Only 2 iodine atoms can be introduced into the pyridine ring or 3 in the benzene ring, if the amino group is attached in the meta position in relation to the carboxyl groups.

Below a list is given of common contrast media together with the chemical formulas, molecular weights, iodine content, official name and commercial name.

Table 1. *Contrast media used for urography*

I. *N-Methyl-3,5-diiodo-4-pyridone-2,6-dicarbon in acid* is used in the form of the di-sodium salt.

Structural formula

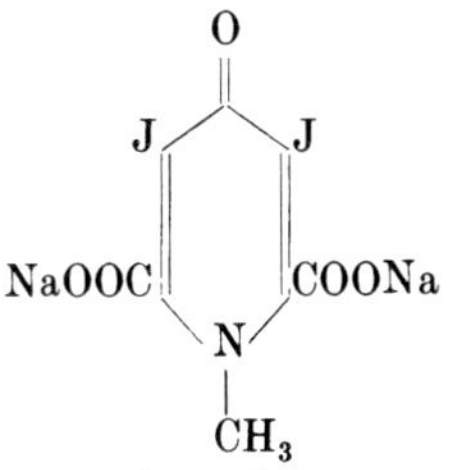

Molecular weight   *Iodine content*
492.9   51.5%

Official names:
Sodium Iodomethamate USP
Iodoxyl BP

Trade marks:
Uroselectan B, Schering AG,
Neo-Iopax, Schering Corp.,
Uropac, May & Baker,
Urombrine, Dagran,
Urumbrine, Boots
Pyelectan, Glaxo

II. *3,5-diiodo-4-pyridone-N-acetic acid* is used in the form of the salt of diethanolamine-(a), diethylamine-(b), morfoline-(c) or methylglucamine(d).

Structural formulas:

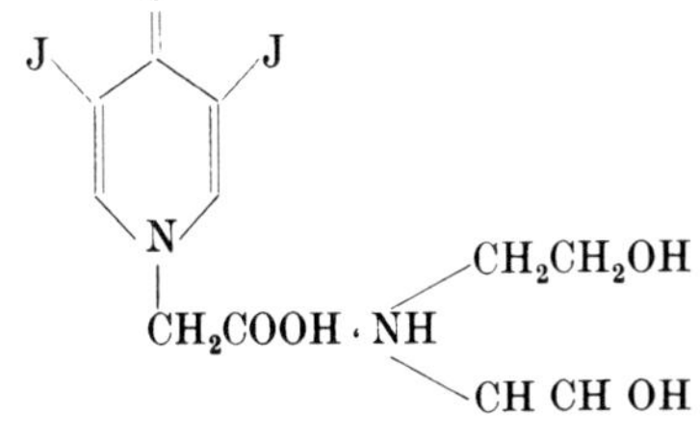

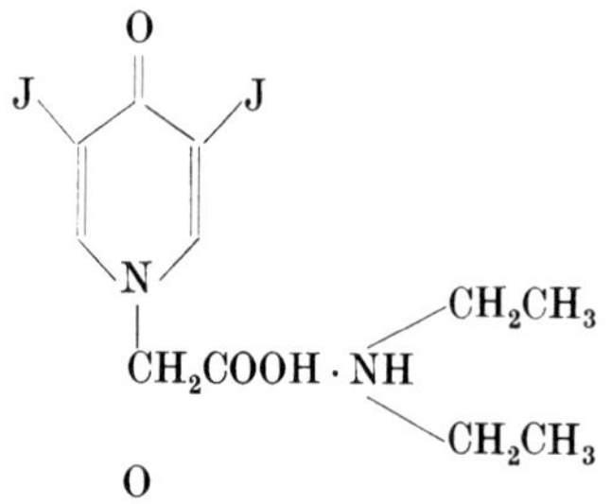

b)

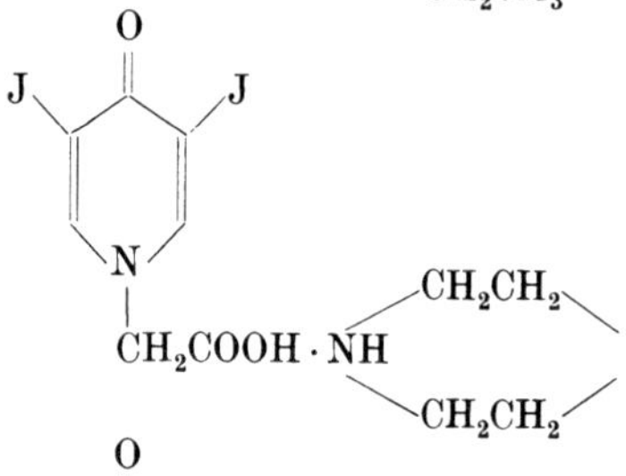

c)

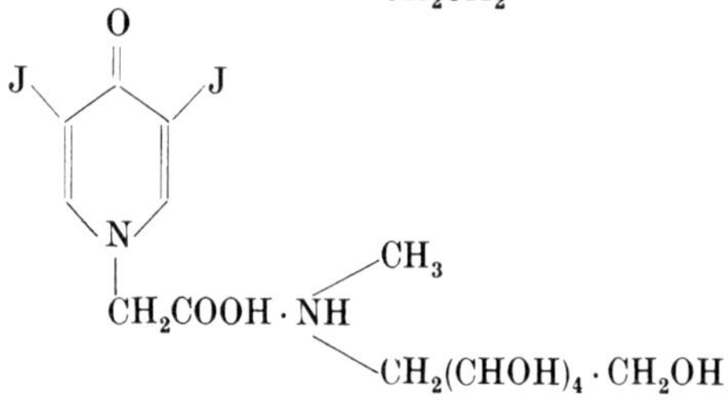

d)

Molecular weight	*Iodine content*
a) 510.1	49.8%
b) 478.1	53.1%
c) 492.1	51.6%
d) 600.2	42.3%

Official names:
Iodopyracet USP
Diodone   BP
Diodonum   NFN

Trade marks:
a) Perabrodil, Bayer,
   Arteriodone, May & Baker,
   Dijodon, Leo,
   Diodrast, Winthrop-Stearns,
   Leodrast, Løven,
   Neo-Ténébryl, Guerbet,
   Nosydrast, Winthrop-Stearns,
   Nosylan, Winthrop-Stearns,
   Nycodrast, Nyco,
   Perjodal, Pharmacia,
   Pyelombrine, Dagra,
   Pyelosil, Glaxo,
   Pylumbrin, Boots,
   Umbradil, Astra,
   Uriodone, May & Baker,
   Vasiodone, May & Baker,
a+b) Iodopyracet compound solution, USP,
   Diodrast compound solution, Winthrop-Stearns,
   Falitrast U, Fahlberg-List,
  c) Joduron, Cilag,
  d) Perabrodil M, Bayer,
   Glucadiodone, Guerbet,
   Hydrombrine, Dagra,
   Pyelombrine M, Dagra.

III. *3-Acetylamino-2,4,6-tri-iodobenzoic acid* is used in the form of the sodium salt or the methyl glucamine salt.

Structural formulas:

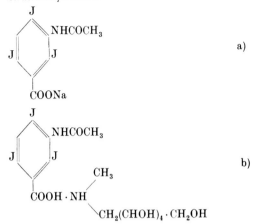

a)

b)

Molecular weight

a) 578.9
b) 752.1

Iodine content

65.8%
50.6%

Official names:

Sodium Acetrizoate NND
Acidum acetrizoicum NFN

Trade marks:

a) Urokon Sodium, Mallinckrodt,
   Acétiodone, Guerbet,
   Diaginol, May & Baker,
   Iodopaque, Labaz,
   Rheopak, Astra,
   Triabrodil, Bayer,
   Trijodyl, Lundbeck,
   Triopac, Cilag,
   Triurol, Leo,
   Urokon, Pharmacia,
   Vesamin, Byk-Gulden,
b) Fortombrine M, Dagra.

IV. *3,5-Diacetylamino-2,4,6-triiodobenzoic acid* is used in the form of the sodium and methyl glucamine salt.

Structural formulas:

a)

b)

Molecular weight   *Iodine content*
a) 635.9   59.9%
b) 809.2   47.1%

Official names:

Diatrizoate Sodium NND
Acidum amidotrizoicum NFN

Trade marks:

a) Hypaque Sodium, Winthrop-Stearns,
   Hypaque, Winthrop
a+b) Urografin (10a + 66b), Schering AG,
   Renografin (10a + 66b), Squibb,
   Hypaque M (1a + 2b), Winthrop.

V. *3,5-Dipropionylamino-2,4,6-tri-iodo-benzoic acid* is used in the form of sodium salt.

Structural formula:

$$CH_3CH_2CONH \underset{\underset{COONa}{J \quad J}}{\overset{J}{\diagup \diagdown}} NHCOCH_2CH_3$$

Molecular weight   *Iodine content*
     663.9   57,4%

Official name:

Sodium diprotrizoate NNR

Trade mark:

Miokon Sodium, Mallinckrodt.

For brevity and clarity these groups of contrast media will hereinafter be referred to as the di-iodine group, and the tri-iodine group (2 iodine atoms respectively 3 in the molecule). The contrast media within each of these groups differ considerably in quality.

For a contrast medium to be acceptable for such a common examination method as urography it must naturally be of low toxicity and it must be well tolerated by the organism. Contrast media of the di-iodine and tri-iodine groups are of low toxicity. The LD 50 for the di-iodine group is, for example, about 3.5 g per kg body weight when used intravenously, while the LD 50 of the tri-iodine group is still lower, namely 10—15 g per kg body weight.

All contrast media have a certain generalized effect on the respiration and blood vessels. Contrast media belonging to the di-iodine group and some of those belonging to the tri-iodine group produce a fairly protracted dilatation of the vessels and sometimes contraction, while others such as diatrizoate sodium belonging to the tri-iodine group have hardly any demonstrable effect on the circulation.

The local tolerance of the tissues to the contrast media is high. This is of importance in the diagnosis of diseases requiring a large amount of contrast medium of high concentration in an organ to be studied *e.g.* in the kidneys for renal angiography. The specific local tolerance of the kidneys will be discussed in the chapter on renal angiography.

Contrast media are capable of causing hypersensitivity reactions. This side-effect will be discussed in association with the description of the injection of contrast medium.

b) Excretion of contrast medium during urography

Contrast media used for urography are excreted in the urine. About $1/2$—1 litre of urine is produced a day, which implies that each kidney excretes $1/4$—$1/2$ ml per minute. The excretion may increase somewhat during urography because of the diuresis produced by the contrast medium.

The contrast medium is excreted partly by ultrafiltration in the glomeruli and partly by excretion from the tubular epithelium. The amount excreted by either way varies from one medium to another. The amount filtrated is directly proportional to the concentration of the contrast medium in the plasma. A high concentration of contrast medium not bound to the plasma protein will thus result in high ultrafiltration. This increased ultrafiltration is, however, accompanied by an increase in diuresis by the diuretic effect of the contrast medium. The increased excretion is thus balanced by the increased amount of urine so that the concentration of the contrast medium in the excreted urine will remain unchanged. This regulation of the concentration of the contrast medium in the urine is known from experience with other diuretics such as para-amino-hippuric acid, which is excreted in the same way as diodrast (RAPOPORT, BRODSKY, WEST & MACKLER 1949).

On dehydration the reabsorption of water is so marked that the concentration of the contrast medium in the urine will be higher than ordinarily. Thus, if the osmotic pressure—if this term should still be used—on the tissue side is high as it is in a dehydrated person, the reabsorption of water in the distal convolute tubuli will be increased to such an extent that the concentration of the contrast medium excreted will be higher than otherwise. A high osmotic pressure on the tissue side will thus permit a higher osmotic pressure on the tubular side, which in turn will result in the possibility of the kidneys excreting a urine richer in contrast medium.

The contrast medium excreted by the tubules is proportional to the blood concentration only if this is low, but since the tubular excretion easily reaches a maximum with the ordinary doses used for urography (this maximum is 25 to 50 mg/min of diodrast iodine/100 ml) the concentration is said not to increase further with increasing dose. Thus a further increase in the dose will, as a rule, not increase the density of the contrast urine in the kidney pelvis because the increase in concentration by filtration is lowered by dilution by the increased diuresis and, secondly, the concentration by tubular excretion depends on the low excretion maximum of the tubules.

This thus implies that the actual maximum molecular concentration of the various contrast media—independently of differences in the way they are excreted—is fairly equal for ordinary doses used for urography. An increased dose leads only to a prolongation of the constant level, which in human beings can be shown during urography simply by determining the specific gravity of the urine (HARROW 1955). Contrast density of the urogram can, as mentioned, be improved to a certain extent by restriction of fluid intake. KEATES (1953) thus found a decrease in di-iodine concentration in patients who had been deprived of fluid for 18 hours when compared with those deprived for 7 hours.

In children below one year of age the concentration is often low due to their large fluid intake (WYATT 1941). It should also be observed that during the first 2 weeks of life clearances in infants show low values, which afterwards increase, but with a wide individual variation (VESTERDAL & TUDVAD 1949).

Owing to the difference in the ways in which the contrast media are excreted, some being excreted mainly by glomerular filtration others mainly by tubular excretion, HARROW (1955) has suggested the use of a mixture of different contrast media.

An important possibility of improving the contrast density of the urogram is to increase the amount radiopaque component of the contrast medium without increasing the osmotic pressure. This can be secured by using contrast molecules containing several iodine atoms. The tri-iodine media represent examples of this. A solution of tri-iodine of given tonicity contains more iodine than a di-iodine solution of the same tonicity (but see below).

As to the contrast density, the literature contains numerous reports of trials with, and the relative value of, new contrast media in comparison with other media. Such comparisons are often of little or no value because the authors appear to have limited knowledge of the way in which the contrast medium is excreted and have not considered the sources of error in the evaluation of the results. MADSEN (1957) has pointed out that subjects to be examined represent such heterogenous conditions for excretion and technique of exposures that these factors alone make any evaluation illusory. It is better, but probably not sufficient, to submit the same patient to urography on two occasions within a short period. The only reliable basis is afforded by precise clinical and laboratory studies. Such an investigation has shown that if the patient is dehydrated the amount of iodine excreted, i.e. the factor of importance, is larger if contrast media of the di-iodine group are used, while in non-dehydrated patients contrast media of the tri-iodine group are superior.

The excretion of contrast media, however, also depends on the secretory pressure of the kidney and on the intrapelvic pressure. If the secretory pressure is lowered owing to a fall in the arterial blood pressure, urinary secretion ceases. WICKBOM (1950) has shown this on urography of human beings in whom excretion ceased when the blood pressure was lowered down to 70 mm Hg. I have seen cases in which excretion ceased on fall of the blood pressure to 80 mm/Hg. This has been investigated experimentally by EDLING, HELANDER & RENCK (1954). An increase in the intrapelvic pressure can also increase or impair the excretion of contrast medium. This is discussed in the chapter on urography during renal colic.

It is difficult to judge the density of contrast medium. This depends not only on the density of the contrast urine excreted but also on the amount of urine in the renal pelvis with which the contrast urine is diluted. In addition the width of the renal pelvis must be considered, the thickness of the layer of contrast urine increasing with the width of the renal pelvis. In the beginning of excretion the contrast density of the urine in the renal pelvis will be lower because the excreted contrast medium will be diluted by the urine in the dead space in the tubules and renal pelvis. Not until this urine has been removed by contrast urine will the density in the renal pelvis increase. If the renal pelvis is contracted or unusually small, the thickness of the layer will be less and the density of the contrast will therefore be accordingly low at a late stage of the examination, while if the renal pelvis is wide, there will be a thick layer and therefore high contrast density. After application of ureteric compression the renal pelvis will increase in width and the contrast density thereby increase. In fact the width is of decisive importance in judging density. This obvious and important point has been clearly illustrated schematically by MINDER (1936).

In addition excretion of contrast medium is also judged by such a crude method as estimating the differences in the density as seen in the film. Despite standardization of the method regarding preparation of the patient, of the contrast injection, of the type and amount of contrast medium used, of exposure, development and viewing and even if it be assumed that the thickness of the layer of contrast medium in the renal pelvis is always the same, there still remains the fact that the film reproduces contrast densities poorly, and the power of the eye to perceive differences in intensity of contrast is low.

As mentioned, modern contrast media have such a high iodine content that often a good contrast density can be secured in the renal pelvis even if a fair portion of the renal parenchyma is no longer functioning. This is demonstrated by the term selective pyelography (OLLE OLSSON 1943), which implies that small portions of the kidney can excrete contrast urine of ordinary density, while other parts excrete urine of low density or no urine at all. This phenomenon can be demonstrated in films taken immediately after a kidney with local lesions has begun to excrete contrast urine. Later during the examination this difference disappears and the renal pelvis can be filled with dense contrast urine coming from only a small portion of the kidney. Even in generalized kidney disease with decreasing capacity of the kidney to concentrate urine, the contrast density may be fairly high for a long time. This explains why the excretion of contrast urine may sometimes be good even in the presence of fairly severe renal damage. With a decrease in capacity of clearance by more than 50% the contrast density in urography may still be good enough for diagnostic purposes.

On the other hand, if the contrast excretion is low, this decrease may vary widely without it being demonstrable in the film or detectable by the examiner as reduced contrast density. Finally, the absence of demonstrable excretion of contrast urine in urography may mean anything between impaired excretion and no excretion at all. The above remarks elucidate the possibility of judging renal function from the density of the contrast urine. It is obvious that this method for judging renal function is very crude. Neither is anything else to be expected, since urography aims at securing an excretion of contrast urine as dense as possible in as short a time as possible, and it must be said to have filled this requirement very well.

Another method for judging the excretion of contrast medium has been suggested by RAVASINI (1935). He determines the time between the injection of contrast medium intravenously and the appearance of the contrast medium in the renal pelvis. According to this method, several films are taken soon after the injection of the contrast medium. In such an evaluation of the excretion the blood pressure must be taken into account. If the blood pressure falls on injection of contrast medium, excretion will be delayed. The amount of contrast medium injected and the concentration of the medium are also important. In my opinion, function can be better evaluated by determining the interval between the time of injection of a small amount of contrast medium and the appearance in the renal pelvis. Such a method, which might be called mini-urography, permits fine assessment of excretion and is not contra-indicated by severe renal disease.

Heterotopic excretion of contrast medium: In this conjunction it might be convenient to mention that occasionally contrast excretion is seen in the stomach (SCHOLTZ 1941). On injection of a relatively large dose of contrast medium the latter might also be excreted in the bile which we have observed in association with renal angiography with injection of contrast medium into the hepatic artery.

We have found contrast medium in the bowel of patients who after having undergone angiography in another hospital have been referred to us because of severe renal insufficiency (accentuated, but not caused by the urographic examination) (see Fig. 34).

During cholegraphy some of the contrast medium is always excreted via the kidneys. In hepatic cellular failure the renal excretion of the medium may be increased and thereby convert cholegraphy into urography. A case has been described by THEANDER (1956) in which such an unintentional urogram revealed a space-occupying lesion in the right kidney, the kidney on the right side always being included in gallbladder survey films.

c) Injection and dose of contrast medium

The patient is prepared for the examination in the same way as for plain roentgenography of the urinary tract. In view of the smallness of many of the pathologic changes that can be seen during urography proper preparation of the patient is important (see chapter D). Some authors recommend dehydration by restriction of fluid intake prior to the examination. This might be useful when di-iodines are used as a contrast medium, but is hardly necessary when tri-iodines are employed, except for patient with a large fluid intake. Withdrawal of fluids should, according to many authors, also imply that water enema should not be given because water can be absorbed from the large intestine. Since such water absorption is slow, a water enema is not contraindicated if given shortly before urography (STEINERT 1952) regardless of the type of contrast medium used.

As a rule, about 20 ml of contrast medium is injected for urography. We generally use 35—50% solutions of the di-iodine media and 30—40% solutions for the tri-iodine. Investigations on the tolerance to contrast media in association with angiocardiography have shown that large amounts can be used and therefore if, for some technical reason, the filling of the renal pelvis during ureteric compression is not satisfactory, the compression may be adjusted and a further dose of 20—40 ml, for example, injected. For children the dose of contrast medium need not be so large, but the dose should not be too small, 12—20 ml usually being suitable. If the dose is too small, contrast may be poor because of the relatively low tubular secretion in infants.

One may, however, if desired, try a small dose of contrast medium for urography. In adults good urography is sometimes possible with such a small dose as 3 ml of a contrast medium in ordinary concentration.

The medium is usually administered intravenously but may be given intra-arterially or intra-muscularly or subcutaneously. On extravascular injection we usually dilute the contrast medium with one or two parts of distilled water and, before injecting it, we prepare the site of injection with hyaluronidase to increase the rate of absorption (OLLE OLSSON & LÖFGREN 1949).

Any extravasation following the intravenous injection of modern contrast media will only cause a reddening and tenderness and requires no special treatment.

Oral and rectal administration of contrast media have been tried but as yet without success.

Contrast medium has also been injected into the medulla of bones, e.g. in the tibia or the sternum. Then the contrast medium must be diluted considerably though large amounts may be injected within a fairly short time (WALLDÉN 1944). This method is, however, not widely used.

Before the injection of contrast medium the patient should empty the bladder, a full bladder interfering with the excretion and transport of urine. As known, filling of the bladder with oil was once used instead of ureteric compression for urography.

d) Reactions

Contrast media are capable of causing untoward reactions. Such reactions may be local or general.

It has often been claimed that urography may be performed independently of the state of renal function (FEY & TRUCHOT 1944, JOSEPHSON 1947, SAND-STRÖM 1953). Two arguments may be raised against this opinion. From a roentgen-diagnostic point of view it is meaningless to do urography when kidney function is very poor because the excretion of urine and the concentration of the contrast medium will be so low that no information can be expected. Experience has shown that with clearance values below 40% the excretion of contrast medium is so poor that it is of no diagnostic value. In addition, if renal function is severely impaired, the injection of contrast medium for urography can increase the impairment. It is true that serious reactions are rare, as are immediate accidents, in association with injection of the contrast medium, but this does not imply that such hazards may be ignored. We have studied renal function before and after urography of patients with impaired renal function and found function to be somewhat poorer after urography. Cases from other hospitals have been referred to our special department for renal diseases because of anuria-oliguria following urography (ALWALL, ERLANSON & TORNBERG 1955).

In this respect patients with myeloma have received particular attention. Renal lesions are very common in myelomatosis. Patients with this disease are therefore often referred for urography, which is performed simply on the basis of the objective urinary findings, e.g. proteinuria. Urography may then be followed by acute or gradually increasing anuria (HOLMAN 1939, BARTELS, BRUN, GAMMEL-TOFT & GJØRUP 1954, KILLMANN, GJØRUP & THAYSEN 1957, PERILLIE & CONN 1958). Anuria in these cases has been ascribed to sudden precipitation in the renal tubules. We have seen cases referred to our hospital because of anuria after urography, in which further investigation showed myeloma to be the fundamental disease.

General reactions to contrast media fall into two groups, namely those due mainly to hypertonicity and specific toxicity of the contrast medium and described above and, secondly, reactions caused by hypersensitivity to the media. The severity of the latter varies from very slight to fatal.

The injection of the contrast medium is sometimes followed by a feeling of burning, reddening, nausea or vomiting, but the reaction is usually transient. Sometimes reactions of another type appear, namely urticaria in the form of single wheals or more widespread changes coalescing to form large regions of edema. Such edema may be serious if it involves the larynx and causes respiratory difficulties. A special type of reaction has been described by SUSSMAN & MILLER (1956). It is iodide mumps and consists of a swelling of the salivary glands occurring some days after the injection of contrast medium. In this connection it might be mentioned that the contrast medium for urography is not excreted in the urine in the form of mineralized iodine but leaves the body without undergoing any chemical change (HECHT 1938).

Occasionally shock develops with the usual signs: imperceptible pulse, pallor and severe drop in blood pressure. Such shock may, though rarely, be fatal. PENDERGRASS, TONDREAU, PENDERGRASS, RITCHIE, HILDRETH & ASKOVITZ (1958) made two large scale inquiries in the U.S. for any deaths during urography. The latter inquiry, which covered 4 million urographies, revealed 31 deaths, of which 25 were classified as immediate. Since then an occasional fatal reaction to contrast medium has been described, but it is very probable that not all cases have been published. To these must be added a certain number with uremia but without a fatal issue. It might be convenient here to point out that urography should not always be blamed for any serious condition arising soon after the examination. This is illustrated by a case described by COUNTS, MAGILL & SHER-

MAN (1957) in which fatal intra-abdominal bleeding was erroneously interpreted as shock caused by the contrast medium for urography.

Owing to the risk of severe reactions to the injection of contrast medium the examination room should always be equipped with an emergency tray with analeptics and antihistaminics and with instruments for artificial respiration, thoracotomy, and heart massage. It might be mentioned that hydrocortisone has been successfully used in the treatment of severe reactions (WRIGHT 1959). Adrenaline should not be used because it may cause ventricular fibrillation.

All steps should, of course, be taken to prevent such reactions. For this purpose certain precautions have been taken, namely testing the patient before the examination for any hypersensitivity to the contrast medium in contemplated urography and, secondly, simultaneous administration of anti-histaminics to try to counteract such reactions. Attempts have also been made to desensibilize hypersensitive patients.

Injections of 1—2 ml intravenously as a provocation test, intracutaneous injection of a small amount of contrast medium or a drop of the medium into the conjunctiva bulbi have been used as a test. Care should be taken that such a test-dose and the examination dose should be of the same type and preferably from the same batch. Since side reactions may occur several hours after the injection, the test-injection should preferably be given the day before the actual examination.

ALYEA & HAINES (1947) have compared the results of such test injections with those of injections for the examination proper. Their study confirmed clinical experience that there is no parallelism between the results of the test injections and reaction to the contrast medium for the examination and that there is no parallelism either between the incidence of allergic symptoms such as asthma and reactions to contrast media. If there is a personal history of asthma, hay fever or drug sensitivity and the skin test is positive, there is a definite possibility that the patient will have a general reaction to the drug, according to these authors. In such cases the performance or non-performance of the examination depends on the indication. On contrast injection of the same type but for definitely different purposes e.g. cerebral angiography, we have often found that patients hypersensitive to the test dose showed no untoward reactions to subsequent angiography, which had to be made for vital indications, and this despite the use of repeated injections.

PENDERGRASS et al. have described a case of death following injection of a test dose. Another case of death following intravenous injection of 1 ml contrast medium has been described by PAYNE, MORSE & RAINES (1956). I have also observed a case of sudden death following intravenous injection of 2 ml of contrast medium as a test injection. Death was due to bronchospasm, which could not be controlled. Emergency therapy including immediate heart massage after thoracotomy was unsuccessful.

Though fatal reactions are rare, the frequency of mild reactions is not insignificant, though it is true that they have become much less common since the introduction of tri-iodine contrast media. Attempts have been made to prevent reactions by using antihistaminics in association with the contrast injection (CREPEA, ALLANSON & DE LAMBRE 1949), or by adding a small amount of antihistamine to the contrast medium injected (OLLE OLSSON 1951). Such an admixture has been found to reduce the frequency of reactions but not to prevent them altogether. GETZOFF (1951), INMAN (1952), GILG (1953) and MOORE and SANDERS (1953) also reported a certain effect of anti-histaminics in association with the injection of contrast medium. Other authors, however, have found such drugs to have no effect. WINTER (1955) and DOYLE (1959) found reactions to

Miokon significantly to diminish when chlor-trimetone was incorporated with the contrast medium (diprotrizoate 30 cc 50% + chlortrimetone maleate 1 cc mixed).

Attempts to desensibilize patients according to allergologic principles have been performed by ARNER (1959) and we have seen patients who first reacted markedly to the contrast medium but after such desensibilization showed no reaction at all. The sensibility may be specific for a certain contrast medium. Recently we had a patient who could not be densensibilized to Hypaque, while desensibilization to Miokon was successful.

e) Examination technique

Urography may be used for studying renal function or renal anatomy or both. The evaluation of function should include not only the capacity of the kidneys to excrete contrast medium, but also of the capacity of the urinary tract to receive and to transport it. The morphologic examination is possible only in a functioning kidney and is thus in reality a combination of a functional and morphologic examination. If only function is to be studied, excretion is assessed on the basis of films taken at suitable intervals from the commencement of the excretion of contrast

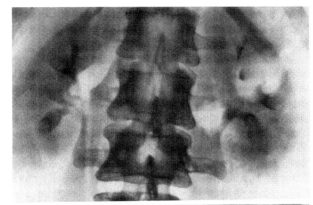

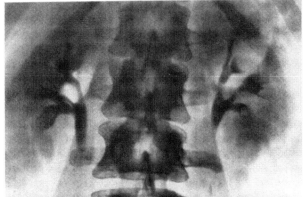

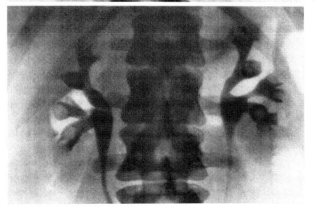

Fig. 26a—c. Urography. a Excretion starting, b maximal filling with free flow, c after ureteric compression for 5 min. Note filling defects caused by arteries in b in two branches on left side. They disappear on slight distension of pelvis by compression

urine, its excretion from different parts of the renal parenchyma, the concentration of the contrast medium, the filling of the renal pelvis and the ureter and further transport of contrast urine.

The first excretory urogram should be taken 1—3 minutes after the injection of the contrast medium. It will show excretion of the contrast medium with collection of contrast urine in the periphery of the renal pelvis, thus in the calyces. The most dorsal calyces will be filled first because of the high specific gravity of the contrast urine. The program of the rest of the examination will vary with the information desired and the findings made in the films as they are developed (Fig. 26).

If drainage of the kidney is not obstructed, the renal pelvis and ureters will never be completely filled. Owing to the rhythmic contractions of the renal pelvis, certain parts will be filled, while others will be contracted. Since diastole is much longer than systole the set of films will be dominated by those taken during diastole with relatively good filling of most of the calyces. The cranial calyces are filled first and then the dorsal, as mentioned, because of the position of the kidney and the high specific gravity of the contrast urine. The caudal and ventral calyces are often not filled or filled only incompletely. Normally the filling of the ureter is never continuous, usually the upper and lower thirds are filled, while the middle third is void of contrast medium, or a filling may be obtained of other segments of the ureter.

Detailed examination of the anatomy therefore requires the accumulation of contrast urine in the renal pelvis by ureteric compression and examination of the entire ureter requires films taken, when the contrast urine, on release of ureteric compression, flows from the renal pelvis down through the ureter.

As mentioned, examination of the anatomy of the kidney requires acceptable renal function. Compression should therefore not be applied until satisfactory excretion has been demonstrated. This can usually be done in a single film, well coned for the kidneys only, and taken 3 minutes after the contrast excretion.

Different methods have been described for ureteric compression. The best results are obtained by the use of a couple of rubber bags placed over either ureter and inflated to a pressure of 0.3—0.4 kg/cm². The pressure should be increased only slowly. A large single balloon placed over the middle of the abdomen often dislocates the ureters laterally and results in poor compression, besides which it increases intra-abdominal pressure with consequent impairment of renal function (BRADLEY & BRADLEY 1947). Some examination tables are equipped with an appliance for the application of compression, but such accessories fixed to the examination table prevent change in the posture of the patient during the examination. Change in posture is important, particularly for taking oblique films for demonstrating details of the renal pelvis. Compression appliances of this type are constructed in such a way that they cause a rapid increase in the pressure, which makes their use still less desirable.

It has been questioned whether ureteric compression really does obstruct flow through the ureters (CARLSON 1946). Such an opinion only serves to demonstrate lack of knowledge of the technique of ureteric compression and of interpretation of the findings when compression is used. In fact flow through the ureter can be completely obstructed, and prolonged compression can produce such an increase in intrapelvic pressure as to cause renal colic. It is also possible in this way to cause distension of the renal pelvis with rupture of the fornix with sinus reflux. The effect of compression of the ureter is best seen on comparison of the flow in the two ureters on compression of one of them.

On occasion, when it is difficult to obtain a filling of the renal pelves because of their being markedly contracted, it might be advisable to inject some antispasmodic drug (SINGER 1947, MÖCKEL 1954). Such antispasmodics should be used only exceptionally, and they do not always produce the desired effect.

Occasionally the injection of the contrast medium or the compression causes a fall in the blood pressure with decreased secretory pressure and cessation of excretion as a result. Injection of ephedrine with consequent increase in the blood pressure will be followed immediately by excretion.

A good filling of the renal pelvis usually requires 5—10 minutes' ureteric compression. Sometimes compression must be adjusted. If necessary, a second dose of contrast medium should be injected. It might sometimes be desirable to prolong compression for a considerable time. It might also be necessary to take films with the patient in different postures possibly including the erect position. In the examination of individual calyces well coned films in different projections are always necessary.

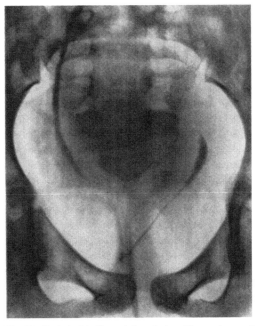

The examination is concluded with films of the ureter and bladder taken on release of compression. The contrast urine then rushes through the ureters which are then filled along their entire length (see Fig. 23a). It is important that the films of the ureters be sharp. Experience has shown that on release of the compression the patient moves and therefore he has to be properly instructed not to do so. Sharp roentgenograms are necessary because examination of the ureters is important for the detection of papilloma, cystic ureteritis etc., the changes often being very slight.

Fig. 27. Ureteric jet. From left ureteric orifice a stream of contrast urine is ejected through the bladder to the base to the right of the midline

On release of compression with flow of contrast urine through the ureter into the bladder, where the contrast urine is diluted, a jet of ureter urine is sometimes seen in the bladder (Fig. 27). This might convey a false impression of the site of the ureteric orifice.

After injection of contrast medium the renal parenchyma becomes denser because the contrast medium is condensed in the excretory system of the kidney. This phenomenon is called the nephrographic effect. It is most striking in a kidney with normal renal parenchyma, which cannot be drained because of increased intrapelvic pressure or low secretory pressure. Normally the nephrographic effect can be increased markedly by loading the kidneys by the injection of a large dose of contrast medium (WEENS & FLORENCE 1947, VESEY, DOTTER & STEINBERG 1950, WALL & ROSE 1951, DETAR & HARRIS (1954). VESEY, DOTTER & STEINBERG (1950) injected 50 ml 70% diodrast within 2 seconds and took films of the kidneys 16—28 seconds later. Satisfactory nephrograms were obtained in 18 of 25 cases by this technique.

The papillae often increase in contrast density owing to stoppage of flow of contrast urine of high concentration in the papillary ducts. This is thus a sign of stasis. This increase in contrast may be extensive or limited to a few papillae and should not be confused with papillary ulcerations. On the other hand, papillary ulceration should not be missed by confusion with this phenomenon. If it is very marked, it can simulate medullary sponge kidney (see chapter T).

It is well known that substances secreted by the tubules can block the excretion of other substances such as phenol red, para-amino-hippuric acid (PAH) and penicillin. In animal experiments EDLING, HELANDER & SELDINGER (1957) showed that the nephrographic effect is reduced if the injection of the contrast medium is preceded by injection of any of these agents.

In the many comparisons of the value of urography and pyelography it is widely believed that urography cannot yield desired information on morphologic problems. In view of what is said above it should be borne in mind that urography is often, if not most often, performed in such a way that the amount of information it gives on the morphology of the kidneys will depend almost entirely on chance. If properly performed urography can, however, as a rule give satisfactory information on the anatomy in addition to the information it yields about the function of the kidney and the urinary pathways.

Some authors disapprove of the use of urography in the investigation of morphologic changes in general or for certain purposes. Thus v. LICHTENBERG and BOEMINGHAUS are often referred to. As a matter of principle, ureteric compression should not be used in an examination of function, which has, of course, been emphasized by pioneers in this field. I would here once more stress that in the examination of physiologic conditions e.g. in the investigation of stasis, compression should not be applied. In other cases and with the advances made in urography together with the availability of contrast media that are excreted in high concentration, it is possible to make combined functional and morphologic examinations with the emphasis on the morphology. This also often makes retrograde pyelography unnecessary, which is an important advantage if check examinations are contemplated that do not in themselves require catheterization. Such a combined examination also often simplifies investigation and gives more richly faceted information. If the excretion of contrast medium is good and the examination technique satisfactory, it is possible, with the use of compression, to judge even details of the morphology.

An investigation by DIHLMANN (1958) produced statistical evidence of the value of compression, but in his investigation the examinations were standardized and therefore do not show the true value of the examination method. I can therefore agree with his results but not with his conclusion when he says that incipient pathologic changes of the calyces can still be recognized best by means of retrograde pyelography. This is not always true. Even incipient changes can often be demonstrated distinctly by urography, and sometimes urography is even superior to retrograde pyelography in this respect. It is, however, important that, as pointed out previously, the examination steps be adjusted to circumstances in the way described above and not in accordance with any strictly standardized procedure.

It is widely accepted as a fundamental rule that films taken during urography should be exposed at certain standardized intervals after injection of the contrast medium. In my opinion, such a procedure is not acceptable, the excretion, filling and emptying of the kidney pelvis and flow of contrast urine through the ureters as well as the pathologic processes of varying appearance, extent and effect on renal function calling for full utilization of all the possibilities of the method. All this makes individual variation of the examination technique necessary. All standardization and *laissez-faire* procedures imply a poor technique. *The films should never be taken according to hard and fast rules. The examination procedure should instead be adjusted according to the requirements of the individual cases and with full utilization of all the possibilities of the method.*

IV. Renal angiography

In renal angiography all the vessels of the kidney can be studied, thus not only the arteries. An examination performed to study the arteries only, should be referred to as arteriography. The veins in the kidney are, however, often of diagnostic importance. They can be studied in the late phase of angiography or in association with cavography or by renal phlebography. The capillary phase is usually of still greater importance. Renal angiography should therefore be performed in such a way as to yield as detailed information as possible on the different phases, which should be considered together in the final interpretation of the findings. Renal angiography should always be properly planned and performed, and nothing should be left to chance.

Renal angiography can be performed as aortic renal angiography, when the contrast medium is injected into the abdominal aorta, or as selective renal angiography, when the medium is injected directly into the renal artery.

A filling of the renal arteries can be obtained by different measures such as direct (percutaneous) aortic puncture, catherization of the aorta or selective catheterization of a renal artery.

a) Aortic puncture

The original method was described by Dos Santos, Lamas and Caldas in 1929. With the patient supine and with a needle 1.2 mm in outer diameter with a stylet the lumbar aorta is punctured laterally from the left side immediately below the twelfth rib with the needle directed ventrally, medially and cranially, in an attempt to puncture the aorta above the origin of the renal arteries. If puncture is successful, arterial blood will flow from the tip of the needle on removal of the stylet. This flow of arterial blood shows that the tip of the needle lies free in an artery, but does not indicate with certainty that it is in the aorta. This is an important point because a dose of contrast medium adjusted with due allowance for dilution with the relatively large volume of blood in the aorta can be injected directly into a mesenteric or a lumbar artery or into a renal artery, for example, if the tip of the needle happens to have pierced that artery instead of the aorta. Dos Santos (1937) tried to avoid injection of contrast medium directly into a renal artery by avoiding puncture of that part of the aorta from which the renal arteries usually arise. He called that section *la zone dangereuse*. In renal angiography, however, it is desirable to deposit the contrast medium as close to the renal arteries as possible. To avoid injection of contrast medium directly into an artery branching from the aorta Bazy, Huguier, Reboul, Laubry & Aubert (1948) modified the method: they fitted the puncture needle with a silver stylet a few centimetres longer than the needle so that they could palpate the opposite side of the vessel wall. If the stylet can be advanced more than 2 cm beyond the tip of the needle the needle must be lying free in a branch of the aorta. A needle based on these principles was constructed (Lindgren 1953) with a movable stop-screw on the stylet and another stop-screw on the needle to prevent displacement of the needle during the injection.

b) Catheterization

Another method is catheterization with its many modifications. They fall into two groups, namely open and percutaneous catheterization. The former method was introduced by Fariñas (1946) who exposed the femoral artery, inserted a catheter up into the aorta and injected the contrast medium through the catheter. It has since been modified in several respects *e.g.* catheterization via the radial artery (Radner 1949) and brachial artery etc.

The percutaneous method was described by PEIRCE in 1953. He punctured the femoral artery with a wide needle and passed a catheter via the lumen of the needle. Needles used for this purpose must have a large bore because the lumen of the catheter should be as wide as possible to diminish the fall in pressure.

In order to avoid having to pass the catheter through a cannula and thereby to permit the introduction of a catheter of the same outer diameter or of even larger diameter than that of the needle used for puncture SELDINGER (1953) devised a valuable modification. Poisseuille's law states that when pressure and viscosity are constant, the rate of flow through narrow tubes is inversely proportional to the length of the tube and directly proportional to the 4th power of the radius of the tube. The cross section of the catheter therefore has a dominant influence on the flow of the injected contrast medium. This is utilized in the construction in the following way. A flexible guide reinforced with a central wire is introduced into the cannula with which the vessels is punctured, after which the cannula is withdrawn completely and a polyethylene catheter is threaded over the guide and fed up into the vessel.

The catheterization method permits examination of the patient in supine position. This is of importance from the point of view of selectivity. The heavy contrast medium flows along the dorsal part of the aorta, and since the renal arteries spring from the aorta more dorsally than the mesenteric artery, it is possible, with the use of a suitable injection pressure, to obtain a filling of the renal arteries without any disturbing filling of the otherwise superimposed mesenteric artery. By placing the tip of the catheter in proper relation to the origin of the renal arteries it is also possible to a certain extent to avoid a filling of the splenic artery and hepatic artery (see Fig. 109). If the tip of the catheter is not in proper position, the bulk of the contrast medium may flow into one side, e.g. if the tip of the catheter faces the orifice of a renal artery or if the contrast medium is injected against the wall of the aorta and flows along it.

A combination of translumbar and catheterization methods has been described by CUÉLLAR (1956). This method has no advantages.

The advantages of the catheterization method over aortic puncture are that the contrast medium can be deposited more correctly, the contrast dose can be kept low, the patient can be examined in the supine position, the object—film distance can accordingly be kept short, and the patient may be turned and tilted during the examination. The only advantage of direct aortic puncture over catheterization is that it usually requires less time.

Further refinement of the catheterization method to secure greater selectivity can be achieved by *selective catheterization* of either renal artery. Methods for performing selective catheterization by exposure or by percutaneous puncture have been suggested. The first method of selective catheterization was devised at our department by TILLANDER (1951). He used a special catheter, the tip of which consisted of small steel links. This flexible steel tip was manipulated by a strong magnetic field so that the tip of the catheter could be passed into the renal artery under fluoroscopic control. BIERMAN, MILLER, BYRON, DOD, KELLY & BLACK (1951) used a radiopaque cardiac catheter with a fixed curve at the tip. The catheter was inserted into the arterial system by exposure of a suitable artery of sufficient caliber and could be advanced into any one of the branches of the aorta.

The percutaneous method is to be preferred. ÖDMAN (1956) uses a polythene catheter, the tip of which can be moulded into suitable shape by immersion in hot water and dipping it immediately afterwards in cold water. The catheter is radiopaque, which is a great advantage when feeding it into the renal artery under fluoroscopic control. It is introduced percutaneously *e.g.* into the femoral artery by the SELDINGER technique. The catheter should be properly curved according to the course of the renal artery. This artery constantly arises from the aorta at the level of the first lumbar vertebra. If plain roentgenography has shown that the kidney is low, it may be concluded that the renal artery springs at an acute angle from the aorta. The catheter should then be bent accordingly. Secondly, the catheter should be formed so as not to be fed too far into the renal artery because then only the ventral branch or the dorsal branch may be catheterized. When studying the films it is important to note where the contrast medium has been deposited.

EDHOLM & SELDINGER (1956) use an ordinary catheter which is bent by warming it cautiously above a match flame. The metal guide is introduced into the lumen of the catheter until it projects beyond its tip, and the curvature of the catheter is then straightened out. The catheter is introduced into the aorta. When the guide is withdrawn, the catheter will again bend and can be manipulated into the renal artery.

GOLLMANN (1957) modified this method, using a suitably bent wire instead of the reinforcing, straight wire. Another modification by the same author was to give the wire a flexible tip to permit passage of the wire also through tortuous arteries (GOLLMANN 1958).

To facilitate catheterization we usually place a lead marker on the back of the patient at the level where the renal arteries usually originate. We use ÖDMAN's catheter. When the catheter has been introduced into the renal artery, we check the return flow through the catheter to make sure that the tip is free in the artery and that the catheter does not occlude the vessel. We therefore never use catheters with side-holes but with a hole at the tip. The tip of catheters with side-holes is liable to be introduced too far into the vessel. If the return flow stops, the catheter is immediately withdrawn into the aorta. In addition, we take care that the catheter is introduced only a very short distance into the mouth of the renal artery. This is important because in 7 % of our material the dorsal branch of the renal artery has an early departure. If, in such a case, the catheter is fed past the origin of a branch departing early, it will enter directly into the ventral artery and give a filling only of the region supplied by this branch, which in addition receives the entire dose of contrast medium that is diluted only slightly by the blood. The catheter may also be pushed directly into the dorsal branch.

If a kidney is supplied by more than one renal artery, selective angiography may lead to misinterpretation if a filling is obtained of only one of them. If such incomplete filling is suspected, angiography should be repeated with injection of the contrast medium into the aorta. To avoid misinterpretation the examiner must be familiar with the normal anatomy and check that all intrarenal arteries are filled and that all parts of the kidney show an accumulation of contrast medium in the nephrographic phase. Reproductions of angiograms in the literature reveal that this source of error has sometimes escaped attention. The selective technique should therefore not be used in cases where there is reason to suspect multiple arteries, such as in double kidney, fused kidney, dystopia or hydronephrosis.

Some authors believe stereo-roentgenography to be useful. The procedure usually requires two injections, which is not advisable with contrast media of the di-iodine type, but may be performed with the best tri-iodine contrast media. It is, however, preferable in such cases to use simultaneous stereography according to FERNSTRÖM & LINDBLOM (1955). We do not use stereography, which we consider unnecessary if the examiner is familiar with the normal anatomy of the renal arteries (see below). In some cases we prefer to take an oblique view with a second injection of the same contrast medium in the small amount we always use for selective examinations.

c) Comparison between selective and aortic renal angiography

Of the methods available for renal angiography then, the examiner may choose between the aortic and the selective method. For some cases in which it is desirable also to examine the aorta and both the renal arteries, such as in arteriosclerosis or, if both renal arteries are to be compared such as for assessing potential renal function (see page 137), the aortic method is to be preferred. This also holds for patients with multiple renal arteries. Otherwise the selective method is to be preferred. The selective method has the following disadvantages: It may incur a risk, though rare, of blood clot formation, there is the theoretical possibility of infarction of some vessel region if it should be obstructed by the passing of the catheter too far (not observed), it requires more time than the other method, it may be necessary to supplement the examination or repeat the examination by the aortic method if multiple arteries are found or suspected.

The advantages of the selective method are that the pictures obtained are superior without any superimposition and that it permits the choice of predetermined contrast density. The examination can be performed with a very small dose of contrast medium and only one kidney is exposed to the contrast medium. We generally use the selective method even in patients with only one kidney. In such cases the range of indications for the examination must of course be kept narrow.

We have had fairly wide experience with both aortic and selective renal angiography. But for the exceptions described the selective technique is, in our opinion, far superior to the aortic. This impression is strengthened particularly in those cases in which the information desired should make the use of the selective technique desirable but in which for some reason the method could not be used, and in those cases examined first by the aortic method and then by the selective. *In renal angiography then, as in all types of angiography, the technique should be as selective as possible.*

d) Angiography of operatively exposed kidney

A special type of examination is angiography of the surgically exposed kidney described by ALKEN (1950). The contrast medium is injected directly into the renal artery or one of its branches at operation. GRAVES (1956) described a special injection needle for this purpose. Films are taken of the exposed kidney (for technique see page 20) and provide a good basis for detailed study of parenchymal changes. It is supposed to be valuable when explorative surgery, for example, reveals changes possibly indicating partial nephrectomy.

e) Injection of contrast medium

In aortic angiography the contrast medium may be injected by hand. If a catheter is used, greater pressure is required, and then a mechanical injector should be used. The injector described by Dos SANTOS is unsuitable because gas is then in direct contact with the contrast fluid. Modifications eliminating this risk have been described by CHRISTOPHE & HONORÉ (1947) and LINDGREN (1953). A more elaborate injector for angiography has been devised by GIDLUND (1956). We find this injector excellent. We have attached a simple accessory in which the syringe can be loaded with a small amount of contrast medium.

Timing of the exposures is important. Well timed exposures are easily obtained by taking films in rapid succession, preferably by cineradiography (GREGG, ALLCOCK & BERRIDGE 1957). We have solved the timing problem in a simple way by a method devised by OLIN (1958) with E.C.G.-control. It consists of a simple device plugged into the circuit film changer—electrocardiograph—electric pressure syringe—roentgen—apparatus with a program selector. Signals from the electrocardiograph pass a transistorized amplifier to a relay, which releases the program (see OLLE OLSSON 1961). It is apparent that this requires an apparatus permitting exposures in relatively rapid succession. Various types of such an apparatus with a program selector are available. We have found a roll film changer satisfactory, but for small size angiograms we use a cut film changer. When this apparatus is started, injection from the pressure syringe is started in association with the next QRS-complex. When the pressure syringe starts, the roll film changer is also automatically started and the program selected is run. Since the pressure syringe has a certain inertia, we do not generally use extra latency after the QRS-complex. With this injection technique 5 ml contrast medium is enough. If the kidney is unusually small, the amount of contrast medium may be decreased still more, while a larger dose is necessary for a differential diagnosis of large expanding lesions in the kidney. This E.C.G.-controlled contrast injector offers a great advantage, it being possible to inject contrast medium during diastole, *i.e.* when the admixture of the blood is small, and a good filling can be obtained of the renal artery with a small amount of contrast medium. The flow in the arteries varies rhythmically with the heart beat, the rate of flow being highest in systole and dropping rapidly immediately afterwards. Thus, to obtain the best possible filling of the arterial branches of the kidney with the smallest possible amount of contrast medium, the latter should be injected in the beginning of diastole when the blood flow to the kidney is lowest.

Many authors state that the examination should be carried out under general anaesthesia. Apnea can be readily secured under anaesthesia, but it can also be achieved without anaesthesia by good co-operation with the patient. We therefore find general anaesthesia unnecessary, like WEYDE (1952) and MALUF & McCOY (1955). A method using reduction of the blood pressure to secure the important nephrographic phase based on WICKBOM's observations referred to on page 42 have been described by LINDGREN (1953). With good timing of the pictures it is not necessary to use this method. Moreover, it may imply a risk of the examination by prolonging the time the vessels are exposed to the contrast medium.

f) Contrast media

For many years the use of renal angiography was severely limited by the toxicity of the contrast media. The method therefore fell into disgrace. The contrast media used were halogen salts, particularly sodium iodide. Yet authors who have not kept abreast of modern advances in the chemistry of contrast media still recommend the use of sodium iodide (RITTER 1955). Though unsuitable contrast media may thus be used here and there, they need not be dealt with here. Suffice it to stress that only the best contrast media should be employed.

Water soluble contrast media superseded the iodides: this implied a considerable advance. Though di-iodine contrast media are going out of use in angiography, they are still used to such an extent as to require brief commentation. Renal angiography is often performed without the examiner having any opinion of the tolerance of the kidney to the contrast media, and many authors even go so far as to say that the method involves no risks at all. Perusal of the literature will, however, reveal that the use of contrast media of di-iodine type has been followed by severe renal injury, occasionally with a fatal issue (collection by OLLE OLSSON 1955). Since then further cases have been described (LANDELIUS 1955, BERG 1956, EDLING & HELANDER 1957, 320 cases with 5 serious reactions). A collection based on a survey of 13,207 abdominal aortograms of all kinds with only 375 by the catheterization method with an overall complication rate of 1.02 per cent and a mortality rate of 0.28 per cent has been published by McAFEE (1957). In 1,732 cases more than 40 cc of contrast medium had been injected.

In a systematic investigation of the NPN, albuminuria, cylindruria and size of kidney after renal angiography with di-iodine contrast medium injected directly into the aorta in a 60 per cent solution IDBOHRN (1956) found signs of slight renal injury in 11 cases out of 39, and in 2 out of 15 in which 50 per cent solution had

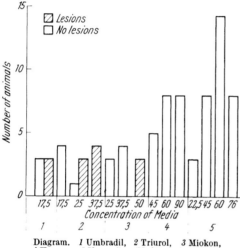

been used under otherwise identical conditions. In an experimental investigation IDBOHRN & BERG (1954) using a refined technique well adapted for investigation of the tolerance of the kidneys to contrast media found that injury can occur at concentrations of di-iodine contrast media above a critical level lying somewhere between 10% and 17.5% concentration in the actual renal artery. The tolerance appears to vary from one individual to another. By studies on renal function and experimental renal angiography on dogs WIDÉN (1958) verified the patho-anatomic findings of IDBOHRN & BERG.

Diagram. *1* Umbradil, *2* Triurol, *3* Miokon, *4* Hypaque, *5* Urografin. (Modified after BERG, IDBOHRN & WENDEBERG)

The tri-iodine contrast media have been studied in the same way (BERG, IDBOHRN & WENDEBERG 1958). It was shown that Urografin and Hypaque produce no histologically demonstrable renal damage. Triurol, however, in a concentration of 25% and more, usually caused histologic changes. Miokon in 50% concentration was also followed by renal injury. Control experiments with Umbradil in 17.5% concentration produced toxic changes in half of the animals studied (see Diagram above). It should be observed that these concentrations refer to the actual concentration in the renal artery, which can be assessed if the experimental design is suitable. In an investigation by IDBOHRN & NORGREN it was shown that renal blood flow was not affected by the best tri-iodine media (see OLLE OLSSON 1961).

In an investigation by EDLING, HELANDER, PERSSON & ÅSHEIM (1958) with 60 per cent Urografin and 50 per cent Miokon in large doses injected through a catheter inserted in the aorta of dogs no renal injury was demonstrable despite the use of very large doses. It should be remembered that contrast medium injected in this way is diluted with aortic blood and does not correspond to the actual concentration in the renal arteries. One can, however, agree with the authors when they conclude that properly performed aortographies, preferably by transfemoral catheterization, will not damage healthy kidneys, though it should perhaps be added: with the use of the best tri-iodine contrast media. It is thus obvious that certain tri-iodine contrast media are the best media hitherto available for renal angiography and that there is no reason to use the di-iodine media. The last mentioned authors also performed an investigation on dogs with selective renal angiography using di-iodine media as well as one of the less good tri-iodine media. This contrast medium produced renal damage when used in a large dose, while a small dose produced no change. This implies that the risks of renal damage are small, but may be are somewhat greater in selective angiography than in aortic angiography.

Dose of contrast medium. For aortic renal angiography we use 25—30 ml Urografin; for selective angiography with injection directly into a renal artery, 5 ml. For lean patients we use 60% solution; for obese patients, 76%.

We keep the exposure time as short as possible with a voltage of about 100 kV. We take films in a series of 6 pictures the first second, then 1 picture a second for 4 seconds and then 1 picture every third second for 9 seconds.

g) Risks

On direct puncture some or all of the contrast medium may be deposited extravascularly. As a rule, this will produce at most slight discomfort. But pleural effusion may occur on the injected side. Pneumothorax may also develop owing to puncture of the pleural cavity if the lung extends far down, such as in emphysema.

Contrast medium may also be accidentally deposited subintimally in the aorta as in the carotid artery in carotid angiography, for example (IDBOHRN 1951), *i.e.* a fairly well defined accumulation of contrast medium will be seen which does not mix with the blood (GAYLIS & LAWS 1956, BOBLITT, FIGLEY & WOLFMAN 1959). The amount of contrast medium deposited subintimally may be small or large. If the amount thus deposited is small, complications will not occur. If the amount is large, symptoms of the type seen in dissecting aneurysms may occur with a fatal issue.

On catheterization as well as on direct puncture haemorrhage may occur at the site of puncture. Such haemorrhage in association with aortography is usually very slight. It is also slight if the femoral artery is punctured. Care should, however, be taken to puncture the artery well below the inguinal ligament, so that any subsequent haematoma may be readily discovered. If the artery is punctured higher up, haematoma may develop retroperitoneally and remain concealed for a long time.

A case report is given by ANTONI & LINDGREN (1949) of an aged, arteriosclerotic man in whom abdominal aortography (prone position, pillow under upper part of abdomen, percutaneous puncture) was followed by a flaccid paraplegia. Without discussing the contrast medium used they believe the lesion to have been caused by the compression of the aorta, thus constituting in reality a Steno's experiment in man.

If the contrast medium intended to be injected into the aorta is injected directly into the renal artery, the concentration may exceed the tolerance of the renal parenchyma with renal damage as a consequence. This might also occur if the flow in the distal part of the aorta is obstructed (BARNES, SHAW, LEAF & LINTON 1955, GROSSMAN & KIRTLEY 1958, McDOWELL & THOMPSON 1959). On accidental injection into a lumbar artery the contrast medium may damage the spinal cord (ABESHOUSE & TIONGSON 1956, McCORMACK 1956, BAURYS 1956, CONGER, REARDON & AREY 1957, HARE 1957). The tolerance of the spinal cord to contrast medium has been studied by HOL & SKJERVEN (1954). They claim that examination of animals in supine position favours damage to the spine because the contrast medium is heavy and will therefore flow dorsally. TARAZI,

MARGOLIS & GRIMSON (1956) state that the large volume of contrast media injected through a site near a major radicular artery and the use of the supine position have increased the frequency and extent of damage to the spinal cord. With the use of the catheterization technique, a small amount of a suitable contrast medium this risk is very small indeed.

Sometimes spasm is seen. The pathologic nephrogram due to spasm produced by traumatization of the arterial wall by the catheter, by occlusion of the vessel by the catheter, and by too large a dose of contrast medium has been described by EDSMAN (1957) and studied experimentally by EDLING & HELANDER (1959). One or more intrarenal branches show no contrast filling and ischemia occurs peripherally in a circumscribed region or around the whole kidney. This gives the nephrogram a characteristic appearance with irregular parts of increased density intermingled with mostly cortical irregular filling defects.

Spasm may also occur in a kidney with multiple arteries if the entire dose of contrast medium is injected into a thin supplementary artery which is occluded by the catheter. LODIN & THORÉN (1955) suggested that the examination might be performed under ganglionic block to counteract the risk of spasm. Under anaesthesia the vessels are occasionally wider than otherwise. In my opinion, neither ganglionic block nor anaesthesia are necessary. Spasm is best avoided by using a small dose of a good contrast medium and proper catheterization technique.

Occasionally small clots may occur at the tip of the catheter and, if the technique is poor, gas bubbles.

In this connection it might be convenient to stress that certain authors claim that renal angiography is of little or no value in the investigation of urologic problems and should therefore not be performed (NESBITT 1955, CONGER, REARDON & AREY 1957). Such a view represents a conservative attitude and is not acceptable, but it is undoubtedly a healthy counter-weight to the postulation by many uncritical authors that renal angiography is a perfectly safe procedure independently of the way it is performed. In my opinion, *renal angiography is an indispensable diagnostic method. But it should be performed in a proper way and for good indications.* It is apparent from reports and illustrations on record that the technique employed often leaves much to be desired.

h) Anatomy and roentgen anatomy

α) Arteries

The two renal arteries arise from the aorta in the sectional mid-plane and usually at the same level, *i.e.* at the lower third of the first lumbar vertebra or at the disk between the first and second lumbar vertebrae. The superior mesenteric artery arises somewhat cranial thereto and from a more ventral aspect. The origin of the right renal artery is, as a rule, somewhat more cranial than that of the left. The right renal artery most frequently runs a horizontal or descending course; the left, a horizontal or ascending course. The renal artery always enters the upper part of the hilum cranial to the renal pelvis and here the artery has its center of divergence. In 68% of all cases the artery divides after it has entered the hilum (HOU-JENSEN 1929). It may, however, divide earlier and in 20—40% two renal arteries occur on eithei side (POIRIER & CHARPY 1923). The renal artery is of end artery type right down to the interlobar branches, so that each branch has its own field of supply and does not anastomose with the other territories at that level. The kidney has an anterior territory and a posterior territory divided by an intermediate region fairly poor in vessels somewhat posterior to the longitudinal plane of the kidney. There is a segmental arrangement of the intrarenal arteries, which is said to be constant. The region of supply of the renal artery has been described as being divided into 5 segments, apical, upper, middle,

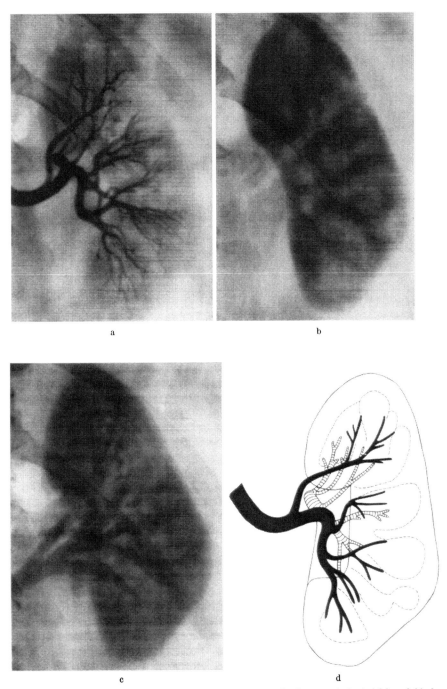

Fig. 28a—d. Normal renal angiography. a Arterial phase [skiagram (d) shows ventral arterial branch black, dorsal branch hatched]. b Nephrographic phase, cortex and columnae Bertini filled, pyramids appearing as defects. c Venous phase

lower, posterior, each of which is supplied by its own artery without any collateral circulation (GRAVES 1954). The artery to the apical segment had the most varying

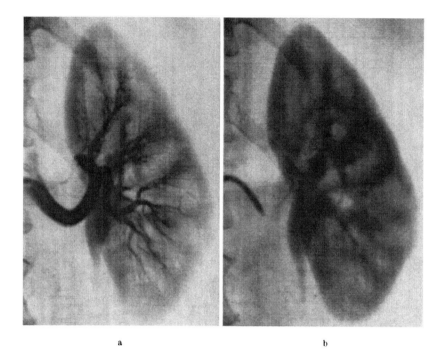

a   b

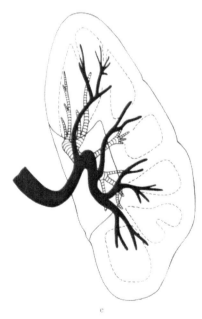

c

Fig. 29 a—c. a, b Arterial and nephrographic
phase, oblique view. c Skiagram

origin. Some kidneys have, as normal variants, branches running directly to the upper and the lower pole (almost 20% and 1% respectively: HELLSTRÖM 1928, BERGENDAL 1936). It should be observed that the arborization does not coincide with the lobation of the kidney (SMITHUIS 1956). It might be very irregular, one branch, for example, dividing within the hilum and running to both poles (CHIAUDANO 1955). (See chapter F.)

Selective angiography will give a clear impression of the anatomy of the vessels, knowledge of which is necessary for proper interpretation of the films. Knowledge of the course of the vessels is likewise of importance prior to any operation on the kidney, particularly if resection is contemplated. The anatomy of the vessels and their segmental distribution should therefore be founded on the angiographic findings. From this starting point BOIJSEN (1959) made an exhaustive investigation of the anatomy of the renal artery and its branches. The segmental distribution was studied in angiograms of autopsy specimens and in our clinical angiograms. The distribution is based on the localization of 7 pairs of pyramids described by Löfgren (1949). In principle, there is a ventral field and a dorsal field supplied by arteries arising from the renal artery. These arteries run ventrally respectively dorsally to the renal pelvis and always supply the intermediate parts of the kidney, namely the fourth and fifth ventral respectively

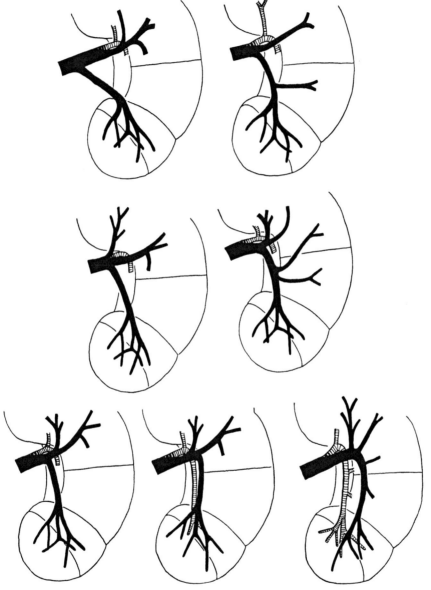

Fig. 30 a. Diagram of left cranial renal pole showing common variations of arterial supply. (After Boijsen)

dorsal pyramids. They often extend cranially and caudally so far as to include all the ventral and dorsal pyramids respectively. More commonly, however, the ventral arteries supply not only the ventral part of the intermediate part, but also the ventral and dorsal pyramids in the inferior part and the dorsal artery, the two uppermost pairs of pyramids in the superior part and the dorsal intermediate part.

Owing to the tilted position of the kidney and the characteristic appearance of the dorsal and ventral branch of the renal artery, a single projection is often sufficient to chart the course and field of supply of these branches. Sometimes an oblique view is helpful (Figs. 28, 29). As a rule, the dorsal branch gives the impression of being the first branch from the renal artery, in most cases it is much narrower than the ventral branch, and, owing to the position of the kidney, it runs more medially than the ventral branch and its field of supply is also situated more medially. Separate arteries from the renal artery sometimes run to the two poles before division into dorsal and ventral branches, though, as a rule, the poles are supplied by the ventral and dorsal branch respectively.

The nutrition of the first two pairs of pyramids varies widely; they are often supplied by several arteries (Fig. 30a). The supply to the pars inferior, on the

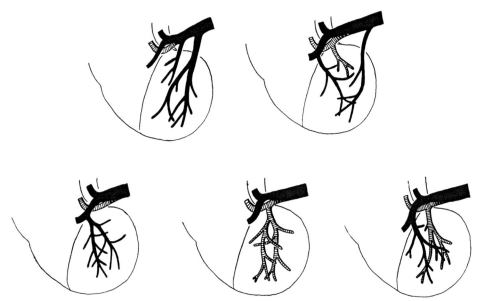

Fig. 30b. Diagram showing common variations in origin, course and field of supply of arterial branches to caudal pole. (After BOIJSEN)

other hand, is more regular, usually with only one artery running to the lower pole (Fig. 30b). In 30% of the cases in our material the dorsal branch supplied the dorsal pyramids; the ventral branch, only the ventral pyramids in the lower pole. In 60% of the cases the entire inferior part was supplied by a lower polar artery arising from the renal artery or its ventral branch (Fig. 31). In these cases the vessels to the lower pole can be ligated in the hilum so that an almost horizontal incision can be made through the lower part of the kidney on resection of the lower renal pole.

The renal arteries are end-arteries, so that examination by the selective technique will be incomplete if the kidney is supplied by more than one renal artery (Fig. 32). Of our series of "normal" kidneys, we found supplementary arteries in 20%. We did not find the number of renal arteries to vary with the normal variation in the shape of the renal pelvis. On the other hand, we did find that double kidneys and kidneys with hydronephrosis due to obstruction of the pelviureteric junction were supplied by multiple arteries in 50% of the cases. Almost all kidneys with a congenital malformation had multiple renal arteries. Therefore in such cases we do not perform selective catheterization of the renal artery.

Multiple arteries will be discussed in association with anomalies (page 92) and hydronephrosis (page 251).

The caliber of the artery is of importance from certain diagnostic points of view. In the anatomic literature it is described as being 6 mm wide. We have found a considerable range of variation of the caliber of the renal artery in normals and a general tendency of the caliber to decrease with increasing age. In a clinical

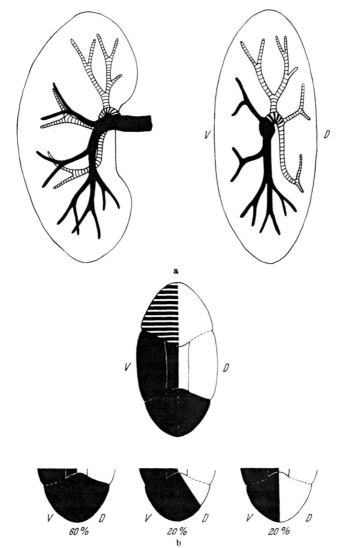

Fig. 31 a and b. Schematic illustration of segmental distribution of ventral and dorsal branch of renal artery

material EDSMAN (1957) found the renal artery, as measured on angiograms, to range between 6.1 and 9.7 mm in the majority of cases, the corresponding figures for women being 4.6—8.2 mm. There was no difference in the luminal diameter of the single renal artery on the right side and the left side in his material.

In selective angiography the capsular arteries, arteria capsularis superior and arteria capsularis media and inferior, will often be filled (Fig. 33). They stand out distinctly because of the relatively slow rate of flow in them and they appear filled with contrast medium longer than the renal artery. These arteries can be displaced by tumours. They may also contribute to the supply of renal carcinoma and occasionally be the main supply.

Renal pelvis arteries can also be observed. They are, however, so narrow that they can, as a rule, barely be discerned except in pathologic processes in the renal pelvis *e.g.* pyelonephritis. This is also the case with the ureteric artery (BOIJSEN 1959).

β) Nephrographic phase (see Figs. 29 and 30)

It has been suggested to call this phase the capillary phase. This is not correct because it represents not only the contrast medium in the capillaries but also that in the excretory system of the kidney. This has been investigated by EDLING & HELANDER (1959) in well designed experiments in which Thorotrast which cannot be excreted by the kidney was injected into one renal artery, and water soluble contrast medium of the type excreted by the kidneys was injected into the other renal artery. Their investigation showed that the capillary filling is only a minor component of the nephrographic phase. The nephrographic effect is initially due to a very slight vascular phase, and mainly to accumulation of the contrast medium in the tubular epithelium of the cortex and in the urine inside the tubuli. If excretion is obstructed, back-diffusion of contrast medium to the blood may occur.

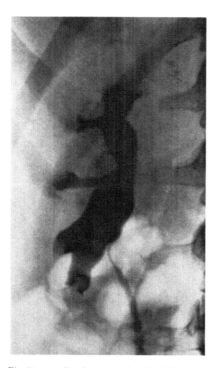

Fig. 32 a—e. Renal angiography. Technical performance. a Urography, malrotated kidney. Renal angiography

About 10 seconds after the injection of the contrast medium the nephrographic phase usually begins to reach a maximum, at which it persists for a period varying with the blood pressure. If the blood pressure is lowered, it may persist for several seconds. In this phase a dense accumulation of contrast medium is first seen in the cortex and columnae Bertini, while the pyramids appear as contrast defects against the rest of the kidney. Then the density of contrast also increases in the pyramids and thereby in the entire renal parenchyma. Because of the different directions of these pyramids in relation to the hilum, the density of the kidney will be irregular. This varies widely with the rate of injection of the contrast medium. If the amount of contrast medium injected is small or if the contrast medium is injected at a slow rate, these differences in the nephrographic phase will be blurred.

The outline of the kidney appears distinctly in the nephrogram and, as a rule, the hilum and the sinus are readily recognized. Any persisting foetal lobation can also be seen. The hilum varies considerably in shape.

γ) Venous phase (see Fig. 29)

The veins, which are wide, about twice as wide as the arteries, lie ventral to the latter and follow them in their course. Like the arteries, they may be duplicated, though less often than arteries (HELLSTRÖM 1928). In the hilum they are formed from 1—4 trunks. In contradistinction to the intrarenal arteries, the veins present no segmental arrangement, there being a free anastomosis of venous

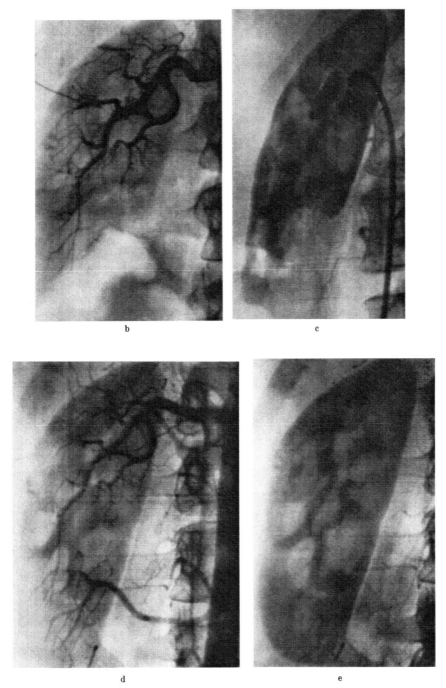

Fig. 32 b—e. b selective catheterization of renal artery. Arteries to lower pole missing. c Nephrographic phase. Irregularly outlined defect in lower pole. Aortic renal angiography. d Supplementary artery to lower pole corresponding to filling defect. e Nephrogram now complete

channels throughout the kidney (GRAVES 1956). The veins usually begin to become visible about 10 seconds after the injection of the contrast medium, but sometimes earlier, and the filling usually reaches a maximum about 20 seconds after the end of the injection. The use of a highly concentrated contrast medium will increase the visibility of the veins because the contrast blood is not cleared completely from contrast medium. This also appears to be the case if renal function is impaired. If the examination is carried out with the patient holding his breath in different respiratory phases, considerable differences can be seen in the course of the veins. According to LINDGREN the best filling is obtained when the blood pressure is so low that renal secretion almost ceases.

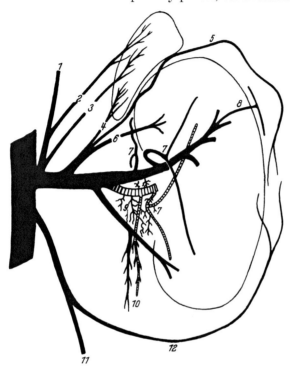

In this connection it might be mentioned that we have sometimes found the gallbladder to be filled after injection of contrast medium into the aorta for renal angiography.

We have also seen contrast medium in the bowel owing to renal damage, which was so severe as to prevent excretion through the kidneys. Fig. 34 shows such a case in which aortic renal angiography in another hospital was done with 50 cc of 50% Triurol on a patient with only one kidney.

Fig. 33. Diagram of arteries arising from the renal artery or its intrarenal branches and supplying extrarenal parts. *1* Inferior phrenic artery. *2—4* Arteries to adrenal. *5* Superior capsular artery. *6* R. sup. pyr. 1 V. *7—8* Middle capsular arteries: Recurrent (*7*) and perforating (*8*) arteries. *9* Pelvic arteries. *10* Ureteric arteries (ventral and dorsal). *11* Internal spermatic artery. *12* Inferior capsular artery, which together with the superior capsular artery forms "l'arcade exorénale" (SCHMERBER). Occasionally, though rarely, the inferior capsular artery departs from the renal artery. (After BOIJSEN)

Renal phlebography

In certain conditions, such as suspected thrombosis of the renal vein or the inferior caval vein by an ordinary thrombus or tumor thrombus, phlebography might be informative. This examination can be performed in association with cavography. Both femoral veins are then punctured and contrast medium injected at the same time on both sides. A catheter may also be passed, on one or both sides, into the iliac veins or farther up the caval vein to the level of the origin of the renal vein. The catheter might also be passed via an arm vein (exposed or percutaneously) the catheter then being fed through the right auricle of the heart down into the inferior caval vein. It is also possible to perform selective catheterization of the renal vein and selective renal phlebography (Fig. 35). GOSPODINOW & TOPALOW (1959) catheterize via the left spermatic vein, which is an unnecessarily complicated procedure.

Cavography is performed with the patient supine and preferably turned slightly to the side to be studied and with the head end somewhat raised. This position facilitates filling of the renal vein because of the high specific gravity of the contrast medium. After manual injection of 15—20 cm³ contrast medium (best tri-iodine medium) into each femoral vein, exposures are made preferably with a cassette changer. During the injection the patient may be instructed to strain when the head of the column of contrast medium has passed the origin of the renal vein. This facilitates the filling of the vein. If the flow in the renal vein is unobstructed, streamlining in the caval vein will be seen. On selective catheterization 10 to 20 ml is injected into the renal vein.

A special type of renal phlebography with catheterization is that performed on patients in whom an anastomosis has been surgically established between the splenic and renal vein because of portal hypertension. In such cases we have been able to catheterize both the renal vein and the anastomosis and pass the catheter into the stump of the splenic vein.

A special form of phlebography with a filling of veins in the direction of flow, thus from the side of the kidney, has sometimes occurred accidentally in association with direct puncture of the kidney and injection of contrast medium directly into the renal parenchyma (Fig. 36). This

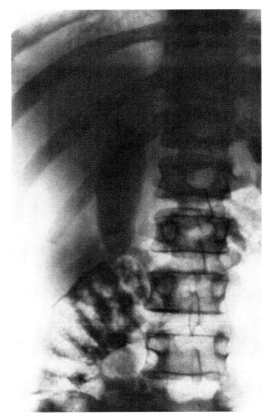

Fig. 34

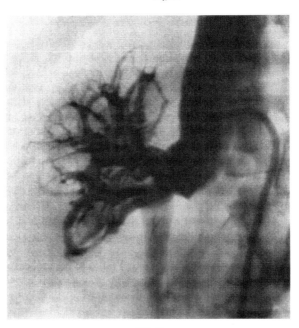

Fig. 35

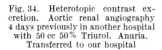

Fig. 34. Heterotopic contrast excretion. Aortic renal angiography 4 days previously in another hospital with 50 cc 50% Triurol. Anuria. Transferred to our hospital

Fig. 35. Renal phlebography. Selective catheterization of renal vein. Filling of renal vein and intrarenal tributaries and of inferior caval vein

5*

has occurred in association with splenoportography in which the needle has accidentally been inserted into the kidney instead of into the spleen. Excellent renal phlebograms were obtained without any side effects of the puncture. Two such cases have been described by LEGER, PROUX & DURANTEAU (1957). We have also had two such cases at our department.

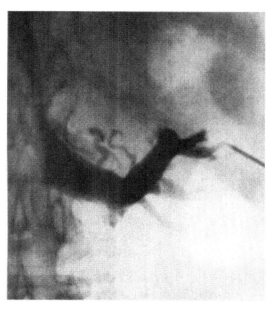

Fig. 36. Accidental puncture of kidney and injection into intra-renal venous branch. Filling of renal vein and of lateral part of inferior caval vein. (Puncture made for splenoportography)

Normal anatomy

The inferior caval vein crosses the right part of the spine. It is fairly straight and has a caliber of 1.5—3 cm. It anastomoses richly with the spinal and other veins which can be observed if the vein is compressed by a pathologic process or artificially. On performance of the Valsalva maneuver, contrast medium injected will enter the renal vein in retrograde direction.

On catheterization of the renal vein and injection of contrast medium directly into that vein, a considerable retrograde filling will be obtained of venous radicles as well as of the main trunks (see above).

F. Anomalies

Anomalies of the kidneys and upper urinary tract are common and represent a major part of all malformations. The normal range of variation of the anatomy of the kidney, urinary tract and renal vessels is so wide that it is sometimes difficult to decide what should be regarded as normal or anomalous in a given case. The shape of the kidney, for example, varies so widely that any deviations must be fairly marked before they can be classified as anomalous. The branching of the renal pelvis and the pattern of the calyces also vary considerably. Description of the anomalies is made all the more difficult by the fact that it is often not possible to say whether an irregularity observed is congenital or acquired, e.g. many of the so-called hypoplasias and of the so-called calyceal diverticula. Deviations referred to as anomalies here and in the literature in general are at any rate marked deviations from the rule. Below, these anomalies will be considered mainly from a roentgendiagnostic point of view.

Anomalies are usually described against the background of the complex but fairly well understood embryology of the kidney. When the anomalies represent conspicuous deviations from well known normal embryologic development and can be referred to certain embryonal stages, this method is very illustrative. But many anomalies are difficult to explain embryologically. It therefore appears more practical to describe these anomalies independently of embryology rather than to try to make them fit into any embryologic model.

A well defined component of the kidney now more accessible to roentgen examinations, *i.e.* by means of angiography, is the vasculature, particularly the arteries. The vasculature of the kidney varies considerably. Some of the variants were described in the preceding chapter. Some of these variants or anomalies are of interest from a clinical and/or roentgen-technical point of view. In addition there is a large group of vascular anomalies occurring only in association with other anomalies of the kidneys and urinary tract. Examples of independent vascular anomalies of clinical interest are supplementary arteries and veins obstructing drainage of the renal pelvis and supplementary arteries stretched by a dilated renal pelvis and thereby causing ischaemic pain (see Chapter Dilatation of the urinary tract). They also represent examples of vascular anomalies of interest in the technical performance of the examination because in the presence of multiple arteries only one of the latter will be filled on selective catheterization. This may lead to an erroneous interpretation of the findings (see Fig. 32).

An anomaly may consist of an abnormality in size or shape of the kidney, or in the position of the kidney in craniocaudal, medio-lateral or axial direction. Anomalous development may also be due to imperfect separation of the primordia of the kidneys and to malformation of the renal pelvis and urinary pathways. The above-mentioned anomalies are often seen in combination. They are also sometimes seen in association with extrarenal anomalies.

The kidney and the urinary tract develop from a ureterogenic component and a nephrogenic component. The kidneys and the upper urinary tract result from the interplay between these two components *i.e.* the ureteric bud and the metanephrogenic blastema. The blastema component, which is the origin of the secretory portion, thus the nephrons, is laid down first. The ureteric bud containing the primordium of the excretory part, thus the collecting tubules of the pyramids, the renal pelvis and ureters are laid down somewhat later. The ureteric part is the formative component (ASK-UPMARK 1929). Those parts of the urinary tract derived from the ureteric bud therefore dominate the anomalies. These parts are best accessible to roentgenology, particularly to urography and pyelography. In contrast to most descriptions of the anomalies, those of greatest importance and most easily accessible to diagnostic roentgenology will be dealt with first.

No attempt will be made here to include all anomalies due to embryologic disturbances. Some will be described in appropriate chapters, *e.g.* polycystic disease in association with renal cyst, stenosis of the pelviureteric junction in association with dilatation of the urinary pathways etc.

I. Anomalies of the renal pelvis and associated anomalies of the ureter

As mentioned in the description of the normal anatomy, the shape of the renal pelvis varies so widely that it is often difficult to decide whether it should be regarded as normal or not. In connection with the description of the anatomy a small process from the confluence or upper or lower branch for instance is described which probably represents a slight inhibitory malformation (Fig. 17). A definite but rare congenital anomaly of the renal pelvis is illustrated in Fig. 37. The commonest of all anomalies is the double renal pelvis with forked ureter or complete double ureter.

1. Double renal pelvis

The embryonal renal pelvis has two parts separated by a sulcus, the so-called primary bifurcation angle (LÖFGREN 1949). If these two parts persist more or less independently in the confluence, it will result in the formation of a deeply cloven renal pelvis which is usually regarded as a normal anatomic variant. If they do not fuse at all, the result will be an anomaly, the so-called ureter fissus or forked ureter. The kidney then has two separate pelves, each drained by its own ureter. The ureters unite, however, and from their point of union, which may occur at variable levels, there extends a common ureter to the bladder. Ureter fissus is regarded by many (cited NORD-MARK 1948) as being due to premature division of the ureteric bud or from an originally double ureteric bud. If this double bud persists, it will result in a double ureter. If the buds fuse partially, they will result in the formation of a forked ureter. Other authors claim that a divided renal pelvis, forked ureter and double ureter are different grades of one and the same anomaly, *i.e.* the ureteric bud divides a varying distance from its attachment to the Wolffian duct.

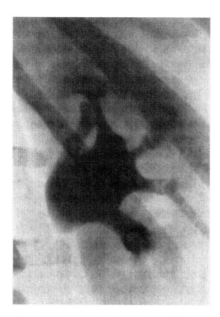

Fig. 37. Strange anatomic anomaly of kidney pelvis

In double ureter the upper renal pelvis is most usually the smaller (Fig. 38, 39). As a rule, it consists of two small groups of calyces corresponding to the upper branch of the ordinary renal pelvis. It may, however, also be much smaller and have only one calyx which drains only a small amount of renal parenchyma. It then forms a transition to a blind ureter (see below). In bilateral double kidney the renal pelves on one side may be very different from those on the other. Thus, the upper renal pelvis on one side may have the common shape described above, while that on the other may have only one calyx.

The lower part of the renal pelvis may resemble a small normal single pelvis. Particularly in children it may sometimes be difficult to distinguish the lower part of a double kidney from the renal pelvis in a normal kidney. This

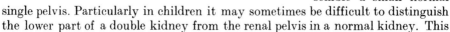

a   b

Fig. 38 a and b. Bilateral double kidney pelvis. On right side large upper part; on left side, small. Lower kidney pelvis slightly impressed bilaterally by upper part

should be remembered in cases where no excretion of contrast urine occurs in the upper renal pelvis during urography. The distance from the calyces to the cranial renal pole is then usually but not always longer. This should lead the examiner's thoughts to the possibility of a second renal pelvis. In addition the distance from the uppermost calyx to the medial surface of the kidney is usually increased. Therefore, in the absence of demonstrable excretion in the upper renal pelvis the presence of a tumor in the upper part may be suspected. The upper calyces of the lower renal pelvis also often appear to be flattened. This anatomic shape of the upper calyces of the lower pelvis with flattening can be thought to be due to pressure by a tumor (see Fig. 38). Thorough knowledge of the shape of the lower renal pelvis, especially the topography of its upper calyces, is therefore imperative if mistakes are to be avoided. The shape of the lower renal pelvis in a double kidney may vary considerably and sometimes represent the smaller part of the total volume of the renal pelvis. The lower part of the kidney is then often small and the changes as a whole may be caused by atrophy due to pyelonephritis (see Fig. 253).

In complete duplicate ureter one of the ureters may have an ectopic orifice. In males it is prone to empty into the prostatic part of the urethra and in females into the urethra, vagina

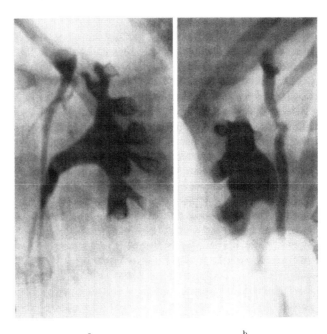

a   b

Fig. 39a and b. Double kidney pelvis with small upper part. In (a) caudal pelvis of ordinary anatomic form, not modelled by cranial part of kidney, which is too small to influence large caudal part. Note pyelolymphatic backflow from uppermost calyx of caudal pelvis. In (b) small pyelogenic cyst at edge of uppermost calyx of caudal pelvis

or vulva. It is usually the ureter draining the upper renal pelvis that has the ectopic orifice. This is readily understood on an embryologic basis. In the course of embryologic development the orifice of the upper ureter is regularly situated further down and closer to the middle of the bladder than the orifice of the lower ureter in complete duplication (Weigert-Meyers rule). Thus since the ureter of the upper renal pelvis is located further down, it will be closely related to the Wolffian duct and organs derived from it.

In double kidney changes may also be observed in the appearance of the actual renal parenchyma. Thus, plain roentgenography will sometimes show two hili or an unusually long hilum in the medial contour of the kidney. The medial contour is also strikingly straight with the hilar lips turned only slightly inwards. Sometimes a marked indentation is seen in the lateral outline between the two parts of the kidneys. The amount of parenchyma belonging to one pole or the other may vary widely. In the absence of lesions localized to either part of the kidney the parenchyma of the upper half is usually the smaller. It corresponds to the pars cranialis of the normal kidney and, as a rule, comprises three pairs of pyramids, while the lower part corresponds to the pars intermedia and caudalis of the normal kidney and contains four pairs of pyramids (LÖFGREN 1949). The line of demarcation between the regions of the parenchyma is not sharp. This may be demonstrated clearly by the nephrographic effect on urography in acute urinary stasis due to stone in one of the ureters (HELLMER 1942) (see Fig. 107). If one part of a double kidney harbours a lesion, e.g. pyelonephritis, it may shrink and the upper part may show hypertrophy with a marked difference between the two parts (see Fig. 253).

The parts of the kidney on one side may also be entirely independent with supernumerary kidneys as a result.

Renal angiography often, though not regularly, shows multiple arteries to kidneys with a double pelvis.

NORDMARK (1948) studied the frequency of double renal pelvis. Of 4,744 urograms he found duplication of the renal pelvis in 201 or 4.2 per cent and duplication of the ureter in 138 or 2.8 per cent. Bilateral double pelvis was seen in 1 per cent of the cases and double ureter in 0.4 per cent. Unilateral incomplete division of the ureter, thus forked ureter, was seen in 60 cases, unilateral complete division of the ureter in 59 cases, bilateral complete division of the ureter in 11, bilateral incomplete division of the ureter in 5, and complete division of one side and incomplete division of the other in 3 cases.

As mentioned, supernumerary kidneys also occur. Thus ureters may not only be duplicated but also triplicated. In all cases of triplication of the ureter on record the anomaly was unilateral. The three ureters may empty separately into the bladder or together with a varying length of the different free ureteric segments. One or more of the ureters may be dilatated and empty ectopically. As a rule, they belong to a composite kidney, which may be caudally ectopic (PERRIN 1927). But a ureter may belong to a free supernumerary kidney (LAU & HENLINE 1931) or it may be a blind ureter (CHWALLA 1935). A good survey of these rare anomalies has been given by GILL (1952). A case of sextuplicitas renum, six functioning kidneys and ureters, was described by BEGG (1953). He gives a critical survey on prevailing theories offered to explain how such an anomaly can arise.

For completion mention might be made of a ureter duplicatus caudalis, i.e. one renal pelvis but with branching of the ureter. This anomaly is difficult to understand.

2. Blind ureter

On double formation of the ureter one of them may cease in the course of its development and never unite with the renal parenchyma. It persists as a blind ureter. It may be as short as 1—2 cm, but it may also be even longer than a normal ureter (ENGEL 1939). The long blind ureter is, in reality, the ureter to the upper part of a double kidney that fails to form and, as mentioned, this malformation approaches that of a double kidney with a very small upper part. The blind part may unite with the lower ureter to form a forked ureter. It may, however, also be free and can then empty ectopically. Though such a ureter does not drain any parenchyma and thus has no real function, contractions may occur in its wall and the contractions may be so severe as to cause pain. Stagnation of urine in the blind ureter favours infection with fever, pain and stone formation which can cause pyuria and haematuria.

A blind ureter is best detected by retrograde pyelography. It can, however, be diagnosed by urography if it opens into the other ureter. It must not be confused with a ureteric diverticulum which is only a pouch adjacent a stricture in a ureter, for instance.

3. Anomalies of the calyces

An important group of anomalies which have received but scanty attention but which are of great importance are malformations of the calyces. These are important not only from a purely diagnostic point of view since they are apt to be mistaken for pathologic processes, but also because they may favour stone formation, for example. It is difficult to draw any definite line of distinction between normal variation and anomaly because, as mentioned, the range of normal variation is so wide and has not been the subject of sufficient systematic investigations. *Microcalyces* (Fig. 19) may be regarded as anomalous. They are very small, 5—10 mm long, calyx-shaped, tiny projections from the border of a calyx or consist of thin branches of a renal pelvis like an ordinary calyx. In these microcalyces stones may sometimes be observed and they may dilate (Fig. 40, see also Fig. 77). They may simulate a well defined sinus reflux.

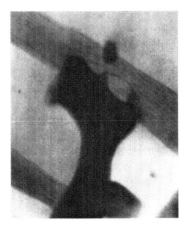
Fig. 40. Dilated micro-calyx

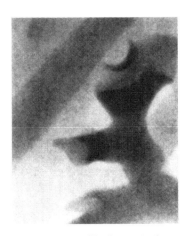
Fig. 41. Calyceal border evagination

Another anomaly consists of more or less distinct local evaginations from the border of the calyx (Fig. 41) usually from several calyces in the same kidney. Such small evaginations sometimes contain minute calculi (see Fig. 78). It is suggested that the term *calyceal evaginations* be reserved for this anomaly. Some of these changes represent borderline cases of a spongy kidney, for instance (see chapter T).

4. Anomalies in the border between calyces and renal parenchyma

Along the border between the two components of the ureteric bud and of the metanephrogenic blastoma, thus the junction between the calyces and parenchyma, anomalies are common. This region is also a common seat of pathologic changes. The diagnosis and differential diagnosis are therefore difficult in the presence of changes in this region. The most important form of anomaly is a cyst. A large number of bewildering names have been given to these formations such as cystes urinaires (RAYER 1841), pyelogenic cyst (DAMM 1932, LJUNGGREN 1942), calyceal diverticulum, Kelchdivertikel (ITIKAWA & TANIO 1939, PRATHER 1941), cyst of the kidney due to hydrocalicosis (WATKINS 1939), calectasia (ENGEL 1947), solitary renal cyst with communication to the renal pelvis (NATVIG 1941), Kelchzyste (ESCH & HALBEIS 1953), diverticules kystique des calices (FEY, GOYGOU, TEINTURIER 1951), ectopic calyx (KENT 1954) etc. This long list is by no means exhaustive. It is, however, sufficient to show that the nomenclature is confusing. These terms have undoubtedly been used to cover many different pathologic conditions. It is obvious that many authors have used the same name for different processes and that other authors have used different names for one and the same condition. This may be explained by the fact that some different pathologic conditions may simulate one another macroscopically, *i.e.* at roentgen examination and at operation and, secondly, various names have apparently been suggested without due consideration.

On roentgen examination the change appears as a cavity connected to a calyx. It is well outlined, more or less oval or round of varying size from a few millimetres to a few centimetres in diameter situated at any height in the kidney and usually connected with the renal pelvis by a narrow or wide, short or long channel. It may communicate with the fornix of a more or less well preserved calyx or with the middle of a calyx or it may originate between two calyces.

The pathologic conditions capable of producing such a roentgen finding may be divided roughly into two groups: 1. changes in the renal parenchyma with formation of a cyst communicating with the renal pelvis and 2. changes in the renal pelvis, particularly a calyx which may intrude upon the renal parenchyma.

Group 1. Various types of papillary ulceration such as renal tuberculosis, pyelonephritis and papillary necrosis may lead to destruction of the papilla and a wide communication or fistulation to a calyx. In long-standing or healed processes the remaining cavity may be smooth and well-defined.

If it is situated near the renal pelvis, a so-called meta-nephrogenic renal cyst which is laid down in the usual way, may rupture into the renal pelvis with which it then communicates. In such cases cysts are usually multiple and dislocate the branches of the renal pelvis. Meta-nephrogenic cysts communicating with the renal pelvis have cubical epithelium. The so-called pyelogenic cyst (see Fig. 39 and 79) may be of similar appearance, but it is usually single and, unlike multicystic changes, it does not deform the renal pelvis. The pyelogenic cyst is as a rule small, 1—2 cm diameter, but may, on occasion, be much larger. It is round or oval and well defined. The cyst often contains calculi, sometimes numerous microliths. Such a case has been described by RUDSTRÖM (1941) with about 2,000 microliths. The communication of a pyelogenic cyst with the renal pelvis may be very narrow. Not until after prolonged compression during urography can a filling be obtained, and sometimes the cyst is situated deep in the parenchyma without any demonstrable connection with the renal pelvis. This is because the duct is so thin that it cannot be seen. The collecting tubules empty into the wall of the cyst, and it is possible that a filling might be obtained from the parenchymal side, which explains why cysts of this type are sometimes not demonstrable by retrograde pyelography. As a rule, however, it must be supposed that even in urography the cysts are filled in retrograde direction by contrast medium which is first excreted into the renal pelvis. Only in one instance have I seen a fairly large cyst communicating with the renal pelvis, which after prolonged compression became filled and then suddenly expanded and dislocated adjacent calyces. Microscopically the pyelogenic cyst has transitional epithelium. Without shedding much light upon this anomaly DALLA BERNARDINA & RIGOLI (1958) ascribed it to "calico-pyramidal dysplasia". Roentgenologically the term pyelogenic cyst undoubtedly covers changes of different origins.

Group 2. The actual border of the calyx is capable of wide variation and, as mentioned, can show bulges which will be referred to here as calyceal evaginations. Most of the changes in this group, however, consist of hydrocalyces. Papillary ulceration often involves both the renal parenchyma and the renal pelvis. This is so in tuberculosis and pyelonephritis. In these diseases edema occurs in the stem of a calyx which may be accompanied by shrinkage resulting in stasis in the calyx with distension, flattening of the papilla and ulceration if infection is present. A common cause of hydrocalicosis is stone lodged in the stem of the calyx.

It has been claimed (WATKINS 1939 and others) that hydrocalicosis may result from achalasia of the muscle in the calyceal wall. The idea is interesting but as yet no supportive evidence is available.

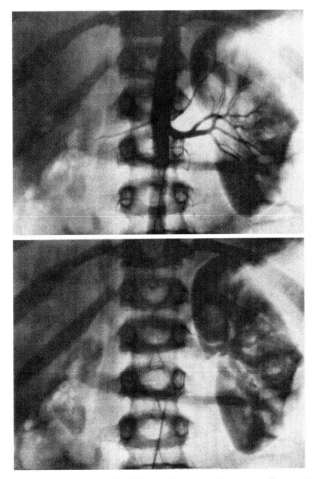

Fig. 42. Aplasia. Right kidney very small. Left kidney fairly large. Urography: No excretion on right side. Normal function and morphology on left side. Aortic renal angiography: Normal conditions on left side. Note separate upper polar branch to dorsal pyramids. Extremely small but otherwise normal kidney on right side. In final stage of renal angiography contrast urine was excreted also from right kidney showing small but otherwise normal kidney pelvis

The changes in juvenile hypertension described by ASK-UPMARK (1929) show anomalies of the calyx as well as of the corresponding part of the renal parenchyma. In these cases the calyx may be club-shaped and extend out to the periphery of the kidney. The appearance of the change simulates that of so-called local hypoplasia. A similar picture is seen in healed papillary necrosis.

Many of the lesions referred to above are difficult to distinguish from one another and undoubtedly a change of a certain type may be the end result of many completely disparate lesions.

II. Anomalies of the renal parenchyma

1. Aplasia and agenesia

Defective development of the kidney may vary from slight hypoplasia to severe aplasia and agenesia. Hypoplasia has been defined as a local or general maldevelopment of a kidney with apparently normal excretory capacity, as judged by urography (see below). The definition is arbitrary. Aplastic kidney is accordingly to be understood as a small malformed kidney showing only slight or no

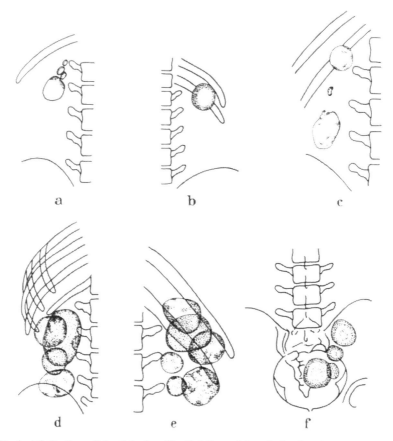

Fig. 43 a—f. Aplasia. Congenital unilateral multicystic kidney. Schematic drawing of some different types of this rare form of aplasia. (After STAEHLER)

excretion during urography. Such a kidney is sometimes seen in plain roentgenography as a small formation resembling a kidney only in outline. Sometimes it does not show up in plain roentgenograms but can be demonstrated by retroperitoneal pneumography. It may be demonstrable by renal angiography and will then be seen as a miniature of an ordinary kidney (Fig. 42). This type of defective formation of the kidney must be remembered in obscure cases of pyuria.

In the gravest form of aplasia one or more irregular cyst-like formations, usually calcified and of different size, are seen in the area normally occupied by a kidney. This is the result of a malformed primordium of the kidney. Such aplasia known as Knollenniere in the German literature and in English as congenital unilateral multicystic kidney (SCHWARTZ 1936, SPENCE 1955) is very rare (Fig. 43). On occasion, such a kidney may have a normal ureter, but it is usually atretic, rudimentary or missing. The vascularity is also rudimentary or missing. The deformed kidney may be ectopic, it might even show crossed ectopy (DEÁK 1956). One of the cases published by LEWIS & DOSS (1958) of calcified hydronephrosis resembles such an anomaly.

2. Hypoplasia

The finding of a small kidney on one side and a normal sized or compensatorily enlarged kidney on the other is not uncommon. The smallness of the kidney may be explained in different ways: it might originally be hypoplastic or it might have shrunk. Shrinkage may be due to different conditions such as tuberculous or non-tuberculous inflammation, stasis due to stone or it may be due to emboli, for example. The most common cause is pyelonephritis. Sometimes neither roentgen examination nor pathologic examination can explain the cause of the small kidney. Only if the shrinkage of a kidney has been followed roentgenographically, is it possible to diagnose the small kidney as a shrunken kidney. Repeated roentgen examination will reveal the course of reduction of a normal-sized kidney and thereby yield definite evidence that the kidney is contracted. The more widely the value of roentgenologic follow-up during conservative treatment of renal disease is realized, the more often will it be possible to ascertain whether a small kidney is the end-result of pyelonephritis, for instance.

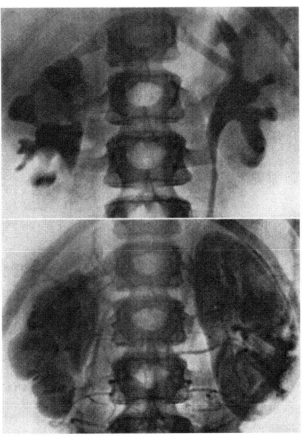

Fig. 44a and b. Local (left) and general (right) hypoplasia. a Urography. Left kidney of ordinary size and shape. Club-shaped calyces in caudal pole. Small right kidney. Dilated calyces in cranial pole extending to surface of kidney. Club-shaped calyx in caudal pole, laterally also extending to surface at site of deep indentation. Fairly good function. b Renal angiography, late nephrographic phase showing marked atrophy and scar-formation of right kidney

Many pathologists have tried to find acceptable criteria regarding the origin of small kidneys. But those suggested are to a large extent contradictory. After a careful study of 183 unilateral small kidneys, of which half were available for pathologic examination EMMETT, ALVAREZ-IERENA & McDONALD (1952) conclude "There is no doubt in our minds that the unilateral 'hypoplastic' or 'atrophic' kidney represents several different and distinct pathological entities. We are sure

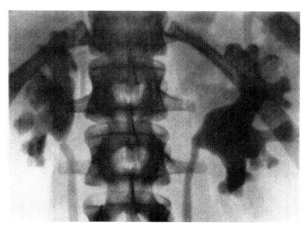

Fig. 45. General and local hypoplasia. Urography. Right kidney small, function somewhat delayed. All calyces deformed.—General hypoplasia. Left kidney: Calyces in cranial and caudal pole deformed. Majority of calyces in middle part of kidney normal.—Local hypoplasia

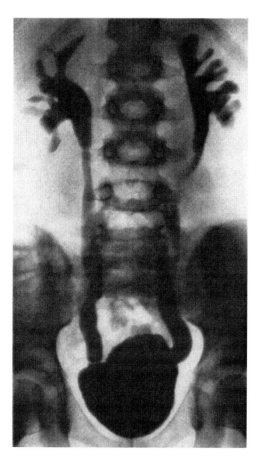

Fig. 46. Bilateral general hypoplasia (pyelonephritis?). Pyelography by reflux from bladder. All calyces in both kidneys deformed

that in some cases the lesion is congenital while in others it is the result of acquired or a combination of congenital and acquired conditions. One of the commonest acquired conditions is infection ('chronic atrophic pyelonephritis'). We feel that in some cases of apparent chronic atrophic pyelonephritis the kidney may have been congenitally small to start with, but we know of no way to decide this problem accurately. For this reason it would seem that it might be more sensible to forego any attempts at classification according to origin and clinical findings and instead to employ some common 'blanket' term, such as 'atrophic kidney' or 'renal atrophy', to describe the unilateral small kidney, the cause of which is not apparent."

In a monograph on hypoplasia EKSTRÖM (1955) presented a material in which kidneys were said to be hypoplastic if one of the two kidneys was small (two third or less than that on the other side) with adequate excretion on urography. Kidneys of this type often show characteristic renal pelvic changes, which can also sometimes be found to a varying extent in somewhat small or normal-sized kidneys. Such cases were also included as local or partial hypoplasia. The material consisted of 156 cases of hypoplasia. Females were more common than males, namely 128 of the 156. In addition, in the females the condition was much more frequently seen on the right side. I feel that the sex distribution and the preponderance of the condition on the right side strongly suggest that the material was biased by non-congenital factors.

It is obvious that neither the size of the kidney nor its capacity of excreting contrast urine is a reliable criterion in the diagnosis of renal hypoplasia. This term therefore simply means unilateral small kidney with good function. Some cases may be congenital, while others are undoubtedly acquired. Changes seen in the so-called hypoplastic kidney are described with due reservation below.

EKSTRÖM (1955) distinguishes three grades of renal hypoplasia, namely general, partial and local. Partial hypoplasia is to be understood as hypoplasia in one half of a kidney with a double renal pelvis. In the series of 156 cases of renal hypoplasia the disease was general in 98, partial in 18 and local in 40. In 35 of the 40 cases of local hypoplasia the entire contralateral kidney was hypoplastic, in 3 cases only part of the kidney was hypoplastic.

In two thirds of the cases with local hypoplasia the condition was localized to the upper pole.

a) General hypoplasia (Figs. 44, 45, 46)

The plain roentgenogram shows a small kidney. It may be so small as to simulate agenesia. It may also occur as a small oblong formation, which closer examination by tomography, for example, or retroperitoneal pneumography, will reveal to be a small kidney. As a rule, however, the kidney is somewhat larger, of ordinary shape and of smooth outline.

Urography and retrograde pyelography will show the renal pelvis to be small for the size of the kidney. The renal pelvis may be of ordinary shape or it may be short, upright and with few calyces. These calyces are, on occasion, elongated and almost reach the surface of the kidney and they may be club-shaped, so-called dysplastic calyces. This implies that the corresponding papilla is missing. In fact, it is this form of calyx that is the most common characteristic feature of so-called hypoplasia. Sometimes the changes closely resemble the anomalies described by ASK-UPMARK in which the recesses of the renal pelvis extended towards an indentation in the outline of the kidney, where they terminated blindly. This last mentioned change is, however, said always to be located in the central portion of the kidney or in the lower pole.

The contralateral kidney is usually hyperplastic. The kidney is then somewhat larger than usual and often rounded and plump, but otherwise of normal shape.

In partial hypoplasia changes of the type described above are localized to one half of a double kidney. Then the upper part is as a rule involved, and, on occasion, it is converted into a small or large hydronephrotic sac with extremely little parenchyma. Malformations such as ectopic ureteric orifice are sometimes seen in association with this condition. The disease may, however, be localized to the lower part of the kidney with hyperplasia of the upper part.

b) Local hypoplasia (see Figs. 45, 46)

Local hypoplasia involves only a part of a kidney. If the change is small, the kidney may be of ordinary size but usually its outline will show an indentation or a reduction in the size of the pole at the seat of the hypoplasia. The calyces in the region involved resemble those described above and thus differ from those in the rest of the kidney. The calyces are short and broad or long and clubbed. Local bulges can sometimes be seen along the border of a calyx resembling calyceal border evaginations or pyelogenic cysts.

All types of hypoplasia can be bilateral with different distribution of the changes on the two sides.

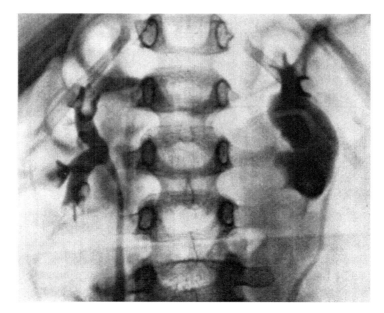

Fig. 47

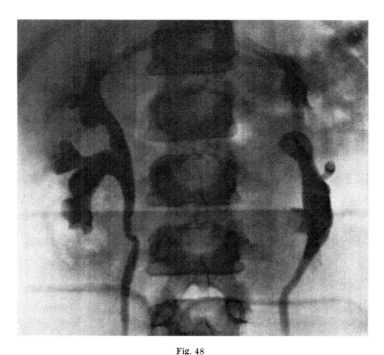

Fig. 48

Fig. 47 and 48. Malrotation. Urography: Different types of unilateral malrotation

It must be noted that roentgendiagnostic features described as characteristic for so-called hypoplasia may be caused by pyelonephritis and represent end-stages of papillary necrosis and parenchymal scar formation.

Renal angiography

In the few cases in which urography showed a small but normally functioning kidney the appearance of the vasculature was a miniature of that of a normal kidney. Severe changes in the size, shape and outline of the kidney may, however, also be seen (see Fig. 44). Experience is, however, too limited to allow of a description of changes seen on renal angiography in cases of hypoplasia.

III. Malrotation

On their ascent up to their definitive position during embryonal life, the kidneys rotate about their longitudinal axis. This may be a true rotation, or

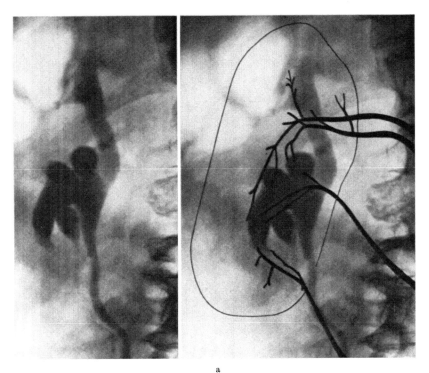

a

Fig. 49a and b. Slight malrotation. a Urography: So-called intrarenal kidney pelvis. Calyces in lower pole directed medially. Urogram and diagrammatic superimposition of arteriogram showing the relation between kidney pelvis and arteries

only apparent and due to different regional growth of the renal parenchyma. From an originally ventral position the kidney pelvis then assumes a medial position. Sometimes this rotation is arrested at an intermediate stage, resulting in malposition of the kidney, which is termed malrotation in accordance with similar inhibitory malformations in the digestive tract. Arrested rotation may be a better term but the term malrotation is widely used. The confluence of the malrotated kidney faces more or less ventrally and, accordingly, one or more calyces are directed medially.

The malformation may be more or less pronounced. In fact, some cases of so-called intrarenal position of the kidney pelvis and diagnosed roentgenologically are in reality a slightly malrotated kidney in which the kidney pelvis has been projected completely within the contour of the kidney. The malrotation may be unilateral or bilateral (Figs. 47, 48, 49, 50; see Fig. 32).

Vascular anomalies are common in malrotated kidneys. Most malrotated kidneys have a short and straight supplementary artery running from a low abdominal segment to the posterior part of its lower pole (Fig. 51). The course and straightness of this artery give the impression that it has arrested further rotation of the kidney (BOIJSEN 1959).

Malrotation is often seen in association with other malformations, such as caudal ectopia and fusion.

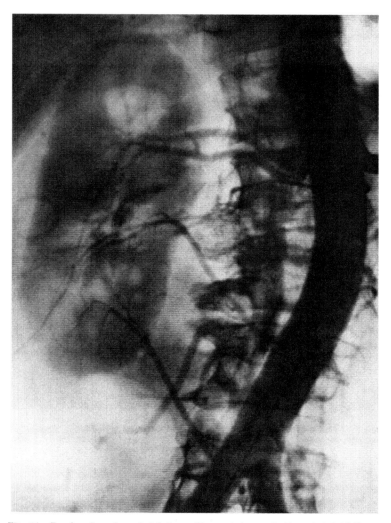

Fig. 49 b. Renal angiography, arterial phase. Three arteries supply the malrotated kidney

IV. Ectopia

Ectopia means displacement or malposition. The term dystopia is sometimes used to designate the condition, but etymologically it implies a more serious condition, for which it should be reserved. It should not be used for the whole group. Renal ectopia means that one or both kidneys are malpositioned owing to defective development. The kidney may be displaced caudally, cranially or medially. Caudal and cranial ectopia are often referred to under the common name of axial

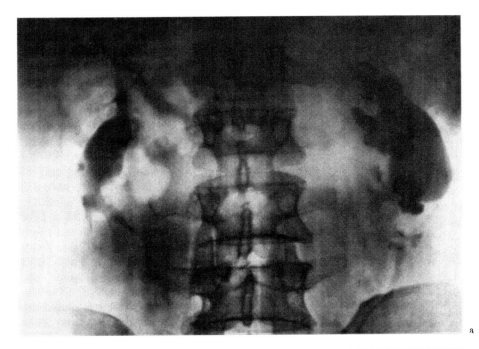

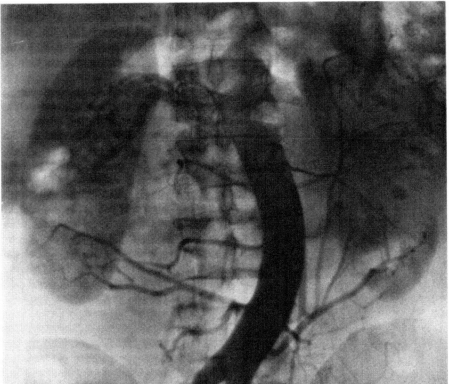

Fig. 50a and b. Bilateral marked malrotation. a Urography. b Aortic renal angiography. Late arteriographic phase. Straight supplementary artery to caudal kidney pole bilaterally. No fusion

6*

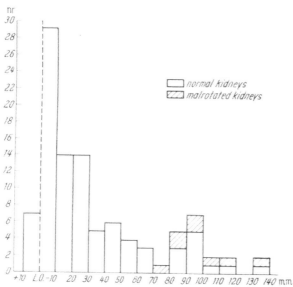

Fig. 51. Variations in distance between origin of supplementary artery to caudal pole and main artery in well rotated and malrotated kidneys with multiple arteries. *L.O.* Level of origin of the main artery. + and − denote origin of the supplementary artery cranially respectively caudally to the main artery. (After BOIJSEN)

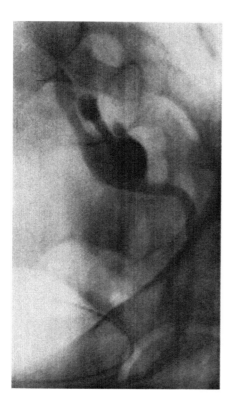

Fig. 52. Caudal ectopia. Pyelography. Malrotation, confluence of kidney pelvis situated anteriorly

or longitudinal ectopia. Caudal displacement of the kidney is the commonest type (Figs. 52, 53 a, b). Various types may be recognized such as the pelvic type, which means that the kidney is located in the true pelvis, the iliac type, where the kidney is found in the iliac fossa or opposite the crest of the ileum, and the abdominal type, when the kidney is fixed below the level of the second or third lumbar vertebra and above the crest of the ileum (THOMPSON & PACE 1937). An abdominal caudal ectopia may be difficult to distinguish from a caudal dislocation of a kidney in an originally normal position, so-called mobile or ptozed kidney. In principle, an ectopic kidney is understood as a kidney that has never occupied a normal position, while a dislocated kidney has attained but not maintained its normal position (HARRISON & BOTSFORD 1946). Of 97 cases of caudal ectopia THOMPSON & PACE found pelvic ectopia in 61, iliac in 8 and abdominal in 28. Of these, 4 were bilateral and in 8 cases the ectopic kidney was the only one. The ectopic kidney may thus be a solitary kidney. A collection of 66 cases of single ectopic kidney from the literature has been published by BORELL & FERNSTRÖM (1954). Pelvic ectopia may be so severe that the renal pole may be situated in a scrotal hernia. Bilateral ectopias are uncommon. COPPRIDGE (1934) collected 21 cases of bilateral pelvic ectopia from the literature, to which he added one of his own.

According to THOMAS & BARTON (1936) and CAMPBELL (1954) renal ectopia has been found more frequently on roentgen examination (one out of 500 according to THOMAS & BARTON 1936) than in autopsy series (one out of 700—1,000). The frequency with which the condition is

seen at autopsy will, of course, vary
with the thoroughness of the examination, the criteria used and the
composition of the material, *i.e.*
whether it consists mainly of urologic cases. An over-representation
may be assumed in urologic cases
because pathologic conditions such
as stone and hydronephrosis are
more common in renal ectopia.

Caudal ectopia is often combined
with malrotation (Fig. 54).

Pelvic ectopy is of obstetric importance because it might complicate
delivery. As a rule, a pelvic ectopic
kidney is pushed out of the pelvis
during delivery, but if the existence
of the anomaly is known, delivery
by caesarean section might be considered (ANDERSON, RICE & HARRIS
1951).

Ectopia may also be cranial
(SPILLANE & PRATHER 1949). In this
rare type of anomaly the kidney is
localized more cranially than normally and may have reached the
level of or passed through the diaphragm into the thorax and be discovered on roentgen examination of
the chest. Its passage through the
diaphragm is due to migration
through the foetal hiatus pleuro-
peritonealis which does not close but
persists as a diaphragmatic defect,
the so-called foramen of Bochdalek.
In fact, in recent years such cases of
ectopia have been discovered in association with mass chest radiography,
particularly when the examination
included lateral views, in which the
kidney is seen as a mass in the posterior part of one of the sinuses. Unless this possibility is borne in mind,
cranial ectopia might be mistaken
for diaphragmatic tumour. Cranial
ectopia occurs on occasion in association with eventration of the diaphragm (BULGRIN & HOLMES 1955).

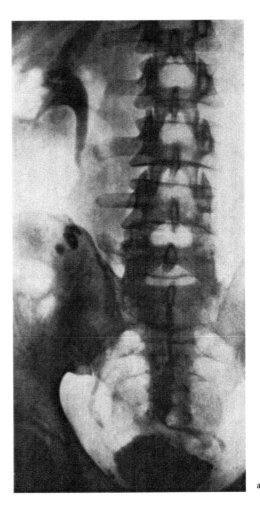

a

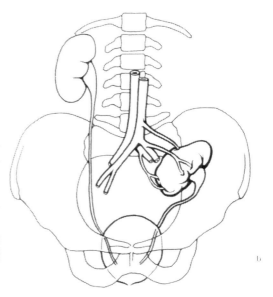

b

Fig. 53a and b. Pelvic ectopia. a Urography. Good
excretion of contrast urine from ectopic kidney to
the left in pelvis. b Schematic representation of
similar case. (After STAEHLER)

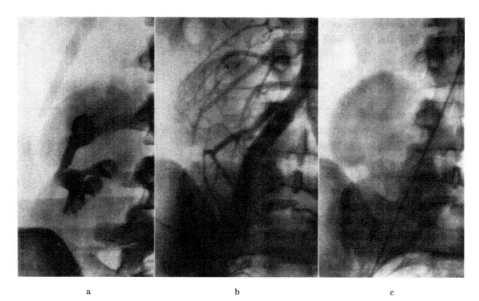

a   b   c

Fig. 54a—c. Iliac caudal ectopia with pronounced malrotation. Examination because of recurrent, severe pains on right side. a Urography: Kidney pelvis occupies a ventral, lateral position. Hilum of kidney points laterally. b Aortic renal angiography: Multiple arteries to right kidney, the most caudal one taking its origin from the iliac artery. c Nephrogram clearly demonstrates position of hilum. At operation the upper $^1/_3$ of the kidney was found to be pressed between an anterior and a posterior artery and vein forming deep impressions in the parenchyma. Resection of this part of the kidney. Patient completely free of pain

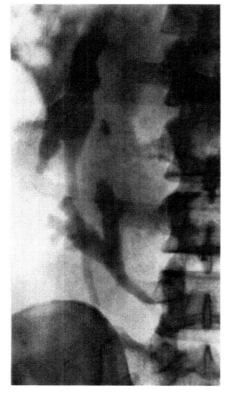

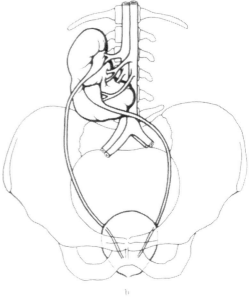

Fig. 55a and b. Medial dystopia (crossed dystopia) and fusion. Both ureters open in the bladder at normal site. Schematic representation of similar case. (After STAEHLER)

Medial dystopia is usually called crossed dystopia. Both kidneys then lie on the same side (Figs. 55a, b, 56). The ureteric orifice is usually not ectopic, the ureter passing across the spine. The displaced kidney may be fused with or separated from the fellow kidney or the ectopic kidney may be the only kidney,

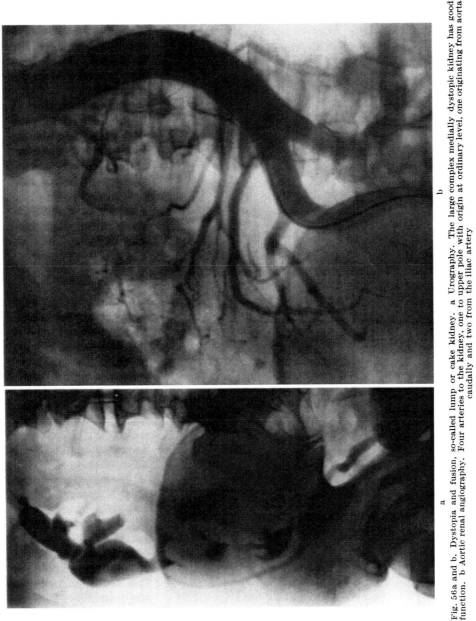

Fig. 56a and b. Dystopia and fusion, so-called lump or cake kidney. a Urography. The large complex medially dystopic kidney has good function. b Aortic renal angiography. Four arteries to the kidney, one to upper pole with origin at ordinary level, one originating from aorta caudally and two from the iliac artery

the fellow kidney being hypo- or aplastic. The ectopic kidney, however, is often small and is usually situated adjacent the lower pole of the normally situated kidney. Only in 7 per cent of the cases is it adjacent the upper pole (DAVIDSON 1938). The kidney is also usually malrotated. According to ØDEGAARD (1946), it is more common in males than in females and the left kidney is more frequently ectopic than the right.

True crossed dystopia, *i.e.* the right kidney on the left side and the left kidney on the right, has been described by HARRIS (1939) under the name of double crossed ureters. He also reported that one of the ureters of a double kidney can cross the midline. The lower portion of a double kidney may thus be crossed. A kidney is then present also on the other side.

In this connection it might also be mentioned that the kidney may be located in a true lumbar hernia. This is a very rare type of hernia, and such a hernia containing a kidney is, of course, a great rarity (KRETSCH-MER 1951).

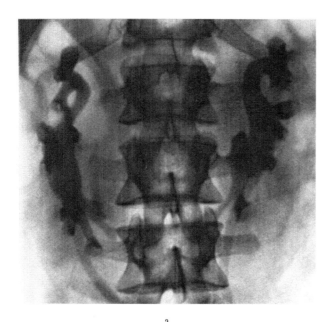

a

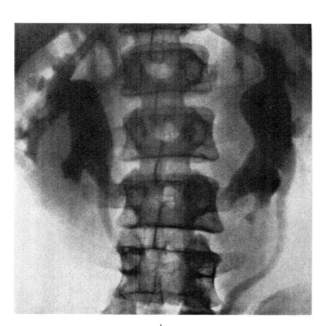

b

Fig. 57a—c. Fusion. Urography: Horse-shoe kidneys of different types

V. Fusion

Fusion means that both kidneys are united. The commonest type is the horse-shoe kidney, in which the two lower poles are united, while the upper poles are separate. On occasion, though rarely, the upper poles of the kidneys may be united and the lower poles separate.

Plain roentgenograms of a horse-shoe kidney will show kidneys with the lower poles directed towards the spine. The longitudinal axes of the kidneys run parallel to that of the body or converge caudally. The kidneys are often situated lower than usual and always rotated with their medial parts anteriorly, and one can often see the outline of one kidney merge with that of the other. In such cases the kidneys are united by a bridge of parenchyma. However, on occasion one or both renal poles are well outlined on either side of the spine, while their position and shape is otherwise characteristic of horse-shoe kidney. In such cases it may be assumed that the two kidneys are united only by a band of connective tissue.

The anatomy of the renal parenchyma of a horse-shoe kidney can be studied best in the renal nephrogram (see Fig. 59). If the kidneys are united by a parenchymal bridge, it will show up distinctly in the nephrogram, while if the kidneys are joined only by a connective tissue bridge, they will appear as separate formations in the nephrogram. Urography will show calyces on either side to be directed medially and the renal pelvis to bend towards the

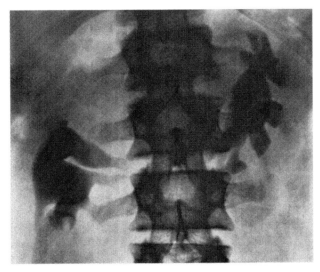

Fig. 57c

midline (Figs. 57 a—c, 58, 59). The course of the ureters varies with the severity of malrotation and deformation. As a rule, the ureters extend from a lateral origin and swing in a fairly sharp bend towards one another.

The degree of anomaly of a horse-shoe kidney varies widely from case to case. It may be slight, and then two kidneys of almost ordinary shape but malrotated may be seen, or it may be severe, one kidney may be small, for example, and the other may be situated on the contralateral side with the course of the ureter resembling that in crossed ectopia (PETROVČIĆ & MILIĆ 1956).

These last-mentioned, less characteristic types of horse-shoe kidney are transitional forms to severe types in which de-

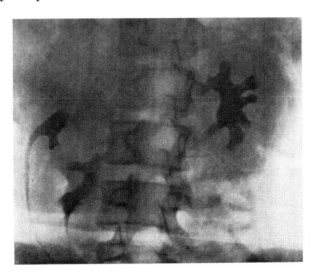

Fig. 58. Fusion. Urography: Complex horse-shoe kidney with three kidney pelves

formed kidneys are fused in various different ways. These types of malformations are referred to as lump kidney or cake kidney. Such fusion occurs, in particular, in caudally ectopic kidneys and therefore pelvic fused kidneys are not so very rare. Such kidneys are markedly lobulated. It has also been claimed (GLENN 1958) that the calyceal configuration is abnormal (which is probably to be understood

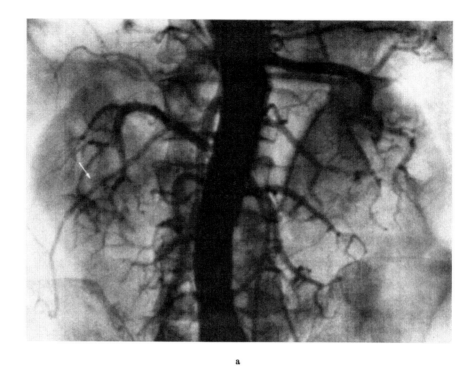

a

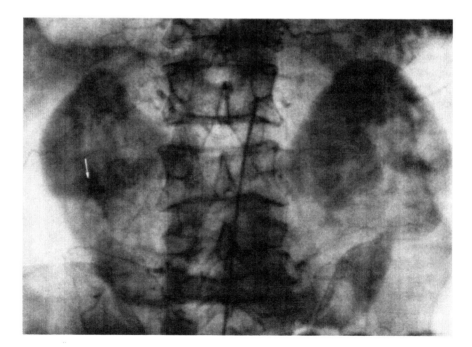

b

Fig. 59a—c. Fusion and carcinoma of right kidney pelvis. Horse-shoe kidney. Aortic renal angiography. a Arterial phase. Multiple arteries. Note pathological vessels in right kidney, corresponding to kidney pelvis tumor. b Nephrographic phase. Parenchymal bridge fuses the kidneys. Irregular tumor in right kidney pelvis with calcifications in part of tumour. Nephrectomy of right part of horse-shoe kidney

as hypoplasia) and that histologic examinations will reveal, among other things, immature glomeruli. Taken together, these anomalies are supposed to show that the development of the kidney has been arrested at approximately the ten-millimetre stage of embryonal development.

The pathologic conditions seen in horse-shoe kidney vary with the severety of the anomaly. Dilatation of the renal pelvis often seen in horse-shoe kidneys may thus vary widely from case to case. The obstructed drainage may result in stone formation and infection. Pelvic fused, like pelvic ectopic, kidney may be of obstetric importance. The reader is referred to a compilation of 91 cases with pelvic kidney and pregnancy by ANDERSON, RICE & HARRIS (1951).

VI. Vascular changes in renal anomalies

As mentioned in the introduction, vascular anomalies are common and important in association with other anomalies of the urinary tract. The more widely renal angiography is used the greater will our knowledge become of associated vascular anomalies. The frequency of vascular anomalies in connection with some of the severe anomalies described above is so high that they appear to be a regular accompaniment of all

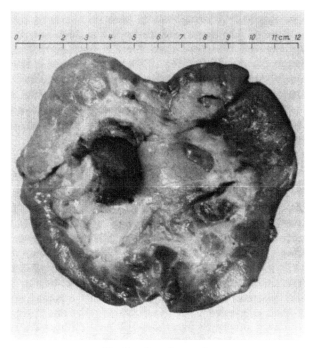

Fig. 59 c. Operative specimen

types of maldevelopment of the kidneys. Vascular anomalies appear to be the rule in malrotated kidneys. They usually consist of multiple renal arteries or of branches of a single renal artery with an anomalous course. The artery need not enter the kidney via the hilum: wide branches may instead pass directly into the renal parenchyma through the capsule from the side opposite the hilum. Both arterial and venous branches may embrace large or small parts of the kidney like tongs. The branches then run along the dorsal and ventral surface toward the hilum. They may enter the hilum or they may pierce the renal capsule and pass directly into the parenchyma. The vessels may then lie so close to the renal parenchyma as to form ridges in it. We have seen a case in our department in which such a vascular tong pressed the kidney so as to cause stasis in the upper part of it with pain as a consequence (see Fig. 54).

Horse-shoe kidneys nearly always have multiple arteries, often a large number of them, arising from the aorta and/or iliac arteries. This might cause hydronephrosis. Ectopic kidneys also often have anomalous arteries usually branching from an abnormally low segment. According to the anatomic literature, in cranial ectopia the artery extends from a high aortic segment.

In less severe anomalies, such as calyceal anomalies and hypoplasia, vascular anomalies are less common.

Multiple renal arteries

Multiple renal arteries represent the most common vascular abnormality.

In the kidney supplied by a single renal artery the pattern of the renal vasculature may, as mentioned, vary widely. The range of variation in the renal blood supply is widened still more by the numerous anomalies. In this respect multiple arteries are of importance.

Vessels deviating from the natural number are referred to in the literature by etymologically different names such as aberrant, accessory, abnormal or supernumerary. The nomenclature is all the more bewildering because some authors use one and the same name for different anomalies, while others use different names for the same thing. This nomenclature is misleading because it suggests the existence of an extra arterial supply to the kidney. But there is no such extra supply. Like other renal arteries, multiple arteries are end-arteries. They often supply a large portion of the renal parenchyma, as a rule between 20% and 50% (McDONALD & KENNELLY 1959). The vessels should therefore preferably be referred to as multiple or supplementary.

a) Anatomic investigations

In the anatomic literature the frequency of multiple arteries is given as 20—25 per cent. In a series of 2,562 kidneys HOU-JENSEN (1930) found multiple arteries in 22.4%. As a rule supplementary arteries arise near the origin of the main renal artery but sometimes a fair distance from it, if it stems from the iliac artery, for example. HELLSTRÖM (1928) found the longest distance to be 70 mm, while SELDOWITSCH (1909) found a vessel to originate 105 mm distal to the other arteries. Multiple arteries may course separately or together with a main artery into the renal hilum or directly into the parenchyma depending on the distance of their origin from the renal artery (GRAVES 1956).

In the anatomic literature opinions differ widely on the regions supplied by multiple arteries. A thorough investigation by GRAVES (1954, 1956) showed that the vessels are normal segmental arteries but arising extrarenally instead of intrarenally. He found multiple arteries coursing to the lower pole to be more common than others and related this to the fact that in 63% of these cases the lower polar artery was given off as the first branch of the renal artery when the latter was single (see below).

b) Angiographic studies

Only few angiographic investigations have been made of the frequency of multiple renal arteries. EDSMAN (1957) found multiple arteries in 21% of 1,240 kidneys. After exclusion of hydronephrotic kidneys the frequency was 20%. Our material (BOIJSEN 1959) consisted of 638 kidneys, of which 152 (23.8%) showed multiple arteries. After exclusion of hydronephrotic kidneys (64), multiple arteries were found in 20.6 per cent.

Multiple arteries are not seen quite so frequently in angiographic studies as in autopsy series. According to BOIJSEN this can be explained by the fact that fine arteries coursing to the two cranial pyramids and supplying at most one renculus do not always show up in the film because they are too thin. The possibility of the existence of fine vessels not demonstrable in the angiogram should be borne in mind in contemplated partial nephrectomy.

As a rule, but not always, multiple arteries are of smaller caliber than the main renal artery.

c) Level of origin

Of 101 kidneys in our material in which the level of origin of the supplementary arteries could be judged, 50 originated at a distance of up to 19 mm from the renal artery, of which 7 arose cranially thereto. Nineteen arose 20—39 mm, ten 40 to 50 mm and four 60—70 mm from the renal artery. Thus, the frequency of multiple arteries decreased with increasing distance from the main artery. After a distance of 80 mm, however, the frequency again began to increase and as many as 18 kidneys were in that group (BOIJSEN).

The distribution of supplementary arteries in our material is:

to the upper pole 14% ;
to the middle ventral segment 5.5% ;
to the middle dorsal segment 14% ;
to the lower pole segment 72.5%.

It is clear from the figures that some kidneys were supplied by more than two renal arteries. Supplementary arteries coursing to the lower pole were most common. Of 134 kidneys with only one supplementary artery, the latter supplied pyramids in the pars inferior in as many as 95 (71%).

GRAVES, as mentioned, ascribed the high frequency of supplementary arteries to the lower pole to the fact that in 63% of his cases it was the first artery to leave the renal artery when the latter was single. This assumption could not be confirmed in our material. The reason for the high frequency of arteries to the lower pole may instead be that all supplementary arteries near the main artery represent persisting mesonephric arteries. These vessels degenerate in cranio-caudal direction so that the vessels situated most caudally are obliterated last and are therefore most likely to persist in adults (BOIJSEN 1959).

On selective angiography special attention must be given to the possibility of multiple renal arteries. This can always be checked by examination of the pattern of the vessels in the arteriogram and by examination of the nephrogram for any defects. This is achieved best by examination of the kidney in more than one projection. Should multiple arteries be demonstrated or suspected, aortic renal angiography should be done (see, for example, Figs. 49, 50, 54, 56, 59).

If the catheter for selective angiography is passed into a small supplementary artery and the entire dose of contrast medium deposited there, it will result in a high concentration of the medium in a small portion of the kidney (LJUNGGREN & EDSMAN 1955) with a pathologic nephrogram as a consequence.

If the tip of the catheter lies in the main renal artery but a supplementary artery is present, branches to a portion of the kidney will be missing in the arteriogram. The absence of such a filling is, however, more obvious in the nephrogram. Then the region supplied by the supplementary artery not filled with contrast medium will appear as a defect in the nephrogram and be diffusely outlined against the rest of the renal parenchyma. Unless the possibility of a supplementary artery be borne in mind, this may result in an erroneous diagnosis. If the artery is very narrow, the region it supplies may be so small as not to show up in the nephrogram. Such fine supplementary arteries sometimes course to the upper pole and escape detection in the arteriogram and nephrogram, as mentioned above. The clinical importance of supplementary arteries is discussed in chapter N. I. 3.

VII. Renal angiography in anomalies

In the investigation of renal and urinary tract anomalies renal angiography may sometimes be helpful. Fusion, double kidneys and malrotations of different types may occasionally offer differential diagnostic difficulties and in plain roentgenography, urography or pyelography may be suspected of representing tumor, for instance. Renal angiography then helps to solve the differential-diagnostic problem. In hypoplasia, particularly if local, as well as in other types of parenchymal malformations renal angiography may be useful in determining more exactly the amount of functioning renal parenchyma and its distribution. Angiography may be valuable for differentiation between aplasia and ectopia.

In contemplated operation for malformation knowledge of the frequently bizarre vasculature is important. As mentioned, multiple arteries arising at different levels from the aorta and/or iliac arteries are common in renal malformations and increase in frequency with the complexity of the malformation.

Horse-shoe kidney may consist of two separate kidneys united only by a narrow neck of connective tissue, or of a true conglomerate kidney. Renal angiography, particularly the nephrogram, can clear up any doubt in this respect and also show the amount of renal parenchyma in different parts of a conglomerate kidney. This is important in contemplated operation for stone or hydronephrosis in part of such a kidney.

As mentioned in the chapter on vascular anomalies, malformations are sometimes dominated by the bizarre appearance of vessels, which makes angiography a rational method in the investigation of many anomalies. Clinically important changes, often combined with multiple vessels, as hydronephrosis, require angiography.

To summarize, it may be concluded that anomalies are common in the calyces, renal pelvis and ureter, and that grave anomalies such as ectopia, fusion, malrotation, hypoplasia are not uncommon. These anomalies are due to disturbances in embryo-dynamics and therefore often appear in combination. The earlier such disturbances occur in foetal life the more complex the anomalies will be. Anomalies of this type are often closely connected to the development of the vasculature. Renal angiography is therefore an important method in the investigation of anomalies.

It cannot be stressed enough that anomalies of the urinary tract are often multiple. It has even been questioned by FELTON (1959) whether it might not be wise to consider urography indicated in all cases of such readily demonstrable anomalies as cryptorchism and hypospadia. Of 61 patients with undescended testes urography showed unsuspected significant anomalies of the upper urinary tract in 13.5%, and in 9% of 45 patients with hypospadia.

It may finally be stressed that grave anomalies of the urinary tract are often seen in association with anomalies in other parts of the organism.

VIII. Ureteric anomalies

Ureteric anomalies have been described under the heading of blind ureter, and a deviating course of the ureter in association with renal anomalies has also been described in connection with fusion, ectopia and malrotation of the kidneys.

1. Retro-caval ureter

Another unusual but often characteristic and important deviation from the ordinary course is that shown by the ante-ureteric inferior caval vein, usually known as retro-caval, post-caval or circum-caval ureter. As indicated by the name, the right ureter passes behind or round the inferior caval vein from a

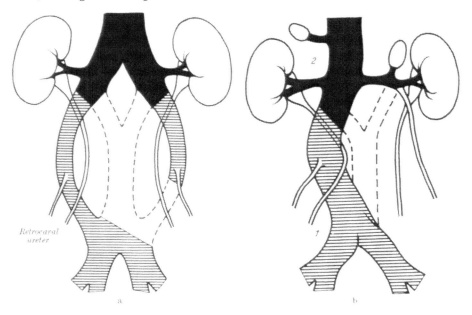

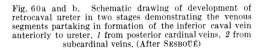

position lateral and ventral to the vein to a point medial to it. Several variants of the course of the ureter in relation to anomalous veins can be seen. It should be observed that this abnormal course of the ureter is secondary to a venous anomaly, which is indicated by the correct name given above.

On occasion, the distal portion of the right ureter contacts the inferior caval vein but is not displaced by it. In the anomaly under discussion the ureter is situated roughly at the level between its upper and middle third behind the vein, and is compressed between the latter and the posterior abdominal wall and aorta respectively. In such cases the ureter will be bent medially and displaced backwards, and its cranial segment and the renal pelvis will be dilated. The impression caused by

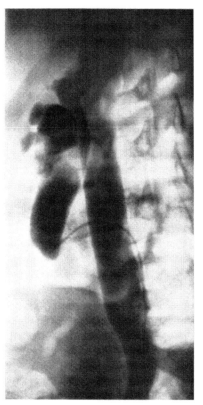

Fig. 60a and b. Schematic drawing of development of retrocaval ureter in two stages demonstrating the venous segments partaking in formation of the inferior caval vein anteriorly to ureter, *1* from posterior cardinal veins, *2* from subcardinal veins. (After SESBOUÉ)

Fig. 60c. Retrocaval ureter. Simultaneous pyelography and cavography. Kidney pelvis and proximal part of ureter markedly dilated. Ureter (catheter) swings behind inferior caval vein. (Courtesy of Dr. ARNE NILSSON)

the vein may be considerable. The medially bent portion of the ureter may cross the midline and the distal two thirds may run relatively close to the midline.

The embryonic development of the caval vein is briefly as follows (Fig. 60). It arises from a venous system originally consisting of 3 different venous trunks on either side of the midline and anastomosing richly with one another. Their arrangement in medio-lateral and dorso-ventral direction and their transverse anastomoses give them the shape of a tunnel through which the kidney passes during its ascent. The postcardinal vein runs anteriorly and laterally to the ureter. During embryonic life that segment of the vein caudal to the kidney atrophies and the inferior caval vein develops from the right and left supra-cardinal veins. The ureter thus lies lateral to the vein. However, in some cases the caval vein is formed from the post-cardinal vein instead, and then the ureter lies behind the caval vein and medially it will follow the anterior aspect of the vein. Thus, the anomalous course of the ureter is caused by a persisting post-cardinal vein forming the inferior caval vein. The anomaly can vary widely with double caval vein, for instance, in which both the post-cardinal and supra-cardinal veins persist and each forms its own caval vein. In one case retro-caval position of the ureter has been found to be bilateral in association with grave renal malformation. All cases on record are otherwise right-sided. A detailed description has been given by SESBOÜE (1952). One case of retro-caval ureter and solitary kidney has been described by LAUGHLIN (1954). It is pointed out by ARNE NILSSON (1960) that the changes in the size and shape of the kidney pelvis and ureter caused by this anomaly can be uncharacteristic. Cavography is a rational diagnostic method (Fig. 60c).

Other common anomalies may cause changes of the same type as retro-caval ureter (DREYFUSS 1959).

2. Ureters with ectopic orifice

An uncommon but important anomaly, which frequently offers diagnostic difficulties is a ureter with an ectopic orifice, i.e. when the ureter empties extra-vesically. The possibility of this anomaly must be considered, particularly in the investigation of incontinence in either sex and in obscure pyuria. Such an ectopic orifice may belong to the only ureter on one side or, in double ureter on one side, to one of the two or to both ureters. Most commonly it is one of the ureters from a double kidney, and then it is the ureter draining the upper renal pelvis that empties ectopically. In males the ectopic orifice is situated in the urethra or genital organs, in females in the vagina or urethra or vulva. Since the orifice is narrow, the flow of urine from the kidney or that part of the kidney drained by the ureter with an ectopic orifice often is impaired. Then dilatation and functional disturbances may occur (see chapter N). The corresponding kidney or part of the kidney is often more or less hypoplastic.

Ureters with an ectopic orifice can be readily diagnosed by retrograde pyelography if the orifice can be observed. Then the ureter is usually dilated and the corresponding renal pelvis is seen as a small sac. The lower ureter may be severely distended and resemble a dilated blind ureter. Urography will sometimes show delayed excretion with poor concentration in the affected part of the renal pelvis. In double kidney excretion can be seen from that half that is drained by an ordinary ureter and then one can conclude or suspect the existence of a second dilated renal pelvis. (A source of error in the diagnosis of suspected ectopic orifice of a ureter by urography is the so-called ureter jet. The stream of contrast medium from the jet should not be mistaken for an extension of a ureter.) The parenchyma can be studied more closely by renal angiography (see chapter N). By catheterization of the orifice of a ductus ejaculatorius in colliculus seminalis in association with urethroscopy and contrast injection a retrograde filling can be obtained via the ductus deferens and possibly via the seminal vesicles (ENGEL 1948). A corresponding filling can be obtained by vesiculography (MEISEL 1952). HAMILTON & PEYTON (1950) and PASQUIER & WOMACK (1953) described a case in which a cystic formation protruding into the urinary bladder was punctured in association with cystoscopy and in which contrast medium was injected. The cystic formation proved to consist of a dilated ureter and the likewise dilated seminal vesicles, into which the ureter emptied.

The occurrence of an ectopic ureteric orifice can easily be explained from an embryologic point of view on the basis of the close relationship between the Wolffian duct and the urogenital sinus. The ureter arises as a bud from the Wolffian duct, from which the posterior urethra, seminal vesicles, ejaculatory duct and vas deferens develop in males. In females Gartners duct, when present, is a rudiment of the Wolffian duct, which also gives rise to the urethra and vestibulum vaginae. The Wolffian duct is intimately related with the urogenital sinus from which the major part of the proximal urethra is formed in males, and of the vaginal vestibule in females. More difficult to explain are those rare cases in which an ectopic ureteric orifice is seen within the uterus respectively in the rectum.

An ectopic ureteric orifice is sometimes seen in association with complex malformations.

3. Ureteric valve

A few cases of a valve in the ureter have been described. It may have the form of an iris with a central opening and be unilateral or bilateral (WALL & WACHTER 1952) and be situated at any level of the ureter. The anomaly causes dilatation of the urinary tract. It may also cause total occlusion with atrophic hydronephrosis (ROBERTS 1956).

G. Nephro- and ureterolithiasis

Stone in the upper urinary tract is a common disease. It is seen not only as an independent clinical entity, but also as a complication in other diseases. The occurrence of urinary calculi in association with infection, long bed-rest, metabolic disorders, malformations, certain genetic characteristics etc. makes the diagnosis of nephro- and ureterolithiasis richly faceted. Acute attacks give the diagnosis a dramatic touch; they limelight fundamental aspects of the pathophysiology of the urinary tract and in addition present important differential-diagnostic problems.

Being a common cause of renal damage, lithiasis is of great practical importance from a urologic point of view. This is clearly stressed by the fact that about one third of all nephrectomies are necessary because of stone (DODSON 1956). The importance of a refined roentgen examination method including evaluation of renal function is obvious, if the disease is to be diagnosed with reliable detailed information on various relevant aspects to permit timely institution of adequate conservative therapy to avoid nephrectomy.

I. Chemical composition of stones

Demonstration of stones in the upper urinary tract in plain radiography depends on their chemical composition, *i.e.* on their content of radiopaque material. Most stones contain calcium and can therefore be demonstrated in plain roentgenograms.

The composition of the stones has been described by many authors. Most data available are, however, based on chemical examination. Since practically all urinary calculi are crystalline, they should preferably be analysed by means of

Table 2. *Components identified in urinary calculi by x-ray diffraction and their frequency of occurrence.* (After LAGERGREN)

Chemical name	Chemical formula	Mineralogical name	Percentage frequency of occurrence		
			Kidney-ureter (460 cases)	Bladder (140 cases)	Total (600 cases)
1. Calcium oxalate mono-hydrate	$CaC_2O_4 \cdot H_2O$	Whewellite	52.4	26.4	46.3
2. Calcium oxalate dihy-drate	$CaC_2O_4 \cdot 2H_2O$	Weddellite	52.0	24.3	45.5
3. Calcium hydrogen phosphate dihydrate (CHPD)	$CaHPO_4 \cdot 2H_2O$	Brushite	2.6	6.4	3.5
4. Tricalcium phosphate (TCP)	$Ca_3(PO_4)_2$	Whitlockite	1.3	1.5	1.3
5. Basic calcium phosphate, "apatite".	$Ca_{10}(PO_4)_6(OH)_2$	Hydroxy-apatite	75.8	68.0	74.0
6. Magnesium ammonium phosphate hexahydrate (MAPH), "triple phosphate".	$MgNH_4PO_4 \cdot 6H_2O$	Struvite	30.2	45.0	33.7
7. Calcium sulfate dihydrate	$CaSO_4 \cdot 2H_2O$	Gypsum	—	0.7	0.2
8. Uric acid.	$C_5H_4N_4O_3$		3.9	24.3	8.7
9. Ammonium hydrogen urate	$NH_4C_5H_3N_4O_3$		0.2	10.0	2.5
10. Sodium hydrogen urate monohydrate	$NaC_5H_3N_4O_3 \cdot H_2O$		—	0.7	0.2
11. Cystine	$[SCH_2CH(NH_2)\text{-}COOH]_2$		1.1	1.4	1.2

physical methods used in the study of minerals, particularly X-ray diffraction. TOVBORG JENSEN & THYGESEN (1938) used this method in their analysis of stones from 111 patients. The largest material studied by the method is that described by PRIEN & FRONDEL (1947). Their series consisted of 1,000 cases, afterwards increased to 6,000. They stated that the crystalline components of urinary calculi are: calcium oxalate monohydrate, calcium oxalate dihydrate, magnesium ammonium phosphate hexahydrate, carbonate-apatite and hydroxyl-apatite, calcium hydrogen phosphate dihydrate, uric acid, cystine and sodium acid urate.

Pure calcium oxalate calculi represented 36.1 per cent of the total; mixed calcium oxalate-apatite calculi comprised 31.0 per cent; together they composed 67.1 per cent of the total. These calculi usually occurred in acid, sterile urine.

Pure magnesium ammonium phosphate hexahydrate, pure apatite and mixed magnesium ammonium phosphate hexahydrate-apatite calculi represented 19.5 per cent of the total. These calculi usually occurred in alkaline, infected urine.

Calcium hydrogen phosphate dihydrate occurred in 1.6 per cent of calculi. Uric acid and cystine existed more frequently in pure than mixed form and occurred in 6.1 per cent and 3.8 per cent, respectively, of the series.

Sodium acid urate occurred but once in the series and then only in microscopic amount. It was the only urate found.

PRIEN (1955) summarized: There are apparently only three important crystalline substances in calcium-containing calculi. They are calcium oxalate monohydrate, calcium phosphate (or apatite as it has been called) and magnesium ammonium phosphate. In addition, uric acid and cystine are of clinical importance.

LAGERGREN (1956) published 600 cases examined by x-ray crystallography, microradiography and x-ray micro-diffraction. His figures agree well with those given above (see Table 2). The survey shows the existence of 11 distinct crystalline substances occurring either in pure or in mixed form. It is clear from the table that 460 of the stones were renal or ureteric calculi and 140 vesical calculi. The percentage distribution of the components present in kidney and ureter calculi differed significantly from that of the calculi recovered from the urinary bladder. Uric acid stones, for instance, were much more common in the urinary bladder than in the kidney or ureter.

The most common component of the calculi was apatite, but only 3.9 per cent of the samples were made of pure apatite. In all cases but one, multiple concrement from the same individual were of identical composition.

Analysis of urinary calculi may be of importance from a therapeutic point of view. WINER (1959) points out that such a chemical analysis may give information as to specific causes of formation of certain types of stone and be a guide to preventing further formation. When the etiology of stone is unknown "the chemical composition indicates the type of isohydruria which permits each particular crystalloid to be precipitated with its associated matrix. Isohydruria may be changed by proper utilization of drug and dietary means".

II. Age, sex, and side involved

On perusal of the records at our department, renal and ureteric calculi were found to be twice as common in males as in females. In males the disease was found to be most common between the ages 40 and 50, in females between the ages of 20 and 30. The disease was, however, roughly equally common in all age groups except in the 0—10 year group, in which it was by far the lowest. Stone in the upper urinary tract is fairly uncommon in childhood, except in association with bed-rest because of fracture. The possibility of calculi, however, should always be considered in children with diffuse abdominal pain.

The frequencies given for urinary calculi in children are usually high, but vary widely. The explanation may be that bladder stones are extremely common in tropical regions, particularly in boys.

Of 900 patients in our material, about 800 had stone on one side only and 100 on both. The unilateral cases occurred equally often on either side. The concrements were much more frequently situated in the caudal calyces and the confluence of the renal pelvis than in the middle and cranial calyces.

III. Size and shape of stones

Calculi vary widely in both size and shape; they range from minute stones, hardly possible to detect, to large stones with branches filling almost the entire renal pelvis.

7*

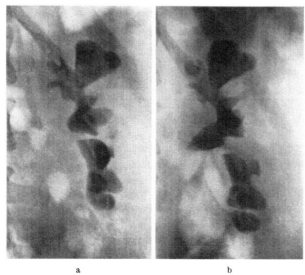

a   b

Fig. 61 a and b. Staghorn calculus with multiple fragments. In (b) one fragment has changed position and plugs pelviureteric junction. (Patient examined because of pain)

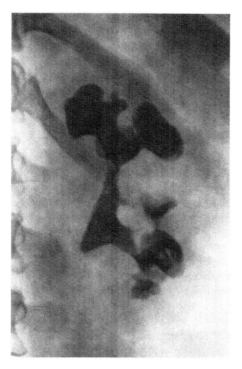

Fig. 62. Staghorn calculus. Shape of stone shows that calyces are dilated, whereas branches and confluence are narrow

Solitary stones are about 3 times as common as multiple stones. It is, however, sometimes difficult to decide whether a stone is solitary or not. Determination of the number of stones or their shape, requires films taken in different projections.

The kidneys may contain very small calculi in a papilla (see Fig. 76) or one stone moulded to a calyx or a calyx with its stem. The cast may fill the entire renal pelvis or one of its branches. In such cases the shape of the stones will usually show that the calyces are more or less severely dilated. These calyxshaped stones sometimes have amorphous calcareous extensions reaching the surface of the kidney and thereby demonstrating severe dilatation of calyces or tissue destruction with calcareous deposits. These milk of calcium renal stones consist of an amorphous mass of calcareous sand and are usually situated in a hydrocalyx or a pyelogenic cyst. The shape of the deposit usually changes with the posture of the patient. The phenomenon is analogous to limy bile in the gallbladder. Lateral to a large stone small calculi may be seen which shift within the kidney on change of posture of the patient. Such stones are situated in hydrocalyces or other spaces formed on obstruction of drainage by the jackstone. One or more stones, often fragmented stag-horn stones, are sometimes seen to shift within a dilated renal pelvis (Fig. 61).

Concrements often completely fill the confluence and assume the original anatomic shape of the latter (Figs. 62, 63). Stag-horn stones vary widely in shape with their site of formation and extent, and any dilatation of the pelvis and calyces. That part of the concrement corresponding to the confluence is often slender, while the peripheral parts formed in the dilated calyces and in regions of parenchymal destruction are plump. The slender part is a cast of the contracted confluence and corresponds to what is said below about the shape of the confluence when it harbours a calculus.

In renal anomalies the site and shape of calculi may indicate the type of anomaly, e.g. double kidney (Figs. 64, 65, 66, 67), horse-shoe kidney, malrotation.

In papillary necrosis tissue shed gathers calcium to form concrements. These stones are often of a characteristic papillary shape and thereby betray the nature of the fundamental disease.

Concrements vary in opacity, but owing to their calcium content they are often rather opaque. The calculi are usually homogeneous, but not always. Sometimes they are irregularly vacuolized or they may contain radiating structures. Distinctly laminated calculi (Fig. 68) occur not only in the urinary bladder but also in the renal pelvis, and in hydronephrosis they may even be very large (SAUPE 1931, KJELLBERG 1935).

A group of calculi of wax-like consistency and with a low calcium content should also be mentioned. These concrements are made up of organic material which has begun to gather calcium deposits. The organic material may consist of a clot or a detached renal papilla. It is sometimes difficult to decide whether such formations should be classified as calculi (MEADS 1939).

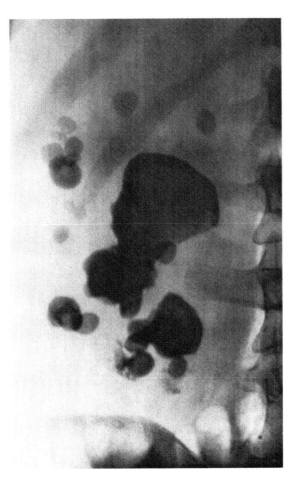

Fig. 63. Multiple stones in pyonephrosis with peripheral stones in dilated calyces

Calculi are capable of changing in size and then usually increase (Figs. 69, 70; see also Fig. 75). The increase is, as a rule, slow but sometimes a small stone may develop into a large stag-horn stone within a month or two. Thus, after surgical removal of a large stone, any small stones or fragments left behind may sometimes be seen to grow rapidly.

Sometimes, however, stones decrease in size because small parts separate and pass with the urine. Stones may also diminish in size in association with antibiotic therapy for infection.

Stones also change in opacity, which usually increases. This may occur very rapidly by the deposition of calcium on organic substance, e.g. a coagulum. The

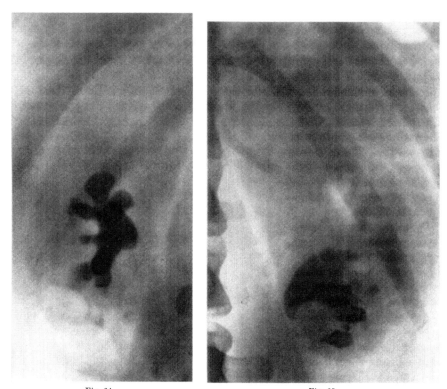

Fig. 64   Fig. 65

Fig. 64. Staghorn calculus filling caudal kidney pelvis in double kidney

Fig. 65. Stone in caudal kidney pelvis of double kidney. Stone in caudal calyx widened towards surface
of caudal pole

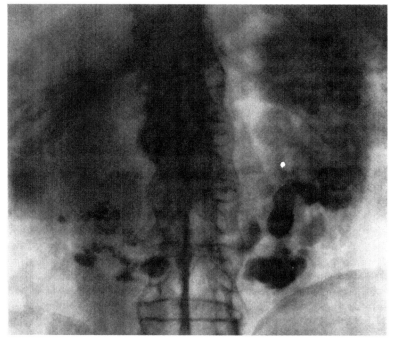

Fig. 66. Horseshoe kidney with stones. Arrangement of stones indicates the anomaly

concrements may decrease in opacity in association with therapy, particularly antibiotic therapy. This, too, may occur rapidly.

Any change observed in the size, shape or opacity of a concrement might be only apparent and due to the stone having rotated or shifted. Rotation of a stone, particularly if it is elongated or flat, can give an erroneous impression of all types of such changes. A supplementary film taken at a different angle will reveal whether any such change is true or only apparent.

Ureteric calculi (Figs. 71, 72) are, as a rule, renal calculi that have been passed down into the ureter. They are usually small or relatively small. Roentgeno-

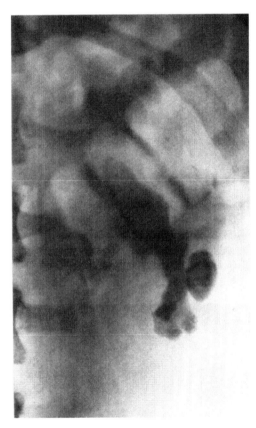
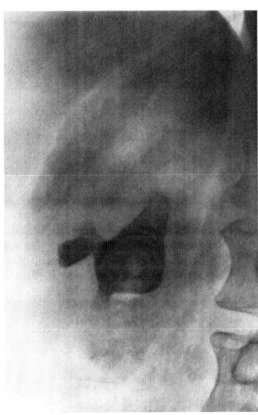

Fig. 67. Malrotated kidney. Shape of stone indicates the anomaly

Fig. 68. Large laminated stone

grams taken with the beam parallel to the longitudinal axis of the small pelvis and with relatively soft roentgen rays will often demonstrate even very small stones in the distal part of the ureter. Ureteric stones are often faceted or spiculated. It should, however, be observed that stones that appear to be spiculated may be smooth: the core may be spiculated but embedded in a less opaque, smooth-surfaced mass. Stones more than a few millimetres in diameter sometimes show a central rarefaction indicating the presence of a lumen or groove permitting the passage of urine.

Small stones lodged in the ureter often move freely up and down. They may also rotate. This should be recollected when judging the size of a ureteric stone. Oblong stones usually lie longitudinally in the ureter, which is sometimes obvious in the lower part of the ureter, which bends medially, sometimes cranially. Large stones may be seen to pass into the ureter. As a rule, they are lodged high up in the ureter, but occasionally they may pass fairly far down. Ureteric stones are on occasion very long and can fracture (BURKLAND 1953).

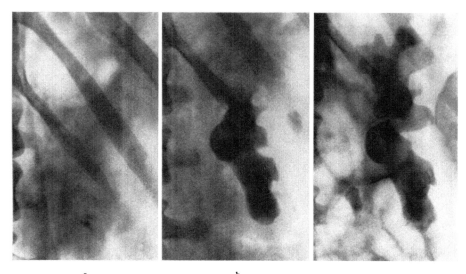

a   b   c
Fig. 69a—c. Development of stone. From (a) to (b) seven years. From (b) to (c) $^1/_2$ year

Stones sometimes form in the ureter, *e.g.* in a diverticulum or more commonly in or above a ureterocele. Such stones may be solitary or multiple. The shape and position of the calculi in plain roentgenograms are often sufficient to show that they are situated in a ureterocele (Figs. 73, 74).

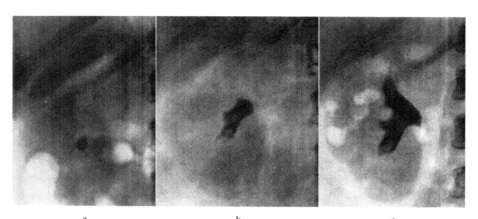

a   b   c
Fig. 70a—c. Development of stone in girl 5 years old, confined to bed because of chronic rheumatoid disease. From (a) to (b) 2 months. From (b) to (c) seven months

The roentgenologic appearance of urinary calculi has undoubtedly not received the attention it deserves. It is true that the density of a calculus, its shape and sometimes its size will permit certain conclusions regarding its chemistry. Thus cystine stones and urate stones can often be recognized as such because of their low opacity and smooth surface. Opaque, spiculated calculi are often oxalate

stones. Large-stag-horn calculi usually consist of phosphate or carbonate (WILD-
BOLZ 1959). However, a more careful chemical diagnosis of the type of stone is
probably often possible if clinically necessary.

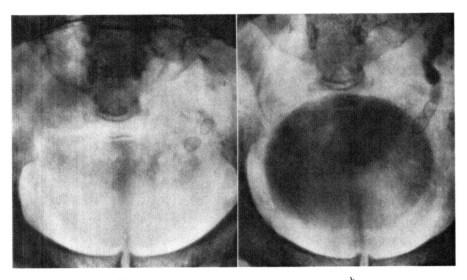

a   b
Fig. 71a and b. Stones in distal part of ureter. a Plain roentgenogram. b Urography

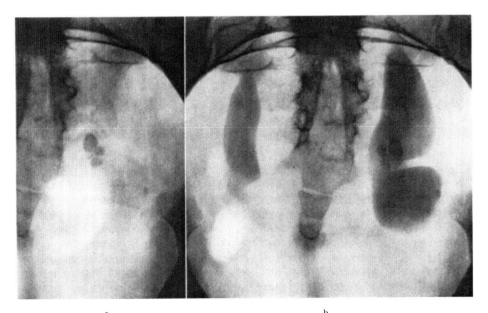

a   b
Fig. 72a and b. Bilateral hydroureter with stones on left side. a Plain roentgenogram. b Urography

IV. Stone in association with certain diseases

Renal calculi are common accompaniments of some diseases, the most well-
known being parathyroid adenoma with ostitis fibrosa cystica generalisata, in
which bilateral renal calculi are common. Intrarenal calcifications and calculi are

often also seen in patients with sarcoidosis. The co-existence of peptic ulcer and urinary tract calculi has been discussed (HELLSTRÖM 1935). The metabolism of oxalic acid is liable to be disturbed in gastro-intestinal diseases. Concerning the combination of peptic ulcer and urinary calculus, reference may be made to experimental investigations performed for other purposes, but which showed that oxalate is absorbed in large amounts in the small intestine in very acid environments.

Urinary calculi are common in association with decalcifying tumours such as myeloma, and skeletal carcinomatosis as well as in leukaemia. In renal osteodystrophy, urinary calculi are also fairly common. This disease is difficult to distinguish roentgenologically from hyperparathyroidism.

Vitamin A-deficiency regularly produces renal stones in experimental animals and it has been shown that patients with urinary stone may also have latent

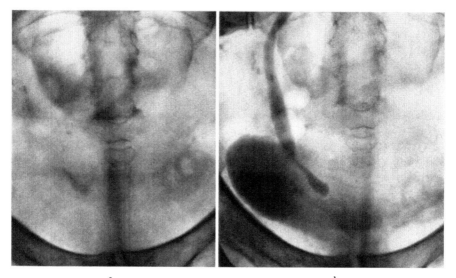

a   b
Fig. 73a and b. Stone in ureterocele. a Plain roentgenogram. b Urography

vitamin A-deficiency (EZICKSON & FELDMAN 1937). The relationship, if any, between vitamin A-deficiency and concrement formation is, however, still obscure.

In the metabolic disorder known as oxalosis or oxalaemia, and occurring mainly in children, calcium oxalate is deposited in the renal tubules, and large concrements sometimes form in the renal pelvis. Oxalate can also be deposited in the bones and in the intestinal wall (OSTRY 1951, ZOLLINGER & ROSENMUND 1952, DUNN 1955). In this disease the oxalate normally excreted in the urine is precipitated and forms calculi. In animal experiments chronic oxalic acid-poisoning has been shown to result in a filling of the tubules with calcium oxalate crystals (EBSTEIN & NICOLAIER 1897). As mentioned, certain metabolic disorders are sometimes seen in association with cystine and uric acid concrements.

Uric acid calculi, although rare, are produced continually because of the metabolic disorder responsible for their formation. In urine of average pH (6 or higher) uric acid is present largely as the soluble sodium and potassium urates, whereas in highly acid urine the relatively insoluble free acid may predominate and may precipitate from solution. ALLYN (1957) for example, described a patient who had passed 2,000 renal calculi, as many as 15 a month,

for about 25 years. As a rule, calculi of this type cannot be seen in plain roentgenograms of even good quality. In leukemia and osteomyelosclerosis such stones are
formed by rapid destruction of protein-rich tissue.

In cystinuria, a familial intermediary metabolic disorder, which appears to be
more common in males than in females, cystine stones are prone to form in the uri-

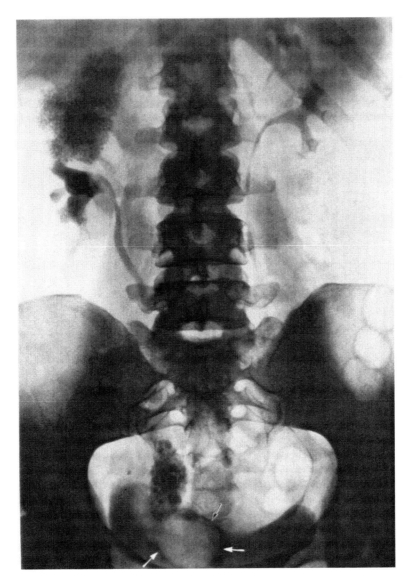

Fig. 74. Innumerable small stones in dilated cranial pelvis of double kidney and in distal part of dilated ureter.
Dilatation due to large ureterocele protruding into bladder and demonstrable as a filling defect (arrows) in
contrast urine in bladder

nary tract. When a cystine stone is found, there is every reason to examine close re-
latives to the patient owing to the familial occurrence of cystine calculi. Such stones
are capable of growing rapidly but also of responding promptly to adequate therapy. If the urinary tract is infected, they may become encrusted with calcium.

Concrements sometimes form around organic material, *e.g.* around tissue shed in papillary necrosis (Fig. 75) and around blood clots. Sometimes, foreign bodies inserted or left at operation or passed into the kidney via the ureter or via perforation become encrusted with calcium to form calculi.

In tuberculosis sand or seed-like concrements form in the renal pelvis. Such microliths may also form in the presence of a tumour, *e.g.* papilloma, in the renal pelvis.

In medullary sponge kidney calculi are common and they are often of characteristic appearance and location (see Fig. 246). The more one is familiar with the appearance of concrements in papillary necrosis and medullary sponge kidney, for example, the more often can these diseases be diagnosed on the basis of the appearance of the calculi.

Long bed-rest is known to favour stone-formation, as is apparent from the term "recumbency stones". In patients lying on their backs, stones will more

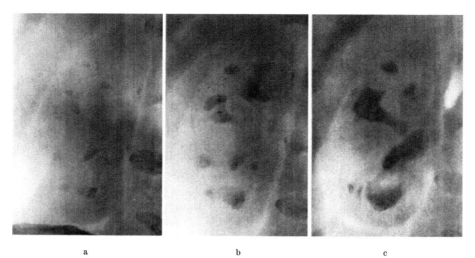

a   b   c
Fig. 75a—c. Stone in papillary necrosis. a Multiple papilla-shaped stones. Development of stones: From (a) to (b) 6 months, from (b) to (c) 11 months

often form in the cranial calyces, but in patients not confined to bed, stones are more common in the caudal calyces. Of 100 patients with fractures of the lumbar spine without neurologic symptoms, urinary calculi formed in 10 (CONWELL). Among 800 patients who had been invalids for a long time KIMBROUGH & DENSLOW (1949) found 15 with urinary calculi that had formed within 74 to 1,200 days. On examination of 1,104 paraplegic patients COMARR (1955) found renal calculosis to be more frequent in patients with lower motor neuron lesions and that the incidence of renal calculosis was higher among patients with complete neurologic lesions than with incomplete lesions. Urinary calculi are common in patients with orthopaedic diseases. Of some 300 patients with different types of spondylitis, about 3% were found to have lithiasis. The incidence of stones in spondylitis is higher in patients with an active inflammatory process such as an abscess, and the incidence of stone formation can be reduced in such patients by regular postural changes (STÅHL 1942).

V. Stones induced by side-effects of therapy

Vitamin D intoxication can cause nephrolithiasis in childhood, because this vitamin facilitates absorption of calcium from the intestine. Formation of calculi in association with treatment of infections with sulphonamides has been seen as deposits of sand in the mucosa of the renal pelvis demonstrable in the roentgenograms as a faint calcification. This type of calculi was common when only less soluble sulphonamides were available. Now that readily soluble preparations are obtainable, such concrements are only of historical interest.

Acetasolamide (Diamox) has been used in ophthalmiatrics, because it reduces the secretion of the aqueous humor in the eye. But it also produces diuresis by a complex process, inhibiting the enzyme carbonic anhydrase in the kidney tubuli. The treatment of glaucoma with this substance is sometimes accompanied by attacks of renal colic due to concrements of low opacity. It is believed that the formation of these concrements is due to a decrease in urinary excretion of citrate, which substance aids in maintaining calcium in the urine in a soluble complex (PERSKY, CHAMBERS & POTTS 1956).

According to HAMMARSTEN (1958), concrements induced by therapy are seen also in conditions with increased precipitation of calcium in the urine, not only vitamin-D intoxication, in patients receiving large doses of parathormone or AT 10, and formation of uric acid ammonium urate stones can be seen on medication with substances producing a strongly acid urine. Mandelic acid is liable to give rise to calcium oxalate concrements by being split to glycolic acid, which can be oxidized to oxalic acid. Finally, antacids containing silicates can cause silicate calculi.

Renal insufficiency together with hypercalcaemia causes the milk-alkali syndrome due to excessive ingestion of milk and absorbable alkali usually taken as treatment for peptic ulcer (BURNETT, COMMONS, ALBRIGHT & HOWARD 1949, KEATING jr. 1958).

VI. Formation of stones from a roentgenologic point of view

Calcifications in the renal pelvis or lower urinary tract are usually called concrements to distinguish them from the many varying types of parenchymal calcifications. In the discussion of the aetiology of calculi, however, calcifications in the renal parenchyma lining the renal pelvis are important. In 1937 RANDALL suggested that the source of renal calculi should be sought in the fornix calycis or in the papillae. In a careful study of autopsy specimens he sometimes observed calcium deposits on the tips of the renal papillae under the epithelium and in one case he found such a calcium deposit to have become detached to form a concrement. On examination, under a magnifying glass, of small stones that had been passed by patients with concrements he found them to have a grooved surface corresponding to the attachment to a papilla. ROSENOW (1940) and VER-MOOTEN (1941) confirmed RANDALL's findings.

CARR (1954) made a further contribution to the theory of the formation of renal calculi. He claims his observations to argue for the assumption that renal calculi form at the edge of the calyx when the lymphatic drainage mechanism breaks down because of overloading of the mechanism by an excessive number of microliths, such as occurs in hyperparathyreoidism and other disorders of calcium excretion, and possibly absence or deficiency of protective colloids etc., and because of impairment of the mechanism of lymphatic drainage due to previous inflammatory changes with subsequent fibrosis. Small calcifications collected outside the fornix calycis have been identified by x-ray diffraction as ordinary types of concrements. CARR's theory includes some of RANDALL's observations.

Roentgen examination provides some support for these views by the demonstration of very small, often multiple papillary incrustations (Fig. 76a and b).

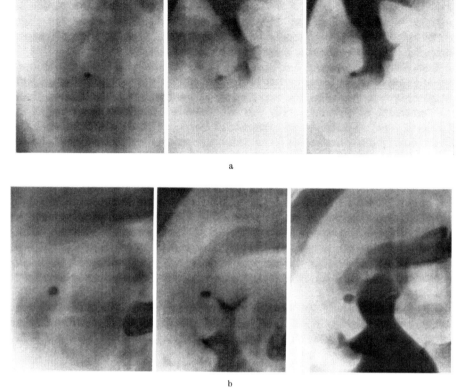

Fig. 76a and b. Formation of stone according to Randall-Carr theory. Small stone in fornical angle of calyx

Sometimes such incrustations are seen by themselves, but they can also be seen in association with concrements moving freely in the renal pelvis. In this connection the hitherto obscure entity, medullary sponge kidney (see page 304), should be borne in mind.

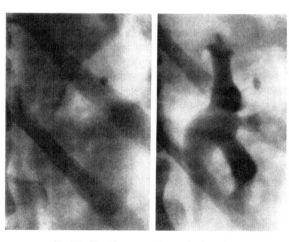

Fig. 77. Stone in narrow-stemmed microcalyx

Since urinary calculi are usually unilateral stone formation can hardly be simply a matter of general metabolism and the urinary crystalloid-colloid balance (TWINEM 1940). Importance must therefore be attached to localizing factors. Such factors have long been known, but those which can be demonstrated explain only a small percentage of the stones. The anatomy of the calyx is one of these localizing factors. Small calyces with small stems may contain stones (Fig. 77), small diverticula-like bulges in the edge of the calyx, so-called calyx border evaginations, and pyelogenic cysts (Figs. 78, 79), may also contain small stones. Such small bulges can occur in many calyces, of which only a few harbour calculi.

In addition, it is known that gross anomalies such as horse-shoe kidney predispose to the formation of calculi as do urinary obstruction and infections.

Against the background of the above remarks renal stones may be classified as primary or secondary, the primary being due to some factor outside the urinary tract, the secondary to a localizing factor in the urinary tract.

I have gained the general impression that stone formation has two principal sources. One is that suggested in the RANDALL-CARR theory with the formation of small stones detached from the papilla and apt to pass in association with an attack of renal colic.

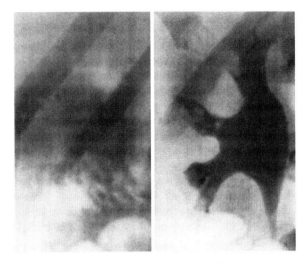

Fig. 78. Stone in calyceal border evagination

The other, and in my opinion more important, is stone formation in organic material in the kidney pelvis. This organic nucleus may be a blood clot, pus or a

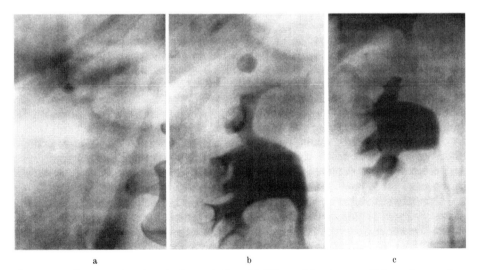

a   b   c

Fig. 79a—c. Stone in pyelogenic cyst. Communication with kidney pelvis not seen. a Plain roentgenography.
b Urography. c After cranial polar nephrectomy

piece of tissue shed from a papilla out into the kidney pelvis, in pyelonephritis, for example. In this connexion it must be mentioned that papillary necrosis is common in pyelonephritis. Stones of this type have a marked tendency to increase in size and to recur after removal.

Recurrence of stone after passage or removal is common. It is favoured by the fact that the localizing factor or the original disorder may be unknown or inaccessible to treatment.

VII. Plain roentgenography

As mentioned, most calculi contain radiopaque material and are therefore demonstrable in plain roentgenograms.

Opinions differ, however, on the possibility of demonstrating cystine stones in this way. It is widely believed that these calculi are not opaque enough to be demonstrated in plain roentgenograms. RENANDER's investigation (1941) of 15 cases, however, shows that these stones always show up in good quality plain films. Photometric examination of urinary calculi showed the following roentgen densities in air: for cystine 3.8, uric acid 1.1, calcium oxalate 4.9, ammonium magnesium phosphate 5.1, calcium diphosphate 7.6, all in relation to water. Without going into the accuracy of the measuring technique, these figures show the relative density of these substances. The value in water, *i.e.* the value corresponding to roentgen examination in practice, was 2.7 or 30% lower than for cystine in air. For ammonium magnesium phosphate it was 3.2 and for calcium diphosphate 5.7.

The possibility of demonstrating calculi depends not only on their chemical composition but also on their size. It is obviously more difficult to demonstrate a small stone than a large one. But an effective technique will often demonstrate even small calculi. However, if the patient is obese and stocky, some small stones and even large ones of certain chemical composition are sometimes not demonstrable by the very best technique owing to poor definition because of low primary absorption and high secondary radiation. In some of these cases roentgen examination of the surgically exposed kidney in association with operation may be important.

Whether a stone will be demonstrable or not naturally depends on the examination technique and preparation of the patient for the examination. As far as the examination technique is concerned, it should be observed that the calculus may be projected onto bone, *e.g.* if a ureteric stone is situated in that part of the ureter passing over the pelvis (see Fig. 100). If the floor of the pelvis is low, as it often is in multiparae, a stone in the lower section of the ureter may be projected onto the lower pelvic bone. The different parts of the pelvic ureter can, however, be projected free by changing the angulation of the beam.

Non-opaque stones sometimes rapidly become encrusted with such a thick layer of calcium as to be demonstrable in plain roentgenograms. I have seen radiolucent stones demonstrated by pyelography to become so opaque within 3 weeks as to be readily demonstrable in plain roentgenograms.

Several authors have assessed the percentage of radiolucent stones. BOEMINGHAUS & ZEISS (1935) thus gave 2—5% of so-called roentgen negative calculi, while KNEISE & SCHOBER (1941), gave 5—10% as more probable, and WILDBOLZ (1959) 10%. It is obvious that anything like an accurate evaluation is difficult because of differences in the technique used by different authors and particularly because it is hardly possible to check the reliability of figures given. Suffice it here to say that a certain percentage of stones cannot be demonstrated in plain films but that this percentage can be markedly reduced by the use of a first-class technique.

1. Differential diagnosis of stone by plain roentgenography

In view of the wide variety of types of calcification in the renal pelvis, and renal parenchyma, in the neighbourhood of the kidney and in regions which may be projected onto the kidney, much space could be allotted to the differential diagnosis of stones in plain roentgenograms. All of these different factors can, however, be reduced to prime factors by a simple examination scheme. On detection of a calcification, that is projected onto the kidney, the first step is to decide whether the calcification is situated in the kidney or outside it. This can be done by taking films at different angulations, usually a frontal view, and one or more oblique views. It is, however, not wise to use two projections at right angles to one another, e.g. a frontal and a lateral view, recommended by SGALITZER (1936). In lateral views the kidneys are not only superimposed on one another but also projected onto the spine. In addition the patient receives an unnecessarily large radiation dose.

It is, above all, not only unnecessary but also indefensible to use complicated methods instead of the very simple and reliable procedure, i.e. oblique views, to solve the problem. A handbook of urology of 1959 gives illustrations and description of a case in which in addition to plain radiography, pyelography, stereoroentgenography, pyelography with gas, and urography were performed to show that some calcifications were situated outside the kidney. The question could have been answered properly, easily, cheaply and safely by simply extending plain radiography to include an oblique film.

If the calcification is found to be within the kidney, the next step is to decide whether it is situated in the renal parenchyma and thus represents a parenchymal calcification or whether it is situated in the renal pelvis and thus represents a stone. This can often be decided by the appearance and shape of the calcifications. If not the decision can be made with use of contrast media, calcifications in the renal parenchyma can then be projected outside the contrast filled renal pelvis. Difficulties are offered only by the above mentioned small calcifications situated at the border between the renal parenchyma and the renal pelvis.

Calcifications close to the ureter and resembling ureteric calculi in shape and size may be difficult to distinguish from concrements in the ureter. This applies in particular to the distal parts of the ureter, where the differential diagnosis may be made difficult by phleboliths. As a rule, however, differentiation offers no difficulties. Often the phleboliths are of characteristic appearance. They are round, laminated, dense, multiple and bilateral. Their size, form, density and number can, however, vary. Sometimes their position is such as to exclude their being located in the ureter. The ureteric stones are as a rule oval, homogeneous, less dense, singular and unilateral. They are oriented in the direction of the ureter. If the phleboliths are not numerous, a differential diagnosis is, as a rule, easy. But if they are numerous, the diagnosis of a possible ureteric stone among innumerable phleboliths might be difficult and require further investigation with contrast medium or insertion of a contrast catheter. The decision then depends on the possibility of showing whether one of the calcifications is situated within the ureter. This can be done by the taking films of the contrast filled ureter in different planes. In urography the urinary stasis might be of diagnostic importance. Calcifications outside the urinary pathways may be situated immediately adjacent the ureter so that large changes in the angles of projection are necessary to demonstrate with certainty that the calcification is situated outside the ureter.

2. Disappearance of renal and ureteric stones

Renal and ureteric stones are often passed spontaneously, frequently while the patient is under observation including roentgenographic follow-up. If the nurse and/or the patient are observant, the passage of the stone is often noticed and the stone can be compared with the roentgen findings. In very many cases the stone passes unnoticed or it is not presented for examination. When a stone has been demonstrated but is no longer detectable on check examination it does not, however, necessarily mean that the stone has passed. Several factors might explain why the stone is not demonstrable in the film.

1. The stone might have shifted. A renal calculus may have been passed into the ureter or the bladder. On check radiography for renal stone it is, of course, not sufficient to examine the kidneys only, if the stone is no longer demonstrable. Examination must include the entire urinary tract. A ureteric concrement may also pass into the bladder or urethra. The possibility of the stone having passed into the urethra should be considered, since in males the urethra is usually not included in plain roentgenograms of the urinary tract.

Sometimes, on the other hand, a ureteric stone may migrate up the ureter. If the ureter is dilated above a concrement, the stone may be dislodged and, particularly if the patient is confined to bed or if the ureter has been catheterized, the stone may be displaced up into the renal pelvis.

2. A calculus might have shifted and might be projected onto bone, e.g. a ureteric concrement lodged in that part of the ureter passing over the pelvic bones. Careful study of these cases will, however, often reveal the concrement. Special projections should preferably be used to project this part of the ureter free. This is possible by turning the patient slightly on the side and using more or less craniocaudally and caudocranially strongly angulated views.

3. The examination technique may be less satisfactory for some reason, or intestinal contents may be abundant.

4. The calculus might have become less opaque. Just as the calcium content of a stone may increase rapidly, it may rapidly diminish during treatment of a urinary tract infection, for instance.

5. The calculus may disappear on suitable medical treatment. This holds in particular for urate concrements (SMITH, KOLB & HARPER 1959).

3. Perforation

Occasionally a stone may cause decubital lesions in the wall of the renal pelvis with perforation as a result (RENANDER 1940). A stone in an occluded calyx may also perforate the renal parenchyma (COUNCILL & COUNCILL 1950). In such cases stones may be seen in uncommon positions or give rise to extravasation of contrast medium on urography or pyelography. Such perforations may also lead to peri-nephritis (see chapter Q).

VIII. Roentgen examination in association with operation

From what has been said above about the size, density, passage and recurrence of stones the importance of roentgen examination immediately before, during and after operation is obvious. As known, calculi are liable to migrate in the urinary tract. As a precaution we therefore always take films of the urinary tract immediately before operation. Such films often reveal that the stones to be removed have shifted within the kidney. We have also observed that a concrement previously demonstrated on various occasions in the ureter has found its way up into the renal pelvis or that a stone regularly seen high up in the ureter on previous examinations has been passed down to the distal part of the ureter or even into the urinary bladder. Such check radiography immediately before operation has often facilitated a better planning of the operation or even made it unnecessary.

Roentgen examination during the actual operation is sometimes necessary to locate stones, find stones of low density and to check the result of extraction.

(Regarding technique see chapter E. II. 3.) To locate exactly the concrements or remnants of them after extraction, it is sometimes necessary to insert needles as indicators into the kidney and to locate the stones in various planes in relation to the needles (QUINBY 1924, PETRÉN 1936). A grid can also be used (PUHL; UEBEL-HÖR 1936).

The patient should always be examined roentgenologically before he leaves hospital to ascertain whether any concrements have been left. Such films may then be used with advantage on any later check examination for recurrences.

Roentgen examination may also be performed in association with extraction of ureteric stones. The introduction and manipulation of the extractor can be controlled under fluoroscopy (preferably with image amplifier using low effect). As a rule, however, this is not necessary. The main purpose of roentgen examination after successful extraction of stone is to check that no stones or parts of a stone have been left. If the stone is not delivered, the purpose of the examination is to demonstrate any change in its position.

IX. Urography and pyelography

The value of urography and pyelography is apparent from the preceeding section. Its purpose is first to decide whether calcifications demonstrated within the kidney in plain roentgenograms are situated in the renal parenchyma or in the renal pelvis. If the examination has shown the calcifications to be concrements, the next step in the examination is to study the shape of the renal pelvis, the functioning capacity of the kidney and position of the stone in the renal pelvis. Attention is also focused on details, *inter alia* the anatomy of the calyces. Reflux phenomena (see chapter O) must be kept in mind. Pyelonephritis may complicate the stone disease and be responsible for marked concomitant impairment of functional capacity and changes in the morphology of the kidney and kidney pelvis (see chapter on Pyelonephritis).

To detect concrements appearing as filling defects in the contrast medium, the concentration of the medium in the renal pelvis must be suitable. In pyelography this can be secured by choosing the right concentration of the contrast medium injected or by choice of a suitable amount of contrast medium. In urography it can be secured by exposing the films at an optimal moment in relation to excretion or to release of ureteric compression.

The voltage of the roentgen tube regulating the wave-length and thereby penetration of the radiation can play a decisive role and must be chosen accordingly. It is often difficult to detect stones in the contrast-filled renal pelvis, even when they have been clearly seen in plain roentgenograms. This stresses the necessity of taking plain roentgenograms before starting contrast radiography (see Figs. 87, 88 for example).

In the differential diagnosis thin stones (Fig. 80, 81) must be distinguished from polypoid tumors of the renal pelvis, gas in the renal pelvis after instrumental intervention or due to fistulation between the digestive tract and the urinary pathways, and gas formation owing to fermentation in the renal pelvis. Such stones must also sometimes be distinguished from polyp-like parts of a nephroma bulging into the renal pelvis. In haematuria clots are liable to form and then may appear as filling defects. The possibility of filling defects in the urinary pathways, renal pelvis, ureter or bladder in patients with haematuria being due to blood clots must always be borne in mind. Check examination after short expectancy will generally decide whether any such filling defect was due to stone or to a clot.

8*

A gas bubble in the digestive tract can be projected onto the renal pelvis and then simulate a filling defect caused by a stone. The examiner must, of course,

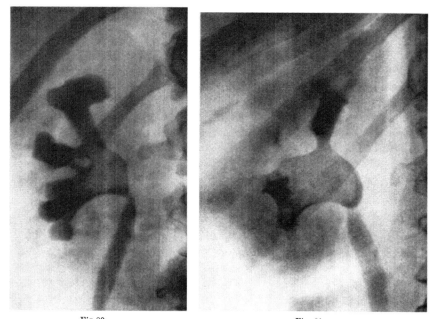

Fig 80   Fig. 81

Fig. 80 and 81. Non-opaque stones. Thin layer of contrast urine around stone. Pelviureteric junction narrow, which is often seen in presence of stones in confluence

check whether any filling defect really is caused by a pathologic process in the renal pelvis by taking films at different angles.

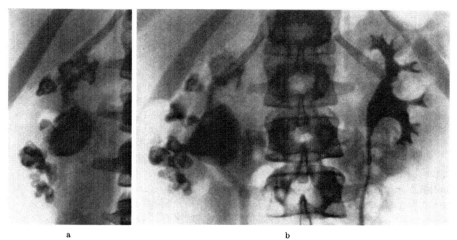

a   b

Fig. 82a and b. Excretion of contrast urine. a Plain radiography. b Urography. Slight excretion

Even if the renal pelvis is full of large stones, contrast medium may nevertheless be excreted during urography. The excretion is usually delayed and of low concentration and often only discernable as a brim around the stone or part of its circumference (Figs. 82, 83, 84). But even large stones do not necessarily always produce stasis (Fig. 85). With optimal filling the film will sometimes show

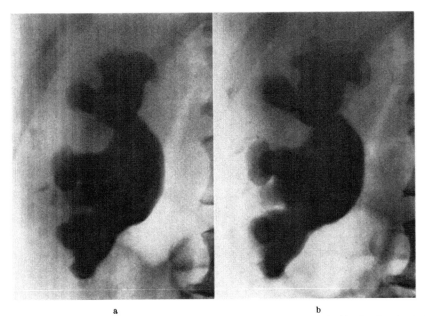

a   b

Fig. 83a and b. Excretion of contrast urine. a Plain radiography. b Urography. Only thin rim of contrast urine of low concentration around stone

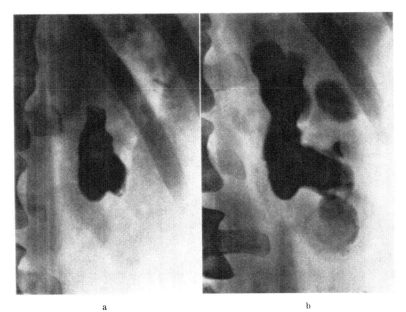

a   b

Fig. 84a and b. Excretion of contrast urine. a Plain radiography. b Urography. Fairly good excretion in dilated calyces

irregular indentations and contraction in the confluence of the renal pelvis due to mucosal lesions and shrinkage (Fig. 86, 87, 88). The possibility of a tumour of the

renal pelvis, which is often a complication of stone, should be borne in mind
(see chapter J).

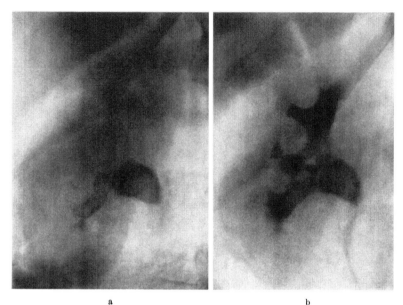

a   b

Fig. 85a and b. Excretion of contrast urine. a Plain radiography. b Urography. Good excretion and no dilatation
despite large stones

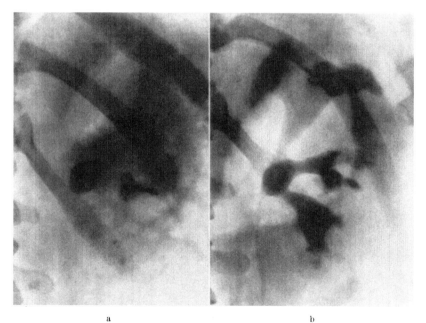

a   b

Fig. 86. Stone in confluence and in deformed calyces in caudal pole. Urography: Marked narrowing of confluence
around stone; dilatation of branches and calyces with papillary necroses

The mucosa of the renal pelvis may be coarse when the pelvis houses stones.
Sometimes the mucosa has a granulated appearance, so-called pyelitis granularis
(Fig. 89; see also Fig. 84).

In the presence of stones in the confluence the latter may be decreased in volume due to contraction and shrinkage. It is striking that the confluence is

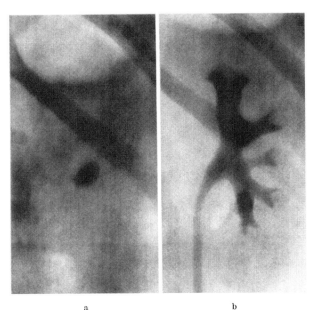

a   b
Fig. 87 a and b. Stone in confluence. Narrowing around stone and slight peripheral dilatation

often narrow and the calyces wide. This is particularly conspicuous in those case in which the shape of the renal pelvis was known before the formation of stone

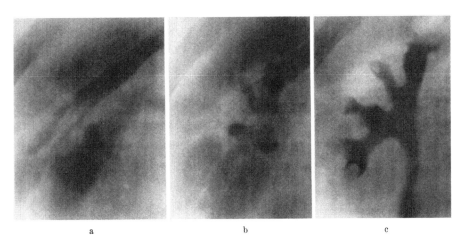

a   b   c
Fig. 88a—c. Stone in confluence with narrowing of latter around stone. a Plain radiography. b Urography at early stage. Contrast urine in cranial (lowermost) calyces. c Ureteric compression. Stone masked by contrast urine. Note coarse mucosa in confluence and cranial part of ureter

(Figs. 90, 91; see also for example Figs. 86, 87, 88). Distal to the thus changed renal pelvis the ureter is usually dilated although no obstruction can be seen in the ureter.

Concrements are capable of obstructing the drainage of a single calyx, a major portion of the renal pelvis or of the entire renal pelvis with the formation of a

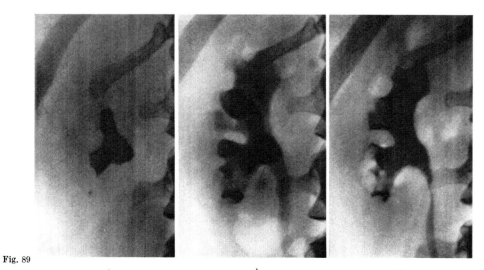

Fig. 89

a   b   c

Fig. 89a—c. Irregular surface of
stone in (a) corresponds to granular pyelitis seen in (c) after release
of ureteric compression

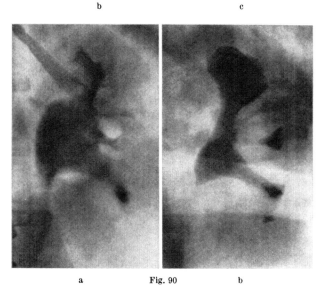

Fig. 90 and 91. Stone in confluence causes marked narrowing.
Compare urography before formation of stone (a)

a   Fig. 90   b

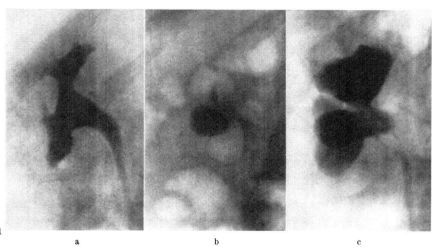

Fig. 91

a   b   c

hydrocalyx or hydronephrosis as a consequence (Figs. 92, 93, 94). The delay of excretion of contrast medium in such blocked parts of a kidney may be temporary

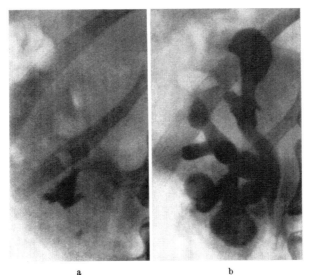

a   b

Fig. 92 a and b. Stone in caudal branch causing hydrocalicosis

or permanent. Oddly enough, as mentioned, even large stones do not always interfere with drainage.

In stone pyonephrosis the kidney is usually changed in size and shape and there is no excretion of contrast medium owing to stasis and parenchymal destruction (Figs. 95, 96).

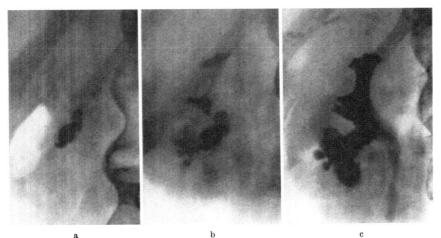

a   b   c

Fig. 93 a—c. Stones in caudal branch causing dilatation of caudal half of kidney pelvis. In (c) (during ureteric compression) stones are masked by contrast urine

Ureteric stones may be situated anywhere between the pelviureteric junction down to the ureteric orifice in the bladder. Small concrements are usually situated in the distal part. Larger concrements are often impacted high up. Large concrements may, however, sometimes pass down to the lower third of the ureter.

The column of contrast urine in the ureter is seen to cease at the level blocked by stone, but usually the contrast medium more or less easily flows past the stone.

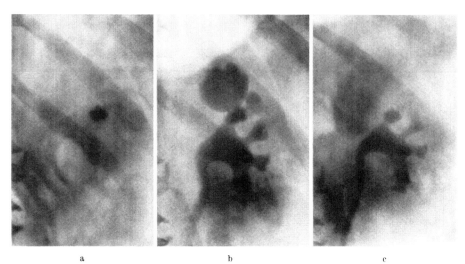

a   b   c

Fig. 94 a—c. Stone in upper branch causing dilatation of cranial calyces (b) and finally complete block. (2 years between b and c.) Note displacement of filled cranial calyx by dilated, unfilled part of kidney pelvis in (c)

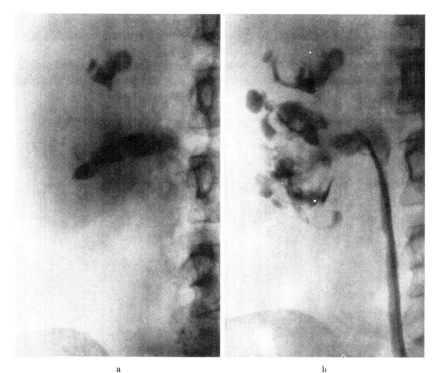

a   b

Fig. 95a and b. Stone pyonephrosis. a Plain roentgenography. Multiple stones. Shape of cranial stones indicates papillary necrosis, the remaining cavities filled with parts of the stone moulded to cranial calyces. b Pyelography: Papillary necrosis. Detritus, partly calcified, in kidney pelvis

The ureter is then often dilated to a varying degree above the stone, while it is of ordinary width below. Contrast medium is sometimes seen to flow around even fairly large stones or through a groove in the concrement. Therefore, if it is not certain whether a calcification really is a stone ureteric compression may sometimes be applied for a while to secure an accumulation of contrast urine, which owing to its volume causes a slight stasis above a stone on release of compression. It should, however, be observed that if compression is applied *below* the level of a high stone, the stoppage of urinary flow and consequent dilatation of the ureter may mask slight stasis.

X. Nephrectomy, partial nephrectomy and ureterolithotomy

Stones may have been left or new stones may have formed and maintain an infection of the ureteric stump after nephrectomy

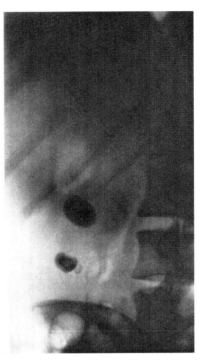

a

Fig. 96a—d. Hydronephrosis with laminated stones. a Urography: No excretion. Renal angiography. b Arterial phase. Arteries thin, stretched and capsular branches stretched along dilated kidney pelvis. c Nephrographic phase. Atrophy of almost entire kidney parenchyma

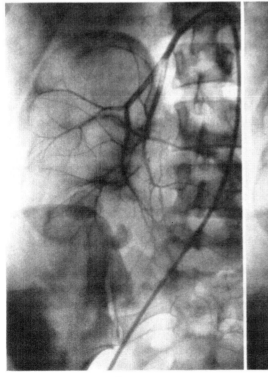

b

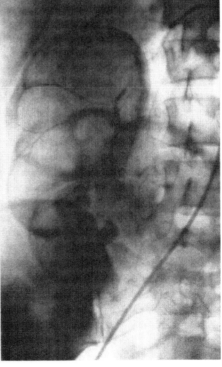

c

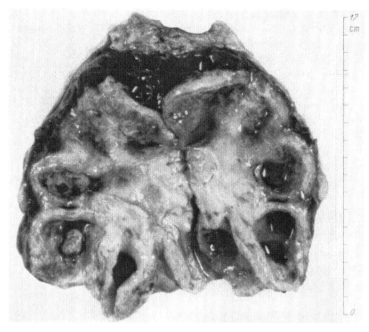

Fig. 96 d. Operative specimen

for stone. It is sometimes possible to obtain a filling of such a stump by catheterization or by reflux from the urinary bladder.

Partial or polar nephrectomy is a common operation for renal stone (Figs. 97,
98). As mentioned in the description of the sites of renal stones, calculi are often
situated in the caudal pole of the kidney. Concrements are also often seen in
malformed calyces, in calyceal border evaginations, pyelogenic cysts, hydrocalicosis etc. The wide use of partial nephrectomy has increased the importance
of detecting such localizing factors roentgenologically. Angiography is useful for
preoperative investigation of the vasculature, particularly in the poles of the
kidney. It may, however, also be of importance for showing any impaired supply
to the region in which the stone is lodged and for demonstrating, in the nephrogram,
parenchymal atrophy around the stone due to stasis and/or infection.

Post-operative check-radiography after partial nephrectomy will usually show
a diminished but well defined kidney. The resected region is usually plump, and
the kidney is often somewhat rotated with the long axis in a straight cranio-
caudal direction. Its outline is sometimes blurred by postoperative fibrosis of the
fatty capsule. Urography shows ordinary excretion of contrast medium and
demonstrates the amputated region of the renal pelvis, varying in size according
to the extent of the operation.

In the event of fistulization perirenal oedema may be seen, and the excreted
contrast medium will fill the fistula respectively show impaired excretion.

After ureterolithotomy the ureter usually rapidly resumes its normal shape
and width. Recovery is as a rule so complete that after one month no change is
demonstrable at the site of the operation. Occasionally, however, a marked
stricture is seen at the site of intervention (Fig. 99). Proximal to such a stricture
the ureter is dilated. In the event of complications such as large decubitus
ulceration in the ureteric wall or infection, large or small fistulae may develop.

On pyelography or urography contrast medium may then be seen to escape into the periureteric tissue. If the fistula is large, it may break into the intestine or out through the skin. In the latter case fistulography may be performed to demonstrate the anatomy of the fistula.

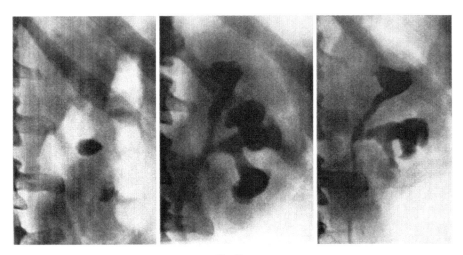

Fig. 97

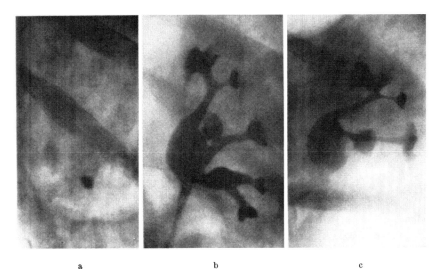

a   b   c

Fig. 97 and 98a—c. Partial nephrectomy for stone. a Plain radiography. Stone in confluence and caudal calyces.
b Urography. c Urography after partial nephrectomy

XI. Roentgen examination during renal colic

Acute renal colic is as a rule a dramatic experience for the patient and often gives rise to important differential-diagnostic problems. From a patho-physiologic point of view the attack is of considerable theoretic interest, since different phases of the attack can be demonstrated urographically.

In acute renal colic urography is therefore of great diagnostic and differential diagnostic value, particularly because of the reliability of the results of the examination during the acute attack.

For reasons given below the examination should be carried out as soon as possible. The patient is taken, so to say, straight from the street to the examination table. There is no time and generally no need for an enema or purgatives. In addition, diseases of differential diagnostic importance such as appendicitis prohibit enema.

1. Plain radiography

In such emergency cases the large intestine often contains fecal material and meteorism may exist, which is sometimes considerable. If the attack is severe, it will often be accompanied by lumbar scoliosis with the concavity facing the side of the attack, and the contracted musculature in the flank will be seen to bulge onto the extraperitoneal fat.

The kidney on the side involved is usually somewhat large and plump

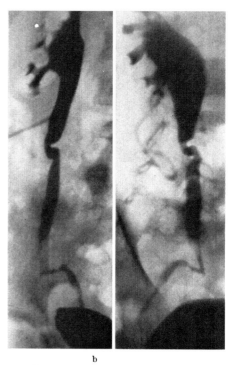

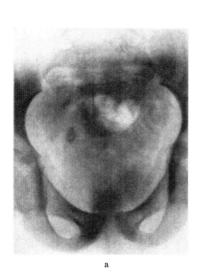

a   b

Fig. 99a and b. Ureteric stricture after ureterolithotomy and ureteritis. a Plain film: Large ureteric stone. b Postoperative antegrade pyelography 4 months after operation. Marked strictures and angulation owing to adhesion

owing to renal stasis. It has been claimed (FELTER) that the dilated renal pelvis is capable of compressing the veins in the sinus and that the increase in size of the kidney is therefore due in part to venous stasis.

The stone responsible for the attack is usually demonstrable. It may be situated at the pelviureteric junction, but most commonly in the ureter, and then most frequently in the distal part. Sometimes, no concrement can be observed because the concrement is so small and/or not opaque enough to be demonstrated, or it might be masked by intestinal contents. It might also be due to projection of the stone onto bone, if it happens to be situated in that part of the ureter crossing the pelvis (Fig. 100). It should also be borne in mind—as mentioned above—that in multiparae the floor of the pelvis is often low. Low ureteric stones may therefore be projected low down and be masked by the anterior portion of the pelvic bone. As mentioned previously, stones may occasionally be lodged in the urethra in males. The stones might also have been passed, but stasis persist.

Finally, the absence of any demonstrable concrements may be due to the attack not having been caused by a stone but a clot, for example (see below).

During the examination a stone may sometimes be seen to shift (see Fig. 102), e.g. a concrement lodged at the pelviureteric junction may be displaced up into the renal pelvis, and the attack may then cease, or a high stone may be seen to pass on distally or a distal stone to pass into the urinary bladder.

Severe retroperitoneal oedema is sometimes demonstrated, and then it might blur the entire outline of the kidney or part of it. This is due to urinary reflux with retroperitoneal uroplania (see chapter O).

2. Urography

After plain films have been taken and examined, contrast medium is injected for urography. The first film should be taken soon, 1—3 minutes, after the injection and further films some minutes later. With these films as a guide the examination may be continued. Ureteric compression is, of course, not applied. The main reason for this is that compression influences the examination findings. Compression causes stasis and should therefore not be used in the investigation of supposed urinary stasis. Another reason is that the examination is often per-

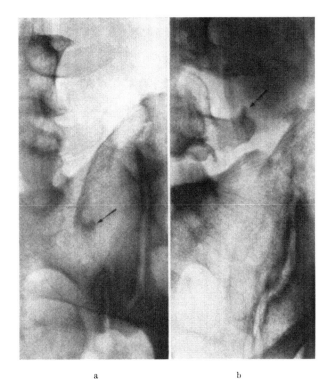

a   b

Fig. 100 a and b. Stone projected onto bone. Plain radiography in two different projections. In (b) the tube is tilted cranially and the stone is projected free. (Arrow)

formed to decide whether the attack is due to stone or appendicitis, for example. Application of compression to the abdomen of a patient with acute appendicitis is, of course, indefensible. In the examination of a patient during an attack, application of ureteric compression is thus a grave mistake.

Examination of the first urogram during the actual attack is usually sufficient to make a differential diagnosis. Absence of excretion on the affected side with ordinary excretion on the other side indicates stasis and it may be concluded that the pain is due to renal colic. If, however, excretion starts at the same time on both sides in a patient complaining of pain, the cause of the attack is not located in the urinary pathways but elsewhere. In other words the attack in this case is not renal colic.

As mentioned, on examination during an attack of renal colic urinary stasis will be demonstrated by delayed excretion of contrast medium (Figs. 101, 102). This delay may be several hours or a day. In these cases renal parenchyma will usually show increased density. The increase might sometimes be considerable. The

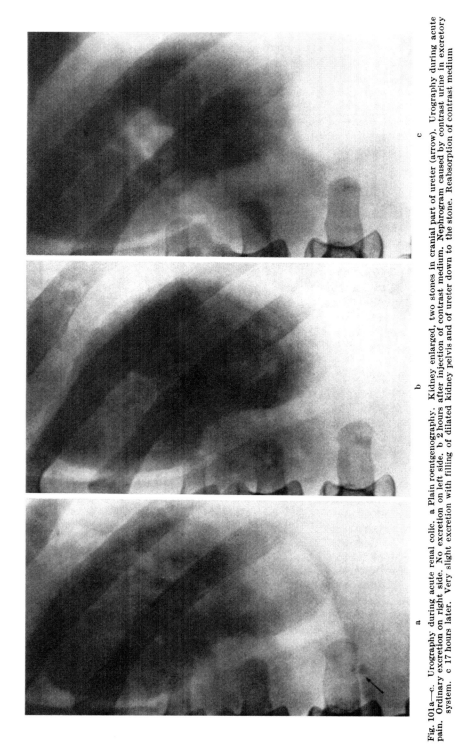

Fig. 101a—c. Urography during acute renal colic. a Plain roentgenography. b 2 hours after injection of contrast medium. c 17 hours later. Kidney enlarged, two stones in cranial part of ureter (arrow). Urography during acute pain. Ordinary excretion on right side. No excretion on left side. Very slight excretion with filling of dilated kidney pelvis and of ureter down to the stone. Nephrogram caused by contrast urine in excretory system. Reabsorption of contrast medium

contrast medium is accumulated in the cells of the tubules and in the urinary ducts and the nephrogram might then not differ essentially from that seen in

renal angiograms in the late nephrographic phase (chapter E IV.). In the enlarged
kidney with increased density, the renal sinus will appear as a distinct, irregular
filling defect in the renal parenchyma (HELLMER 1942).

The accumulation of contrast medium in the renal parenchyma may persist
for a short while or for one or several days if the stasis persists. The density of

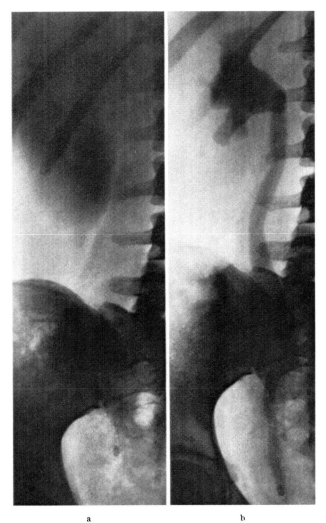

a   b

Fig. 102a and b. Right-sided renal colic. Stone in distal part of ureter. a Plain roentgenography. Urography.
Excretion of contrast medium delayed. Filling of dilated kidney pelvis and ureter down to stone, which has
moved distally 2 cm. b Four days after contrast injection

the kidney will gradually decrease with re-absorption of the contrast medium.
More often, however, the density decreases rapidly. As soon as the attack sub-
sides and the excretion of contrast medium into the renal pelvis starts, the contrast medium in the kidney empties into the urinary pathways.

As a rule, even in severe stasis, small amounts of contrast medium will gradually
flow into the renal pelvis in which contrast medium of very low concentration can
be demonstrated. First some of the dorsal and cranial calyces are filled because

the heavy contrast medium collects most readily in these calyces when the patient
is supine. The calyces use to be markedly dilated, but sometimes the dilatation
is surprisingly small.

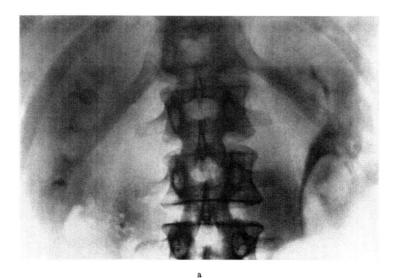

a

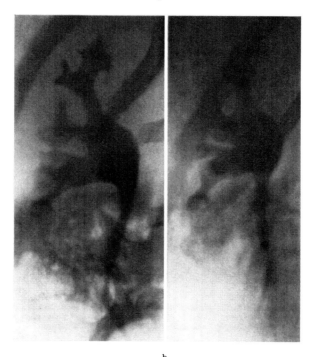

b

Fig. 103a and b. Examination during acute pain on right side. Urography during slight pain without preparation
of patient. Plain roentgenogram: Right kidney plump. Small stone in cranial part of ureter. a Urography 6 min.
after contrast injection. Slightly dilated calyces filled. Analgetics given. b 20 min. later (frontal, oblique view).
Slightly dilated pelvis. Cranial part of ureter also slightly dilated down to concrement. Contrast urine flows
past stone in ureter of ordinary width

As soon as the diagnosis is established, and, as mentioned, this is usually
possible after examination of the first urograms, and it has been shown that the

attack is due to urinary tract disease, the patient might be given an anaesthetic and the examination continued at leisure. It is believed (HERZAN & O'BRIEN 1952) that a glass of ice water will produce immediate relief and induce the excretion of contrast medium. We have tried this and found that it is sometimes, though only occasionally, effective.

As soon as the pain has ceased, contrast medium will be excreted. The last step of the examination is to demonstrate the stone (Figs. 103, 104, 105). It may be useful to follow the excretion until it is well under way and the contrast urine has filled the ureter down to the site of the stone. The interval between the exposures is dictated to some extent by the findings but mainly by rule of thumb. The patient should preferably walk about to promote the flow of the heavy contrast urine down into the ureter towards the obstructing calculus. If the concrement is close to the bladder, the contrast urine in the bladder covers the region (Fig. 106). Then the patient should urinate in order to permit a completely free projection of the lower ureter and the concrement. If several calcifications are demonstrable and a differential-diagnosis is to be made between concrements and phleboliths, oblique films must decide which calcification is the concrement.

During or immediately after a less severe attack the excretion of contrast medium may be only moderately or very slightly delayed. In addition, the renal pelvis is usually slightly dilated and the ureter is filled down to the level of a stone, if any, and the emptying of the renal pelvis and the ureter is delayed.

Symptoms of obstructed drainage in renal colic are the same on obstruction of one half of a double kidney. Thus, in the presence of obstruction of one part of a forked ureter or in one of the ureters in the presence of double ureter stasis is limited to that part of the kidney drained by the ureter in question (Fig. 107). In severe stasis pronounced accumulation of contrast medium may be seen in the corresponding part of the kidney (HELLMER 1942). The possibility of a double kidney, which is not an uncommon anomaly, must therefore always be borne in mind on examination of a patient during an acute attack.

It cannot be stressed enough that in the performance of urography for such a differential diagnosis e.g. renal colic-appendicitis, ureteric compression should never be applied.

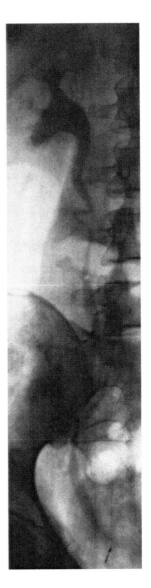

Fig. 104. Renal colic. Pain subsided during examination. Slight stasis with continuous filling of ureter down to very small stone at ureteric orifice (arrow)

3. Discussion of signs of stasis

HELLMER (1935), who described the above described signs of stasis, stressed, like WULFF (1936), that the frequency of positive roentgen findings decreases with increasing interval after the attack has passed off. If the patient is examined

9*

during the attack, stasis will be demonstrable in almost all cases. Signs of stasis will be detectable in only 88%, if the examination is done within 3 hours of the

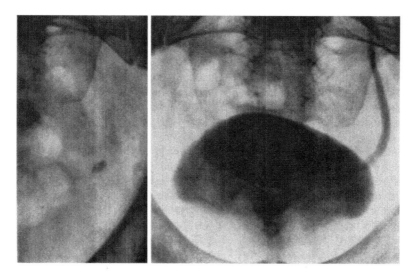

Fig. 105. Left-sided renal colic. Examination after pain has subsided. Slight stasis with filling of entire ureter. Contrast urine passes stone in extravesical part of distal end of ureter

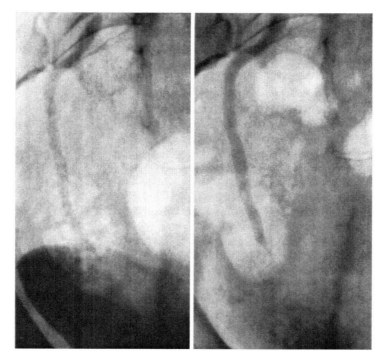

Fig. 106. Stone in distal ureter. Urography. Continuous filling of ureter down to stone. Distal end of ureter shows up better after voiding of contrast urine from bladder

cessation of the attack, after 6—12 hours in 80% and in only 50% after 24 to 48 hours. Since the examination yields most information if it is performed during the attack, the examination should be done as soon as possible while the attack is still in progress. Since the roentgen examination under such circumstances gives clear-cut information, the diagnosis can be made in a very early stage of the examination. The first or second urogram is usually enough to decide whether stasis is present or not, and thus whether the pain is due to renal colic. Thus, if the first urogram shows stasis, it may be concluded that the attack is due to urinary tract obstruction and the differential diagnostic problem is solved. These remarks apply in particular to the differential-diagnostic problem caused by appendicitis. It has been claimed (ARNESEN 1939) that in acute appendicitis the urogram will show characteristics that might be confused with the signs of urinary

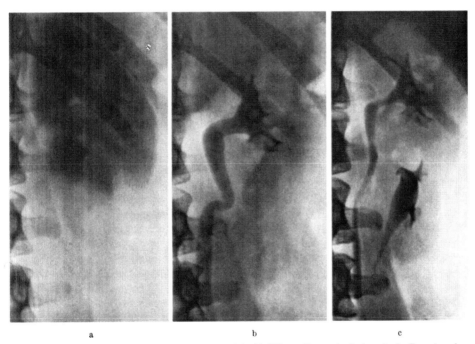

a   b   c

Fig. 107a—c. Renal colic left side. Stasis upper part of double kidney. Urography during attack. Low stone in left ureter. 3 min. after contrast injection normal excretion right side and caudal kidney pole left side. a 1¼ hour later. Nephrography of kidney parenchyma belonging to cranial part. Note irregular border to caudal part. b 2¼ hours later. Excretion into dilated cranial pelvis and corresponding ureter. c Urography after pain has subsided. Ordinary excretion

stasis seen during renal colic. ARNESEN's opinion cannot be accepted. No signs of stasis of any type have ever been observed in the many hundred cases of appendicitis examined at our department. In appendical abscess, in which the ureter might be involved, the flow in the ureter may, of course, be impaired, but never in acute appendicitis.

The signs referred to above represent different grades of stasis, the markedly delayed excretion of contrast medium and the pronounced accumulation of contrast medium in the renal parenchyma representing signs of severe stasis. Repeated urography during one and the same attack will never show an increase in the severity of stasis (ARNESEN 1939). The longer the interval after the onset of attack, the more the appearance of the roentgenogram will be dominated by signs of mild stasis, such as slight dilatation of the ureter and a continuous filling of the ureter with contrast medium down to a small stone near the ureteric orifice.

Urography during an attack of renal colic will not always demonstrate a concrement. This might be due to the stone being situated at a site where it is capable of remaining concealed, *e.g.* it might be projected onto bone. The stone might also be too small to be detected, or it might not be opaque enough. But, as pointed out by ARNESEN, it might also have passed. Thus, on occasion, the stone might have passed despite persistent stasis, such stasis being of functional origin or due to oedema of the ureteric orifice.

Another possibility, which must always be kept in mind is that the absence of a demonstrable concrement might be explained by the renal colic not having been caused by a stone but by a clot, for example. It should be emphasized that signs of stasis are signs of renal colic and not of urinary stone. The colic is most often caused by stone, but this does not mean that the colic is always caused by stone. A diagnosis of urinary calculus can only be made if the concrement has been demonstrated on the roentgenogram or if it really has been passed. In the presence of stasis without a demonstrable concrement, the examination must be repeated after a few days when the patient is free of pain and can be prepared for the examination. This re-examination then has to be done as a morphologic examination with ureteric compression. The reason for this is that certain diseases can cause renal colic without stone. This may occur, for example, in renal tuberculosis and in renal tumour. ROSENDAL (1948), on examination of a series of renal tuberculosis, found that as many as 7 out of 59 cases had colicky attacks in their history. A renal tumour may bleed and consequent clot formation may cause colicky pain. Urinary stasis in such a case is demonstrable on examination during an acute attack, but since meteorism is often present, and ureteric compression cannot be applied, the morphology of the renal pelvis cannot be properly investigated. Therefore, in such cases examination of the anatomy of the kidney pelvis must be postponed until repeat urography after the pain has ceased (OLLE OLSSON 1949).

The pathophysiology of renal colic is reflected most strikingly by urography. The predominant feature in the early phase of the attack is the increased pressure in the renal pelvis and ureter. This increase in pressure can be so severe as to rupture the fornix calycis, and then urine or contrast medium will pass out into the renal sinus and, via the hilum, far out into the retroperitoneal space (see Fig. 215). Such cases have been described by OLLE OLSSON (1948 and 1953) and have also been observed since (see chapter O). In all of the cases in which this was seen the patient had been examined relatively soon, within 2—2$^{1}/_{2}$ hours, of the onset of the colicky pains. The renal pelvis was but slightly distended and the backflow was visualized already in the early phase of the examination, which suggests that the contrast medium followed a path prepared beforehand by the urine. The contrast medium usually spread far into the retroperitoneal space and was rapidly absorbed. Plain films without excretion of the contrast medium during colicky pains did not infrequently show retroperitoneal changes of the same type as those seen in cases with demonstrable backflow of contrast medium.

The cases are interesting from a pathophysiological point of view, because they show the striking increase in the pressure in the renal pelvis during the early stage of the attack. The demonstration of these phenomena is also of interest to the clinician. Our case records in these cases with retroperitoneal changes showed the regular occurrence of usually moderate fever for a day or two after the onset of the attack. The attacks were also usually followed by an increased erythrocyte sedimentation rate, which reached levels of about 20—50 mm/l hour and which gradually returned to normal. Palpation usually revealed tenderness over the area of the kidney and down along the ureter. These observations suggest that certain clinical features of renal colic may be explained by the above-described type of backflow.

To summarize, in renal colic the roentgenologic characteristics as reflected in urography fall into two groups. The first group represents signs during dramatic symptoms, due to high pressure in the renal pelvis, *i.e.* enlarged kidney, markedly delayed excretion of contrast medium, accumulation of contrast medium in the renal parenchyma, rupture of the fornix and sometimes reflux of contrast medium out into the retroperitoneal space. The second group represents the less severe phase of the attack and the signs are due mainly to impaired drainage of the contrast medium. They are reflected in the urograms by dilatation of the urinary pathways, uninterrupted contrast filling of the ureter and delayed emptying.

When the pressure in the renal pelvis exceeds the secretory pressure, the kidney is no longer able to excrete contrast medium. In shock, which is not uncommon in renal colic, the blood pressure may drop. This is accompanied by a fall in the secretory pressure of the kidney, and then stasis is prone to appear. The variation in the urinary excretion with blood pressure on one hand and intrapelvic pressure on the other has long been known.

Since the fundamental investigation by BOEMINGHAUS (1932) of the pathophysiology of renal colic, especially of the increase in pressure, the problem has been studied widely in animal experiments. EDLING et al. (1954) made a thorough study of the variation in the intrapelvic pressure and the influence of such variation on renal secretion of contrast medium. HICKEL (1946) produced an increase in the intrapelvic pressure in human beings by injecting morphine and by increasing the pressure via a ureteric catheter. In this way he was able to reproduce the findings in urinary stasis, even the accumulation of contrast medium in the renal parenchyma. We have also produced such an increase in pressure by means of a Dourmashkin catheter, *i.e.* a catheter with a rubber bag that can be inflated to block the ureter. (It should be kept in mind that the use of such a catheter with a rubber bag involves a risk of ureteric rupture.) RISHOLM (1954) showed that a very moderate rise in pressure (33 mg Hg) in the renal pelvis in man is sufficient to produce pain simulating renal colic. He also found that the upper urinary tract is in a state of hypomotility in renal colic and that the increased pressure in the renal pelvis is the essential cause of the typical pain. Cases have, however, been described by SCHIFFER (1936), for example, in which pyelography during an attack of renal colic shoved a pronounced contraction of the renal pelvis.

WICKBOM (1954) has shown that a nephrogram can be obtained if the blood pressure is low.

In this connexion an interesting case may be reported. On urography of an elderly patient I once saw urographic evidence of severe stasis, namely accumulation of contrast medium in one kidney, the other showing ordinary excretion. The patient had no pain and reported that he had never had any pain previously either. RISHOLM in his above mentioned study reported that as high a pressure in the ureter as 150—190 mm Hg did not invariably produce pain.

4. Reflex anuria

Reflex anuria is to be understood as reflex cessation of urinary excretion on the side involved. More commonly, however, it is used to designate the non-excretion of urine on the contralateral side. As pointed out previously, the pathophysiology of the excretion of contrast medium during renal colic has been clarified experimentally and clinically. It is generally due mainly to the secretory pressure in the kidney on one hand and the intrapelvic pressure on the other.

Thus, no reflex cramps in hypothetic sphincters or elsewhere need be supposed to explain this condition.

Much has been written about this reflex cessation of the excretion on the contralateral side. The many hundred cases of urographic examinations during renal colic at our department alone is sufficient to dismiss the term reflex stone anuria from the medical dictionary. We have never seen any absence of secretion on the contralateral side in cases with unilateral stone. In stasis—also of severe degree in one part of a double kidney—we have never seen reflex cessation of the contrast excretion even in the half of the kidney, whose ureter had not been obstructed.

In animal experiments WULFF (1941) also showed that the possibility of reflex stone anuria may be ignored.

5. Cessation of pain

Cessation of pain usually indicates that passage is restored, which in turn can be due to passage of the stone. Nevertheless stasis might persist. It is believed that such lingering stasis is due to spastic contraction of the distal part of the ureter. But here, too, it is not necessary to assume more or less hypothetical sphincter activity. As a rule, the narrowing is simply due to edema of the mucosa at the site of the stone. As to the distal part of the ureter, the contrast filling is sometimes seen to terminate somewhat short of the concrement. This is often ascribed to spasm around the calculus. It is, however, often due to edema of the mucosa round the stone.

Detrusor spasm on the same side of the urinary bladder as the concrement has also been described in low concrements, and is manifested by assymmetry of the bladder, which is better filled on the opposite side (ENDFEDJIEFF 1958). The phenomenon corresponds to the so-called Constantinescus symptom, which is ascribed to reduced supply of urine from a kidney with impaired excretory capacity.

6. Passage of stone

Stones are often passed during or soon after renal colic. Sometimes, however, they remain impacted. A question that then unsought presents itself is: Is there any reasonable chance of the stone being passed spontaneously or is surgical intervention necessary? In a material of 541 cases of ureteric stone of our department, SANDEGÅRD (1956) made the following observations:

In the absence of indications for active intervention for reasons other than size, shape or localisation of the stone, the actual situation is influenced by the following facts:

a) Small stones (roentgenographic width < 4 mm) in the lower half of the ureter will usually (93 per cent) be passed spontaneously.

b) Small stones in the upper half of the ureter will usually (81 per cent) be passed without serious complications. Sometimes (19 per cent) these stones persist in the upper half and then they can produce considerable obstruction.

c) Medium-sized stones (roentgenographic width 4 > 6 mm) in the lower half of the ureter will often (53 per cent) be passed spontaneously.

d) Medium-sized stones in the upper half of the ureter often (in 14 of 27 cases) migrate down to the lower half within a few months. As long as the stone is in the upper half, it involves a definite risk of serious complications.

e) Large stones (roentgenographic width ≥ 6 mm) in the lower half of the ureter may (in 2 of 9 cases) pass spontaneously.

f) Large stones in the upper half of the ureter seldom (in 1 of 24 cases) migrate down to the lower half. As long as the stone is in the upper half, it involves a considerable risk of serious complications.

XII. Obstructed ureteric flow and kidney function

If a concrement has been demonstrated in the ureter and the stone does not pass spontaneously, the question arises as to how long it can be allowed to obstruct the flow of the urine during expectation that it might pass spontaneously, in other words, how long can operation be postponed without undue risk of definite damage to kidney function. Experimental investigations at our department by WIDÉN (1958) suggest that total obstruction of the urinary flow soon impairs renal function and after 30—40 days complete obstruction, renal function can no longer be recovered.

The finding of a concrement in the ureter permits no direct conclusions concerning the duration of the obstruction. Obstruction may be partial or intermittent and even fairly large stones may, as mentioned, be grooved or channeled and permit the passage of urine. In such cases urography should be done at regular intervals during expectancy to check renal function. As a rule, the excretion of urine will appear normal and the urinary pathways will be at most slightly dilated, even if the concrement is fairly large. In some cases, however, signs of stasis appear, sometimes of severe stasis, and then intervention is indicated. If renal function is markedly impaired or absent, the question is to decide whether the impairment is permanent or temporary. This question is important, particularly in cases in which the onset is not acute and in which it is therefore not possible to estimate how long flow may have been obstructed. Renal angiography can help to decide this point.

XIII. Renal angiography

Renal angiography is of less value in the diagnosis of stone, but it may be very valuable in the evaluation of the condition of the renal parenchyma in stone with complicating infection and in urinary stasis due to stone. In urinary stasis and in infection the entire parenchyma or only part of it may be affected. Thus, in contemplated partial nephrectomy because of stone renal angiography may be useful for judging the state of vascularization of the kidney, the extent of involvement of the parenchyma and for planning of the operation. The method is, however, of still greater value in the estimation of the time drainage has been obstructed and of secondary impairment of kidney function.

It is well-known that prolonged urinary stasis is accompanied by atrophy of the renal parenchyma with gradual loss of renal function. Even if stasis is relieved in such cases, renal function may be definitely impaired. In experiments on rabbits IDBOHRN (1956) at our department showed that in complete unilateral ureteric stasis, pathologic-anatomic changes occurred with destruction of parenchyma proceeding parallel to the length of the stasis during the first 11—12 weeks. After 11—12 weeks' stasis the interstitial tissue had undergone fibrosis-hyalinosis and the tubules were markedly atrophied. After a period of stasis of more than 11—12 weeks the changes progressed only slightly. In further experiments at our department (WIDÉN 1958) on dogs in which urinary stasis had been induced for periods of 7 to 79 days and afterwards released, examination 3 to 7 months after release showed that the kidneys were atrophic, the degree of atrophy varying with the period the ureter had been ligated. As a rule, the tubules were more atrophic than the glomeruli. Atrophy of the parenchyma was accompanied by a

narrowing of the renal artery and changes in the parenchyma as judged by urography and examination of the renal blood flow by physiologic methods (IDBOHRN
& MUREN 1956) showed flow of blood through the kidney to be reduced.

If a ureteric concrement completely obstructs the ureter, and it is not known
how long it has done so, absence of excretion in urography may depend either on

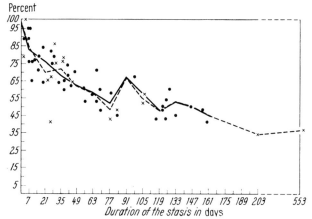

Fig. 108a. Caliber of renal artery in rabbits after ligation of corresponding ureter. Fairly even decrease in caliber
of artery until the 11—12th week, when the caliber is about 50% of original width. (After IDBOHRN)

such long-standing obstruction that the kidney is no longer able to function
because of atrophy of functional elements, or on the pressure in the renal pelvis
being so high as to prevent excretion. In the former case, removal of the obstruction will not be followed by return of function, but in the latter it will give the
kidney the possibility of recovering. In the former case renal angiography may

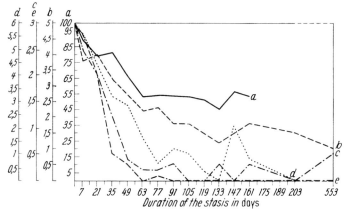

Fig. 108b. Comparison between caliber of renal artery (a), intrarenal arteries (b), nephrographic effect (c), function
after ureterostomy (e) and histologic changes (d). (After IDBOHRN)

show decrease in the width of the renal artery and reduction of the capillary bed
of the kidney as a sign of atrophy, while in the latter the renal artery will be of
normal or nearly normal width and thereby indicate good potential renal function.

Many authors claim that there is a parallelism between the degree of atrophy
of a kidney and the decrease in the width of the renal artery. This conception is,
however, not correct. To clarify the question, IDBOHRN studied the angiographic
changes in animals a varying interval after complete unilateral ureteric obstruction

and WIDÉN studied the same question a long time after stasis had been relieved (Fig. 108). Both investigators showed that patho-anatomic changes with atrophy

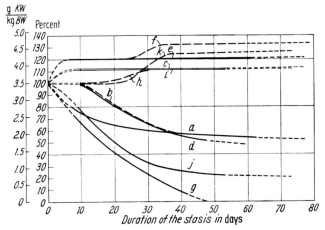

Fig. 108c. Renal angiography in dogs after varying length of time after ligation of corresponding ureter and 3—7 months after release of ureteric occlusion and reestablishment of passage in ureter. The caliber of the renal artery on the ureter-ligated side recovers its original value when the ureter had been completely blocked less than 10 days. Angiographic, functional and morphologic changes in relation to duration of stasis. *a* Caliber of renal artery on ligated side during ligation period. *b* Caliber of renal artery on ligated side during post-release period. *c* Caliber of renal artery on contralateral side during ligation period and post-release period. *d* Size of kidney on ligated side during post-release period. *e* Size of kidney on contralateral side during ligation period and during post-release period after ligation of less than 30 days duration. *f* Size of kidney on the contralateral side during post-release period after ligation period of more than 30 days. *g* Inulin and PAH clearance on ligated side during post-release period, in per cent of half the total preoperative value. *h* Inulin clearance on contralateral side during post-release period, in per cent of half the total preoperative value. *i* PAH clearance on contralateral side during post-release period, in per cent of half the total preoperative value. *j* Weight of kidney (g/kg body-weight) on ligated side. *k* Weight of kidney (g/kg body-weight) on contralateral side. (After WIDÉN)

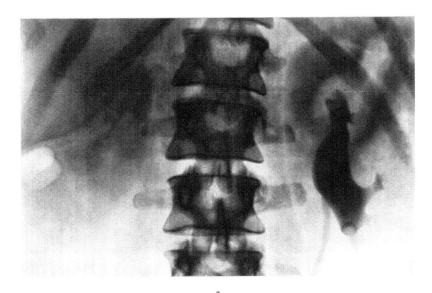

a

Fig. 109a—d. Kidney atrophy due to ureteric obstruction. Gynaecologic operation some years previously. Afterwards "silent kidney". a Urography: No excretion from small right kidney. (See next page)

of the renal parenchyma increased rapidly; the caliber of the artery, however, decreased only slowly. When the caliber of the renal artery had diminished by 50%, all renal function had permanently ceased. Only after complete ureteric occlusion of less than 30 days was any recovery of renal function noted. After 30 days' complete obstruction the artery showed no tendency to recover. The investigations showed that renal angiography with determination of the width

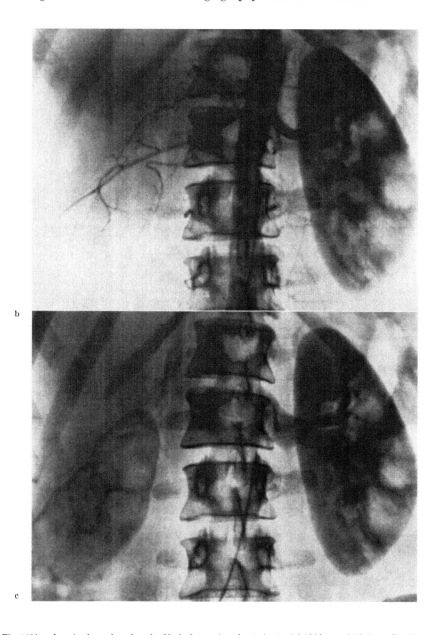

Fig. 109 b and c. Angiography: b and c Marked atrophy of arteries to right kidney, which is small, of irregular outline and has no parenchyma left. Nephrectomy

of renal artery and its branches and evaluation of the renal parenchyma by the nephrogram provides a good method for judging potential renal function. If the caliber of the renal artery has diminished to half its normal width, in practice to half the width of the contralateral renal artery, removal of the obstruction will not result in recovery of renal function (Fig. 109). It is not only the width of the main branch of the renal artery that should be considered but also the appearance of intrarenal branches and, as mentioned, of the nephrogram.

XIV. Nephrocalcinosis

In the discussion of renal stone it has been pointed out that certain diseases predispose to stone formation and in addition are often associated with calcifications in the parenchyma. In parenchymal calcifications smaller calcifications may become detached and appear as concrements.

Nephrocalcinosis is not a clear-cut clinical entity. It is used in the literature to designate calcifications in the kidneys as seen at autopsy or at roentgen examination. Here we are concerned only with the roentgenographic appearance.

Since it appears so often in the literature it will be dwelt on here, but reference is made to the different diseases associated with concrement formation and parenchymal calcifications and described elsewhere. In addition, it is

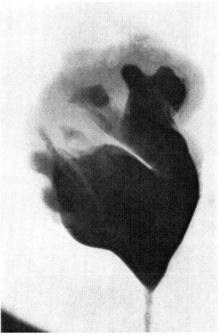

Fig. 109 d. Pyelogram of specimen

stressed that nephrocalcinosis is not a disease *sui generis* and that every single case should be examined and evaluated individually in the light of the fundamental disease.

Renal calcifications are generally classified as metastatic calcifications when they are due to hypercalcaemia in otherwise normal kidneys, and as nonmetastatic or dystrophic calcifications, when a primary renal lesion is present. The division may be useful for purposes of classification, but it is not always possible to make a distinction in a given case, because the renal parenchyma is often damaged, even in cases classified as metastatic.

Nephrocalcinosis is, generally speaking, a roentgen diagnosis. Diagnosis of the condition depends according to MORTENSEN, EMMETT & BAGGENSTOSS (1953) upon the following roentgenographic characteristics: 1. Location of deposits of calcium in the renal parenchyma. 2. The diffuse distribution of such deposits. Obviously the description is diffuse and is worded so as to cover many widely different conditions.

Parenchymal calcifications occurring in association with renal tuberculosis and renal tumor, for example, are usually not included under the name of nephrocalcinosis. This term instead embraces such renal changes as those seen in osteitis fibrosa generalisata. This condition was the first in which the term nephrocalcinosis was used by ALBRIGHT, BAIRD, COPE & BLOOMBERG 1934. It also includes parenchymal changes in sarcoidosis and in some generalized diseases of the renal parenchyma, but only if the disease produces renal calcifications. The term also embraces certain conditions associated with changes in the blood chemistry,

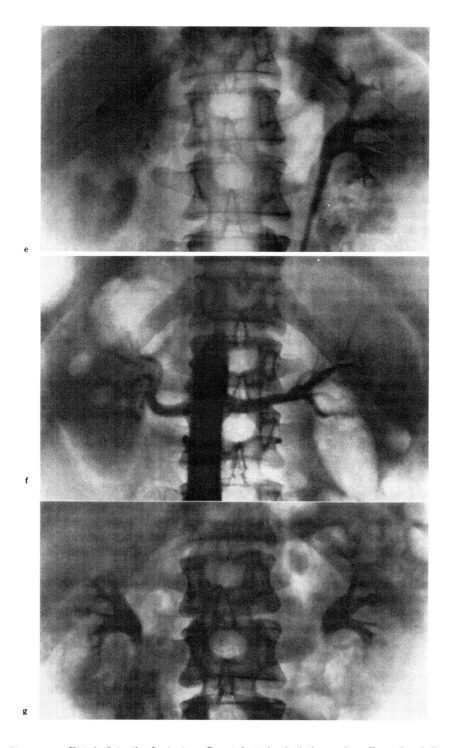

Fig. 109e—g. Ureteric obstruction due to stone. Repeated attacks of pain for months. e Urography. Ordinary excretion left side. No excretion right side. f Renal angiography: Renal arteries have ordinary caliber. Nephrographic phase shows normal conditions. Potential kidney function good. Removal of ureteric stone. g Urography: Normal conditions

particularly hypercalcaemia. Some cases described in the literature under the heading of nephrocalcinosis should have been assigned to other groups such as medullary sponge kidney.

1. Hyperparathyroidism

Hyperparathyroidism, usually due to adenoma of a parathyroid gland, is often accompanied by nephrocalcinosis and renal concrements. The renal changes are the most serious organic complication in this disease. Therefore, in all cases of hyperparathyroidism the kidneys must be examined just as the possibility of hyperparathyroidism should always be considered in all cases of urinary calculi and nephrocalcinosis. HELLSTRÖM (1955) stated that in 56 of his 70 cases of hyperparathyroidism renal concrements were found roentgenologically, namely in one third of the cases stones only, in one third parenchymal calcifications only, and in one third both in combination. According to ALBRIGHT & REIFENSTEIN (1958), on the other hand, hyperparathyroidism is the cause in 5% of all cases of urinary stone. The concrements and calcifications vary widely from case to case and from side to side. One or both kidneys are often reduced in size.

Renal lesions can occur without bone lesions, the former being an index of the severity of the disease; the latter, an index of its duration (ALBRIGHT, BAIRD, COPE & BLOOMBERG 1934).

It is assumed that the roentgen pathology of the bone lesions characteristic of hyperparathyroidism and the method for diagnosing parathyroid adenoma are known and they are therefore not described here.

2. Sarcoidosis

The term sarcoidosis is to be understood here as the obscure disease, also known as Besnier's, Boeck's, or Schaumann's disease, or lymphogranuloma benignum if the changes are localized to the glands, or ostitis multiplex cystica Jüngling when the lesions are seen in the bones.

It is common knowledge that autopsy has revealed calculi and parenchymal calcifications in a high percentage of patients with sarcoidosis. The calcareous formations may involve only a small part of the kidney or renal pelvis or the major part of the kidney. A few descriptions of the roentgen anatomy in this disease are on record. DAVIDSON, DENNIS, McNINCH, WILLSON & BROWN (1954) described the largest series (7 cases) illustrating bilateral nephrocalcinosis; the lesions were irregular and they varied in extent from case to case and from side to side in one and the same patient. The kidneys are also sometimes reduced in size (SCHÜPBACH & WERNLY 1943). Calcium deposits in the soft tissue and resembling the changes seen in peritendinitis calcarea may also occur.

It is presumed that the reader is familiar with the changes of roentgen-diagnostic importance in sarcoidosis outside the urinary tract.

3. Hypercalcaemia

The findings described above in nephrocalcinosis resemble those in other conditions of hypercalcaemia such as bone-destroying tumors.

The largest series of these conditions consists of 91 cases (MORTENSEN & EMMETT 1954: 48 from the literature and 43 personal cases), of which almost half had hyperparathyroidism. Two thirds of the remaining cases consisted of hyperchloric acidosis and chronic pyelonephritis in equal proportion. The group hyper-

chloric acidosis included cases of the type described by BUTLER, WILSON &
FABER (1936) and by ALBRIGHT, CONSOLAZIO, COOMBS, SULKOWITCH & TALBOTT

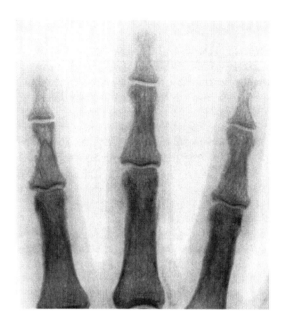

(1940), who called the disease
nephrocalcinosis with rickets
and dwarfism.

Nephrosclerosis occurring in
association with sulphonamide
therapy has been described by
many authors (GREENSPAN 1949,
ENGEL 1951).

4. Glomerulonephritis, pyelonephritis, and tubular nephritis

Glomerulonephritis, pyelonephritis, and tubular nephritis
are sometimes associated with
nephrocalcinosis. Widespread
calcifications have been observed on occasion in chronic
glomerulonephritis (ROSEN-
BAUM, COGGESHALL & LEVIN
1951). In pyelonephritis calcifi-

a

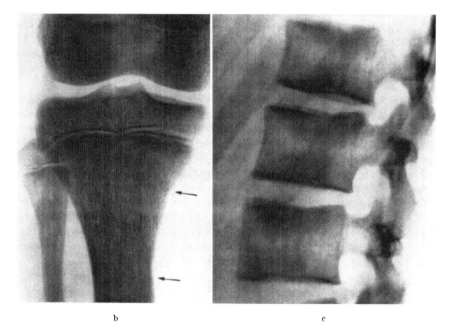

b   c

Fig. 110a—c. Renal osteodystrophy. Characteristic type and localization of bony lesions. a Cortical erosions in
phalanges, especially middle phalangs and (b) in proximal end of tibia medially (between arrows). c Irregular
sclerosis of vertebral bodies

cations may be seen in the pyramids (ALBRIGHT, DIENES & SULKOWITCH 1938)
(papillary necrosis must here be kept in mind). In tubular nephritis cortical

calcifications have been observed by MOËLL in some of our cases. In this conjunction cortical calcifications in gross renal cortical necrosis should be remembered.

In fact, nephrocalcinosis will prove to be fairly common in generalized diseases of the renal parenchyma if the examination aims at demonstrating diffusely spread, fairly thin calcifications.

The group of diseases under discussion is sometimes associated with bone lesions of somewhat varying type, so-called renal osteodystrophy, osteonephropathy etc. The fundamental diseases are of two different types. A smaller group consists of rare cases with selective tubular disturbances, and a second, larger group of cases with chronic renal insufficiency due to glomerulonephritis, pyelonephritis or malformations of the kidneys and urinary tract. The roentgendiagnostic findings consist partly of skeletal changes, partly of changes of the type metastatic calcifications and arterial calcifications. The type and severity of roentgenologic osseous changes vary with the patient's age and severity of renal insufficiency and the duration of such insufficiency. Bone lesions are partly changes of the type seen in rickets and partly changes resembling those occurring in osteitis fibrosa cystica. The former type is seen before the closure of the epiphyseal lines, the latter in adult age. In some cases osteosclerosis is predominant and involves the major part of the skeleton, though it is sometimes limited to the spine, particularly the lumbar portion. These last-mentioned changes can often be detected at plain roentgenography of the urinary tract and then indicate roentgen examination of the entire skeleton or places of predilection (Fig. 110) (CRONQVIST 1961).

Young patients show changes, which in localization and type resemble those seen in rachitis. In adults the most characteristic changes are seen in the phalanges, in the medial part of the proximal third of tibia, in the corresponding part of the humerus and in the clavicle, the acromion and the ulna. In these bones diffusely outlined zones of cortical rarefaction are seen in the cortex.

In advanced cases the skeletal changes are the same as in hyperparathyroidism and can be differentiated from this disease only by blood studies. I doubt whether a differential diagnosis is always possible since hyperparathyroidism is often complicated by renal insufficiency.

H. Renal tuberculosis

Roentgen examination for renal tuberculosis is not only an important field of urologic diagnostic radiology but also of particular interest in so far as fundamental changes in our concept of this disease and its treatment are reflected by the roentgen methods used through the years in the investigation of the condition. Formerly nephrectomy was the rule for unilateral renal tuberculosis regardless of the extent of the lesion in the kidney and then demonstration of the lesion was all that was required. Advances since made in the treatment of the disease necessitate more detailed information and place high demands on diagnostic radiology.

Patho-anatomically the tuberculous infection of the kidney may assume various forms, of which the so-called ulcero-cavernous type is most important from a clinical point of view. One of the purposes of roentgen examination is to detect this ulcero-cavernous tuberculosis and to distinguish it from other types of tuberculous infection of the kidney. Roentgen examination is also important in

the assessment of the extent of the process within the kidney and urinary tract
and of the effect of conservative treatment.

Ulcero-cavernous renal tuberculosis is also often called surgical renal tuberculosis because in this particular type nephrectomy was the rational therapy
before specific antituberculous chemotherapeutics came into use. It is characterized by the fact that in the course of their development the lesions are transiently
or permanently in open communication with the renal pelvis, where they can
deposit infectious material. This explains the clinical picture with so-called aseptic
pyuria and bacilluria. This type of tuberculosis is associated with the risk of
canalicular infection of the entire urinary tract and—in males—the genital organs.

I. Remarks on pathology

Ulcero-cavernous renal tuberculosis usually begins as a focus in a papilla. Communication is established between the focus and the renal pelvis either by fistulation of the lesion into the renal pelvis, if the lesion is located deep in the papilla,
or by a broad ulceration of the papilla toward the renal pelvis, if the caseation is
superficial. The process may in this way involve one or more papillae, often all of
the papillae in the kidney. The ulceration can be localized to the tip or side of a
papilla or up in the fornix, or it might result in caseation of the major part of a
papilla or papillae. The earliest patho-anatomic form of ulcero-cavernous tuberculosis to be met with in roentgen examination is ulceration of a single papilla.
In more widespread changes ulceration of several papillae can occur and cavities
may be formed in the renal parenchyma. They may be small and solitary or
represent complete destruction of the kidney in tuberculous pyonephrosis.
Edema and ulceration occur in the mucosa of the renal pelvis, in the ureters and
in the mucosa of the urinary bladder.

Regressive changes may occur in the renal parenchyma as well as in the urinary
tract. They are manifested by demarcation of necrotic tissue, part of which is
often calcified. Fibrous tissue is formed, which, as in all forms of tuberculosis, is
characterized by a pronounced tendency to shrink. This gives rise to local scars
in the renal parenchyma with local scar formation in the surface of the kidney
or contraction of the entire kidney. Regressive changes, located in the renal pelvis,
may lead to occlusion of small or large parts of the kidney, usually at the level
of the originally narrow parts, such as the stems of the calyces, the pelviureteric
junction, or ureteric orifice in the urinary bladder. This shrinkage due to scar
formation may thus result in various types of obstruction and in considerable
distortion of various parts of the renal pelvis.

II. Roentgen examination

In the light of the gross pathology of ulcero-cavernous renal tuberculosis
outlined above the roentgen findings can be readily understood. The pathologic
changes can be demonstrated by various methods, namely plain roentgenography,
pyelography, urography and angiography. Urethrocystography and occasionally
vesiculography are also important. These examinations are described in part II.

1. Plain roentgenography

The size and shape of a kidney can be changed by a tuberculous process. Plain
roentgenograms will also sometimes show calcifications.

If the kidney is considerably shrunken, it may be very small yet its outline
might be more or less regular and fairly sharp. The final stage of such a process

is the so-called tuberculous contracted kidney. The shrinkage may also be local and limited to one of the poles, for example, or it may only produce local indentations in the outline of the kidney. The kidney may, on the other hand, also be of ordinary size or enlarged with an irregular bulgent outline due to cavities or calyces dilated as a result of strictures. The change may be local with formation of one or more adjacent caverns causing a single bulge in the surface of the kidney.

Calcifications are often seen in the parenchyma (see Figs. 3, 6, 7, 13, 15). They may involve the entire kidney and even the ureter and produce the characteristic putty kidney (see Fig. 113). Sometimes only part of the kidney will assume the appearance of a putty kidney (see Fig. 119 b). On auto-amputation of the upper branch of the renal pelvis, for example, the corresponding portion of the kidney may calcify in the same way as a putty kidney. Irregular calcifications may be widespread. The tuberculous calcifications are usually, however, only seen in small regions. They may appear as amorphous masses in a well-defined area corresponding to a bulge or indentation in the contour of the kidney and then represent calcium deposits in the caseous contents of a cavity. They may also be localized to the wall of a cavity and then give an outline of it. More often they are seen as calcified necrotic areas (see for example Figs. 117, 120, 132). The calcifications are usually dense and of irregular shape. They may be small or large and local or scattered in the kidney. They are most commonly unilateral or at any rate much more marked on one side. Tuberculous cavities sometimes contain multiple concrements resembling those seen in so-called pyelogenic cysts.

The frequency given for parenchymal calcifications varies from one author to another. Of our material, we found such changes in as many as 50 per cent. They vary widely in type and form from minute calcifications, hardly detectable, up to massive formations of the type seen in putty kidney. The difference in the frequency with which these changes have been observed in various series may be due in part to differences in examination technique, differences in the composition of the material and differences in the character of the infection.

In putty kidney and partial putty kidney the roentgen findings are pathognomonic. Other types of calcification in renal tuberculosis are usually not characteristic and may not differ from parenchymal calcifications of other origin.

Calcifications in tuberculous material are sometimes seen in the ureter, particularly in the ureteric stump after nephrectomy, in the seminal vesicles in the prostatic gland, and on occasion in the wall of the urinary bladder. They are very rare in a tuberculous epididymis.

Calcification is, of course, a late pathologic sign, yet it may be seen in patients with only a short history or no history at all. We have not infrequently seen calcifications as part of advanced lesions in patients who not even remember ever having had any urinary symptoms. It is also well known that a putty kidney is often an incidental finding in patients who have no history at all or only slight non-characteristic symptoms. This thus implies that also advanced tuberculous infection of the kidney may sometimes be completely asymptomatic.

In all roentgen examinations for renal tuberculosis due attention should be given to those parts of the skeleton included in plain roentgenograms of the urinary tract. Since renal tuberculosis and skeletal tuberculosis belong to the same phase of infection, they often appear together. Sometimes spondylitis in the lumbar spine with or without abscess can be seen (see Fig. 131). The abscess may displace one or both kidneys. Ileosacral tuberculosis may also be demonstrated. Pleural changes in the base of the thorax are often seen in plain roentgenograms of the kidneys. It is taken for granted that the reader is familiar with the roentgen findings in extrarenal tuberculosis e.g. chest, bone and joints.

As to the localization of extrarenal tuberculosis and the position of renal tuberculosis in the course of the tuberculous infection as well as indications for examination of the kidney for suspected tuberculosis, reference is made to the volume on renal tuberculosis by Ljunggren in volume IX/2 of this encyclopedia.

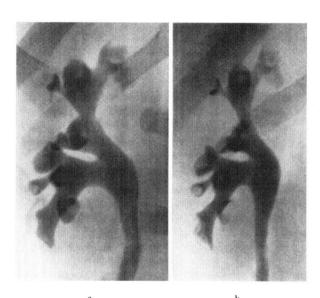

a   b

Fig. 111a and b. Solitary papillary ulceration. Urography. a Small cavity in the uppermost medial part of right kidney and in adjacent papilla. b Oblique view. The lesion is located in the dorsal part of the upper pole

2. Pyelography and urography

Ulcero-cavernous renal tuberculosis can be diagnosed by pyelography or urography because of the fact that the foci are in open communication with, or cause changes in, the renal pelvis. This holds also for the earliest form of renal tuberculosis, *i.e.* ulceration of a single papilla. Contrast urine in the renal pelvis will fill the ulceration. This often has the appearance of a small round or oval cavity with a somewhat irregular outline and in more or less wide communication with the calyx (Figs. 111, 112; see also Fig. 116). The connection might on occasion consist only of a fine duct. A more superficial ulceration of the papilla will be seen only as an irregularity in the outline of one calyx. In more extensive lesions a filling will be obtained of sometimes large cavities of more or less irregular outline in the renal parenchyma (Figs. 113, 114, 115; see also Figs. 117, 118, 129, 131, 132). In some cases a filling may be obtained of only a small cavity, while the pyelogram will show displacement of the adjacent calyces indicating more extensive involvement. This discrepancy might be due to the cavity being very thick-walled or being filled with necrotic material permitting the inflow of only a small amount of contrast medium into it. Sometimes no filling at all is obtained of the cavity,

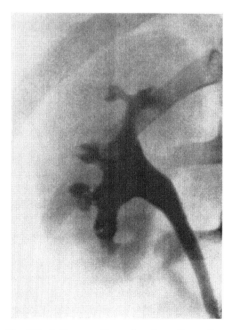

Fig. 112. Solitary papillary ulceration. Urography. Small cavity next to lowermost papilla communicating with calyx

which then appears only as an expanding process by the displacement of the calyces (see Fig. 131) or it may even remain concealed. Cases are on record

(OLLE OLSSON 1943) in which fairly large intrarenal tuberculous foci were shut off from the renal pelvis by stenosis in a branch in such a way that the roentgen anatomy of the renal pelvis appeared normal.

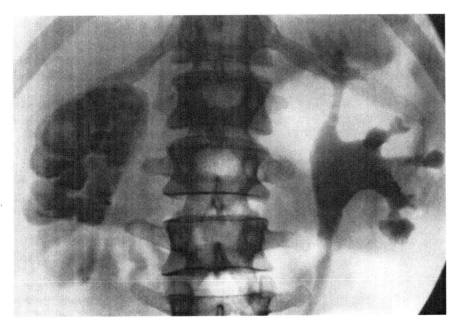

Fig. 113. Bilateral tuberculosis. Urography: Calcified tuberculous pyonephrosis on right side, putty kidney. Small, mainly irregular cavities in most pyramids of left kidney. Slight irregularity of outline of kidney pelvis due to tuberculous pyelitis

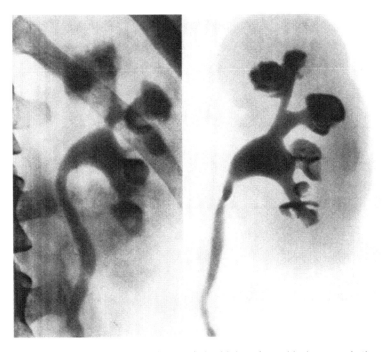

Fig. 114. Widespread, unilateral chronic renal tuberculosis with irregular cavities in communication with most calyces. Urography: Density of contrast urine somewhat decreased. b Pyelogram of operation specimen for comparison with urogram

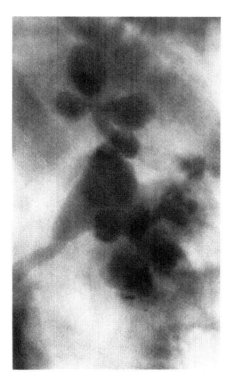

Fig. 115. Large cavities throughout remaining kidney. Urography: Fairly good density of excreted contrast urine in spite of widespread changes

A special type of ulceration is that in which several, sometimes all, papillae are the seat of small relatively superficial ulcerations. This type of ulceration must be distinguished from medullary sponge kidney (see chapter T). In long-standing processes the wall of the cavern may be quite smooth, and such a cavity may contain one or more concrements.

Even such an early change as ulceration of a single papilla may be associated with a narrowing of the calyx draining the papilla. This stenosis is initially due to edema but in more advanced cases, to granulation tissue and finally to shrinkage. Then the calyx often becomes dilated and the obstruction of the flow results in increased destruction of the parenchyma. When the stenosis involves an entire branch the latter often terminates in a series of more or less well defined cavities in the parenchyma. The narrowing may make it difficult to obtain a filling and make prolonged ureteric compression necessary during the urographic procedure. Experience has also shown that urography with prolonged compression is a better method than retrograde pyelography for obtaining a filling of cavities almost completely occluded.

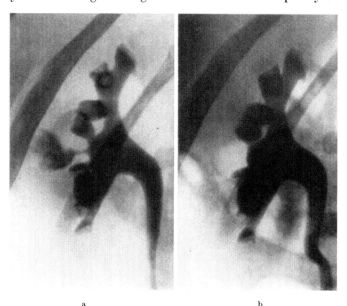

a   b

Fig. 116a and b. Irregular cavity in communication with micro-calyx in middle of kidney (a). b One year later, chemo-therapy. Complete blocking of calyx

By severe narrowing one (Fig. 116) or more calyces (Fig. 117) may be occluded or even an entire branch (Figs 118, 119, 120), so-called auto-amputation of part

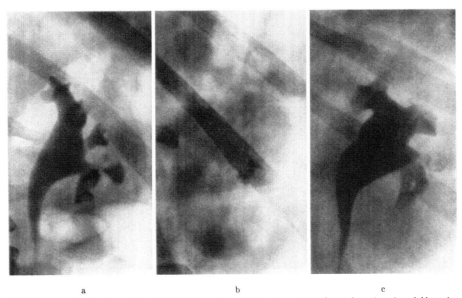

a   b   c

Fig. 117a—c. a Cavity in caudal part of left kidney, stenosis of corresponding calyx and pursing of caudal branch. Chemo-therapy. b Five years later. Plain roentgenogram. Irregular calcification at the site of the cavity. Indentation in the lateral contour of the kidney corresponding to the calcification. c Urography. Blocking of calyx at site of calcification. Pursing of lower branch

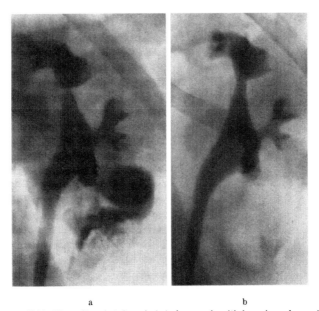

a   b

Fig. 118a and b. Rapid blocking. Chronic tuberculosis in lower pole with large irregular cavities (a). b Three months after institution of chemo-therapy. Complete blocking of caudal branch. Shrinkage of caudal kidney pole

of the renal pelvis. A calyx or a branch may, as mentioned, be shut off completely in such a way as to prevent demonstration of the lesion in the pyelogram. Particularly on check examination during chemo-therapy the films must be carefully

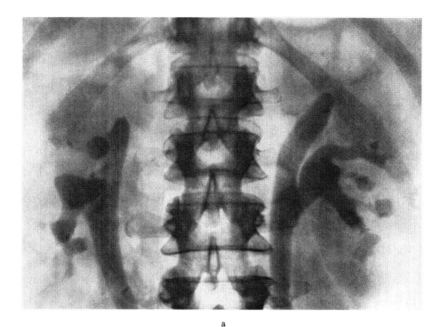

a

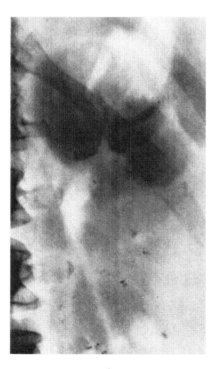

b

Fig. 119a and b. Widespread bilateral long-standing renal tuberculosis. a Urography. Complete auto-amputation of cranial branch bilaterally and of middle calyx group on right side. Multiple small and larger cavities in communication with most calyces on both sides. b Plain roentgenogram 8 years later. Partial putty kidney. Left cranial pole completely calcified

compared with those taken previously in order to permit detection of any occlusion of a minor part of the renal pelvis.

Distortion of one or more calyces by cicatrization of tuberculous tissue usually produces characteristic pyelographic changes in advanced renal tuberculosis (Fig. 121).

It is important to take films in different planes in order to ascertain in what part of the kidney a tuberculous process is located, in particular whether it is situated in the ventral or dorsal part of the kidney (FRIMANN-DAHL 1955). This is of importance in contemplated partial nephrectomy and can be determined easily during urography by turning the patient in suitable projections on the examination table if the compression bandage is fixed to the patient and not to the table. Sometimes it may be advisable to examine the patient also in prone position in order to obtain a filling of cavities situated in the ventral part of the kidney.

A method suggested by FRANZAS (1954) for securing better contrast *i.e.* having a layman, who is specially trained to observe even slight differences in contrast fill in the roentgenograms, is not only non-roentgenologic but also incompatible with medical practice. If artificially increased contrast in a film is for some reason desired, it should be secured by logetronography, for instance, by or under the supervision of the roentgenologist.

In the literature the appearance of a typical pyelogram in renal tuberculosis is often described as resembling a marguerite, a brush, a sod or by some other fanciful name. Such pictorial descriptions based on single cases or projections are dilettantish and their use is unjustified. Roentgen diagnostics with the use of appropriate methods and adaptation of the technic to meet the requirements of the individual case aims at recognizing changes that can be described in patho-anatomic terms.

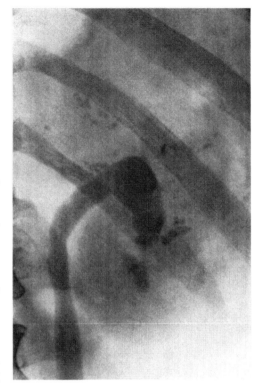

Fig. 120. Disseminated irregular calcifications in necrotic material throughout the kidney. Urography. Entire cranial branch and most calyces are amputated. Caudal pole has small cavity in communication with lowermost calyx. Good density of contrast urine despite widespread changes (contralateral kidney functionless)

Fig. 120

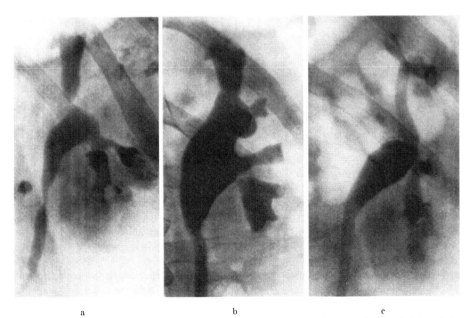

a   b   c

Fig. 121a—c. Examples of marked shrinkage tendency of kidney pelvis in long-standing chronic tuberculosis. a Complete exclusion of middle calyces. Distortion of stem of adjacent calyces and almost complete obstruction of base of cranial branch. b Blocking of small calyx belonging to middle part of kidney and severe obstruction of base of caudal branch. c Blocking of calyces to middle part of kidney. Cavities in communication with filled calyces. Severe distortion of confluence laterally. Pursing of branches

a) Ureteric changes (Fig. 122)

Even relatively small tuberculous foci in the kidney are capable of causing dilatation of the ureter. Such a change has often been regarded as being of functional origin. It is, however, usually due to edema around the ureteric orifice with slight obstruction and stasis as a consequence. Early ureteritis, with edema of the mucosa, then, is seen in the roentgenogram as a slight dilatation of the ureter and a slight irregular outline. Strictures are more common causes of dilatation. They are prone to occur at those levels where the ureter is normally narrow *i.e.* at the pelviureteric junction (Fig. 123) and in the ureteric orifice in the urinary bladder (Fig. 124 a—c). The strictures may be short or long, single

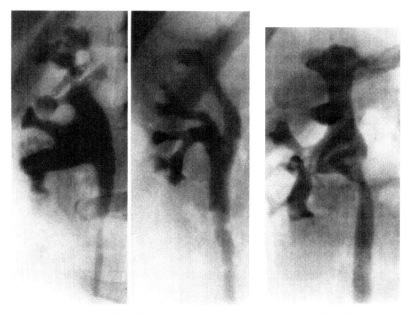

Fig. 122   Fig. 123

Fig. 122. Different types of tuberculous ureteritis. Slight irregular outline of kidney pelvis and of part of ureter. Cavities in cranial kidney pole in both cases

Fig. 123. Tuberculous stricture at pelviureteric junction

or multiple. In the beginning the narrowing is due to edema, later to granulation tissue and eventually to shrinkage. Particularly changes in the lower ureter and in the bladder around the ureteric orifice can cause severe ureteric dilatation. Ureteritis may be confined to the actual ureteric orifice, just as it may extend a fair distance up the ureter with pronounced narrowing of the lumen as a consequence. Ureteric changes may be caused by trauma sustained during catheterization, for example. A very well verified case has been described by ERICSSON & LINDBOM (1950) in which neither urography nor subsequent retrograde pyelography showed any evidence of a pathologic condition in the ureter. Four months later, however, edema was demonstrated at the level to which the tip of the catheter had been passed during the previous pyelography, and another 6 months later examination showed a stricture at the same level with dilatation of the ureter proximal thereto.

The examiner should always be on the watch for ureteric changes, and many urologists are of the opinion that if nephrectomy is indicated, the operation should always be extended to include ureterectomy. On review of 7 patients who had definite tuberculous involvement of the ureter at the time of nephrectomy SENGER, BELL, WARRES & TIRMAN (1947) found the ureter to be sclerotic in 5, in one it was dilated and in one there was empyema of the stump. Inflammation of the lower ureter or the urinary bladder (Figs. 125, 126, 127) can cause destruction in the remaining kidney by increasing the intrapelvic pressure. This mechanism has often been the cause of death in uraemia after nephrectomy although the remaining kidney was free of tuberculosis. Note the French expression "la mort du rein restant" (CIBERT 1946).

Nephrectomy in cases with a shrunken bladder may be followed by marked dilatation of the ureteric stump which then serves, so to say, as a supplementary bladder (Fig. 128).

b) Excretion of contrast medium during urography

The changes described above can be demonstrated not only by pyelography, but also by urography if the excretion of contrast medium is good. In our renal tuberculosis material, in which every case was examined urographically, the excretion of contrast medium was as follows: in about half of

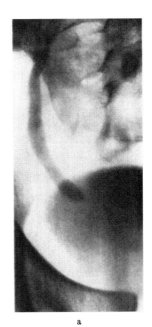

a

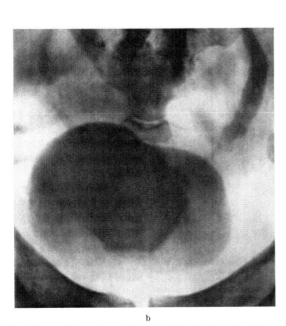

b

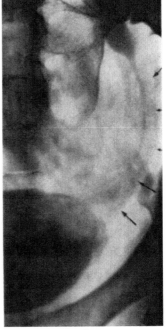

c

Fig. 124 a—c. Tuberculous stricture at distal ureteric end. In (b) and (c) tuberculous cystitis around the ureter orifice. Note in (c) outline of thick ureter wall (arrows)

the cases the contrast urine excreted was of good density and in about two thirds of these cases the density was excellent. In the other half the density was low, and in about one tenth of the whole material there was no excretion at all.

A certain agreement was found between the density of the contrast urine and the amount of non-functioning renal parenchyma. When the lesions were small the density of the contrast urine was normal or only slightly decreased, but when the lesions had involved most or all of the kidney, the density was very poor or no contrast urine was excreted. Despite large changes the density was, however, often good because that part of the renal pelvis draining the affected portion of the kidney was shut off. The pelvis was then filled with urine of ordinary density excreted from unaffected parts of the kidney.

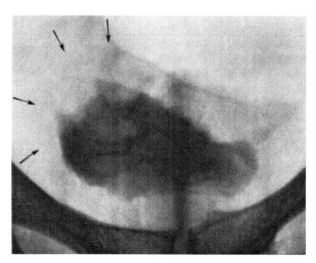

a

Small lesions can thus, as a rule, be diagnosed under optimal contrast conditions. All of our cases with ulceration of a solitary papilla could be diagnosed urographically. Large lesions, on the other hand, can be observed even when the excretion of contrast medium is severely impaired. In cases with no excretion pyelography might be useful, but then associated changes in the bladder and/or ureter often make catheterization impossible.

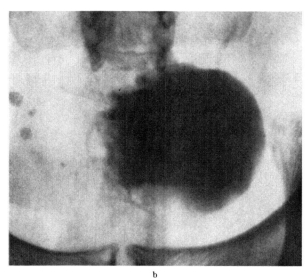

b

Fig. 125a and b. Bladder tuberculosis. a Left-sided long-standing kidney tuberculosis with marked dilatation of kidney pelvis and ureter on "normal" right side. Marked edema in bladder mucosa except small part on the right side. Thickening of bladder wall. Dilatation right side caused by bladder changes. b Left part of bladder free of changes. Right-sided renal tuberculosis

It should be observed that a kidney showing poor excretion of contrast medium may still have some reserve capacity. We have seen a case with widespread tuberculous lesions in one kidney and no demonstrable excretion of contrast medium. The patient had an attack of pain because of stone in the ureter on the "normal" side. Urography during the attack showed no excretion at all on this side but slight excretion by the tuberculous kidney, from which no excretion could be demonstrated before.

Low density of contrast medium excreted has often been ascribed to some toxic effect involving the whole kidney. It is, however, apparent from the remarks set

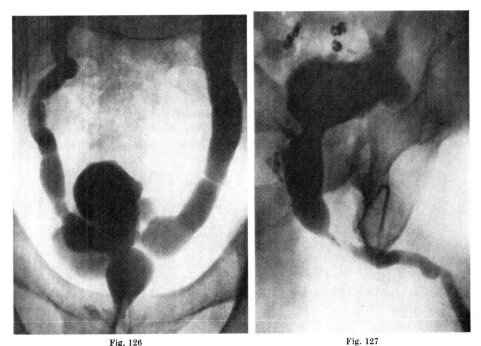

Fig. 126   Fig. 127

Fig. 126. Irregularly contracted bladder. Marked dilatation of ureters. Prostatic abscess

Fig. 127. Urethrocystography. Irregular contracted bladder. Prostatic abscesses. Calcified seminal vesicals. Multiple urethral strictures

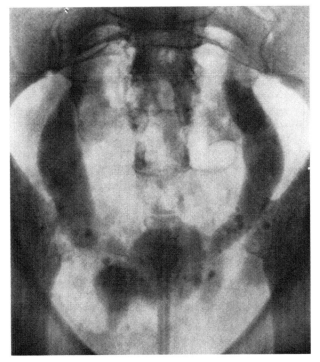

Fig. 128. Contracted bladder with dilatation of ureter to remaining left kidney and of right ureter stump after nephrectomy. Ureter stump increases capacity of contracted bladder

forth above that the density of the contrast medium is to some extent proportional
to the amount of functioning renal parenchyma. An observation arguing against
a general toxic effect being responsible for poor concentration of excreted contrast
medium is that in double kidney with tuberculous lesions only in one half, the
density of the contrast urine in that half will be low but excellent in the other half.
This is borne out still more distinctly by the phenomenon described under the
name of selective pyelography (OLLE OLSSON 1943): In films taken immediately
after injection of the contrast medium, the latter will be first excreted only in
normal calyces draining unaffected renal parenchyma. After these calyces have
been filled the renal pelvis will be filled from them in retrograde direction. The
entire renal pelvis is thus filled with contrast urine excreted by unaffected parts

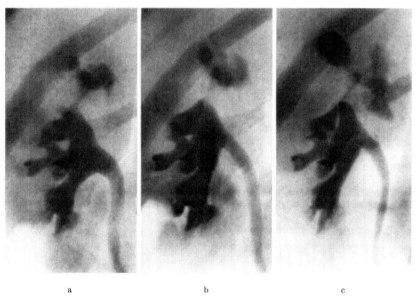

a   b   c

Fig. 129a—f. Tuberculosis in cranial pole of right kidney. a Papillary ulceration and edema in mucosa of
cranial branch. b One year later. Increased cavitation. Stricture of cranial branch. c Another year later increased
cavitation. Pursing of stems of adjacent calyces. Renal angiography. (Fig. 129 d—f see next page)

of the renal parenchyma. Sometimes urine of low contrast density may appear
simultaneously in calyces draining affected parts of the renal parenchyma. The
contrast density of the urine coming from unaffected parts of the kidney is normal.
When this urine is afterwards diluted with urine in the major portion of the renal
pelvis the density of all the contrast medium accumulated in the renal pelvis may
be low, but the fact that urine of ordinary contrast density can be excreted from
one or more unaffected papillae in a kidney harbouring widespread tuberculous
lesions definitely argues against any general toxic effect on the renal parenchyma
influencing the excretion of contrast medium. It should be stressed that the
general toxic effect on the renal parenchyma is discussed here only concerning its
influence on the excretion of contrast urine.

c) Renal angiography

In the discussion of angiography it must never be forgotten that urography
and particularly pyelography have their greatest value in the investigation of
open tuberculosis, which sheds bacilli into the urinary tract with the risk of the
disease spreading to the ureter and bladder. These methods show lesions in the

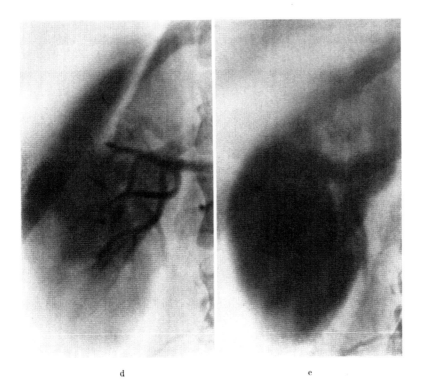

d   e

renal pelvis and ureter and parenchymal changes only
if they are in open communication with, or distort,
the renal pelvis. They do not yield detailed information on lesions within the actual renal parenchyma
shut off from the renal pelvis. Recent therapeutic advances have created an ever-increasing demand for
information on parenchymal involvment. Chemotherapy leads to blockage owing to shrinkage of single
calyces or major parts of the renal pelvis and then the
extent of a process can no longer be judged from the
contrast filling of the renal pelvis. Therefore conservative therapy makes information on the kidney parenchyma necessary. Knowledge not only of the anatomy of the vessels but still more of the extent of the
disease, in particular within the renal parenchyma, is
desirable if partial nephrectomy is contemplated. Renal angiography is valuable not only because it demonstrates the vasculature of the kidney and any
vascular changes in the region of tuberculous foci but
also because the nephrograms show the state of the
renal parenchyma. As yet only few investigations of
this possibility are on record (WEYDE 1952, 1954,
FRIMANN-DAHL 1955, OLLE OLSSON 1955). The arteriogram will show dislocation of vessels around an
inflammatory focus, variation in size or irregularity in
outline of vessels and any abrupt termination of vessels

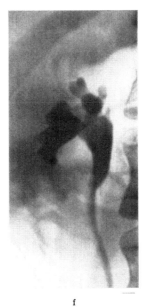

f

Fig. 129 d—f. d Arterial phase.
Endarteritic changes. e Nephrogram shows fairly well defined
destruction in cranial pole. f Partial nephrectomy. Operation confirmed the roentgen findings.
Postoperative check urography
showing ordinary conditions in
remaining part of right kidney

by thrombi or by endarteritis (Fig. 129a—f). On the basis of autopsy studies
AMBROSETTI & SESENNA (1955) have endeavoured to refine the diagnosis by
means of arteriography. Their investigation is of particular interest in the

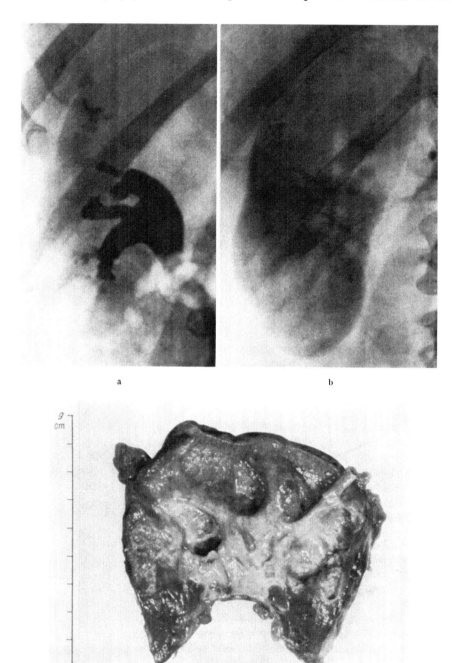

Fig. 130a—c. Long-standing right-sided tuberculosis. a Urography. Complete blocking of cranial branch.
Increased volume of cranial kidney pole. b Renal angiography. Nephrogram. Large thin-walled cavity in cranial
pole. Partial nephrectomy of upper half of right kidney. Specimen. Resected part of kidney is completely cavernous with caseation and widespread fresh tuberculous granulation tissue. c Operative specimen

discussion of so-called tuberculous infarctions in the kidney due to tuberculous endarteritis. But they have also contributed to our knowledge of fine vascular changes in tuberculosis. As yet, however, the findings in the nephrogram are in my opinion the most important. The nephrogram yields most information on the extent of the tuberculous process in the kidney and its exact localisation (Fig. 130a—c). It must be remembered, however, that owing to disturbances in the circulation around the tuberculous focus the nephrogram may suggest a pathologic process to be larger than it really is and in other cases with small changes it may not be possible to assess the full extent of the process because of a relatively thick overlying mass of normal renal tissue.

In my opinion, the best information should be obtainable by combined angiography and simultaneous multiplane body section radiography.

Renal angiography will also show any reduction in the caliber of the renal artery and thereby the reduction in amount of functioning renal parenchyma. This adds renal tuberculosis to diseases with those fundamental problems related to potential renal function which can be solved by means of renal angiography. These problems are discussed in chapter G XIII.

3. Differential diagnosis

It cannot be emphasized enough that hardly any of the roentgen findings in renal tuberculosis are pathognomonic. The wide variation in extent, age, and form of tuberculous changes calls for caution in the interpretation of the roentgen findings. Many non-tuberculous processes can cause changes similar to those seen in different stages of renal tuberculosis. It has also been claimed that the only truly pathognomonic change in renal tuberculosis is that of putty kidney. Pronounced irregular cicatrization and distortion of the renal pelvis are also fairly characteristic. A diagnosis of renal tuberculosis can, however, as a rule, not be made on the basis of roentgen examination only. It will permit a probable diagnosis, but a firm diagnosis requires demonstration of tubercle bacilli.

If the lesions are small, they must be differentiated from fornix reflux described by OLLE OLSSON (1943 and 1948) and LINDBOM (1943). Urograms will often show small sinus refluxes simulating papillary ulcerations. Should such a change appear during an examination, ureteric compression should be prolonged. The reflux will then spread and the contrast medium ooze down along the stems of the calyces and possibly further into the sinus. If the examination cannot be prolonged, the patient may be re-examined after an interval of 1—2 weeks by when the reflux will have healed. The so-called tubular reflux in retrograde pyelography, which can also be demonstrated on urography during ureteric compression and is then due to tubular stasis, usually offers no differential diagnostic difficulties. Pathologic processes of differential diagnostic importance are also papillary necrosis, pyelogenic cyst, calyceal border evagination, calyx hypoplasia with spherical calyces and hydrocalyx caused by calculi, for example. If the process is more advanced, secondary changes in a kidney due to stone and various stages of pyelonephritis might offer differential diagnostic difficulties. The differential diagnosis can ultimately be established by bacteriologic examination.

4. Follow-up examinations

Conservative treatment has made knowledge of the roentgenographic course of renal tuberculosis imperative. The course varies widely. If the vital resistance is low, the process may progress rapidly, while cases detected accidentally, such

as renal tuberculosis in males discovered in association with epididymitis, show
that it can run a very slow and insidious course, with increasing cavitation or
with healing with cicatrization, blockage of the calyces and calcification. Blocking

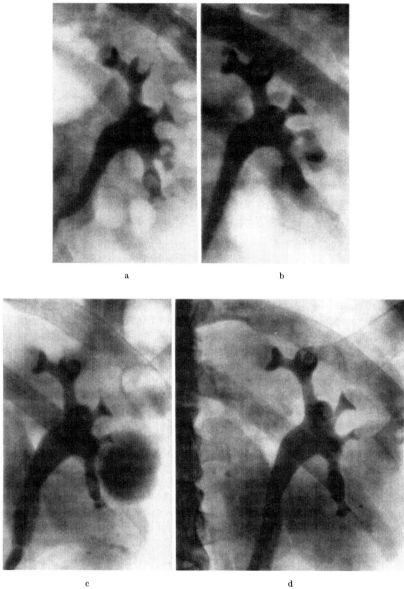

a   b

c   d

Fig. 131a—d. Check examinations during conservative treatment of left-sided tuberculosis. The patient had
many tuberculous lesions in the chest, spine, pelvis etc. and her vital resistance was low. She responded slowly
to conservative therapy, is now well. a Slight irregularity of edge of next to lowermost calyx. b One year later
small cavity formation. c Another three years later large cavity with displacement of nearby calyces. Wall of
cavity fairly smooth. d Five years later. Complete exclu·ion of cavity. Note spondylitis with abscess displacing
kidney laterally. Calcifications in abscess

of a single calyx or of a major part of the renal pelvis can run a course of many
years. On the other hand, such blockage may sometimes progress rapidly and be
complete within 3—4 months, even without chemotherapy. This variation in the

course should be remembered in the roentgenologic evaluation of the effect of conservative treatment, particularly chemotherapy. It should also be borne in mind that renal tuberculosis does not heal with *restitutio ad integrum* but with some type of definite deformation of the renal pelvis (Figs. 131, 132; see also Figs. 116, 118).

A question of great importance formerly was, and to some extent still is, whether the disease is unilateral or bilateral in a given case of renal tuberculosis.

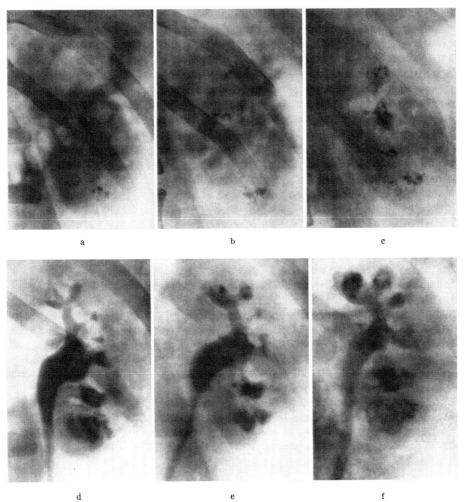

a   b   c

d   e   f

Fig. 132a—f. Bilateral tuberculosis refractory to chemo-therapy with progression in left kidney. Plain roentgeno-grams of left kidney. a Slight calcifications in caudal pole. b Five years later. Small irregular calcifications in middle of kidney and cranial pole. c Another three years later. Wide-spread calcifications in most pyramids. d, e, f Urography at corresponding intervals. Progressive changes with caseation, blocking and decreased function

Now that it is widely accepted that infection occurs on both sides simultaneously, but that it may develop in different ways in both kidneys, it appears that the conservative attitude adopted towards renal tuberculosis in recent years is well founded. This provides a possibility of following the course with repeated roentgen examinations for a long period. Such repeated control is, of course, necessary— especially for assessment of the effect of therapy, and then chemotherapy, in particular. As a rule, renal tuberculosis thus requires roentgen follow-up.

After nephrectomy the patient should be examined at long intervals mainly for any progression of tuberculous lesions known to exist in the remaining kidney. for the development of any lesions in the remaining kidney, for any vesical or ureteric obstruction causing ureteric stenosis with hydronephrosis and impairment of renal function as a consequence. It is, however, the use of chemotherapy that has made check examinations so necessary in renal tuberculosis. All check examinations should be performed in the same way as the original examination. Thus, if prolonged ureteric compression was necessary to demonstrate a cavity, it should also be applied on check examination.

Repeated examinations will show that untreated renal tuberculosis runs a variable course and that the process may remain stationary for several years or it may even regress with stricture and distortion of part of the renal pelvis. As mentioned, this must be recollected in the evaluation of the effect of therapy. In cases with chemotherapy scar formation at the pelviureteric junction or in the ureter may develop rapidly and cause complete obstruction. It may also be local in any part of the kidney pelvis (GAY 1949, CAVAZZANA & MENEGHINI 1956). Such occlusion may, as mentioned, occur rapidly after institution of therapy with tuberculostatics, and HANLEY (1955) stresses the importance of check radiography as early as a few months after the institution of conservative therapy to detect any obstruction of drainage of the renal pelvis.

Pathologically such occlusion is a sign of regression, but clinically it may sometimes be considered a progression. Scar formation and shrinkage may result in a stricture of a calyx or a branch of the renal pelvis. Behind this closure, however, the process may be florid (see Fig. 130). Such shrinkage may also be localized to the pelviureteric junction or to the ureterovesical junction and then give rise to hydronephrosis with all the risks thereby entailed.

In some cases the obstruction is not due to scar formation but to edema and specific granulation tissue and should not be mistaken for a sign of healing. Calcifications in the parenchyma demonstrable in plain radiograms, a sharp outline of the process in the nephrogram or no further changes in the rest of the kidney since the foregoing examination are signs of regression. Any regression of papillary ulceration will be manifested by sharper definition of the previously irregular outlines of the papillae against the renal pelvis and by a smoothing out of the ragged outline of filled cavities.

As mentioned, many urologists consider partial nephrectomy indicated in the treatment of well defined local lesions, usually located in the poles of the kidney. The appearance of the kidney in check roentgenograms after partial nephrectomy will be the same as after the same type of operation for other diseases. It has been described in chapter G.

III. General considerations on examination methods in renal tuberculosis

Much has been written about the relative merits of pyelography and urography in the diagnosis of ulcero-cavernous renal tuberculosis. Both methods are useful and often supplement one another. Pyelography requires catheterization, which is sometimes not possible owing to changes in the urinary bladder or to ureteric stricture, for example. On the other hand, a necessary condition for successful urography is that the kidney still possesses some functional capacity. Urography should, however, first be tried since experience has shown that both cystoscopy and catheterization of the ureter are attended by risks, particularly if these examinations must often be repeated for check examination, such as during chemotherapy. In addition the injection of contrast medium may cause pyelo-venous reflux with spread of tubercle bacilli into the blood stream. A well verified case has been described by LINDBOM (1944) in which such reflux caused fatal miliary tuberculosis. As mentioned, urography may also cause reflux but then it is, as a rule, a sinus reflux and extremely seldom a pyelovenous reflux (see chapter O). As pointed out previously, urography will not only permit establish-ment of the diagnosis but also yield the detailed information required by modern methods of treatment. The importance of urography was brought into sharp focus by OLLE OLSSON (1943) on the basis of a large tuberculosis series. It has been emphasized by CIBERT (1946), ERICSSON & LINDBOM (1950), FRIMANN-DAHL (1955) and others.

The roentgen examination methods used have varied with the advances made in the treatment of tuberculosis. The history of the treatment of renal tuber-culosis falls into three periods. The first period is characterized by Albarran's law: Unilateral renal tuberculosis = nephrectomy. For such cases retrograde pyelography was a good diagnostic method. Then came the period of conservative therapy, which required repeated check radiography. After systematic investiga-tions had confirmed the value of urography the procedure became the method of choice. Urography permits check examinations at fairly short intervals with hardly any risks and only slight inconvenience to the patient. (During such check examinations proper shielding for ray protection of the patient's gonads is of course imperative.)

The third period is characterized by a combination of conservative and surgical therapy namely partial nephrectomy or cavernostomy in association with con-servative medical treatment. This type of treatment requires knowledge of the extent of the process in the actual parenchyma. Renal angiography, particularly the nephrogram, yields valuable information on this point and is therefore now an important diagnostic method in renal tuberculosis.

J. Renal, pelvic and ureteric tumours

I. Kidney tumours

Renal tumours offer many diagnostic and differential diagnostic problems frequently requiring mobilization of all diagnostic methods available. In the examination renal angiography plays an ever-increasing rôle because it yields information on the actual renal parenchyma, and sometimes also demonstrates biologically important characteristics of the tumour.

Renal tumours may be malignant or benign.

The predominant type of malignant renal tumours in adults is different from that in children. The types of tumour occurring in adults are described in the literature under various names such as hypernephroma, nephroma, Grawitz' tumour, renal sarcoma, renal carcinoma etc. Patho-anatomically the commonest malignant tumour is renal adenocarcinoma, which RICHES, GRIFFITHS and THACK-RAY (1951) found to represent 75 per cent of all tumours of the kidney, renal pelvis and ureter in a series of 2,314 tumours. The incorrect name hypernephroma is being superseded by the more neutral term nephroma, but it is becoming the rule to designate the tumour according to its cell type as renal carcinoma.

The commonest type of tumour in children is the embryoma or nephroblastoma, also known as WILMS' tumour. It represented 8% of the series referred to above.

Renal tumours can be diagnosed by different roentgen-diagnostic methods, particularly plain roentgenography, urography or pyelography. The main purpose of roentgen examination is to demonstrate the presence of a tumour and, if a space occupying lesion can be shown, to contribute to the differential diagnosis, and if plain roentgenograms and pyelograms show no signs of a pathologic condition in a patient in whom tumour is nevertheless suspected, to demonstrate or exclude the possibility of such a growth by other roentgen-diagnostic methods.

1. Renal carcinoma

The tumour can vary considerably in size and it may be well defined or show signs of invasion. Sometimes it may infiltrate the entire kidney including the renal pelvis and encroach upon neighbouring tissues. The tumour may often show signs of previous haemorrhages and different sized necrotic foci with cystic formations as a consequence. In some cases only small parts of the tumour show such cysts, while in others—though seldom—the entire kidney may be converted into a cyst or cysts with specific tumour tissue occurring only in the form of a protrusion in the wall of the cystic formation.

All roentgen-diagnostic methods may be used in the diagnosis and differential-diagnosis of renal tumours.

a) Plain roentgenography

A small tumour situated deep in the renal parenchyma need not cause any change in the size or shape of the kidney. If it is situated near the surface of the kidney, it might cause a small bulge in its outline, often seen only in tangential projections. Such a bulge may resemble a persistent fetal lobation, for example. A tumour situated in a hilar lip, may make the latter appear somewhat thicker than usual, a change which cannot always be classified as clearly pathologic owing to the wide normal variation in the anatomy of the kidney, particularly of the lower hilar lip. In our material of verified tumours some 5% produced no sign of a pathologic condition in the plain roentgenograms.

A relatively large tumour will produce a distinct local enlargement of one of the poles of the kidney, for example. The tumour may be round, oval, or lobulated but nevertheless well defined, or it may be well outlined in one part and diffuse in another. Large tumours sometimes infiltrate the entire kidney, and then the kidney is seen as a nodose mass.

The tumour may assume considerable proportions and compress adjacent organs. The liver may, for example, appear as a cap over the tumour and the diaphragm may be displaced upwardly and its mobility may be reduced. We have seen such a tumour weighing 3.4 kg, which had been regarded as inoperable at another hospital after explorative operation, but was successfully removed in our hospital.

The kidney may be displaced in cranio-caudal and medio-lateral direction by the tumour or rotated around different axes. A large tumour in the upper pole of the kidney will often tilt the kidney. A tumour situated dorso-medially to the kidney will rotate the latter in such a way that the hilum will face anteriorly.

A renal tumour may also cause a generalized increase in the volume of the kidney. The kidney becomes plump and large, but is of otherwise normal shape and well outlined. We have found such generalized enlargement in some 15% of our cases of tumour.

Renal carcinoma, regardless of size, sometimes contains calcifications—in 10—15 per cent of our cases (Fig. 133). They vary widely in number, appearance and size, from punctate calcifications to calcium skeletons in the entire tumour. In 50 out of 67 cases of renal mass lesion seen in roentgenograms of varying quality ETTINGER & ELKIN (1954) recognized the mass in 48 cases because of the changed outline of the kidney, and in 2 because of calcifications. In addition to the irregular central calcifications of the tumour, crescent shaped calcifications of the type occurring in cysts or tuberculous cavities are sometimes seen in minor or major parts oft he periphery. The calcifications in the renal tumour are sometimes characteristic, but they may also be non-characteristic and not distinguishable from other calcifications in the renal parenchyma and the renal pelvis.

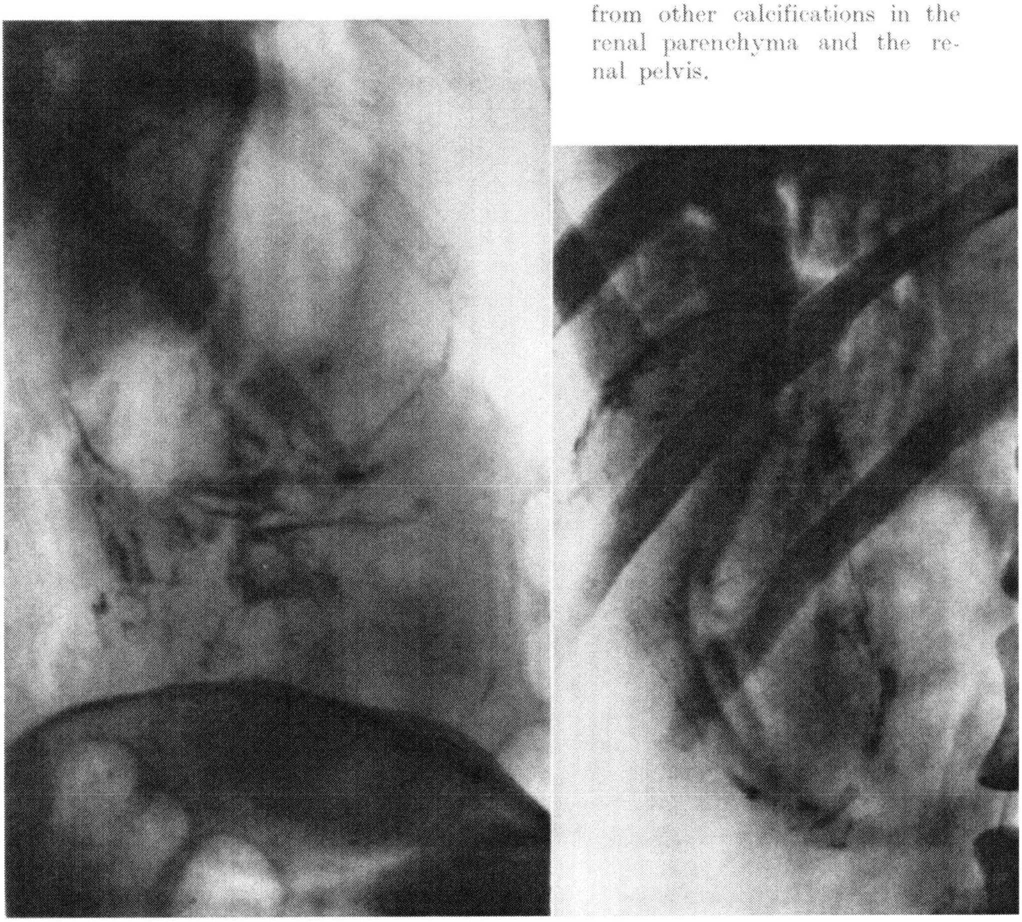

a   b

Fig. 133 a—d. Calcification in renal carcinoma. a, b and c Different types of combined peripheral and central calcifications indicatory of solid tumours. a and b Practically pathognomonic of renal carcinoma

The finding of a renal mass is often accidental in association with other examinations, such as of the gallbladder, particularly if the examiner has made it a rule to pay attention to the appearance of the right kidney, which is included in survey films of the gallbladder.

If the kidney outline is difficult to demonstrate, tomography, possibly combined with retroperitoneal pneumography, may sometimes be useful. This method in the diagnosis of renal tumour (COCCHI 1957) is, in my experience, however, of very limited value.

The changes seen already in plain roentgenograms are sometimes sufficient to permit a diagnosis of renal carcinoma, particularly if the tumour is large and irregular and/or if it contains characteristic calcifications.

On occasion, a large renal carcinoma may encroach directly upon and destroy parts of the skeleton. One or more metastatic foci are not infrequently seen in skeletal parts included in plain roentgenograms of the urinary tract. Such changes in combination with the finding of a space-occupying growth in the kidney permit a diagnosis of tumour. If a space-occupying lesion has been demonstrated in a kidney, we always examine the chest, particularly because the demonstration of metastases there will make the diagnosis of tumour firm.

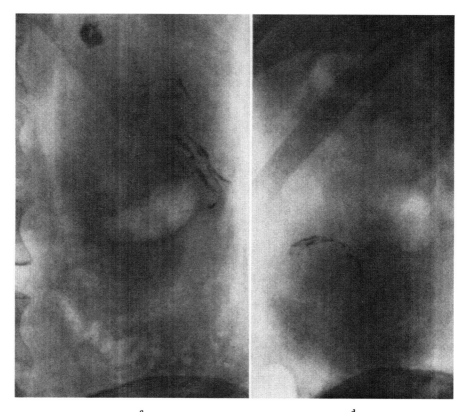

c   d

Fig. 133c and d. d Calcification in tumour periphery not indicative of solid tumour, calcifications of this type also being seen in simple cysts

Large tumours can encroach upon the diaphragm and give rise to metastases in the pleura, demonstrable by the presence of fluid in the corresponding pleural cavity.

It is a well-known fact that on occasion lung changes of the type multiple metastases disappear entirely after nephrectomy. Such cases have been described by BUMPUS (1928), BEER (1937), MANN (1948), ARCOMANO, BARNETT & BOTTONE (1958), KESSEL (1959). The metastases had not been verified pathologically. In this connexion it may be convenient to call attention to a case published by ANDRESEN (1936) from our department. Roentgen examination of the chest of a man, aged 43, revealed changes suggestive of metastases. On examination of the kidneys a space-occupying, well defined lesion was found in one kidney. Renal carcinoma with lung metastases was assumed. The lung changes, however, diminished and operation on the kidney mass was decided upon. It disclosed a benign cyst!

A case has been described by LJUNGGREN, HOLM, KARTH & POMPEIUS (1959) in which histologically verified widespread bilateral pulmonary metastases disappeared completely *before* nephrectomy, which was done afterwards and disclosed a renal carcinoma.

b) Urography and pyelography

With the use of an ordinary dose of contrast medium in urography more than half of our patients showed ordinary excretion permitting detailed study of the morphology of the renal pelvis after ureteric compression. In a further number of cases excretion was impaired but nevertheless sufficient to study the anatomy of the kidney pelvis. Only in about 10 per cent of our cases of malignant renal

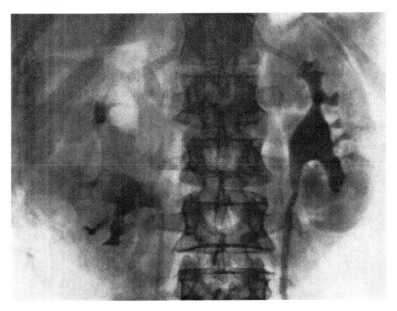

Fig. 134. Renal carcinoma, definite diagnosis possible at urography. Right kidney pelvis irregularly enlarged, contrast excretion diminished, kidney pelvis wall infiltrated

tumour was no excretion of contrast medium demonstrable. On the other hand, in most of these cases considerable changes were demonstrable already in the plain films.

Parts of the renal parenchyma not involved by the tumour will often show a somewhat increased density on ordinary urography, while those parts harbouring a tumour will retain their original density. This difference in density between normal and changed parts of the kidney can be enhanced by the modification of the method with a much larger dose of contrast medium known as nephrourography (see chapter on Urography).

Both retrograde pyelography and morphologic urography will show deformation of the renal pelvis by a space-occupying growth (see Figs. 134—136, 138—144, 147). If the tumour is small and near the surface of the kidney, the deformation might be only slight and consist of a flattening or dislocation of a single calyx. In central tumours the change may consist essentially of a separation of the stems of the calyces, while if the tumour is larger, the calyces may be severely compressed and, if the tumour is very large, the renal pelvis may assume a grotesque shape with extension or shortening by considerable compression of its branches. A single expanding process is capable of producing all types of deformations in different combinations depending on the direction of the pressure the expanding growth

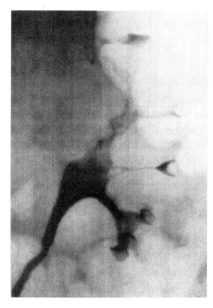

Fig. 135a

exerts in relation to the direction of the branches. The tumour may shorten a calyx stem and cause a flattening of the calyx itself if the tumour exerts its pressure in the longitudinal direction of the calyx. A nearby calyx perpendicular to the direction of pressure of the same tumour may be elongated and compressed, for example. Rotation of the kidney also produces typical changes in the shape of the renal pelvis. A tumour situated in the lower pole of the kidney, particularly in its medial part, will press against the ureter and displace it. Compression of the ureter may cause a dilatation of the renal pelvis. This dilatation deserves a few comments. The deformation of the renal pelvis by a tumor producing only a slight compression may be masked entirely if the renal pelvis is dilated. Therefore, in tumour-suspected cases with a dilatation of the renal pelvis, it is most important to take films from different angles and to use a suitable concentration of the contrast medium. This can be secured in retrograde pyelography with the

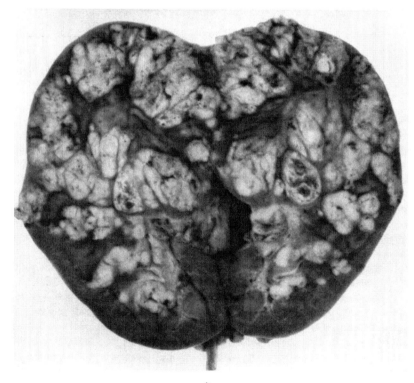

b

Fig. 135a and b. Renal carcinoma infiltrating kidney pelvis. a Pyelography. b Operative specimen

injection of only a small amount of contrast medium or by allowing some of the contrast medium injected to flow back through the catheter. Desired concentration of the contrast medium in the renal pelvis can be achieved in urography by taking the films early during the excretion or after release of ureteric compression.

The deformation of the renal pelvis as seen in the pyelogram is due in part to the fixation of the kidney, which permits only a limited amount of movement. An expanding process in or beneath the kidney is prone to cause deformation of the kidney and the renal pelvis in an early stage because the kidney can only give way to a certain extent. In addition the intrapelvic pressure is ordinarily low and is easily overcome by a growth pressing upon the pelvis. This is conspicuous on comparison between clinical pyelograms and pyelograms of autopsy

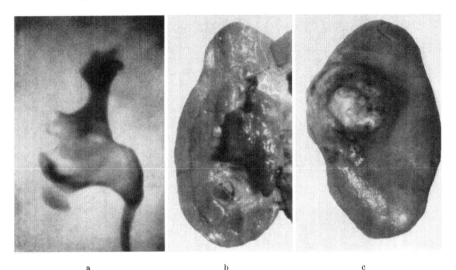

a   b   c

Fig. 136a—c. Small renal carcinoma infiltrating and with a large protuberance projecting into the kidney pelvis. a Pyelography. b and c Operative specimen

specimens, the deformation due to rotation and stretching being much less pronounced in the latter.

Certain features in the pyelogram argue distinctly for tumour and against other types of space-occupying process.

1. When, besides generalized deformation of the renal pelvis, a more local inward bulge is seen due to an irregularly bulgent shape of the space-occupying lesion.

2. Encroachment of the lesion onto the wall or into the lumen of the renal pelvis. In the former case single calyces or large parts of the renal pelvis may be irregularly narrow and their wall rigid, as a sign of invasion, by a malignant tumour, of the wall of the renal pelvis (Figs. 134, 135; see also Fig. 139). In the latter case a more or less irregular filling defect is seen in the renal pelvis (Fig. 136). These defects resemble those produced by papilloma of the renal pelvis or by radiolucent stones. Such a defect in a patient with a space-occupying lesion therefore does not necessarily mean that the lesion is a tumour encroaching upon the renal pelvis. Stones, for instance, may be co-existent with any type of space-occupying parenchymal lesion. The filling defect may also be due to a blood clot.

3. Sometimes, though rarely, both retrograde pyelography and urography will show reflux of contrast medium in pathologic vessels belonging to a tumour or in the outer layer of a tumour, owing to distension of a calyx into the tumour capsule (OLLE OLSSON 1948) (see Fig. 219).

c) Incidence of renal pelvic deformity

Most tumours produce a more or less characteristic deformity of the renal pelvis.
Sometimes the deformity is very slight. The demonstration of the changes in the
renal pelvis depends to a certain extent on the original shape of the renal pelvis.

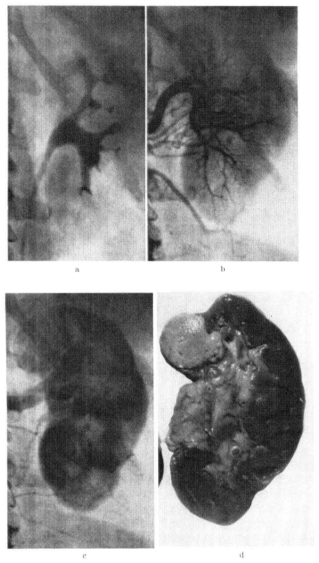

Fig. 137 a—d. Renal carcinoma not detectable without angiography. a Urography. No definite changes. b and
c Renal angiography, arterial and nephrographic phases. Small renal carcinoma with pathologic vessels in
medial part of cranial pole. d Operative specimen

If it has well formed branches, even a slight dislocation will be more conspicuous
than if the renal pelvis has a large confluence and short calyces (OLLE OLSSON
1943).

It is sometimes claimed that no deformity of the renal pelvis may be demonstrable despite changes in the outline of the kidney having been seen in the plain
roentgenogram. Two such cases have been described by ETTINGER & ELKIN (1954).

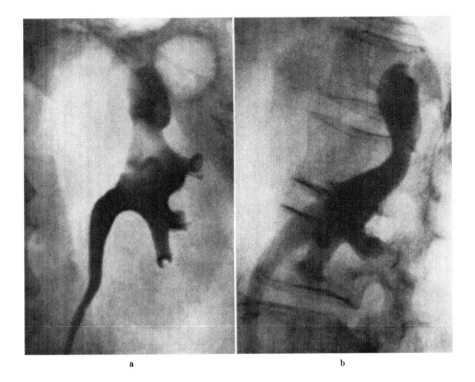

a   b

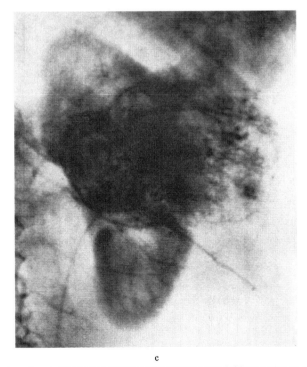

c

Fig. 138a—c. Renal carcinoma. Renal angiography gives much more detailed information on tumour than pyelography. a and b Pyelography. c Renal angiography

Cases have also been described in the literature as "hypernephroma too early to diagnose". Accompanying illustrations, however, show that the examinations were not properly performed and were therefore inconclusive. It is obvious that

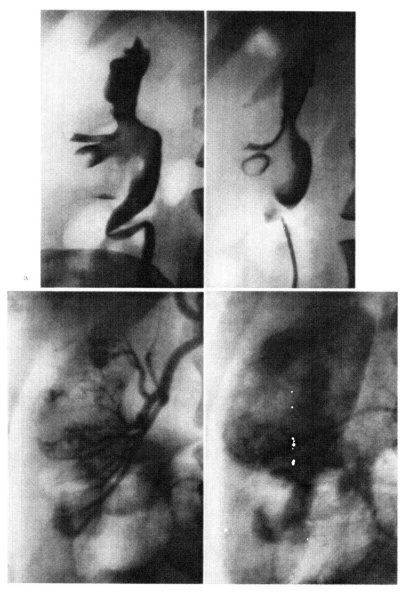

Fig. 139a and b. Renal carcinoma. a Pyelography. Tumour infiltrating kidney pelvis. b Renal angiography. Arterial and nephrographic phase. Well defined tumour, rich in pathologic vessels

the demonstration of changes in the shape of the renal pelvis depends largely on the examination technique. If the technique is slipshod, or standardized without necessary variation in examination technique, urography and pyelography will miss many changes. Only an adaptable technique with suitable projections will demonstrate the deformation to its full extent.

However, cases are on record in which careful and complete examination and check examinations showed no signs of tumour in plain roentgenograms or complete urography or pyelography, but in which further examination by renal angiography (see below) gave the diagnosis (LÖFGREN, OLHAGEN 1954) (Fig. 137).

Morphologic changes in the renal pelvis due to a space-occupying lesion may be studied by pyelography or urography. It is sometimes advisable to supplement urography by retrograde pyelography by which it might be easier to secure suitable projections, particularly true lateral projections. In addition, retrograde pyelography permits fine adjustment of the concentration of contrast medium for special purposes. Urography, on the other hand, has the advantage that it shows the functional capacity of the kidney. Another advantage of urography is that nephrography and nephrotomography, if desired, can be performed during the same session and contribute to the diagnosis or differential diagnosis.

d) Renal angiography

In the presence of a large richly vascularized tumour the renal artery on the side involved by the tumour is usually wider than ordinarily. The main artery and its branches are prone to be displaced in various ways by the expanding process. If the tumour is very large, the lumbar aorta may be displaced laterally. Sometimes fine, stretched vessels form a thin ring about a rounded, well defined tumour.

The region occupied by the tumour usually shows changes in the pattern of the vessels, which run an irregular course and vary abruptly in width. Numerous fine or markedly irregular tortuous vessels with aneurysm-like dilatations or irregularly out-lined accumulations of contrast medium (so-called pooling or laking) are common

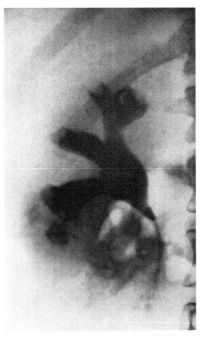

Fig. 140 a

findings. The contrast medium frequently passes rapidly into the veins via arteriovenousf istulae within the tumour. Such fistulae, which were known long before angiography, are capable of producing the same clinical symptoms as large arteriovenous aneurysms. The polycythaemia frequently seen in renal carcinoma has been ascribed to this direct shunting from the artery to the vein (Figs. 137—144; see also Fig. 149).

WOODRUFF, CHALEK, OTTOMAN & WILK (1956) claim that less than one third of all renal tumours will not show pathologic vessels. EDSMAN (1957) found pathologic vessels in 75 of 80 cases of malignant renal tumours. Of the 5 without pathologic vessels, in 3 the nephrogram showed the growth to be a solid tumour of irregular outline against the renal parenchyma. One case showed no pathologic vessels and no accumulation of contrast medium in the nephrogram and was therefore diagnosed as a cyst. The fifth case was a very small tumour described as coffee-bean sized, situated cortically and accidentally found at operation on the kidney.

As a rule, the pathologic vascular pattern is best seen in the arterial phase. In the nephrographic phase the density of normal parenchyma is usually high.

Within the area occupied by the tumour patches of low density may be seen alongside irregular areas of increased density. On occasion the tumor may receive a scanty blood supply from capsular arteries only (see Fig. 143).

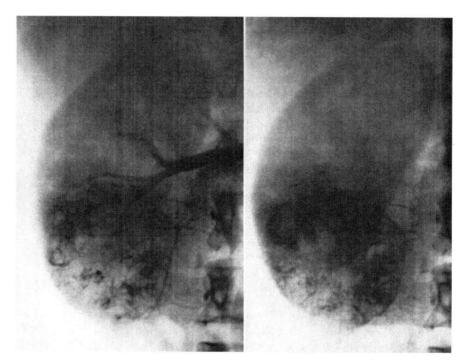

Fig. 140 b

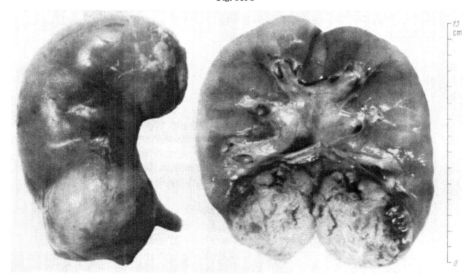

Fig. 140 c. Legend see Fig. 141

BILLING & LINDGREN (1944) described the appearance of the arteriogram on the basis of post mortem angiography and patho-anatomic examination of 14 kidneys with renal carcinoma. The appearance of the arterial tree differed markedly from the normal pattern, and the branches anastomosed richly. Otherwise normal branches of the renal artery terminated in aneurysm-like dilatations giving off several pathologic twigs. The widest pathologic vessels were barely 4 mm in diameter. The irregular caliber and course of the vessels is due to the fact that pathologic vessels have no elastic lamellae, which are always present in dislocated but otherwise normal vessels.

Renal carcinoma is prone to become necrotic partly because of arterial thrombosis. This has been studied from a patho-anatomic point of view by BARTLEY & HULTQUIST (1950), who found fibrosis and other regressive changes. Vessels are never seen within the necrotic parts. This thus implies that some carcinomas are very poor in vessels and have no pathologic vessels at all. In autopsy material LASSER & STAUBITZ (1957) found arterial thrombosis to be capable of preventing the passage of contrast medium to a tumour.

Other types of malignant tumours show essentially the same characteristics as renal carcinoma (see Fig. 153 a).

Avascular tumours can offer differential diagnostic difficulties because the most characteristic feature *i.e.* pathologic vessels, is missing (ABOULKER 1955, OLLE OLSSON 1956, MACQUET, VANDENDORP, LEMAITRE & DU BOIS 1957) (Figs. 147, 148). LINDBLOM & SELDINGER (1955) described huge avascular malignant renal tumours in 3 of their 16 cases. Some authors claim that renal angiography is a less reliable method for demonstrating renal tumour because of their frequently poor vascularization. This is incompatible with our experience. We have found that pathologic vessels are common, that even in the presence of massive necrosis part of the tumour shows pathologic vessels, and that even a poorly vascularized tumour will never produce angiographic changes of the type that is most characteristic of cyst (see below). Even small tumours of clinical significance have pathologic vessels, and in these cases renal angiography is sometimes the only diagnostic method capable of yielding information (see Fig. 137).

The angiographic findings will, of course, vary largely with the technique used. EDSMAN points out that, as a rule, pathologic vessels are observed only in the arterial and in the early nephrographic phase and this phase thus must be well represented in the angiographic series. In addition, the dose of contrast medium used must be of suitable size and concentration to secure a good filling of the arteries and suitable density of the nephrogram. Most important, however, is the use of a selective angiographic technique avoiding superimposition of irrelevant vessels. *A good technique, i.e. good selectivity and timing, is necessary for full utilization of the possibilities of angiography to diagnose malignant renal tumours.*

Perusal of the literature and the descriptions of accompanying illustrations will show that the technique employed often leaves much to be desired. One might

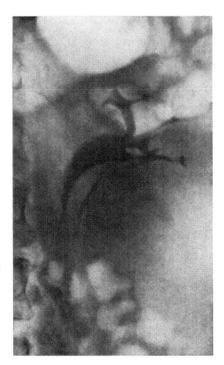

Fig. 141 a

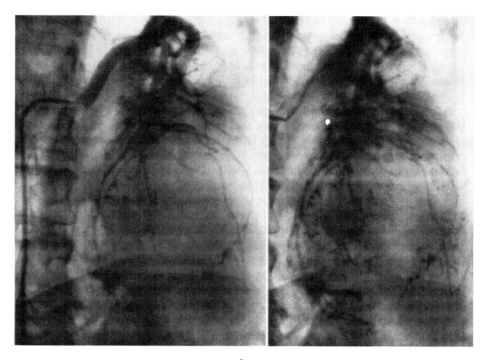

b

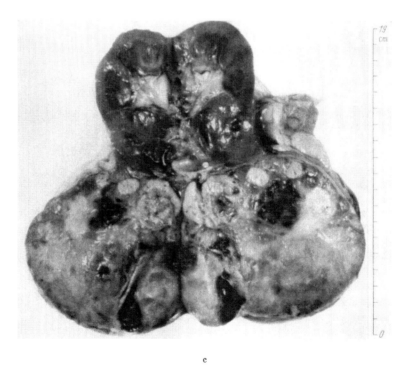

c

Fig. 140 a—c and 141 a—c. Urography shows displacement and deformity of kidney pelvis indicative of space-occupying lesion but does not show whether it is a tumour or simple cyst. a Urography. b Renal angiography. Well defined tumour with pathologic vessels—renal carcinoma. c Operative specimen

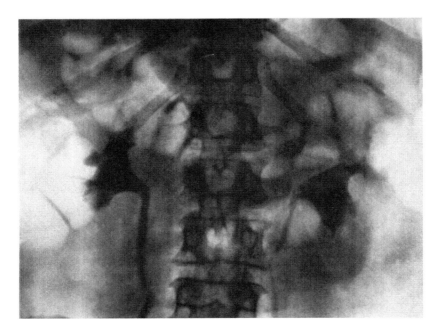

a

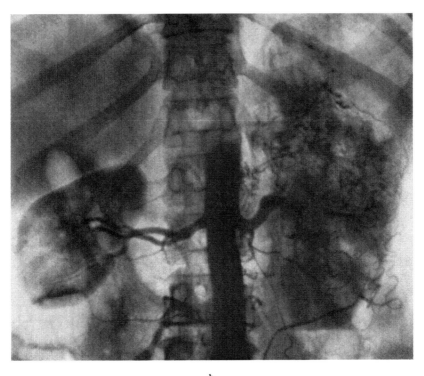

b

Fig. 142a—d. a Urography. Space-occupying lesion upper part, left kidney. b—c Renal angiography. Huge tumour with pathologic vessels—renal carcinoma. b Arterial phase

12*

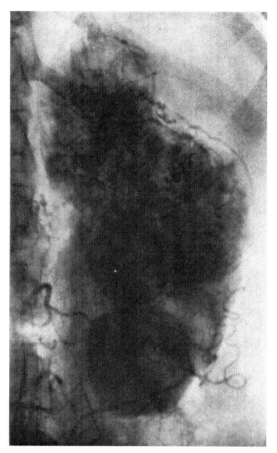

Fig. 142 c.
Nephrographic phase

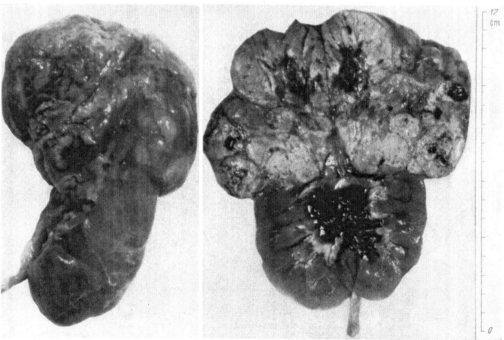

Fig. 142 d. Operative specimen

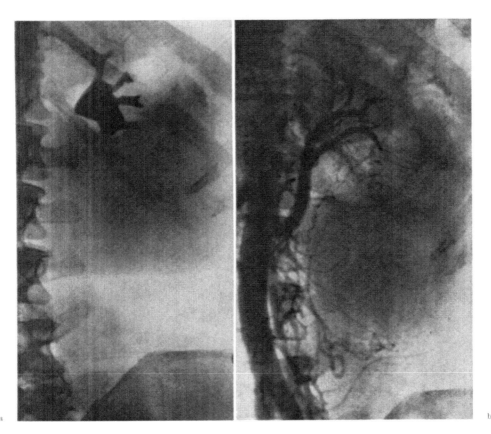

Fig. 143a and b. Renal carcinoma with unusual angiogram. a Urography. Huge space-occupying lesion in caudal part of the kidney with displacement and slight deformity of kidney pelvis. Good excretion of contrast medium. b Renal angiography. Displacement of aorta and main renal arteries. Tumour outlined by capsular arteries forming pathologic vessels in tumour periphery

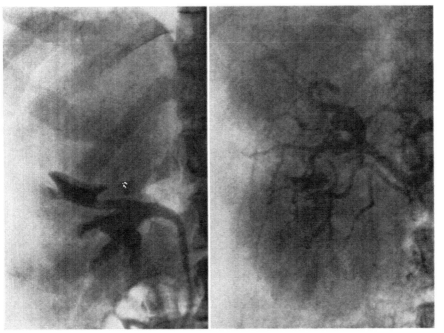

Fig. 144a and b. a Urography. b Renal angiography. Intrarenal branches widened with fusiform aneurysms. Pathologic vessels in cranial pole—renal carcinoma

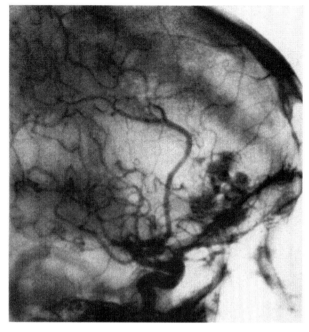

a

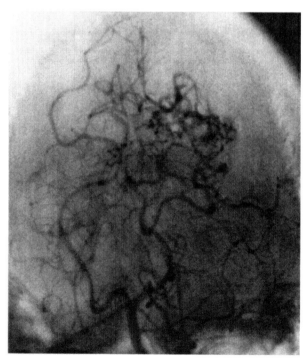

b

Fig. 145a and b. Richly vascularized metastases. Cerebral metastases from renal carcinoma diagnosed by angiography. a Carotid angiography shows one tumour in frontal lobe. b Vertebral angiography shows one tumour in occipital lobe

even go so far as to say that many of the examinations referred to in the literature are not worthy of the name renal angiography. Often they do not represent
a roentgen examination but simply a roentgenogram and often a very inconclusive
one. In my opinion, this is the most important reason why many authors under-
estimate the value of renal angiography in the diagnosis of tumours. It should
therefore be stressed once more that the value of renal angiography depends on
the technique employed. In other words, full utilization of the possibilities of

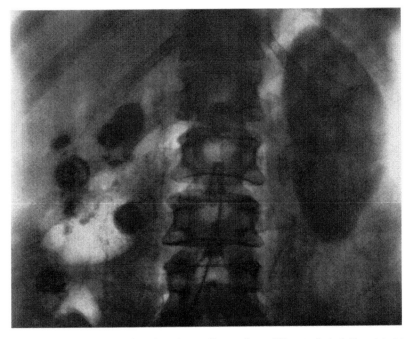

Fig. 146. Local recurrence of operated renal carcinoma. Tumour tissue richly vascularized, like original tumour.
(Courtesy of Dr. HOLM)

angiography requires that the examiner is really familiar with all types of angiography.

Remote metastatic growths in the brain, for example, have the same characteristics (Fig. 145). Angiography sometimes shows metastases close to the kidney
or local recurrences after nephrectomy with vascular patterns resembling those
seen in the primary tumour (HOLM 1957) (Fig. 146).

EVANS (1957) and co-workers (SOUTHWOOD & MARSHALL 1958, POST and
SOUTHWOOD 1959) used so-called nephrotomography in a large material, a method
which is sometimes informative in the diagnosis of tumour, since it shows accumulation of contrast medium within a tumour but no such accumulation in a cyst.
The method is simple, but the information it yields is by no means comparable to
that obtainable by renal angiography.

e) Phlebography

Renal carcinoma has a tendency to invade the renal vein. This tendency does
not indicate renal phlebography in all cases of renal tumour. Sometimes, however,

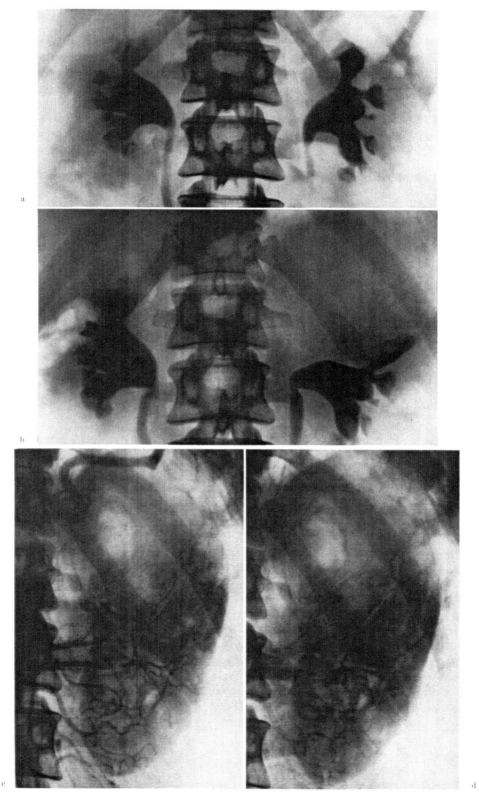

Fig. 147a—d. a Urography for other resons 4 years prior shows no pathologic changes. b Large space-occupying lesion left kidney. Differential diagnosis tumour—cyst not possible. c and d Renal angiography: Space-occupying lesion, definitely solid tumour. Though poorly vascularized the tumour shows some pathologic vessels

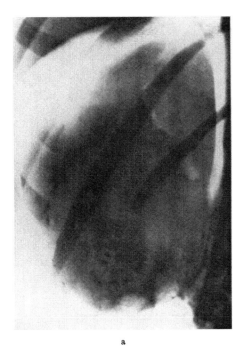

a

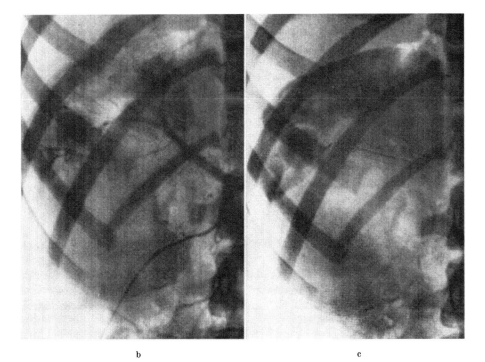

b   c

Fig. 148a—d. Renal carcinoma in 14 year old girl. a Retroperitoneal pneumography. Peripheral scattered calcifications in well defined round expansive lesion in caudal kidney pole. In urography dilatation of kidney pelvis and marked displacement upwards. b Renal angiography, arterial phase: Sparse vascularization in region of expansive lesion. This is definitely a solid tumour. c Nephrographic phase. No changes characteristic of cyst

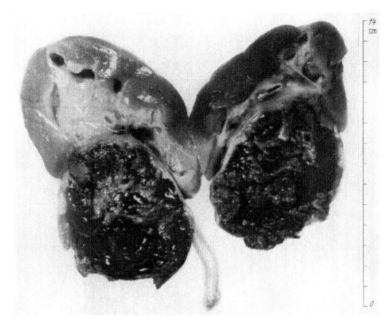

Fig. 148d.   Operative specimen

tumour growth and thrombosis are so massive as to cause stasis in the region
drained by the inferior caval vein. This may occasionally dominate the clinical
picture to such an extent as to be the indication for roentgen examination with
the discovery of the renal tumour as a consequence.

In complete obstruction of the inferior caval vein the normal filling of the vein
is missing and a filling is obtained of the usually numerous collateral veins instead.
If obstruction by thrombosis is not complete, the vein may be dilated distally,
but it may also be distended by the tumour masses. These appear as massive, well
circumscribed filling defects which may assume considerable dimensions. The
tumour may have grown along one of the walls of the vein and obstructed a fair
length of the lumen. Small changes will produce well defined filling defects caused
by protuberances encroaching upon the lumen of the renal vein or from the renal
vein into the caval vein (Fig. 149).

The actual tumour or metastases to the lymph nodes may displace or compress
the renal veins and/or the caval vein.

f) The growth of renal carcinoma

The growth of a renal tumour is demonstrable in cases that have for some
reason or other not been operated upon (see Fig. 147). It varies widely from case
to case. JOHNSSON (1946) described 4 cases examined during expectancy. In 1 case
the tumour grew only 3 cm in diameter in the course of 5 years but retained its round
shape and was well defined. Another 5 years later the patient was examined again
but not operated upon. The tumour had now broken through the capsule, invaded
contiguous tissue and metastasized to the lungs. In another case examination was
repeated after an interval of one year. An increase in diameter of only 0.5 cm was
demonstrable and the tumour was well defined. Two patients were re-examined after
8 and 5 months, respectively. No further roentgen changes could be demonstrated

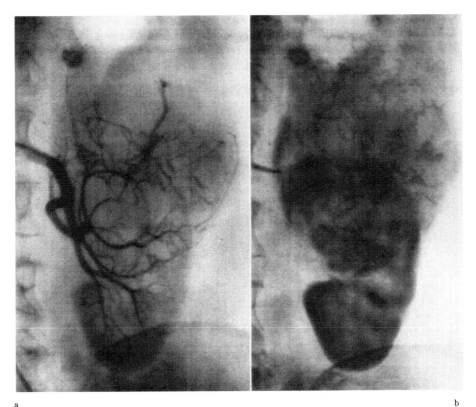

a   b

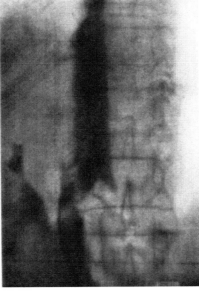

c

Fig. 149a—c. Patient, aged 64 years. Renal carcinoma with tumour invading renal vein and inferior caval vein. At urography slightly decreased concentration of contrast urine. Displacement of kidney pelvis. a and b Renal angiography: Large irregular, richly vascularized tumour. Displacement of arteries. Pathologic vessels. c Cavography. Left renal vein could not be catheterized: Defect in left part of caval vein at level of renal vein—tumour invading vein

between the two examinations. Many cases on the other hand, show a rapid progress. A short while ago we saw a case from another hospital where a renal carcinoma had been examined repeatedly without its nature having been detected. At the first examination the tumour was small and contrast excretion was adequate.

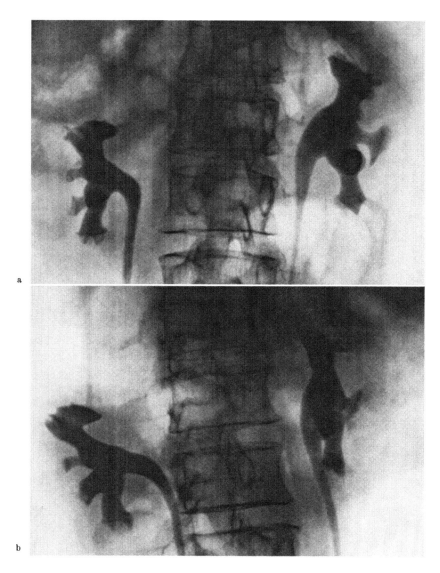

Fig. 150a—d. Liposarcoma in right kidney, simple cyst in left kidney. Urography: a and b Good excretion of contrast medium. Displacement of cranial calyces on right side caudally—expansive lesion in cranial pole. Displacement of middle and caudal calyces on left side—expansive lesion caudo-laterally. (See oblique projection.) Urography cannot reveal the nature of expansive processes

Two months later the growth had increased in size and the excretion of contrast medium was delayed. Another 6 months later the patient came to our hospital bnd then the tumor was very large and the kidney no longer functioning. These aases stress the fact that expectancy is not justified in the differential diagnosis cetween malignant renal tumours and benign lesions. A renal tumour may show

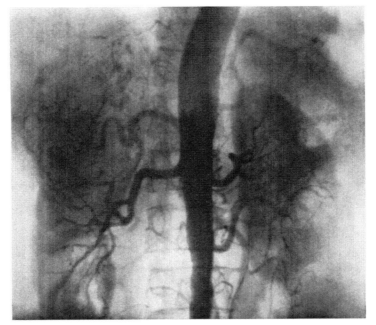

c

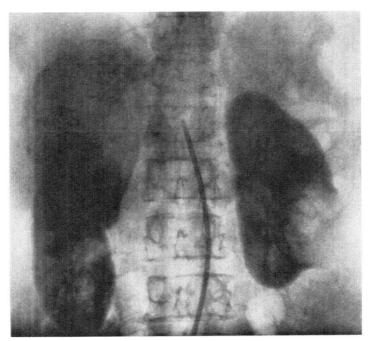

d

Fig. 150 c and d. Renal angiography: c Arterial phase. d Nephrographic phase. Right side large tumour with pathologic vessels. Left side typical cyst. Operative verification. (Courtesy of Dr. BRODÉN)

only very slow progression and be encapsulated for a long time. On the other hand when the tumour breaks through the capsule and appears in the roentgeno-

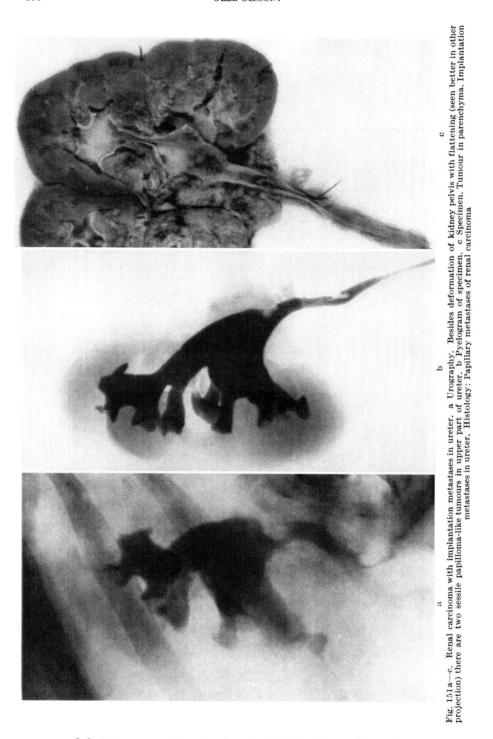

Fig. 151 a—c. Renal carcinoma with implantation metastases in ureter. a Urography. Besides deformation of kidney pelvis with flattening (seen better in other projection) there are two sessile papilloma-like tumours in upper part of ureter. b Pyelogram of specimen. c Specimen. Tumour in parenchyma. Implantation metastases in ureter. Histology: Papillary metastases of renal carcinoma

gram as a definite tumour, an invasion has started. The change that makes the differential diagnosis possible by expectancy thus means a worse situation for the patient.

Though regressive changes are so common in tumours I have observed a renal carcinoma to decrease in size in only one single instance.

g) Multiple tumours

Sometimes renal carcinoma is bilateral. BAILEY & YOUNGBLOOD (1950) described such a case and referred to 11 others from the literature. They stated that it is not possible to decide whether each tumour was primary or whether one was a solitary secondary growth.

Multiple dissimilar tumours sometimes occur in one and the same kidney. Most of the cases on record were, however, probably not dissimilar tumours but represented different patho-anatomic evaluation of different parts of one and the same tumour arising from the same mesenchymal tissue but differentiated to a varying extent in different parts of the tumour. Co-existence of malignant and benign tumours and of tumours of the renal parenchyma in association with tumour of the renal pelvis have also been described. A survey of cases of this type has been given by PENNISI, RUSSI & BUNTS (1957).

Coexistence of tumour and cyst is not uncommon (Fig. 150).

A patient is sometimes referred for roentgen examination for a tumour, which proves to be a metastatic growth. Particularly if a glandular mass is found in a lung hilum, the kidney should be suspected as an origin of primary tumour and the hilar lesions as metastases. Also skeletal and cerebral metastases should direct the examiner's attention to the kidneys as a possible source of a primary tumour. This also holds in cases of unexplained fever, particularly periodic fever and in polycythaemia. Metastatic growths from renal carcinoma are, as mentioned, often characteristic with large arterio-venous fistulae like those in many of the primary tumours. They are therefore well demonstrable by angiography. This applies to local metastases in lymph nodes and retroperitoneal tissue, lung metastases and cerebral metastases.

A renal carcinoma may, though rarely, metastasize to the ureter (Fig. 151) or the urinary bladder and produce symptoms simulating a bladder tumour.

Malignant tumours elsewhere can, though seldom, metastasize to the ureter or to the kidney. AGNEW (1958) reported a metastatic melanoma in a kidney.

2. Malignant renal tumours in children

Renal carcinoma is not strictly limited to adults. In the material of RICHES *et al.* referred to in the beginning the youngest patient was 11 years old. Cases of renal carcinoma in childhood have also been described by HEMPSTEAD, DOCKERTY, PRIESTLEY & LOGAN (1953) and BEATTIE (1954), for example. In their series the youngest patients were 8 and 7 years old respectively.

The commonest malignant renal tumour in childhood is, however, that usually known as Wilms' tumor after Wilms, who was the first to give a detailed description of this previously unknown tumour in 1899. The tumour is known under various names such as adenosarcoma, adenomyosarcoma, dysembryoma but it is usually called embryoma or nephroblastoma. Half of the cases occur in children between the ages of 2 and 4 years. Sometimes it is present already at birth. SALLER described such a case in which the new-born had not only such a tumour but also metastases and LATTIMER, MELICOW & USON (1958) reported nephrectomy of a 4-day old child. The tumour can be of roentgen-diagnostic interest during the prenatal period, tumours of this type often having been observed at autopsy of fetuses, and they are known to be a cause of dystocia.

Apart from the eyes, the kidneys are the commonest seat of tumours in children.

As pointed out by DEUTICKE (1931), for example, tumours of the embryonal type have been known to occur in several members of the same family.

The embryoma usually metastasizes to the liver and lungs but not to the skeleton. It might also spread to the other kidney. Then large space-occupying processes are seen in both kidneys. A case of this type has been described by AGERHOLM-CHRISTENSEN (1939) in an 8 month old child. True double-sidedness may also occur (CAMPBELL 1948) (see Fig. 152). In such cases it may not be possible to distinguish it roentgenologically from polycystic kidney (Fig. 152).

Since the tumour appears at such an early age the diagnosis is usually based on objective findings. Haematuria is rare, and the patients are usually referred for roentgen examination because of a palpable tumour.

a) Plain roentgenography

By the time the patient is referred for roentgen examination the tumour is, as a rule, large, irregular, and often not well outlined. Smaller well defined tumours

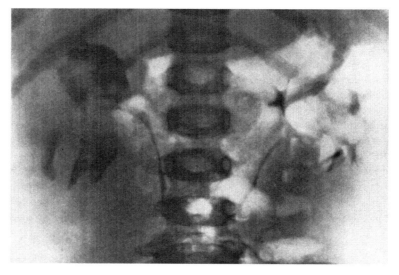

Fig. 152. Bilateral embryoblastoma in 18 month old girl. Urography: Good contrast excretion bilaterally. Large expansive lesions bilaterally. The pyelogenic changes are the same as in bilateral polycystic kidney. Operation with nephrectomy on right side showed embryosarcoma. Patho-anatomic diagnosis on both sides

are, however, also seen. The tumour often contains irregular calcifications. These calcifications may be limited to a small part of the tumour or may be scattered throughout the entire growth.

b) Urography and pyelography

Both urography and pyelography show deformation of essentially the same type as that seen in renal carcinoma in adults (Fig. 153).

In the differential-diagnosis particularly hydronephrosis and polycystic kidney are important, which may also occur in children, and extrarenal expanding processes such as an enlarged spleen. The most important lesion from a differential-diagnostic point of view, however, is another growth, namely sympathico-blastoma. If the growth contains calcifications, the differentiation between these two types of tumour is particularly difficult. In contrast to embryoma, sympathicoblastoma often metastasizes in a typical way to the skeleton.

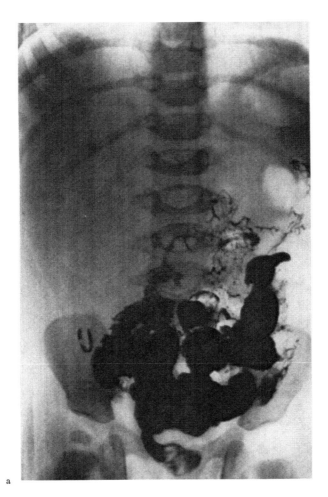

a

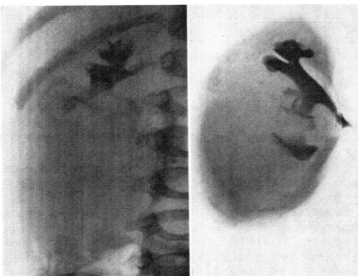

b   c

Fig. 153a—c. Embryoblastoma in 10 months old boy. a Plain roentgenogram. Right kidney large but well defined. Displacement of contrast-filled bowel to the left and downwards. b Urography: Good contrast excretion. Displacement and deformity of kidney pelvis by large tumor in caudal part. c Pyelogram of specimen

c) Renal angiography

Renal angiography of the few cases of embryoblastoma we have examined with this method shows essentially the same features as those of renal carcinoma (Fig. 154).

3. Benign renal tumours

Benign renal tumours of clinical interest are rare. As a rule, these tumours are small and are nearly always found accidentally on patho-anatomic examination of a kidney removed for some other reason or on routine pathologic examination of the kidneys at autopsy. The above mentioned material by RICHES *et al.* consisting of 2,314 cases of renal and ureteric tumours included only 12 benign tumours of the

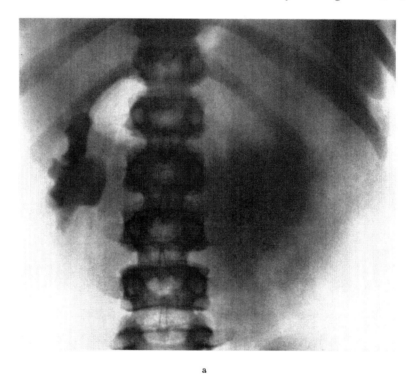

a

Fig. 154a—c. Embryoblastoma in 14 year old boy. a Urography: Right side normal. No contrast excretion on left side, where a large mass can be seen

renal parenchyma, namely 5 adenomas and 3 haemangiomas. In 1956 FOSTER reported that a perusal of the literature on all benign kidney tumours large enough to be of clinical significance revealed a total of 135, namely 57 adenomas, 24 lipomas, 22 myomas, 17 fibromas, 7 angiomas and 8 mixed tumours.

The majority of benign tumours of the renal parenchyma are thus adenomas. Small solitary cortical adenomas are common in arteriosclerotic kidneys (TWISS 1949), but they are of no roentgen-diagnostic interest. Like some fibromas, lipomas and mixed tumours, adenomas can be shown by plain roentgenography and urography or pyelography. The findings are the same as in a well outlined renal carcinoma (BAUER, MURRAY & HIRSCH 1958). In the angiogram the adenoma appears as an avascular tumour which cannot be distinguished from a well demarcated avascular renal carcinoma. It increases in size very slowly. MISHALANY & GILBERT (1957) described a case of probably ossified cortical adenoma which simulated hydatid cyst in the plain roentgenogram and in the pyelogram and which was therefore diagnosed as such. MEISEL (1954) described a case in which both kidneys were studded with small adenomas so that the pyelogram simulated that of a polycystic kidney.

Fibromas are usually very small but may sometimes be very large. Thus Foster (1956) described a case of a tumour in an 8 year old child in whom the tumour weighed 43 pounds, while the patient together with the tumour weighed 94 pounds.

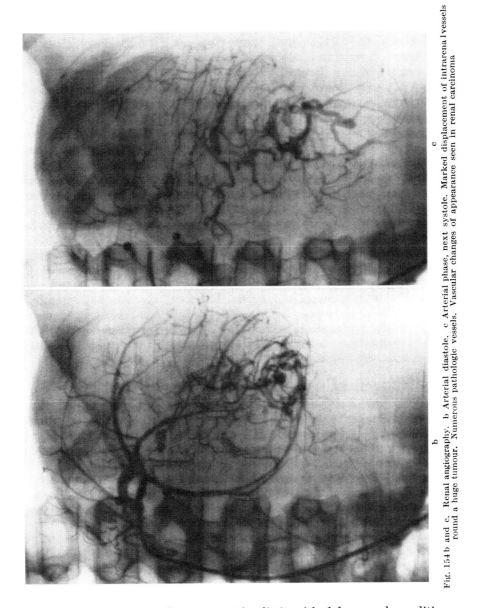

Fig. 154 b and c. Renal angiography. b Arterial diastole. c Arterial phase, next systole. Marked displacement of intrarenal vessels round a huge tumour. Numerous pathologic vessels. Vascular changes of appearance seen in renal carcinoma

The fairly uncommon lipoma must be distinguished from such conditions as replacement lipomatosis (see chapter U. 8). Lipomas are true tumours and often appear as mixed tumours, angiomyolipomas, so-called hamartomas, fibromyxolipomas etc. These tumours are often seen in association with tuberous sclerosis and may then be situated in the brain, for example, or in the heart or kidneys. They may be multiple and bilateral (BECK & HAMMOND 1957, TAYLOR & GENTERS 1958) and they often calcify. WEAVER & CARLQUIST (1957) described such a growth in a 12 year old girl. The tumour was twice as large as the actual kidney and had a circumscribed protuberance growing into the renal pelvis. The tumours sometimes become malignant and then they resemble renal carcinoma roentgenologically. On occasion it is possible to make a diagnosis of lipoma from the striking radiolucency of the expanding process. It has been seen in association with a pararenal lipoma, as described by BRODY & LIPSHUTZ (1955) who also give a detailed survey of the literature. In plain roentgenography these lipomatous tumours do not differ from any other expanding process, such as a circumscribed renal carcinoma. Only if the growth is very large and if it contains calcifications, as in tuberous sclerosis, or if it has a high fat content diminishing the density, can it be diagnosed as a lipoma.

A very rare renal tumour, which may assume a considerable size, is neurinoma, also known as schwannoma, neurilemmoma or neurofribroma (PHILLIPS & BAUMRUCKER 1955).

Haemangiomas are very rare. BELL (1938) reported that he found only one case of haemangioma in a total of 30,000 autopsies. They vary in dimension: they may be very minute or anything up to more than 1 dm in diameter. Haemangioma is usually cavernous, but it may also be capillary. It is sometimes bilateral and can become malignant. A survey of the cases on record in the literature has been made by WALLACH, SUTTON & CLAMAN (1959). The diagnosis is not specific. The reason why such tumours have not been diagnosed angiographically must be due mainly to their rarity.

In this connection mention might be made of the extremely rare cholesteatoma in the kidney, usually in a pyonephrotic renal pelvis. The renal parenchyma may, however, also be invaded. Cholesteatoma is associated with extensive leukoplakia.

A case of multiple eosinophilic granuloma with a well circumscribed expanding process in one kidney was described by AHLSTRÖM & WELIN (1943). The tumour was believed to be a granuloma in the kidney. Verification was not available at the time of publication. Later pathologic examination of the growth, however, has shown it to be a simple cyst.

4. Differential diagnosis of a space-occupying renal lesion

Expanding processes involving the kidney may be of varying origin. They may be due to changes in the actual kidney, or to pararenal or extrarenal processes. Splenomegaly, a conglomerate of lymph nodes, and various types of retroperitoneal tumours and abscess from spondylitis are examples of extrarenal processes capable of simulating a space-occupying process in the kidney. By such a process the kidney may be markedly dislocated or deformed. Urography, pyelography, retroperitoneal pneumography and angiography in a combination chosen according to conditions in a given case can always solve the problem and decide whether such an expanding process is extrarenal or not.

Processes with a pararenal position may be difficult to distinguish from expanding renal processes. In plain roentgenography and urography inflammatory pararenal processes may resemble renal tumours. Paranephritis often originates from a renal carbuncle, which is itself a space-occupying intrarenal lesion. Even without such expansiveness paranephritis may be so local as to simulate a space-occupying lesion in the kidney. Pararenal lipomas, solitary or multiple, can as a rule be readily identified. Pararenal sarcoma is often not well outlined against the kidney, but the margin of the kidney can be recognized in angiograms since the vessels are of normal appearance within the kidney, which is well defined in the nephrogram, while pathologic vessels are located outside the kidney. Adrenal tumours often stand out distinctly against the kidney, which is often deformed in a characteristic way by such tumours, i.e. with a flattened upper pole in which sometimes also an impression is made by the tumour, which in addition displaces the kidney caudally. Sometimes, however, the outline is less clear. Angiography

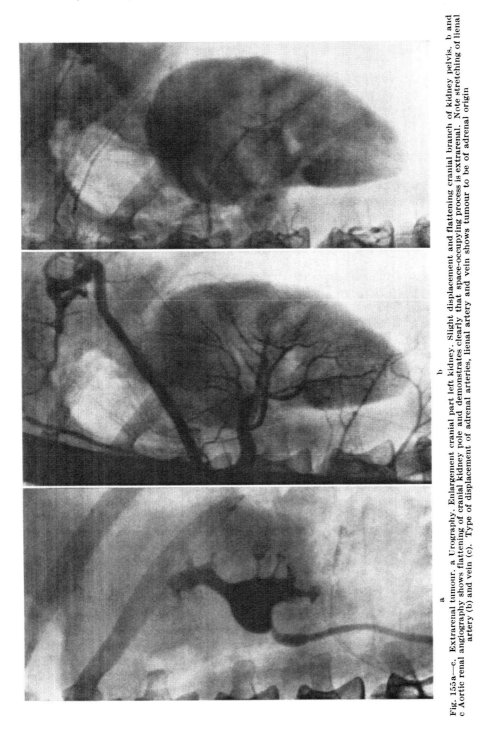

Fig. 155a—c. Extrarenal tumour. a Urography. Enlargement cranial part left kidney. Slight displacement and flattening cranial branch of kidney pelvis. b and c Aortic renal angiography shows flattening of cranial kidney pole and demonstrates clearly that space-occupying process is extrarenal. Note stretching of lienal artery (b) and vein (c). Type of displacement of adrenal arteries, lienal artery and vein shows tumour to be of adrenal origin

decides the diagnosis except in a few cases in which the patho-anatomic diagnosis is also doubtful (Fig. 155).

Intrarenal expanding processes may consist of tumours of different types, cysts, partial or total hydronephrosis, or inflammatory changes. All of these possibilities should be borne in mind in the evaluation of the roentgen findings. Experience has shown that this applies, above all, to the differentiation between a tumour and a large hydronephrotic kidney. It also holds if the upper pole of the kidney is enlarged. It may be due to hydronephrosis of one of the renal pelves in a double kidney or to hydrocalicosis. If no excretion is seen during urography, renal angiography will clarify the situation. If one branch of the renal pelvis is occluded and the rest of the pelvis dislocated, the possibility of an inflammatory process, particularly tuberculosis, must be considered. Irregular calcifications in the occluded part seen in plain roentgenograms often suggest the diagnosis.

The most common differential-diagnosis is that between renal carcinoma and simple renal cyst. Much space has been given to this differential-diagnosis in the literature. I once heard a prominent urologist state that differentiation is always possible by palpation. Such a statement must be rejected on the grounds that changes may be small and that a cyst might be embedded completely in renal parenchyma. It is widely believed that other clinical examination methods will permit a differential-diagnosis. Thus reference is made to the importance of haematuria, raised E.S.R., fever, possibly periodic fever, generalized symptoms of malignant disease etc. In the differentiation under discussion, however, these symptoms are of limited value in a given case. It must be borne in mind that the patients are often referred for roentgen-examination because of symptoms that might be due to renal carcinoma but that might also be explained by something else. In such a material a certain number of simple cysts must be expected. We have also seen renal cysts in patients referred for roentgen-examination because of raised E.S.R., periodic fever and other symptoms of malignancy. On the other hand, a space-occupying renal lesion may be discovered accidentally in a kidney that has produced no symptoms or signs, but which closer investigation shows to be a carcinoma.

It has also been stressed in recent years that certain laboratory studies are of significance in the diagnosis of renal cancer. Thus an increase in the alpha$_2$-globulin fraction in the electrophoretic pattern of the serum has been described as a sign of renal carcinoma. Judging from our experience, the diagnostic value of this method is small.

Many authors recommend surgical exploration for differentiation between cyst and renal tumor. Before deciding upon such an operation, however, the possibilities of making a differential roentgen-diagnosis should be considered. It is clear from the special chapter on renal carcinoma and on simple renal cysts that a differential diagnosis sometimes offers difficulties independently of the method used. The findings in these diseases are therefore discussed below.

a) Plain roentgenography

Tumours and cysts may closely resemble one another in both size and shape. Thus a round, well circumscribed space-occupying process may be due either to a cyst or a pseudo-encapsulated renal carcinoma. If the expanding process is irregular in outline, it argues for carcinoma. However, it should not be forgotten that on occasion cysts can be multiple and lie adjacent one another and produce a polycyclic border.

During expectancy both tumors and cysts may increase in size. If the outline becomes irregular during such expectancy, a tumor may be assumed. Unlike a tumour, a cyst may decrease in size or disappear entirely.

Peripheral calcifications may be seen in cysts and in tumours. Central calcifications which, of course, cannot occur in a cyst, are not uncommon in tumours. Occasionally the tumour may show characteristic calcifications in the form of a calcium skeleton pathognomonic of tumour.

On examination of plain roentgenograms of the kidneys attention must also be paid to the skeletal parts included in the films. If bone destruction is demonstrable, the space-occupying lesion in the kidney is a tumour. This also holds for other extra-renal metastases.

b) Pyelography and urography

Most pyelographic changes are common to both tumour and cyst. A tumour can, however, be diagnosed with certainty if it has infiltrated part of the wall of the renal pelvis or if a tumor protuberance has grown into the renal pelvis. A calculus or a blood clot should not, however, be taken for such a protuberance.

A tumour might interfere with the excretion of contrast urine during the examination. If the excretion is normal, it permits no decision as to whether the enlargement of the kidney is due to a tumour or cyst. If excretion is delayed or absent, it suggests a tumour.

c) Puncture

An expanding process can be punctured percutaneously. A cyst contains clear fluid. After aspiration of the fluid contents of the cyst or part of it, contrast medium can be injected and it can then be checked whether the contrast filled cyst occupies the entire region of the space-occupying process. If the cyst fluid is blood-stained, or if the wall of the cyst is uneven, or if the cyst does not correspond to the entire space-occupying lesion, a tumour must be suspected. On injection of contrast medium into a tumour a filling will be obtained of the interstitial spaces. Such a filling can be so irregular as to permit a diagnosis of tumour. But it might cause diagnostic difficulties if the contrast medium is injected into the normal renal parenchyma outside the wall of the cyst. Puncture is therefore decisive only if it produces positive signs of a cyst. (Cyst fluid should always be sent for patho-anatomic examination for tumour cells as an extra precaution.)

d) Renal angiography

Most tumours show pathologic vessels. The outline of the expanding process is also often irregular. A cyst will produce a region free of contrast medium with a sharp border against normal parenchyma. In the free periphery of the cyst no vessels are seen. If the cyst is surrounded by renal parenchyma, the diagnosis may be difficult and the cyst therefore not easy to distinguish from an avascular tumour. In such cases puncture should be resorted to. The frequency of cases requiring puncture will, however, decrease with improvement of the technique and experience. With reference to the chapter on the technique of renal angiography and to the description of the findings in renal angiography in tumour and in cysts it must be stressed that the value of angiography depends largely on the technical performance of the examination.

e) Metastasis

Sometimes the tumour has metastasized by the time the patient is referred for roentgen examination. As mentioned, those parts of the skeleton included in plain roentgenograms of the urinary tract must receive attention. For the same reason we always examine the chest in patients with a space-occupying lesion in a kidney. Lung metastases confirm the diagnosis of tumour. Owing to absence or neglect of symptoms renal carcinoma has often metastasized by the time the patient is examined.

To summarize, it may thus be stated that the following factors are of the greatest importance in differentiation between malignant tumour and benign cyst.

Irregular outline of the growth argues decidedly for tumour.

Characteristic tumor calcifications may occur.

Infiltration of or growth into the renal pelvis are signs of tumour.

Encroachment upon the skeleton or metastases are signs of tumour.

Severly impaired excretion of contrast medium as seen during urography argues for tumour.

Pathologic vessels in renal angiography are pathognomonic of tumour.

Failure of puncture to aspirate fluid suggests tumour.

If these factors—with reservations given above—are considered in the order given in the various examinations, differentiation between tumour and cyst will nearly always be possible. Establishment of a differential diagnosis should very seldom require surgical exploration.

II. Tumours of the renal pelvis and the ureter

In the collection of RICHES *et al.* of 2,314 tumours of the kidney and ureter, 336 were tumours of the renal pelvis and ureter. Twenty-one were primary tumours of the ureter.

1. Tumours of the renal pelvis

Of the 315 tumors of the renal pelvis, 241 were malignant, the majority transitional cell papillary carcinoma, and less than half as many were squamous cell carcinoma. The youngest patient was 9 years old. Simple papillomas of the renal pelvis were found in 24 cases. Almost one third of the cases of squamous cell carcinoma had renal calculi. This type of tumour is often seen in patients with chronic inflammatory changes and sometimes with co-existent leukoplakia in some parts of the mucosa of the renal pelvis. An important observation of roentgendiagnostic interest is also that the operable cases of transitional cell papillary carcinoma involve the ureter and/or bladder or both in some 50 per cent of all cases. STRICKER (1926 cit. MACLEAN & FOWLER) found that in 47% of 175 cases of papillomatous neoplasms of the renal pelvis neoplasm were also present in the ureter and urinary bladder. Simultaneous involvement of the renal pelvis, ureter and urinary bladder is liable to occur and is characteristic of all the papillary tumours. If this type of tumour is suspected, it is thus necessary to investigate the entire urinary tract. Of 26 cases of primary carcinoma of the ureter WHITLOCK, MCDONALD and COOK (1955) found one third of the tumours of the ureter to be situated in the lower third. In half of these cases where the tumour occupied the lower ureter, a portion of the tumor could be seen protruding from the ureteric orifice at the time of cystoscopic examination. Tumours of the bladder prior to or after operation for a primary carcinoma of the ureter were seen in 14 out of 33 cases and multiple ureteric tumours in 17.

Papillary tumours are often multiple with several tumours in the renal pelvis and tumours may, as mentioned, also occur in the ureter and/or in the urinary bladder. Carcinogenic substances excreted by the kidneys can cause tumour growth at various sites, but tumours lower in the urinary tract may also have been implanted there by material shed from growths higher up.

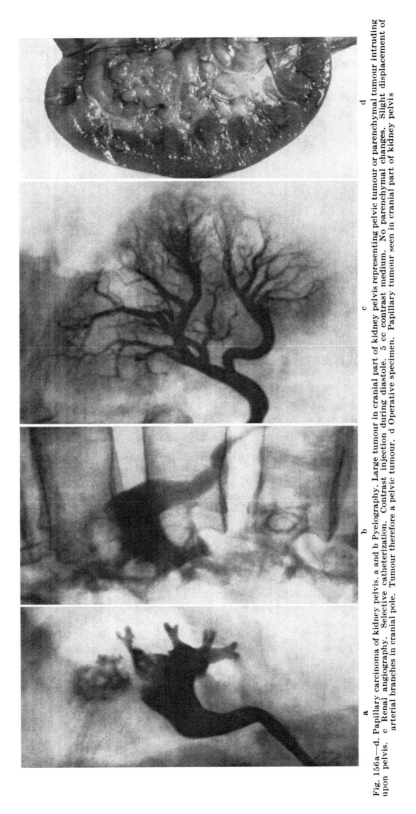

Fig. 156a—d. Papillary carcinoma of kidney pelvis. a and b Pyelography. Large tumour in cranial part of kidney pelvis. c Renal angiography. Selective catheterization. Contrast injection during diastole. 5 cc contrast medium. Tumour therefore a pelvic tumour. d Operative specimen. Papillary tumour seen in cranial part of kidney pelvis representing pelvic tumour or parenchymal tumour intruding upon pelvis. No parenchymal changes. Slight displacement of arterial branches in cranial pole.

Another type of tumour of the renal pelvis should also be mentioned. PLAUT (1929) described a case of stone-producing tumour of the renal pelvis. Since then other cases of this type have been described, the latest by ARCADI (1956) and BRØNDUM NIELSEN (1957). These tumours may be benign or malignant. They

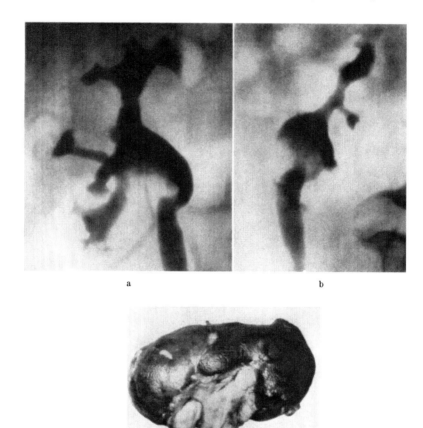

a   b

c

Fig. 157a—c. Malignant papilloma of kidney pelvis. a and b Pyelography. Irregular broad-based malignant tumour of kidney pelvis. c Operative specimen

may be associated with calculi and be difficult to distinguish from stone pyonephrosis.

MacLEAN and FOWLER (1956) described a case of primary liver cancer that had metastasized to the renal pelvis.

Urography and pyelography

With reference to what was said above these two types of examination should include the entire ureter and urinary bladder.

Cancer of the renal pelvis may appear roentgenologically as an infiltration of the renal pelvis wall and as a polypoid tumour bulging into the renal pelvis (Figs. 156, 157, 158, 159). It may invade the renal parenchyma and then it will be difficult or impossible roentgenologically to distinguish the lesion from a primary renal carcinoma encroaching upon the renal pelvis. The infiltration into the wall of the renal pelvis results in deformation with irregular decrease in the lumen and rigid walls. Strictures produced by such infiltration can lead to dilatation of single calyces, groups of calyces or of the entire renal pelvis depending on the

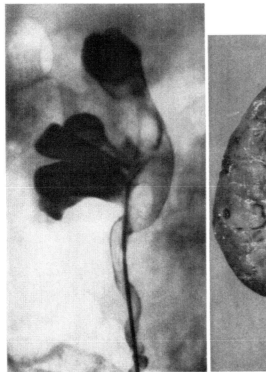 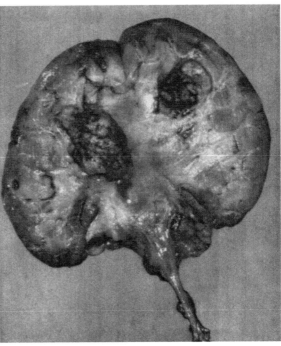

a   b

Fig. 158a and b. Papillary renal pelvis carcinoma. a Pyelography. Dilated kidney pelvis which is almost completely filled with a large blood clot extending down into the ureter. Broad-based tumour with uneven surface can nevertheless be seen filling major part of cranial branch. b Operative specimen. Blood clot removed

level of the stricture. One or several calyces may be destroyed. Stenosis of the stem of a calyx or a branch may resemble that seen in tuberculosis (HEIDEN-BLUT 1955).

Certain types of carcinoma of the kidney pelvis may initially or later resemble pyelonephritic changes with or without stone (Fig. 160). Pyelonephritis may also be coexistent with tumour and complicate the roentgen-symptomatology.

Papillomas appear as filling defects in the contrast medium (Fig. 161). On observation of such a filling defect it must first be decided whether the defect is localized to the kidney pelvis and not outside it, simply representing an intestinal gas bubble superimposed upon the renal pelvis. This can be readily checked by using oblique projections.

Filling defects in the renal pelvis may be due to a wide variety of factors. As mentioned in the chapter on normal anatomy, vessels and the border of the kidney parenchyma may cause impressions in the outline of the renal pelvis with

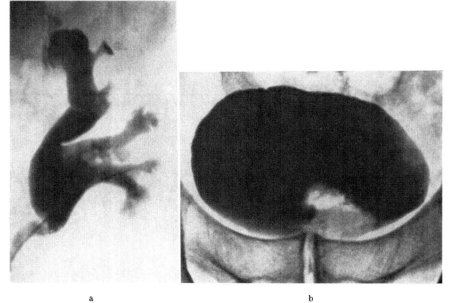

a   b

Fig. 159a and b. Papillary carcinoma of renal pelvis and of bladder. Pyelonephritis. a Pyelography. Irregular tumour with clefts on surface in kidney pelvis laterally at base of middle branch and middle cranial branch. Changes in most papillae characteristic of pyelonephritis with papillary necrosis. b Cystography. Irregular papillary tumour in base of bladder

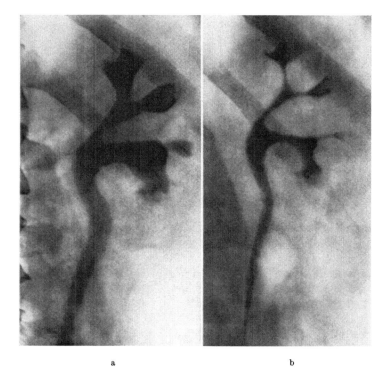

a   b

Fig. 160a and b. Pyelonephritic changes with malignant degeneration. Pyelonephritis for 5 years. Urography: Granular to papillary changes in mucosa of kidney pelvis and ureter. Plasticity of wall normal. (Note distension during ureteric compression [a] compared with [b] after removal of compression.) Two years later pain and haematuria left side. Nephro-ureterectomy. Histology: Chronic pyelonephritis and secondary malignant degeneration in kidney pelvis and ureter. Another 2 years later bladder carcinoma

a filling defect as a result. Such defects are, however, fairly characteristic and are seldom difficult to distinguish from tumours of the renal pelvis. Calculi, blood clots, gas bubbles etc. are all capable of causing filling defects resembling tumours in the renal pelvis. Even if they are of fairly low density calculi can, as a rule, be diagnosed already in plain roentgenograms of good quality, but, as stressed in the chapter on renal calculi, some stones may be of such a low density as not to show up in plain roentgenograms. Tumours cannot be seen in plain roentgenograms except in very rare cases when a papillomatous tumour of the renal pelvis has collected a layer of calcium on its surface. Calculi tend to assume the shape of the renal pelvis and are surrounded by a thin layer of contrast medium. Since patients with suspected tumours are often referred for roentgen examination because of haematuria,

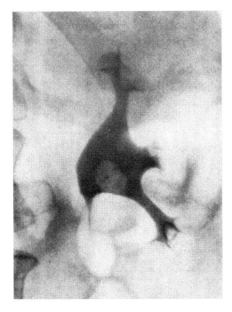

Fig. 161. Small papilloma in kidney pelvis with fairly broad attachement to pelvis wall. Patient previously operated on for bladder papilloma

blood clots are of great importance in the differential diagnosis of changes in the renal pelvis, ureter and urinary bladder. Check-examinations for any change in the shape or size of the defect may sometimes be necessary before a differential diagnosis is possible.

Renal angiography is not widely used for the diagnosis of tumours of the renal pelvis. According to the literature, these tumours produce no angiographic changes. Really selective angiography will, however, though not in all cases, show pathologic changes in tumours of the renal pelvis because in selective angiography the arteries to the renal pelvis and to the ureter can be studied (BOIJSEN

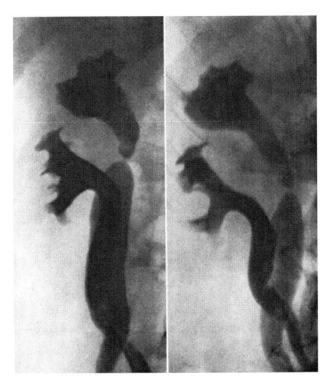

Fig. 162. Ureteric carcinoma. Pyelography: In proximal part of ureter to cranial pelvis in double kidney broad-based, small polypous tumour and marked stricture

1959). Renal angiography can thus contribute to the diagnosis and differential diagnosis of tumours of the renal pelvis (see Fig. 59). We have had 7 cases of tumour in the renal pelvis with positive findings in angiography.

In some cases where ordinary roentgen methods show a tumour in the renal pelvis it is impossible to decide whether the tumour is primary in the kidney pelvis or whether it represents an invasion into the pelvis of a small renal carcinoma (see Fig. 156). Renal angiography in such cases solves the problem.

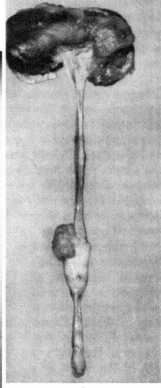

Fig. 163a—d. Ureteric papillomas with incipient malignancy. a and b Pyelography. Large polyp, 3 × 1¹/₂ cm distending but not dilating ureter. c Specimen. Tumour has broad attachement to thickened ureteric wall. Histology: Cancer ureteritis. Papilloma with slightly infiltrative character. d Ureteric papillomas. Two small, sessile papillomas in caudal part of ureter. Papillomas also in bladder

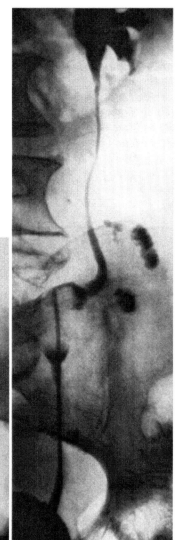

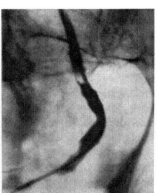

a   b   d

2. Tumours of the ureter

Tumours of the ureter may be malignant or benign. The malignant tumours may be primary or secondary. Owing to the length of the ureter and its intimate relation to several other organs, tumours of the latter are apt to encroach upon the ureter, *e.g.* tumours of the colon and rectum, uterine and ovarian carcinoma. Metastasizing tumours in the retroperitoneal space also often involve the ureters. This is the case, for example, in metastases from seminoma testis to the retroperitoneal lymph nodes or in lymphogranulomatosis. The enlarged lymph nodes often only displace the ureters and sometimes cause indentations in them, and sometimes compress them along a varying length.

Changes of the same type occur in the same diseases in another long transport channel, namely the inferior caval vein, and can be seen on cavography.

Primary malignant tumors of the ureter are rare. ABESHOUSE (1956) has collected 454 cases from the literature. The malignant tumours produce an ill-defined narrowing along a varying length of the ureter or complete obliteration. The obstruction may be abrupt or gradually increasing along a length of a few centimetres. In the region of the infiltration by the tumour the lumen of the ureter is very irregular and superficial ulcerations can be seen, but the infiltration may also be seen as an increasing stricture. The roentgen anatomic findings in cancer of the ureter are of the same type as those well known in other types of malignant infiltration of other ductal organs (Fig. 162). In malignant papillomas the tumour may have the same appearance as a benign papilloma. A broad base and signs of infiltration must make the examiner suspect malignancy (Fig. 163a—d).

The severity of the dilatation above an obstruction varies from case to case and with the duration and severity of stasis. There may be no dilatation at all, or it may be very slight.

The development of carcinoma of the ureter may be slow. One case described by GLENN (1959) was still of identical roentgen appearance on examination after an interval of 8 years.

In strictures of the ureter the possibility of malignant tumour must always be borne in mind.

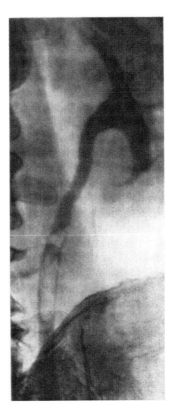

Fig. 163e. Benign ureteric papilloma. Urography: $4^{1}/_{2}$ cm. long polyp surrounded by contrast urine and with thin base attached to ureteric wall cranially-laterally. No dilatation of urinary pathway. Histology: Polypus adenomatosis ureteris

As a rule, primary malignant tumours of the ureter affect only one of the ureters. Cases of bilateral primary carcinoma of the ureter are on record (RATLIFF, BAUM & BUTLER 1949, FELBER 1953, GRACIA & BRADFIELD 1958). Multiple carcinomas of the ureter may also be multiple in one and the same ureter.

Secondary malignant tumours of the ureter are, as a rule, growths from malignant processes in surrounding organs. As mentioned, this is common in rectal cancer or gynecologic cancer, for example. While, as mentioned, the primary malignant tumour in the ureter is, as a rule, unilateral, secondary growths usually involving both ureters and often at the same level. The other type of secondary malignant tumours of the ureter is malignant metastasis to the ureter, which is rare. One case has been described (ROBBINS & LICH 1958) in which carcinoma from the uterine cervix metastasized to the proximal part of the ureter. A renal carcinoma may metastasize to the ureter (see Fig. 151).

Primary benign tumors of the ureter are still rarer than malignant ones. ABES-HOUSE's above mentioned collection included 138 primary benign tumours of the ureter. They are of the same type as tumours of the renal pelvis and tumours occurring elsewhere in the urinary tract. Papillomas and polyps are thus the most common. They are round or oval, usually pedunculated, assume the form of the ureter, and are sometimes very long. They may be very small to very large. HOWARD (1958) thus described a case of a pedunculated ureteric polyp, which measured 10×3 cm and which distended and filled a large part of the ureter but nevertheless permitted good passage of urine and thereby spared renal function which proved to be good, as judged by excretion urography. The renal pelvis was moderately dilated.

It is well known and has been stressed previously that papillomatous tumours have a marked tendency to form multiple and recurrent growths in the entire urinary tract. Papillomas may thus be multiple or solitary. If multiple, they may be seen crowded together at the same level or they may arise at different levels of the ureter.

Roentgenologically, these tumours appear as an obstruction in the ureter. The obstruction is often manifested by a concave outline of the end of the column of contrast medium in contradistinction to the abrupt termination or the tapering of the contrast column in ureteric stricture. The tip of the papilloma may simulate a concrement in the ureterogram. Sometimes the contrast fluid flows around the tumour, whose size and shape can then be assessed (Fig. 163e). The ureter may be markedly widened by the tumour *per se*, in other words, the actual tumour mass distends the ureter. A tumour blocking the ureter causes dilatation of the ureter proximal to the tumour, and of the kidney pelvis. On the other hand, large ureteric tumours may sometimes cause only slight or no dilatation of the renal pelvis.

A ureteric tumour can also prolapse out into the bladder if it is pedunculated. An haemangioma, 6,5 cm long, of this type was described by BRODNY & HERSHMAN (1954) in a patient in whom urography showed ordinary excretion and a filling defect in the distal part of the ureter. Sometimes, though rarely, it may cause intussusception of the ureter (HUNNER 1938, MORLEY, SHUMAKER & GARDNER 1952).

K. Renal cysts

Renal cysts are common and of many patho-anatomic types. They have been classified according to various criteria such as macroscopic characteristics, histologic appearance, clinical significance, site, appearance of fluid content, multiplicity etc. Of the various types of cysts, the pyelogenic and aplastic have been described in the chapter on Anomalies and cystic degeneration of renal carcinoma in the chapter on Tumours. The common small retention cysts situated in the outer part of the cortex are, broadly speaking, of no roentgenologic interest. They may sometimes be demonstrated in the nephrographic phase of renal angiography. This leaves three groups of roentgen-diagnostic importance, namely serous cysts, hydatid cysts and polycystic disease.

Serous cysts

Serous cysts fall essentially into three groups: simple cysts, peripelvic lymphatic cysts and multilocular cysts.

1. The simple cyst

Simple cysts are usually solitary and unilateral. Multiple cysts of this type can, however, occur in one or both kidneys. The name solitary cyst, which is commonly used in the literature is therefore sometimes misleading. Simple cysts occur in all ages, but they are uncommon in childhood. They are often found incidentally to examination of the urinary tract or abdomen for some other reason. In our material a great many cysts have been detected accidentally on routine urography of patients with prostatic hypertrophy. In children positive palpatory findings often lead to the discovery of such cysts.

A simple cyst may be a so-called capsular cyst and be situated almost entirely extrarenally. It may also be partly or completely embedded in renal parenchyma. It can vary widely in size.

a) Plain radiography

The findings made on plain roentgenography vary from case to case depending on the size and site of the cyst. If the cyst is situated mainly outside the kidney, it will be seen as a round or oval, usually very well defined smooth surfaced formation, adjacent the kidney. If the cyst is partly embedded in renal parenchyma, a bulge will be seen in the outline of the kidney. Sometimes the cyst is embedded in parenchyma near the surface of the kidney, and then the bulge may be almost circular. Sometimes the cyst is seated deeper in the parenchyma and then causes only a slight bulge in the outline of the kidney. Exposures should, of course, be taken at different angles in order to secure a projection of the cyst in profile for judging its attachment and size. If the cyst is situated entirely within the kidney, it may cause a generalized enlargement of the latter. A small cyst intrarenally may produce no pathologic changes demonstrable by plain roentgenography.

In the event of multiple cysts, similar changes may be seen in two parts of the kidney. If the cysts are close together, they will cause a coarse lobulation of the outline of the kidney. Sometimes the whole kidney undergoes cystic degeneration and then a well defined lobulated mass, often of considerable size, will be seen instead.

It has been claimed that cysts may be detected in plain roentgenograms as an area of less density than the kidney and that this is sufficient to make a diagnosis of cyst. For this to be possible the density of the normal tissue would have to be increased or the contents of the cyst would have to consist of fat. But, as a rule, neither of these conditions are satisfied by a simple cyst. Such claims are based mainly on non-roentgenologic reasoning.

Sometimes, though very seldom, however, a cyst can be diagnosed because its content is fatty. We have seen this type of cyst only once in our large material of simple cysts. It has also been stated that even large cysts sometimes escape detection in plain roentgenograms. This may be true, but is not due to any specific roentgen-diagnostic character of cysts. It can only happen if the patient is not properly prepared or if the examination is not properly performed. Plain radiography has to be performed efficiently, and such an examination must always be carried out preliminary to urography or pyelography.

Sometimes a cyst may be seen to grow during long expectancy. Of 16 patients with cyst re-examined in our material (JOHNSSON 1946) the cyst was found to increase in size in 6. In one the cyst attained fairly considerable proportions. In one case the cyst had become smaller. A cyst can also disappear completely by rupturing and emptying into the renal pelvis or the retroperitoneal tissue.

The wall of the cyst may calcify. In such cases more or less opaque calcifications are seen in the periphery of the cyst, occasionally as a ring encircling the entire cyst, though more commonly as small bow-shaped calcifications correspond-

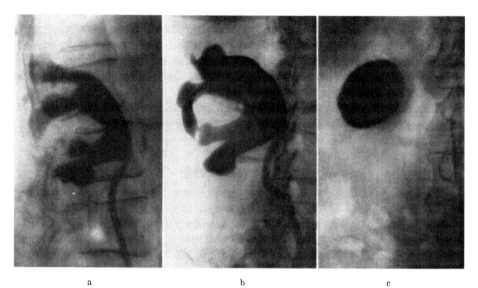

a   b   c

Fig. 164a—c. Simple cyst. Pyelography. a, b Spaceoccupying lesion dorsally. Percutaneous puncture. Clear fluid.
No cells. Injection of contrast medium into cyst. c Contrast filled cyst

ing to parts of the periphery of the cyst. In simple cysts as well as in other types
of cysts heterotopic ossification occurs, though rarely.

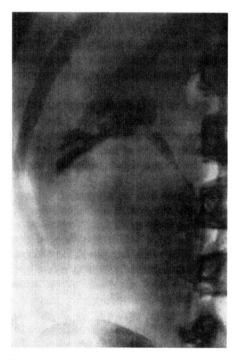

Fig. 165. Simple cyst in 12 year old boy. Cyst diagnosed at 4 years of age. Patho-anatomical verification

b) Urography and pyelography

The shape of the renal pelvis varies
with the position and size of the cyst.
In principle the changes are of the
same type as those seen in well defined
solitary tumor and described above
(Figs. 164, 165, 166; see also Figs. 167,
170). As mentioned, the deformation
will vary to a large extent with the
primary anatomic shape of the renal
pelvis. It has been stated by BRAASCH
& EMMETT that in most cases of cysts
the normal terminal irregularities of
minor calyces involved will be well retained". Although I am not quite sure
what is to be understood by "normal
irregularities" I feel that a cyst and a
well defined nephroma of the same
size and position will produce the same
deformation. Under such conditions
it is not possible to make a differential diagnosis on the basis of the
findings in the plain roentgenogram,
pyelogram or urogram. A guess is
never a diagnosis.

It is often to be read in the literature that cysts do not cause any changes in
the shape of the renal pelvis. This is not true. On the contrary, cysts nearly

always produce demonstrable changes in the shape of the renal pelvis. The more
the cyst is developed in the periphery of the kidney the less it will deform the
pelvis, and sometimes it will only cause a slight flattening or displacement of a
single calyx. This holds especially for the above-mentioned encapsulated cysts.
A necessary condition for demonstrating changes in the renal pelvis, particularly
small changes, is the use of projections capable of demonstrating the changes.
Examinations consisting only of standard frontal projections cannot be regarded
as satisfactory. The urographic and pyelographic technique should always be
adjusted according to the findings of plain roentgenography.

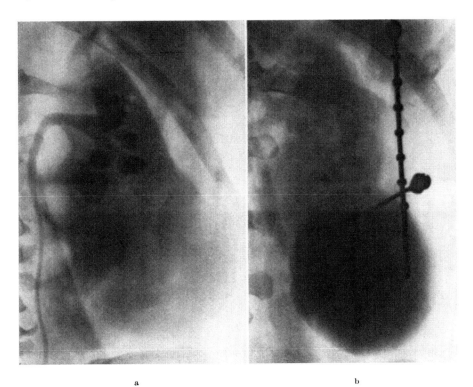

a   b

Fig. 166a and b. Simple cyst. a Urography. Large well-defined spaceoccupying lesion caudal kidney pole. Nephrographic effect in part of kidney with fairly well outlined lesion. Function and type of expanding lesion indicates
puncture. b Percutaneous puncture produced clear fluid. No cells. Contrast filling

On urography and pyelography it may sometimes be necessary to vary the
density of the contrast medium to demonstrate small space-occupying lesions.
It should also be observed that dilatation of the renal pelvis by a pathologic
process or by the examination procedure may mask a small impression in the renal
pelvis.

Specific of urography is excretion of contrast urine. Only if a major portion
of the renal parenchyma has been replaced by cysts will impairment of renal
function be demonstrable urographically. Function might then be completely
lost. Small cysts and even many large cysts without complicating urinary stasis
will, however, produce no demonstrable impairment of excretion. Sometimes the
density of the renal parenchyma in the nephrogram will be increased, while the
region involved by a cyst will show no such increase in density. This nephrographic effect can be increased by injection of a large amount of contrast medium
or by protracted ureteric compression.

14*

On check examination of a patient at intervals of years, the cyst may, as mentioned above, be observed to change in size (Fig. 167). This may cause a marked change in the pyelogram, particularly if a cyst has collapsed (see Fig. 170).

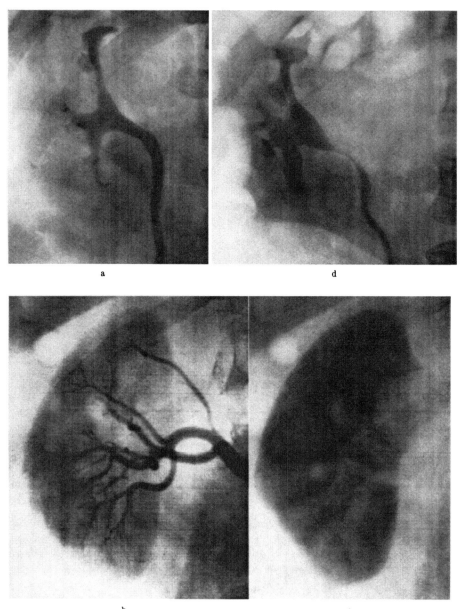

Fig. 167a—d. Simple cyst. Increase in size. a Urography. Displacement of cranial branch by rounded space-occupying lesion in medial part of kidney. Renal angiography. b Arterial phase. Arterial displacement. Avascular part corresponding to space-occupying lesion. c Nephrographic phase. Characteristic cyst. Note lifted paren-chymal border. d Urography. 4 years later. Cyst has increased. Puncture. Clear fluid. No cells

Urography and pyelography will sometimes show filling defects in the renal pelvis due to stone or blood clots in association with haematuria. It is important not to take such filling defects for tumor growing into the renal pelvis with an erroneous diagnosis of renal carcinoma as a consequence.

c) Renal angiography

The arteriogram will show the arteries to be displaced and thin arterial branches will extend around a cyst if the cyst is situated intrarenally. In the venous phase the cyst is often well outlined by fine, stretched veins. If the cyst is mainly extrarenal, such vessels will seldom be seen in the free periphery of the cyst. The most important phase is the nephrographic phase, which should include a sufficiently large number of films. A cyst appears in the nephrogram as a filling defect. Since part of the cyst bulges outside the kidney, the filling defect will be seen as a pit in the renal parenchyma. This is best demonstrated in profile projections of the filling defect. Characteristic of cysts is that this filling defect is bordered by parenchyma which will be beak-shaped in the different projections. This is because the cyst pushes aside and lifts the edge of the parenchyma. The edge of the defect may be somewhat irregular, but it is always sharp in suitable projections (Figs. 168, 169).

If a cyst is small and surrounded by renal parenchyma, it may be difficult to detect.

It is important to perform the examination by the selective technique. Superimposition of vascular branches not belonging to the renal arteries may make it impossible to establish a diagnosis and an avascular region may then appear vascularized. It may also be necessary to use an additional projection to demonstrate the above mentioned pitting in the renal parenchyma due to the cyst and to avoid superimposition of gas bubbles in the gastrointestinal tract.

d) Puncture of cyst

For diagnostic and therapeutic purposes the cyst may be punctured and its contents aspirated. Contrast medium such as gas (FISH 1939) or water-soluble contrast medium (JOHNSSON; LINDBLOM 1946, AINSWORTH & VEST 1951) may be injected (see Figs. 164, 166, 168). The method has been elaborated in detail by LINDBLOM (1946, 1952) and has been used in a large number of cases.

With the guidance of the urography, which may be done in association with puncture, the expanding process is punctured percutaneously from behind. If fluid is produced, it is aspirated and a small amount of contrast medium is injected. If the cyst is large, contrast medium should be injected before all the cyst content has been aspirated. If too much fluid is aspirated, the cyst will collapse and then the needle may slip out and thereby make it impossible to inject contrast medium. The next step is to take films in different projections to ascertain the size of the cavity, its shape and any mural growths. It should be carefully checked that the image of a contrast filled cavity coincides with the filling defect seen in the nephrogram, since part of a tumour can undergo cystic degeneration, and a kidney may harbour both a tumour and a cyst.

It may be difficult to puncture a very small cyst or a ventrally located cyst percutaneously. Puncture is thus useful as a differential diagnostic measure against tumor only if it proves the existence of a cyst. If puncture yields no cyst fluid, it may mean that the expanding process is a solid tumor, but it can also be due to the cyst not having been properly punctured, the tip of the needle having been passed into normal renal parenchyma.

Puncture and injection of contrast medium will often show that the cyst has a somewhat irregular outline. It may be more or less distinctly lobated or be dumb-bell shaped. The wall, however, is quite smooth and the filling complete. Should any mural growth be observed, the lesion cannot be diagnosed as a simple cyst. According to GORDON (1958), all cysts containing blood or heavily blood-

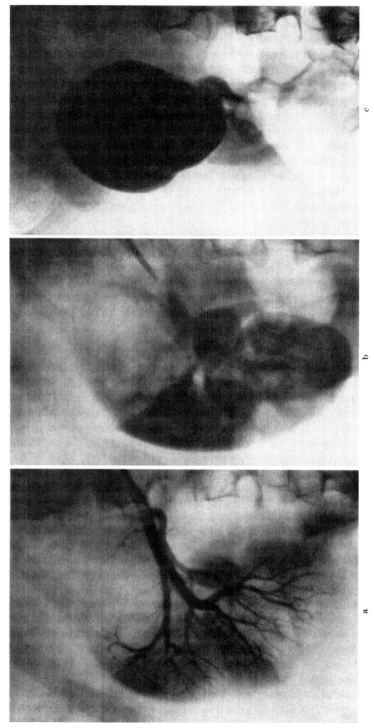

Fig. 168a—c. Simple cyst. Urography: Space-occupying lesion. Normal excretion. Selective renal angiography. a Arterial phase: Main renal artery and cranial branches including fine capsular branches displaced. No vascularization of cranial pole. b Nephrographic phase: Well defined defect. c Percutaneous puncture. Contrast filling of cyst. Completely contrast filled cyst with smooth inner surface coincides exactly with defect in nephrogram and kidney outline

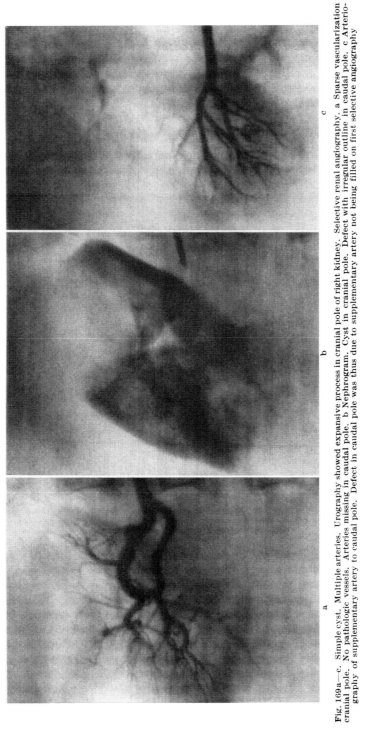

Fig. 169a — c. Simple cyst. Multiple arteries. Urography showed expansive process in cranial pole of right kidney. Selective renal angiography. a Sparse vascularization cranial pole. No pathologic vessels. Arteries missing in caudal pole. b Nephrogram. Cyst in cranial pole. Defect with irregular outline in caudal pole. c Arteriography of supplementary artery to caudal pole. Defect in caudal pole was thus due to supplementary artery not being filled on first selective angiography

stained fluid must be regarded as potentially malignant and accordingly should be surgically explored. As an extra precaution we have the fluid examined histologically for neoplastic cells.

Puncture may sometimes cause mild local pain or a sensation of pressure. A slight rise in temperature may also occur.

The most important differential diagnosis is renal carcinoma versus simple cyst; which is discussed in a special chapter (page 196). Renal abscess, though rare, might also be taken into account. The appearance of such an abscess may simulate that of a simple cyst on plain radiography, urography and pyelography as well as on renal angiography (see Fig. 234).

2. Peripelvic lymphatic cysts

A special variant of renal cyst is the so-called peripelvic lymphatic cyst. This type of cyst, as indicated by its name, is localized to the sinus and hilum of the

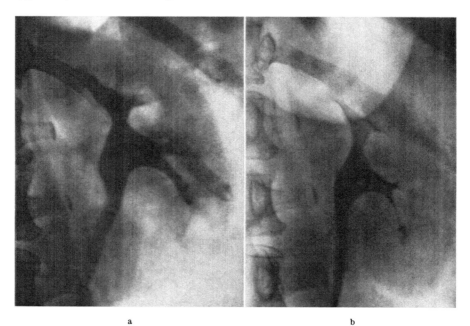

a   b

Fig. 170a and b. Probably peripelvic cyst disappearing spontaneously. a Urography: Expanding lesion medially in caudal pole displacing kidney. Renal angiography showed the space-occupying lesion to be a cyst. b Check urography two years later. Cyst has disappeared

kidney and can protrude out through the hilum. It varies widely in size from a small cystic process to a large formation prolapsing through the hilum. It consists of one or more thin-walled cystic formations related to the lymphatics and is conceived as a lymphatic retention cyst. DUBLIER & EVANS (1958) described the roentgen findings in this disease as characteristic. In plain roentgenograms, in urograms or pyelograms, however, the findings cannot always be distinguished from those produced by simple cysts or tumour (Fig. 170). Renal angiography can distinguish them from tumour. In contrast to the simple cyst, the peripelvic cyst does not produce demonstrable changes in the renal parenchyma. Thus, an extrarenal process situated near and deforming the hilum but producing no angiographic signs of involvement of the renal parenchyma can be diagnosed as a peripelvic renal cyst.

3. Multilocular cysts

Another variant is the multilocular cyst. It consists of a well defined cyst in a firm capsule occupying a major portion of the kidney. The capsule encloses numerous cystic cavities with a mucin-like fluid. This type of cyst is extremely rare but has been described under the same headings as other unilateral cystic processes. It is important because it occurs in childhood and because it has been confused, clinically and roentgenologically, with Wilms' tumour (FRAZIER 1951).

4. Hydatid cysts

Hydatid cyst or echinococcus cyst is a parasite cyst of interest mainly in those countries where the parasite is common. With increasing international traffic, however, the disease must be borne in mind in other countries. It has also been called *une maladie cosmopolite*. On the whole, it follows the industry of sheep and cattle-raising. The dog is the host of the tenia echinococcus granulosus, while man and various ruminants are intermediary hosts for the cystic stage of the worm. The infestation is caused by ingestion of the ova. Hydatid cyst is commonest in the liver, then in the lungs, but it may also occur elsewhere in the body. It is usually solitary. The hydatid cyst consists of a cystic sac surrounded by a fibrous capsule formed as a reaction of the host. The cyst is usually round but may be irregular in shape. It can grow but can also shrink or rupture and empty itself. Infection of the cyst is not uncommon. The connection between the actual parasite and the surrounding fibrous capsule may be more or less firm. The capsule often calcifies.

Plain radiography shows the same findings as those in simple cysts. Capsular calcifications are common. They are irregular and fragmentary but arranged in the form of a spheric shell.

The urographic and pyelographic findings are the same as those produced by a simple cyst or a well defined solid tumour. If the fibrous capsule is not intact, contrast medium can escape in between the latter and the parasite cyst. Reproductions given to illustrate this, however, usually show only a strongly distended calyx whose fading edge has been erroneously regarded as representing contrast medium inside the fibrous capsule. If the cyst perforates into the renal pelvis, contrast medium may enter the actual cyst.

If the calcifications are characteristic the diagnosis is easy. Otherwise it must be differentiated from the same conditions as simple cysts. Clinical serologic findings specific to hydatid cysts can, of course, decide the differential diagnosis.

L. Polycystic disease

Polycystic disease is a bilateral congenital hereditary disease in which both kidneys may be full of cysts of varying size.

The cystic formation on one side may differ considerably from that on the other. Polycystic disease may undoubtedly also occur on one side only. This is, however, uncommon and naturally seen less frequently post mortem than on roentgen examination, because small changes on one side may escape detection or produce non-characteristic and inconclusive changes.

Double-sidedness is thus not a *conditio sine qua non* of this disease. Congenital or hereditary occurrence is often a significant characteristic. However, IVEMARK & LINDBLOM (1958) distinguish a special group adult polycystic kidney, which as a rule, occurs late in life, generally in the fourth decade and with renal colic as its first symptom. On the basis of various observations they suggest that the cysts might be intrarenal haematomas due to rupture of aneurysm-like formations, which they claim to have shown both histologically and by micro-angiography.

Definite proof of the existence of such a group is, however, not yet available. One might also well imagine that the vascular changes and haemorrhage are not primary but secondary, that the vascular changes due to polycystic disease in association with hypertension, for example, might cause the bleedings with consequent changes. Personally, however, I believe that bleeding plays a role in the symptomatology and that the progress of the disease with increasing size of the cysts is due to a mechanism resembling that underlying the increase in the size of a subdural haematoma, namely the breaking down of haemoglobin molecules into several smaller ones with an increased osmotic effect in the cyst.

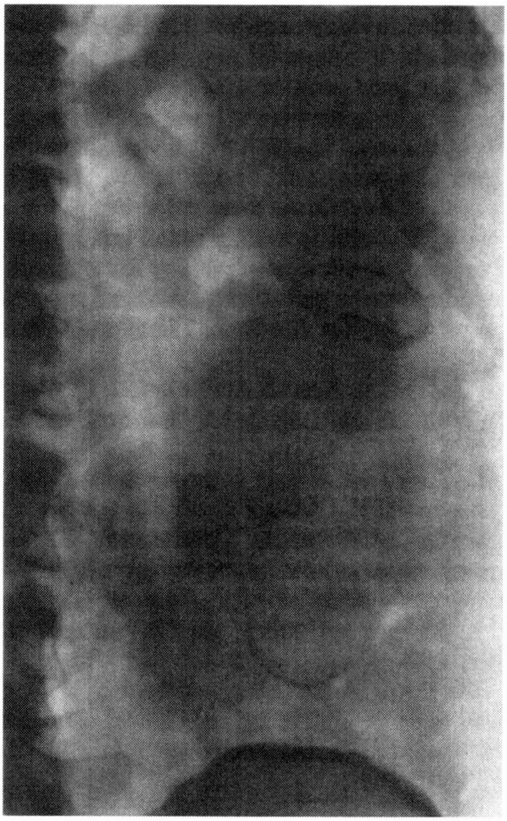

Fig. 171. Polycystic kidney. Very large bulgent kidneys. Multiple cyst-wall calcifications in left kidney. Calcified cysts partly deformed by impression from noncalcified adjacent cysts

a) Plain radiography

Both kidneys are enlarged and their surface is bulgent. Sometimes the enlargement is enormous and equally severe on both sides. Sometimes it is less marked, and sometimes the kidney on one side may be much larger than that on the other.

Calcifications are often seen partly as a thin shell around single cysts and partly as small irregular calcifications (Fig. 171).

b) Urography and pyelography

The characteristic changes in the renal pelvis are multifocal bulges (Figs. 172, 173, 174; see also Fig. 176). In severe cases the findings might be completely characteristic with grotesque deformation of the renal pelvis by different sized multiple, space-occupying processes. The calyces may be severely elongated or one or more calyces may be flattened. The confluence may be compressed or show small impressions. The changes may, however, be slight and on one side the only change may be a single flattened or slightly elongated calyx. Even if the changes are small, their occurrence on both sides is of diagnostic importance. On cyst formation the distance between the periphery of the kidney and the nearest calyx increases. While the distance seldom exceeds 2—2,7 cm in a normal kidney, except in the renal poles, in cystic kidneys it may be more than 3 cm (BILLING 1954).

Single cysts may be in open communication with the renal pelvis and be filled in association with urography or pyelography, or they may be perforated by the catheter or they may rupture (Fig. 175).

On repeated examination at long intervals cystic kidneys will be seen to increase in size and to change in shape (Fig. 176). The deformation of the renal

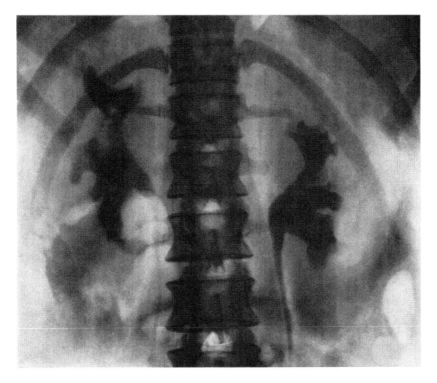

Fig. 172

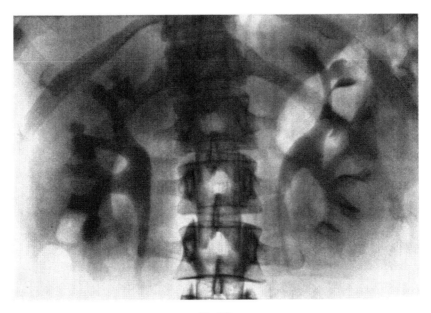

Fig. 173

Fig. 172 and 173. Polycystic kidneys. Enlarged kidneys with bulgent outline. Urography: Good excretion of contrast medium. Marked deformity of both kidney pelves. Increased distance kidney pelvis—kidney surface

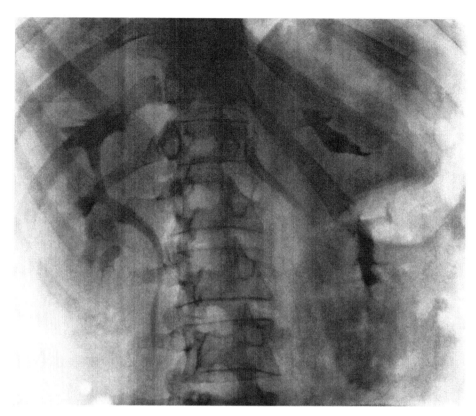

Fig. 174. Polycystic kidneys, fairly large. Double kidney left. Urography: Fairly good excretion. Deformity of kidney pelves

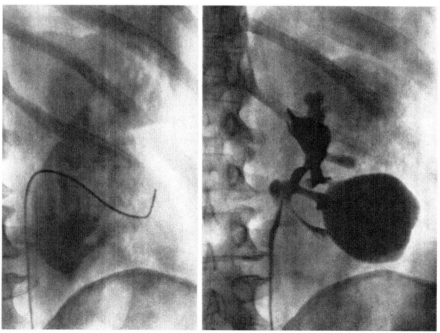

a

b

Fig. 175a and b. Polycystic kidney. One cyst communicating with kidney pelvis. Ureteric catheterization: Blind catheterization: no resistance. a Plain film: Catheter in kidney. Withdrawal of catheter 10 cm. Contrast injection. b Pyelography: Deformed kidney pelvis. Large cyst communicating with calyx. Tracing of plain film with catheter onto pyelogram will demonstrate penetration of catheter into cyst and bending of tip of catheter along lateral cyst wall

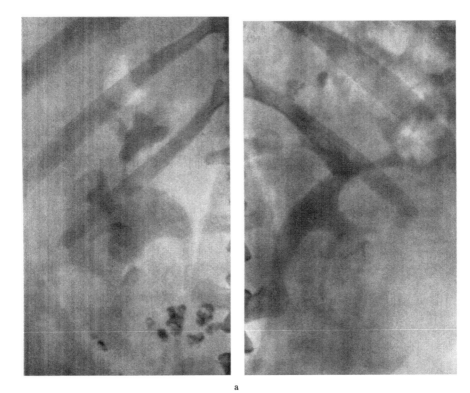

a

b

Fig. 176a and b. Polycystic kidneys. Progression. Urography: a Bilateral moderate changes. b 9 years later. Advanced changes. Another 4 years later uremia. Plain roentgenography demonstrated enormous kidney enlargement

pelvis also changes on development of new cysts and collapse of others. The change may be considerable, from slight or relatively slight to grotesque deformations.

In urography the contrast density is often reduced owing to poor concentrating power of the kidneys. As a rule the density is, however, sufficient for diagnosis.

c) Renal angiography

In advanced cases the intrarenal arterial branches are distended, sometimes they are severely stretched and narrow. The nephrogram shows filling defects resembling those seen in simple cysts. Characteristic of the disease, however, is that the cysts are multiple and of different sizes. A particularly characteristic, pathognomonic angiogram is seen in patients with numerous small cysts. Then the entire cortex of the kidney shows small filling defects giving the kidney an irregular notchy outline in the nephrogram (BILLING 1954) (Fig. 177).

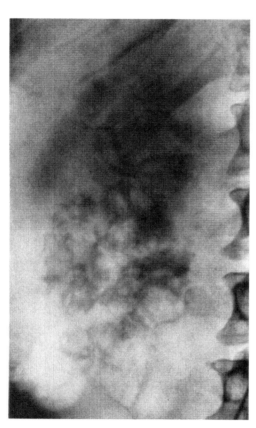

As a rule, however, the diagnosis can be made without renal angiography. The examination may be of prognostic value in so far as it gives a much better impression of the extent of the cystic process and of the amount of functioning renal parenchyma than pyelography or urography. Since renal function is often impaired in polycystic disease the range of indications for renal angiography in this disease must be kept very narrow, and when the examination is indicated, it should be performed by the selective technique, only one kidney should be examined during a single session and the method used should be such as to require only a very small amount of contrast medium.

Fig. 177. Polycystic kidney. Renal angiography. Nephrographic phase. Defects throughout kidney by innumerable cysts. (Courtesy of Dr. BILLING)

Sometimes a kidney with polycystic disease may be the seat of a tumour. Cases have been described with bilateral cancer (BORSKI & KIMBROUGH 1954, PUIGVERT 1958).

It should also be observed that polycystic kidney disease may be only one manifestation of several in Lindau's disease. ISAAC, SCHOEN & WALKER (1956) have described such a case with cystic disease of the kidneys and pancreas with renal and cerebellar tumours. RALL & ODEL (1949) pointed out co-existent cystic degeneration of other organs. Finally, ASK-UPMARK & INGVAR (1950) and others have pointed out that intracranial aneurysms seem to be common in patients with polycystic renal disease.

M. Primary vascular lesions

Renal function is intimately related to the blood supply to the kidneys. Investigation of the renal vasculature is therefore important in many conditions. Changes occur in the pattern of the renal vessels in a variety of renal diseases. Characteristic abnormalities may then be demonstrated by angiography. When this is the case, the appearance of the pathologic findings is described in association with the underlying disease, *e.g.* vascular atrophy in the chapter on stone and on hydronephrosis, pathologic vessels in renal carcinomas in the chapter on renal tumours etc., usually under the sub-heading of renal angiography. These vascular changes are secondary to a primary renal disease.

Certain primary vascular changes are also of great roentgen-diagnostic interest.

I. Arteriosclerosis

Senile changes in the renal arteries are of the same type as those seen in arteriosclerosis elsewhere. The large vessels become more tortuous, often markedly so, deposits of calcium occur in the media and intima, local aneurysm-like widenings may occur with more or less extensive narrowings. In aneurysm of the lumbar aorta attention should be given to the relation of the renal arteries to the aneurysm in case extirpation of the aneurysm and substitution by a vessel transplant should be contemplated.

Calcifications of the type common in the lumbar aorta, namely irregular plaques of varying size, can be seen on plain radiography of the renal artery and then often in the wall of the abdominal aorta and/or in other aortic branches

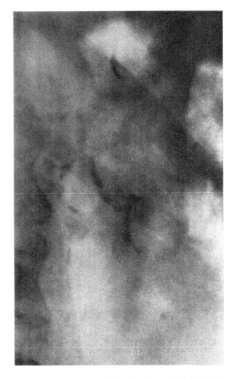

Fig. 178. Intimal calcifications in arteriosclerosis localized to wall of lumbar aorta, main renal artery and large intrarenal branches

(Figs. 178, 179). They are typical intimal calcifications. Sometimes more or less continuous calcareous tubes are seen localized to the media of vessels of apparently normal caliber and course (Fig. 180). Vascular calcifications demonstrable in plain roentgenograms are, however, fairly uncommon. Particularly calcifications in the intra-renal branches are rare, but occasionally a fragmented cast of the wider intrarenal branches may be seen (MOLDENHAUER 1959).

Tortuous, wide vessel branches can cause an impression in the renal pelvis, which may occasionally resemble a small expanding process pressing against the renal pelvis.

Angiography shows the tortuous vessels. Wide differences are seen in the caliber of the arteries or their branches owing to a varying degree of narrowing by intimal thickening of different lengths of the vessels. Locally the arterial wall may give way with the development of an aneurysm-like formation as a consequence (Fig. 181). Narrowing completely obstructs the lumen. In local narrowings the Goldblatt mechanism may be considered. Arteriosclerosis can lead to infarction of parts of the kidney (Fig. 182). Cicatricious contractions can then be observed, and in advanced cases one or both of the kidneys may be severely reduced in size. In polyangiitis nodosa similar changes can occur.

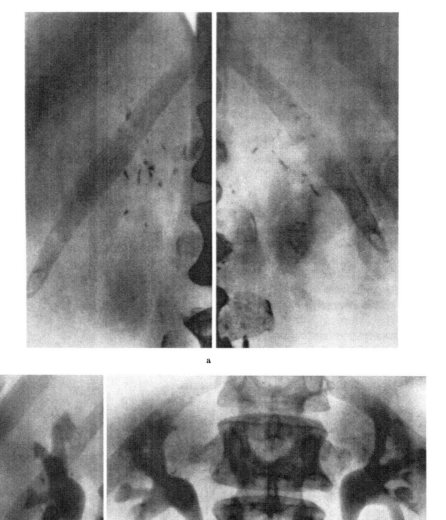

a

b

Fig. 179a and b. Intimal calcifications in arteriosclerosis. a Plain roentgenograms of both kidneys. Calcifications in intrarenal arterial branches. b Urogram including oblique view, right kidney. Calcifications immediately outside kidney pelvis

In this connexion it might be convenient to stress a few facts concerning roentgen examination of the kidneys in hypertension. Without going into the discussion about the rôle of the kidneys in the pathogenesis of hypertension it is obvious that plain radiography of the kidneys and pyelography and urography undoubtedly can reveal important changes. Nevertheless it must be remembered that these examinations delineate the outer and the inner surfaces of the kidney. Urography is the only one of these methods that yields information on renal function. It was pointed out previously (page 43) that urography is a crude method for judging kidney function and that, in spite of a marked decrease in unilateral or bilateral renal function, urography may still show good excretion of

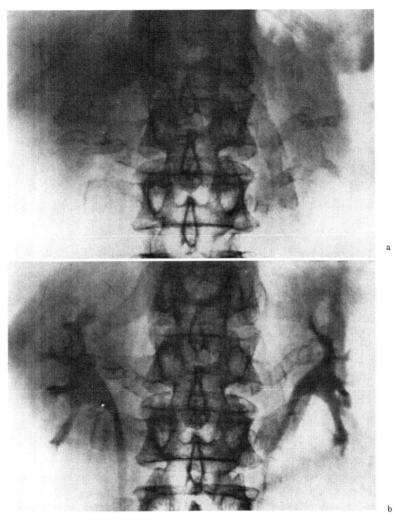

Fig. 180a and b. Calcifications in main renal arteries in intrarenal branches and in supplementary arteries to caudal pole bilaterally. a Plain roentgenography. b Urography

contrast urine. Another method yielding information on kidney function is renal angiography. Lesions responsible for hypertension often produce vascular changes well demonstrable by the angiographic technique. Renal angiography is therefore recommended in the search for renal vascular changes in hypertension.

II. Arterial aneurysms

Arterial aneurysms may be true or false. The latter are due to rupture of an artery and consist of haematomas in a connective tissue capsule, and they may

assume considerable proportions. True aneurysms consist of local widening
involving the entire arterial wall. They are small, usually less than one centimetre
in diameter, most frequently rounded, but sometimes fusiform. These aneurysms
are often bilateral and may occur even in fairly young people, but are most
common in middle age. They are relatively rare and much less common than
aneurysms in the splenic artery, for example. Their incidence, pathologic anatomy
etc. have been discussed thoroughly by ABESHOUSE (1951), for example. "Although
renal artery aneurysms are rare, the prognosis of the untreated case is so extremely
grave that the practicing urologist should acquaint himself with the entity"
(NESBIT & CRENSHAW 1956).

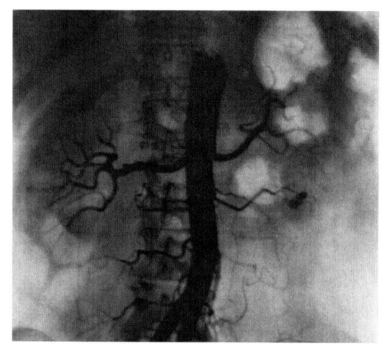

Fig. 181. Arteriosclerosis. Irregular, multiple, small aneurysms in right main renal artery

Plain radiography, urography and angiography

Aneurysms often calcify and then appear as irregular more or less distinct
crescent shaped or circular calcifications 1—3 cm in diameter. The calcifications
are seen as a ring, often with a small defect corresponding to the neck of the
aneurysm, *i.e.* its connection with the renal artery. Other types of fragmentation
may, however, also occur since the wall of the aneurysm is irregularly calcified,
and calcium plaques lying in different planes can be partly superimposed upon one
another. The calcifications are usually situated outside, but close to, the kidney.
Sometimes, however, they are seen within the kidney. They may occasionally be
fairly long and assume the shape of irregular tubes. A calcified aneurysm in the
renal artery has the same appearance as a calcified aneurysm in the splenic artery,
which is much more common and therefore well known to the radiologist. Co-
existent aneurysm calcifications may be seen in the renal artery and in the splenic
artery. In the presence of aneurysm arteriosclerotic calcifications are often seen
also in other vessels, usually in the lumbar aorta. On suitable projection, it is

always easy to determine the relation of the calcifications to the kidney. Stereo-scopy, like tomography, is unnecessary.

In urography and pyelography the calcifications will be seen adjacent the renal pelvis and will often cause an indentation in the latter, usually in the upper

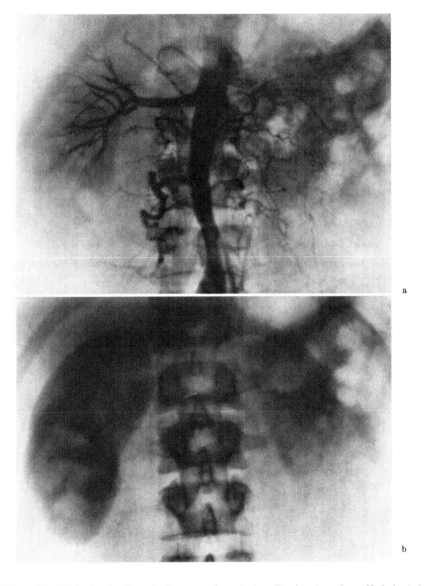

a

b

Fig. 182a and b. Arteriosclerosis. Long-standing, severe hypertension. Renal angiography: a Marked arterio-sclerotic changes in aorta. Left renal artery almost completely occluded at origin. Slight changes in proximal part of right renal artery. b Nephrogram: Normal parenchyma in somewhat large right kidney. Very small, irregular, atrophic kidney. Operation: Small, contracted kidney. Organized thrombus in renal artery

medial part of the renal pelvis because the renal artery always enters the sinus in this region.

Renal angiography will show an occasionally eccentric widening along a short length of the renal artery, which may be of ordinary width distally thereto.

15*

Sometimes the widening may extend to or even involve several peripheral branches. It may appear as a fusiform dilatation at a bifurcation, though it is more commonly

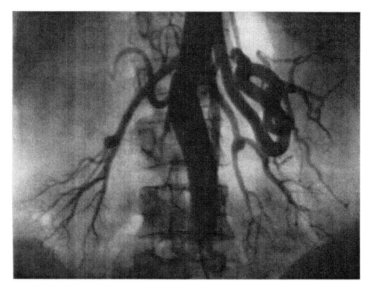

Fig. 183. Arterial aneurysm bilaterally. Aortic renal angiography: Ptosed kidneys. Saccular aneurysm bilaterally at bifurcation. (Courtesy of Dr. EDSMAN)

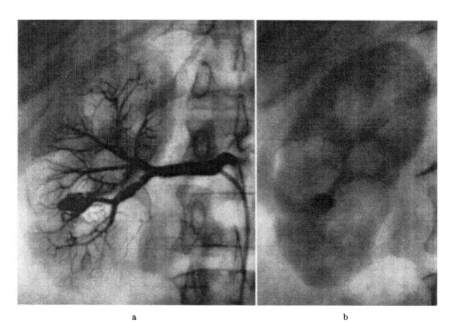

a   b

Fig. 184a—c. Arteriovenous aneurysm. Acute urography because of right sided renal colic and haematuria showed stasis on right side and large coagulum in bladder. Pyelography: Blocking of lower branch of kidney pelvis. Tumour was suspected. a, b Arterial and nephrographic phases. Selective renal angiography. Dorsal branch somewhat widened. Filling of an arteriovenous aneurysm in caudal half of kidney. Long-standing venous filling of aneurysm. Partial nephrectomy

sacculated with a more or less distinctly outlined neck projecting from one side of the renal artery or one of its wider branches (Fig. 183). An aneurysm must be distinguished from a post-stenotic dilatation, which can occur in the renal artery as in any other artery. This is sometimes called a jet aneurysm.

As mentioned, aneurysms are often calcified. This is, however, by no means always the case. Arterial aneurysms not demonstrable in plain roentgenograms or producing no filling defect in pyelograms are sometimes discovered accidentally on renal angiography done for some specific reason. As mentioned, aneurysms are not seldom bilateral. In a material of 7 patients with arterial aneurysm of the renal artery EDSMAN (1957) found the lesion to be bilateral in 5. Of 7 patients with saccular aneurysms, POUTASSE (1957) found bilateral aneurysms in only one. All aneurysms except one in this last mentioned material were calcified. From the illustrations it is clear that a diagnosis of aneurysms on both sides could not always

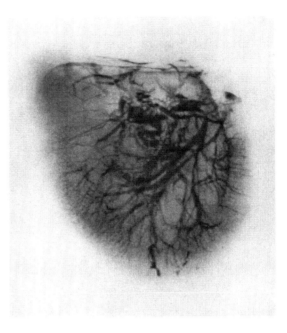

Fig. 184c. Arteriography of specimen showing arteriovenous anomaly

have been made, and that aortography had been performed mainly to obtain information on calcifications resembling aneurysms in plain roentgenograms. This explains why the aneurysms found were so often calcified. Of EDSMAN's 12 aneurysms, only 3 had undergone mural calcification demonstrable in plain roentgenograms. All 3 patients with a calcified aneurysm on one side had an uncalcified aneurysm on the other side and detected on angiography. These ratios undeniably confirm the value of renal angiography in the diagnosis of arterial aneurysm in the planning of surgery.

It may thus be concluded that an aneurysm need not be calcified and that a calcified aneurysm on one side may be accompanied by an uncalcified aneurysm on the other side, and that renal angiography is, of course, the most rational diagnostic method. Aortic renal angiography or bilateral selective angiography is thus always indicated if arterial aneurysm is suspected because of pain or haematuria or if a calcified aneurysm is found on one side.

III. Arteriovenous anastomoses and aneurysms

Arteriovenous anastomoses can occur in kidneys just as well as in other parts of the body following trauma. Two such cases with a pre-operative angiographic diagnosis have been published. SCHWARTZ, BORSKI & JAHNKE (1955) thus described a case with an arteriovenous connection between the stump of the renal artery and the renal vein 5 years after nephrectomy. GARRITANO, WOHL, KIRBY & PIETROLUONGO (1956) also described a case of arteriovenous fistula due either to an aneurysm of the renal artery that had caused erosion into the renal vein, or to trauma. The patient had fallen from a height and sustained severe trauma, and secondly he had sustained a wound which could have caused the arteriovenous anastomosis. Severe changes with a filling of markedly widened venous branches were observed over the ventral surface of the kidney as well as over the entire ventral surface of the spleen.

The type of vascular malformation called arteriovenous aneurysm also occurs in kidneys, but it is very rare. The literature contains 4 such cases, namely one described by SCHULZE-BERGMANN (1954), one by LJUNGGREN & EDSMAN (1956), one by SLOMINSKI-LAWS, KIEFER & VERMEULEN (1956) and the one by BOIJ-SEN & JÖNSSON; the last mentioned from our department and illustrated here (Fig. 184).

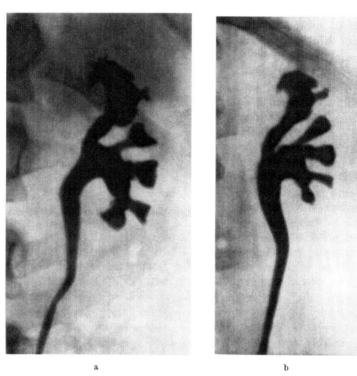

a   b

Fig. 185a—c. Infarction of kidneys. 5 days after acute attack of embolism including renal arteries. Urography: No function of left kidney. a Pyelography: Normal. b Pyelography 3 month later. Kidney pelvis has decreased [markedly in size. Kidney very small and functionless. Contracted kidney

Since arteriovenous aneurysms can be large, and plain roentgenograms and pyelograms may show signs of expansion of the kidney. The nature of the changes is diagnosed by angiography. The angiographic appearance of an arteriovenous aneurysm is the same as that of such aneurysms elsewhere in the body, especially the well-known intracranial aneurysms. One or a few arterial branches may be of increased caliber and lead to a large or small cluster of vessels in which the contrast blood rapidly passes into one or more wide veins (Fig. 184).

The aneurysms may be large and the amount of contrast medium may be rapidly shunted over from the arterial to the venous side to give a filling also of the inferior caval vein.

From a differential-diagnostic point of view, certain types of malignant renal tumours may be mentioned, which may show considerable arteriovenous shunting (see chapter J). In this respect they resemble arteriovenous aneurysms in the brain, which are sometimes difficult to differentiate from malignant tumour, especially glioblastoma multiforme with pronounced arteriovenous fistulae.

IV. Emboli in the renal artery

Autopsy studies have shown that emboli in the renal artery are not uncommon in mitral stenosis, for example. The infarction is usually small and causes only mild clinical symptoms. When the embolus is somewhat larger, especially if it obstructs the entire renal artery, acute symptoms occur. In such cases roentgen examination in the acute stage is sometimes performed because the clinical picture of the patient is that of an acute abdominal attack of unknown origin or of renal colic. The kidney may be enlarged and surrounded by edema. Contrast excretion during urography is impaired or has ceased.

If the infarction is small, the outline of the kidney after the lesion has healed will sometimes show an indentation at the site of the infarction (Fig. 185c). On renal angiography small indentations in the outline of the kidney are seen in the nephrographic phase due to scarring after the infarctions. If the infarction involves the entire kidney, the roentgenologic course is characteristic: the kidney, which is initially somewhat enlarged, decreases succesively to become a small shrunken kidney. Urography will show impaired excretion. Pyelography will show the renal pelvis to be of ordinary shape and to diminish with the reduction in size of the kidney (Fig. 185). On the basis of a case from our department LIEDHOLM (1944) described a pathognomonic triad allowing diagnosis of complete block by embolus of a renal artery, namely, no excretion of con-

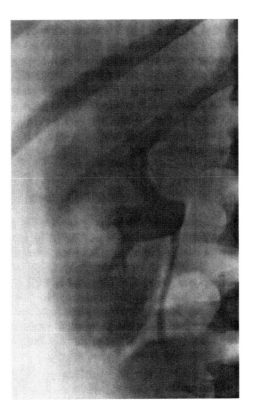

Fig. 185c. Right kidney: Marked indentation below middle of kidney—probably due to local shrinkage caused by infarction

trast urine, progressive reduction in the size of kidney and normal pyelogram. It should be pointed out that infection often supervenes and causes considerable changes in both the kidney and the renal pelvis.

In these cases renal angiography will show complete obstruction of the renal artery.

Since the arterial supply to the kidney can only be occluded for a relatively short time, an hour or so, without definitive loss of renal function, embolectomy must be performed very soon after the onset of the attack, if it is to be successful. Occasionally renal angiography during the acute attack might be helpful.

V. Thrombosis of the renal vein

Obstruction of the renal vein by tumour has been described in chapter J.
Renal vein thrombosis may develop in the same way as thrombosis elsewhere.
It is very uncommon. When it occurs, it may be unilateral or bilateral and is then
usually a serious complication to an already serious disease. It is more common
in children than in adults and is associated with infarction of the kidney. This
infarction has sometimes been demonstrated on roentgen examination during the
acute attack by the finding that the kidney was enlarged, that in urography the
excretion of contrast urine was absent or delayed and that the pyelogram showed
large filling defects in the renal pelvis due to blood clots (EIKNER & BOBECK 1956).
This type of thrombosis is said to indicate immediate nephrectomy.

Angiography has revealed other types of renal thrombosis with a less acute
and less serious course. Thus, cavography may show partial thrombosis of the
inferior caval vein extending into the renal vein, which may be completely obstructed. Sometimes a filling is obtained of collateral veins. In renal angiography
the arterial phase is followed by a venous phase differing from the ordinary type.
If the renal vein is obstructed, contrast medium passes to the caval vein through
collaterals, such as the spermatic vein (see Fig. 200). Knowledge of the different
types of renal vein thrombosis and their appearance in the angiogram, however,
is still very limited.

N. Dilatation of the urinary tract

Dilatations of the urinary tract are common and occupy an important position
in surgical diseases of the kidney. In few urologic conditions is it so difficult to
draw a line of distinction between what should be regarded as normal and pathologic. This is not surprising in the light of the wide normal variation of the width
of the renal pelvis and its parts as well as of the ureter and its various segments.
On the other hand, the nomenclature increases the difficulties, one and the same
name, particularly hydronephrosis, often being used to designate a clinical entity
characterized by a blockage at the pelviureteric junction as well as more or less
marked dilatations of the urinary pathways in many diseases in which the drainage
of the urinary tract is affected.

Dilatation may be unilateral or bilateral. It may involve the renal pelvis
and the entire ureter or part of it. It may also be limited to only part of the renal
pelvis. As mentioned, border-line cases are common, and then it is difficult to
decide whether a dilatation is pathologic or not. It is also sometimes difficult to
decide whether a demonstrable local narrowing really is pathologic and capable
of causing obstruction. In addition, the degree of dilatation might vary widely
with the examination method and technique, and the circumstances under which
the examination is performed, the kidney pelvis being markedly dilated on one
occasion and of largly normal appearance on another, for example. Furthermore,
opinions on the origin of the dilatations vary and are often vague, besides which
knowledge of the significance of the dilatation in renal function and renal infection
is not yet complete. The above-mentioned factors encountered in daily work are
sufficient to make a diagnosis of dilatation of the urinary tract difficult in many
cases. The value of the different roentgen-diagnostic signs must therefore be
judged with caution.

The roentgen findings in the types of dilatation of the urinary tract most
commonly encountered in routine work are described below. If the dilatation is
due to well known changes, such as stone, tumour, or anomalies, the roentgen

findings will be described in association with these conditions or they will be analogically evident from one of the following sections.

I. The obstructed pelviureteric junction

In this book the junction between the renal pelvis and the ureter is called the pelviureteric junction instead of ureteropelvic junction. The latter term is probably based on the instrumental pyelographic procedure, whereas the term "pelviureteric" is consistent with the direction of the urinary flow.

Obstruction of the pelviureteric junction can cause intermittent or permanent dilatation of the renal pelvis. Such dilatation is usually known as hydronephrosis. The name pyelectasis (BRAASCH & EMMETT 1951) is regarded by some authors as being better than hydronephrosis, but the latter term is preferred because it is so deeply rooted. In my opinion, the term hydronephrosis has the advantage that it draws attention to the fact that it is the entire kidney that is affected and not only the renal pelvis. The effect of the obstructed drainage on the kidney is the most important factor.

The normal anatomy of the pelviureteric junction varies widely (see page 26). The junction between a severely or only slightly dilated renal pelvis and a ureter of ordinary width will usually show a marked and short narrowing. The upper portion of the ureter may be fixed to the renal pelvis along a length of 1—3 cm by more or less loose adhesions. These may cause a sharp, more or less rigid bend in that part of the ureter fixed to the renal pelvis. This fixation can be accentuated by a vessel crossing the pelviureteric junction. Such a vessel running before the ureter will then press the bent ureter against the dilated renal pelvis. The fixed ureter can also be hooked and strangulated by the vessel.

Another component of the obstruction is diminution of the lumen of the pelviureteric junction by a more or less regular intrinsic stenosis varying in length from one case to another.

The different forms of obstruction described above, adhesion, compression by a vessel and intrinsic stenosis may occur separately, though more often to a varying degree in combination.

The obstruction caused by these factors is greatest when the renal pelvis is dilated, e.g. in marked diuresis. That part of the ureter adherent to the renal pelvis will then be stretched still more and be compressed, and drainage of the renal pelvis will consequently be poorer and poorer or cease.

In the beginning the obstruction may occur intermittently if for some reason or other the renal pelvis is dilated and drainage impaired. After such an attack of intermittent hydronephrosis a certain degree of dilatation may persist. It may be accentuated further after repeated attacks, and the dilatation may become permanent. The wider the renal pelvis becomes and the more it expands ventrally, the more it will obstruct drainage. Such urinary stasis leads to atrophy of the renal parenchyma and favours infection.

The purpose of the roentgen examination is to demonstrate the site of the obstruction responsible for the hydronephrosis, its severity and nature, its effect on the renal parenchyma and any complications such as stone formation. Considerable information can be required from the roentgen examination, and the diagnostic problems it is called upon to solve are important. This necessitates full utilization of all the diagnostic possibilities of the various examination techniques.

1. Plain radiography

The findings obtained on plain radiography depend upon the severity of the hydronephrosis. If the dilatation is only slight, the examination will reveal no signs of a pathologic condition; if moderate, the kidney will appear enlarged and the hilum wider than ordinarily; if severe, the dilated confluence of the renal pelvis will appear as a soft tissue mass at the hilum of the kidney and the kidney may be displaced laterally, and its lower part rotated laterally. Dilatation of the calyces may also manifest itself as an irregular plump bulging of the outline of the kidney. If the dilatation is still greater, a more or less well-defined soft tissue mass will be seen at the site of the kidney. It may fill half of the abdomen

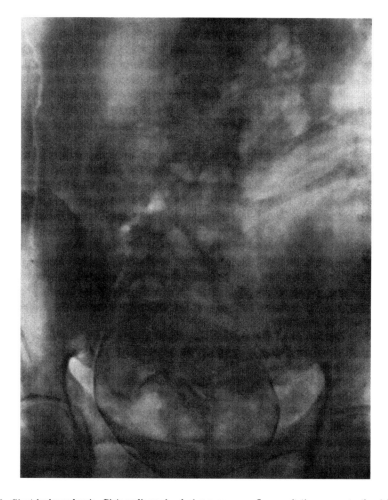

Fig. 186. Giant hydronephrosis. Plain radiography during pregnancy. Large soft tissue mass to the right, displacing uterus with foetus and gas-filled large bowel. Post partum operation disclosed a hydronephrotic sac containing 8 liters of fluid

and even extend beyond the midline. A corresponding displacement, particularly of the stomach, small intestine and large intestine is then demonstrable. I have also seen a uterus towards the end of pregnancy to be displaced severly to the left by a right-sided hydronephrotic sac containing 8 litres of fluid (Fig. 186).

Hydronephrosis is an important differential diagnostic possibility, which must be remembered when a retroperitoneal space-occupying lesion at the site of the kidney has been found. Thus plain radiography may show a large, more or less regularly outlined kidney, while urography may reveal absence of excretion. In such a case the possibility of hydronephrosis should always be borne in mind.

2. Pyelography and urography

Of other examination methods available, pyelography is that used most. Since, however, urography yields largely the same information as pyelography, it is gradually superseding pyelography. The part of the urinary tract on which pyelography will give the most valuable information is the pelviureteric junction. However, the more the examiner is familiar with the different types of obstructed pelviureteric junction and the more renal angiography is used in the diagnosis, the more the combination of urography and renal angiography will be used instead of pyelography. From the small field of vision over the pelviureteric junction, whose detailed anatomy is of minor importance in advanced cases once the site and severity of the obstruction has been established, the examiner has widened his interest to embrace morphology and function of the kidney as a whole, so that evaluation of indications for operation and choice of surgical method can now be made on a broader anatomic and physiologic basis.

a) Pyelography

Judging from the literature, there is more or less general agreement that pyelography should not be performed on a patient with hydronephrosis, particularly because of the risk of infecting an organ whose drainage is blocked. If retrograde pyelography is done, the patient should be turned in different directions in order to obtain a filling of all parts of the renal pelvis. Examination in the prone position is important because the heavy contrast medium flows to the declivous parts of the renal pelvis, *i.e.* in prone position the ventrally situated region including the pelviureteric junction. This region is most important and retrograde pyelography will often elucidate the anatomy there better than urography. It might also be worth while examining the patient in the erect position, because an obstruction *e.g.* by a supplementary vessel, may be more marked when the patient is standing than when he is lying. ROLLESTON & REAY (1957) found a horizontal lateral view with the patient supine to be particularly important because in that position the kidney is dragged posteriorly tending to place it on the stretch with resulting compression of the fixed upper portion of the ureter.

During injection of the contrast medium into the renal pelvis a compensated hydronephrosis may be converted into an acute manifest hydronephrosis. Occasionally a renal pelvis of relatively normal appearance may suddenly expand during retrograde pyelography. If a large amount of contrast medium has been injected into the renal pelvis, the catheter should be left *in situ* for a while to facilitate drainage after the end of the examination.

Here, too, the findings will vary with the severity of dilatation. If obstruction is intermittent, the finding may be quite normal, although a narrow pelviureteric junction may suggest the possibility of obstruction. Even in slight dilatation and especially in cases with persistent slight dilatation after longstanding, fairly marked dilatation the so-called psoas edge sign (HUTTER 1930) may be demonstrated. This sign consists of the medial part of the renal pelvis being pressed against the lateral surface of the psoas muscle so as to appear with a sharp, even outline instead of the usual rounded, medial outline. The phenomenon is due to the renal pelvis being more readily moulded by surrounding tissue than otherwise and thereby being deformed by the firmer psoas muscle and, secondly, by the layer formation occurring between the contrast medium in the urine, a phenomenon described in the chapter on retrograde pyelography. This layer formation plays an important rôle in the examination of hydronephrosis. Thus, the contrast medium will accumulate in the lowest calyces, *i.e.* the dorsal, and cranial if the patient is examined in supine position. To form an opinion of the other calyces, and above all, of the confluence of the renal pelvis, one must either use a large amount of contrast medium to secure a filling of the entire renal pelvis, or one can turn the patient over into prone position so that the confluence of the renal pelvis, which is directed ventrally, will then lie lowermost and thus receive the heavy contrast medium. Layer formation is also demonstrable on examination of the patient in the erect position (Figs. 187, 188, 189).

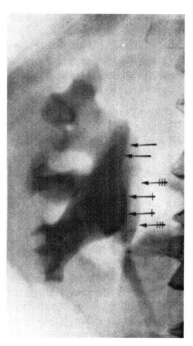

Fig. 187. Layer formation in urography in slightly dilated kidney pelvis. Release of ureteric compression. Three steps of impression into kidney pelvis by oblique lateral part of psoas muscle are seen. The upper branch of dorsalmost part is impressed by most lateral part of muscle, which is most dorsal (←). At ←+ lower branch, situated somewhat more ventrally, is impressed by middle position of muscle. At ←‖ confluence, situated most ventrally, is only slightly impressed

The renal pelvis becomes wider also in that part bordered by the parenchyma, which results in an increase in size of the renal sinus and a flattening of the papillae, so that the calyces become plumper (Fig. 190). This sign has been utilized for determining whether the kidney should be regarded as hydronephrotic or not. O'CONOR (1954) pointed out that a hydronephrotic kidney always has minor calyces showing distortion from the usual umbilicated outline, thus the papillae are flattened and the calyces blunted.

The renal pelvis empties slower than usually, so that examination at an interval of an hour, so-called delayed picture, might be of value.

Dilatation may be mainly intrarenal or extrarenal. If intrarenal, the effect on the renal parenchyma will appear sooner and be more severe with striking widening of the sinus. If the dilatation is mainly extrarenal, large extrarenal hydronephrosis may develop sometimes without appreciably impairing renal function.

At the pelviureteric junction the upper part of the ureter will be situated close to the dilated renal pelvis, which it follows ventrally, cranially and then bends off sharply in caudal direction (Fig. 191). The ureter will often show an extra bend or a small transverse band-shaped filling defect caused by the crossing of a vessel. These changes can be recognized best by turning the patient to a varying extent during fluoroscopic control. If the patient is supine, a filling defect due to an obstruction may be confused with layer formation in the ureter owing to a sharp bend so that its ventral, uppermost part does not contain contrast medium but shows a short filling defect (see Fig. 21). Judging from illustrations in various journals and manuals, such confusion is common. Another common misinterpretation is due to the fact that in a kidney situated somewhat lower than usual, the dilated renal pelvis, even if the dilatation is only slight, will be pressed against the ureter which will show a gentle kink that will not be filled with contrast medium. When the kink is straightened out by change in position of the kidney e.g. by change in the position of the patient, a good filling will be obtained and show no obstruction. A transient contraction of the pelviureteric junction must not be conceived as a stricture either.

Another source of error should be observed: if contrast medium is injected under fairly high pressure near the obstruction, it may be forced through the latter into the fluid in the renal pelvis like a stream (compare the jet phenomenon from a ureteric orifice into the bladder). This should not be interpreted as an obstruction of corresponding length (Fig. 192).

If obstruction is complete, so that it is not possible to inject contrast medium into the renal pelvis via a catheter or if for some reason catheterization is not possible, antegrade pyelography may be resorted to.

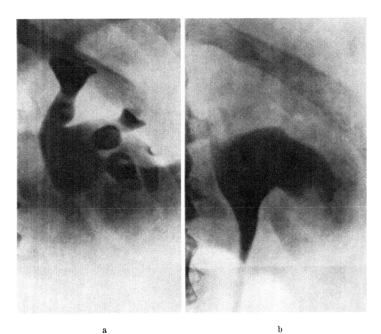

a   b

Fig. 188a and b. Layer formation and its influence on examination technique. Slight obstruction of distal part of ureter. a Supine position: Dorsal calyces and dorsal part of confluence filled. No filling of pelviureteric junction. b Prone position: Ventral parts including pelviureteric junction now contain contrast urine

b) Urography

If contrast urine is excreted, urography offers largely the same diagnostic possibilities as pyelography, but, in addition, information on the function of the kidney. If a complete filling of the renal pelvis is desired, one can inject contrast medium repeatedly until the renal pelvis flows over into the ureter or it can be secured by postural change *i.e.* prone position, as above (see Fig. 195). Ureteric compression is unnecessary and often contraindicated. The diuresis produced by the contrast medium can, like the contrast injection for pyelography, be sufficient to convert a case of hydronephrosis from a compensated to an incompensated condition. In this connection it might be mentioned that in the presence of intermittent hydronephrosis or suspected intermittent hydronephrosis the examination should preferably be performed during an attack of pain (Fig. 193). While the anatomic conditions may show only slight abnormality during remission, examination during an attack—if this is due to hydronephrosis—will show the renal pelvis to be widened and the contrast excretion to be impaired owing to increased intrapelvic pressure.

The examination may also be performed under such conditions as usually produce pain. If pain occurs when the patient has drunk much, one may give

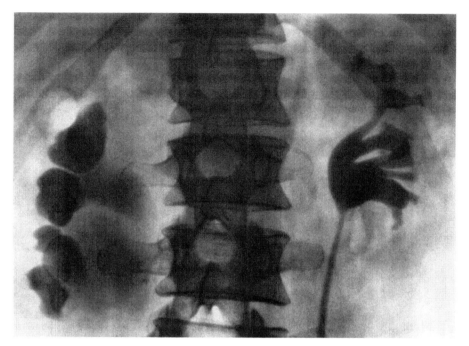

a

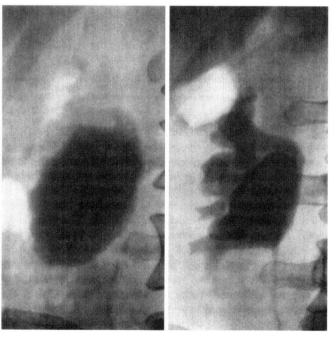

b

Fig. 189a—c. Hydronephrosis. a Urography. Dilatation of right kidney pelvis by obstructed pelviureteric junction. b Prone position. Marked narrowing of junction on contralateral side, but no dilatation. Pyeloplasty a.m. Fenger. c Postoperative check urography. Slight regression of dilatation

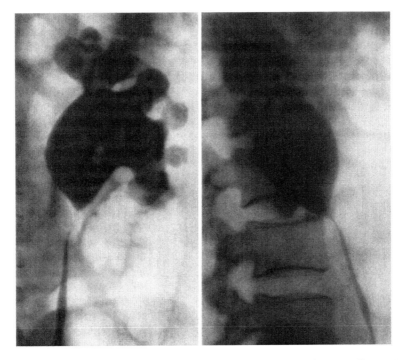

Fig. 190. Hydronephrosis through intrinsic stenosis in pelviureteric junction. Pyelography. Extrarenal pelvis. Marked atrophy of papillae. Note position of calyces and confluence in lateral view

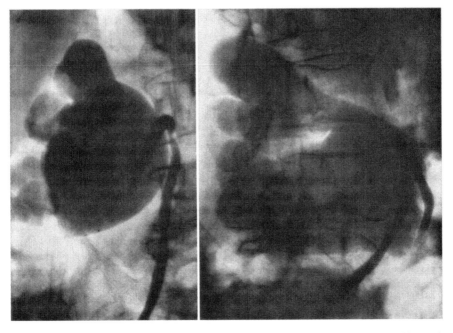

Fig. 191. Dilatation of kidney pelvis and sharp angular fixation of ureter to confluence by adhesions. No vascular anomaly

him a large amount of liquid before urography. We often give fluid by infusion or by mouth (with the patient lying, this enhancing secretion) in such cases. We call the procedure "water-loaded urography" (see chapter Urography technique). In one case described by COVINGTON & REESER (1950) consumption of 1500 cc fluid produced pain. Urography showed severe hydronephrosis, while previous examination had revealed no signs of a pathologic condition.

We have used "water-loaded urography" for evaluation of the pelviureteric junction in doubtful cases. In patients with slight to moderate narrowing, or a narrow pelviureteric junction and data suggesting intermittent hydronephrosis, we have tried to test the function in the narrow junction. The contrast medium is injected when diuresis has started after water loading. On marked diuresis the renal pelvis and the ureter and often also the narrow pelviureteric junction, will be seen to widen.

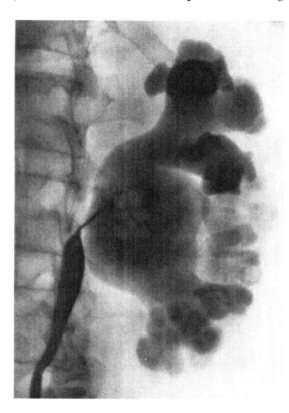

The junction can often be studied with advantage cineradiographically with an image intensifier. A narrow junction may then sometimes be seen to widen to ordinary caliber for a short time. This part of the urinary tract lends itself well to cineradiography. However, neither the normal nor pathologic behaviour of the pelviureteric junction has as yet been properly investigated.

It cannot be stressed enough that narrowing of the pelviureteric junction, as demonstrated by pyelography or urography, is often bilateral. The narrowing need not, however, be of the same severity on both sides. It may be severe on one side and only slight on the other. In the investigation of a given case, however, it is of importance, as will later be apparent, to determine whether the changes are unilateral or bilateral. This is important in the judgement of the prognosis.

Fig. 192. Hydronephrosis due to short intrinsic stenosis. Pyelography. Contrast medium injected under pressure into ureter passes through obstructed pelviureteric junction as a long jet into the confluence giving the impression of long stenosis. Multiple stones. Marked papillary atrophy

Urography offers a possibility of judging renal function, including estimation of the rate at which the renal pelvis is drained, and of the condition of the renal parenchyma. The drainage rate is influenced by the position of the patient, the concentration of the contrast medium and the size of the dose injected, the degree to which the bladder is filled etc. and must therefore be judged with caution and preferably compared with the contralateral kidney if conditions there are normal.

The state of the renal parenchyma can be crudely judged from the excretion of contrast urine; i.e. whether it is ordinary, of low density or whether excretion has ceased.

In the evaluation of the condition of the renal parenchyma the following considerations merit attention. If excretion of contrast urine is good, it indicates good, though not necessarily normal, renal function. If the excretion is impaired or not demonstrable, it may be due to temporary high intrapelvic pressure preventing secretion, the kidney recovering function as soon as the pressure has

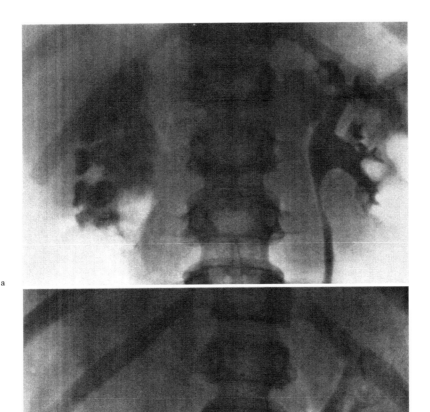

a

b

Fig. 193a and b. Intermittent hydronephrosis in 8 years old child. a Urography in compensated stage: Slight dilatation of right kidney pelvis, atrophy of papillae. b Urography during attack of pain. Kidney markedly enlarged. No excretion of contrast urine by right kidney. Nephrographic effect. Large filling defects caused by dilated calyces not filled with contrast medium

been released. But it may also depend on the renal parenchyma having suffered from protracted high intrapelvic pressure or on infection with consequent permanent loss or impairment of function. In such cases urography will not produce sufficient information for solving this problem. This should also be borne in mind on comparison of results at pre-operative and post-operative

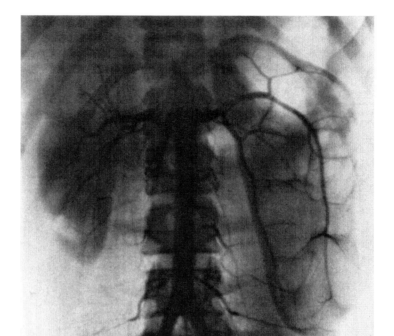

a

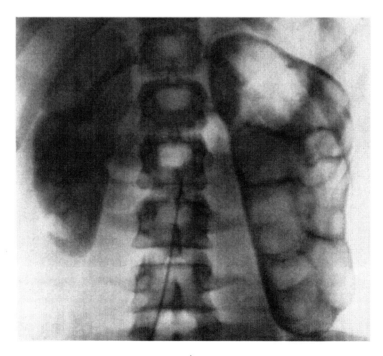

b

Fig. 194a and b. Hydronephrosis. Only very slight excretion of contrast urine in left dilated kidney pelvis. Renal angiography. Marked distension of kidney, sinus and arteries. No anomalous vessels.
a Arterial phase. b Nephrographic phase

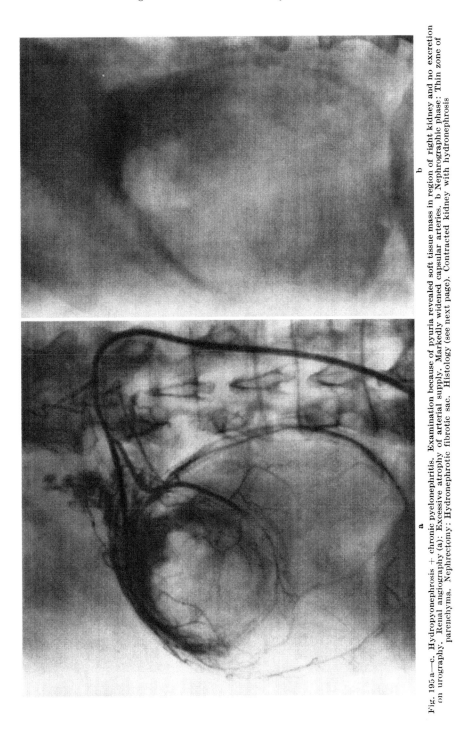

Fig. 195 a—c. Hydropyonephrosis + chronic pyelonephritis. Examination because of pyuria revealed soft tissue mass in region of right kidney and no excretion on urography. Renal angiography (a): Excessive atrophy of arterial supply. Markedly widened capsular arteries. b Nephrographic phase: Thin zone of parenchyma. Nephrectomy: Hydronephrotic fibrotic sac. Histology (see next page). Contracted kidney with hydronephrosis

examination. Urography cannot show whether cessation of function is temporary or permanent.

The literature contains many articles in which this dilemma has not been observed. Absence of excretion of contrast urine has been taken as evidence that

16*

the kidney is destroyed and nephrectomy has been performed. GIBSON (1956) for example writes: "Following nephrectomy, I was nonplussed on finding that the kidney exhibited good parenchyma of almost normal thickness." It is important

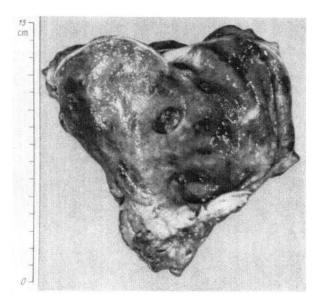

Fig. 195c. Operative specimen

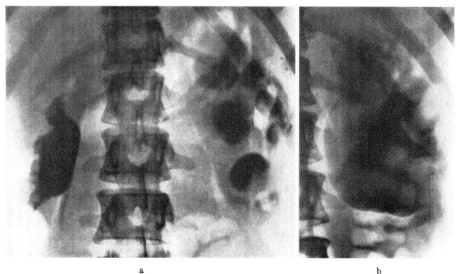

a   b

Fig. 196a—h. Hydronephrosis caused by supplementary artery. a Urography supine position. Marked dilatation of left kidney pelvis. Dorsal calyces filled. b Prone position. Severely dilated confluence filled. Renal angiography. (See next page)

to be familiar with the influence of the secretory pressure and the intrapelvic pressure on the urographic findings if erroneous diagnoses are to be avoided. Definitive evaluation of the amount of functioning parenchyma, *i.e.* potential renal function, requires renal angiography.

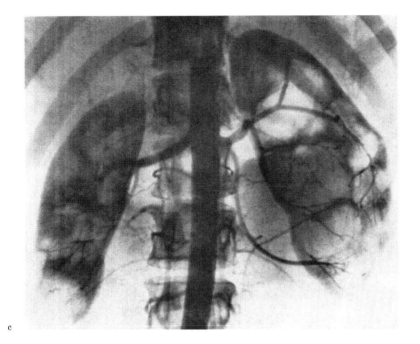

c

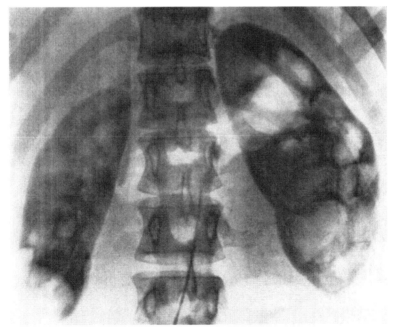

d

Fig. 196 c and d. c Arteries displaced by widened renal pelvis. Fairly good caliber of all branches. Supplementary artery to caudal pole, stretched around dilated pelvis. d Nephrographic phase. Kidney enlarged. Sinus markedly enlarged by dilated calyces. Operation with transposition of supplementary artery. (See next page)

e) Renal angiography

In the arterial phase the intrarenal arteries can be seen to be distended and displaced around the dilated renal pelvis (Fig. 194). The main renal artery and even the aorta may be pushed aside by a markedly dilated pelvis. The interlobar arteries are displaced in wide arches over the branches of the renal pelvis. The narrowing of the arterial branches is due not only to their distension but also to atrophy. It can be extremely marked (Fig. 195). The findings in the presence of atrophy and the principles of interpretation were described in chapter G XIII. Attention should be given not only to the caliber of the renal artery but also to that of its intrarenal branches and the amount of renal parenchyma, as judged in the nephrogram. Knowledge of the width of the intrarenal branches is essential, particularly because atrophy begins in the renal parenchyma and thus involves the intrarenal branches first.

The amount of functioning renal parenchyma can be assessed from the nephrogram. A generalized or local atrophy of the parenchyma may be seen and a corresponding pronounced dilatation of the renal sinus. An irregular reduction

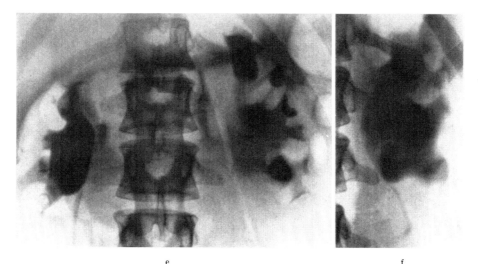

e   f

Fig. 196 e—h. Corresponding examinations. Regression of dilatation. Arteries no longer displaced. Normalization of size of kidney and sinus

in the accumulation of contrast medium or irregular hypervascularization and indentation in the surface of the kidney may be seen as a sign of pyelonephritis. Proper evaluation of the renal parenchyma requires a sufficient number of films taken during the nephrographic phase. A single film may, for example, be taken at such a moment in relation to the initial accumulation of contrast medium that no nephrographic effect can be expected.

In the venous phase the renal vein may be displaced in the same way as the renal artery.

It is obvious from what has been said that renal angiography properly performed and critically judged forms a sound basis for assessing potential kidney function. The decision whether conservative therapy should be tried in a given case or whether nephrectomy should be resorted to is facilitated to a great extent by the information obtained from renal angiography.

Renal angiography also offers a possibility of detecting supplementary arteries and veins (Figs. 196, 197). Almost half of our series of renal angiograms of patients with hydronephrosis showed multiple arteries. This frequency is consistent with that found by others (ANDERSON 1953, EDSMAN 1954). The importance of a supplementary artery in a given case of hydronephrosis varies. Sometimes its

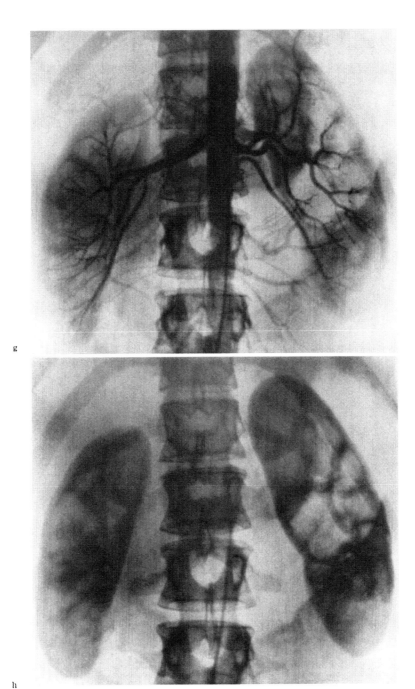

g

h

Fig. 196 g and h

course is such that the possibility of it being the cause of obstruction of the pelviureteric junction can be dismissed. In other cases the vessel may run close to the site of the narrowing. As a rule, the vessel then originates close to the main renal artery, runs in a curve corresponding to the periphery of the dilated renal pelvis, and crosses the junction. The vessel is narrow and distended, and that

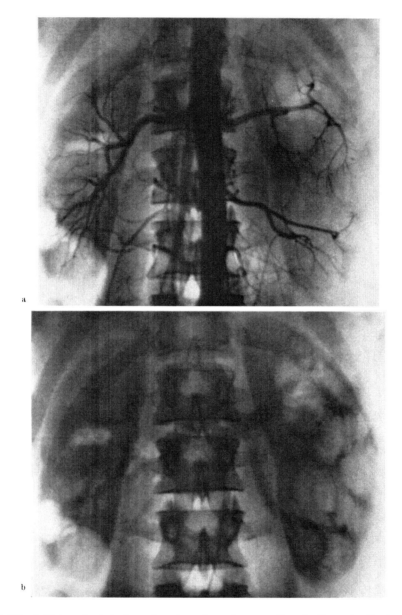

Fig. 197a—f. Hydronephrosis due to supplementary artery and corresponding vein. Urography: Scanty excretion on right side and marked dilatation of kidney pelvis. Obstruction at pelviureteric junction. a Renal angiography. Two arteries to left kidney displaced apart. b Kidney enlarged and sinus widened. Displacement of vein from caudal pole around dilated pelvis. Operation. Transposition of obstructing artery and vein. Loosening of adhesions. Urography. Marked regression of dilatation. Free flow into ureter

segment crossing the pelviureteric junction will correspond to a possible transverse filling defect observed in a previous pyelogram. The situation can be more easily judged if renal angiography is followed by urography with the patient in the same position. It is then possible to form an accurate opinion of the relationship between the artery and the renal pelvis by tracing the arteriogram onto the urogram.

Sometimes the density of the nephrogram will be decreased in that part of the renal parenchyma supplied by the distended supplementary artery.

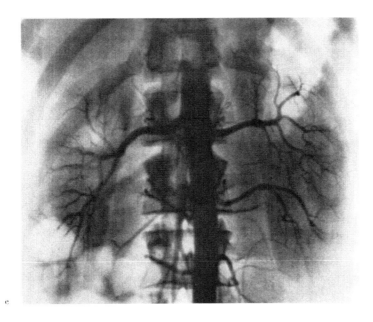

c

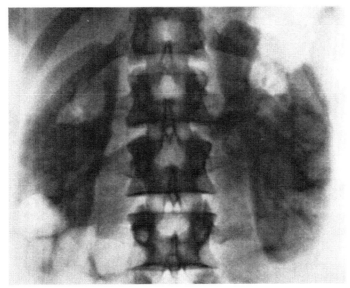

d

Fig. 197c and d. Postoperative renal angiography. No displacement of arteries or veins. Kidney size reduced. Urography. (See next page)

Even if the artery does run along the border of the dilated renal pelvis, it does not necessarily imply that the vessel is the cause of the hydronephrosis or even partly responsible. Occasionally even a distended artery may not interfere with drainage. More frequently, however, such a vessel may be a contributory factor and not the only cause. Operation reveals, in addition to such a vessel, an adhesion, for example, outside the renal pelvis and ureter as well as reduction in the lumen of the ureter. It is sometimes not possible to decide to what extent a supplementary artery is responsible for the obstruction until operation, when attempts are made to widen or empty the renal pelvis.

Supplementary veins often accompany the arteries and may contribute to such obstruction or be entirely responsible for it, while the supplementary artery may be of no importance.

If operation shows a supplementary artery to be responsible for the obstruction, it should not be severed because the operation would result in atrophy of the

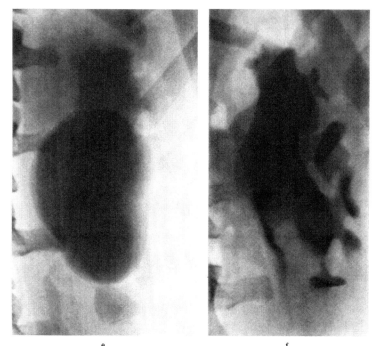

e   f
Fig. e and f. Left kidney (e) before and (f) after operation

part of the renal parenchyma supplied by it. Cases are on record in which such resection has resulted in hypertension. The vessel should be transposed in such a way as not to disturb drainage.

The adjusted course of the vessel can be checked after operation by angiography. If the operation is successful, the nephrogram will show that the renal parenchyma supplied by the supplementary artery and of decreased density when the vessel was distended before operation, is now of normal appearance.

Anomalous vessels may also obstruct drainage by compressing the distal part of the ureter. Two cases of this rare type have been described by GREENE, PRIESTLY, SIMON & HEMPSTEAD (1954).

d) Check roentgenography after operation for hydronephrosis

As mentioned, on check roentgenography to assess the result of the operation it is important that the examination be performed under the same conditions as before the operation. Any difference between the findings on pre- and post-operative urography can then be ascribed to the operation and the possibility of differences in the examination technique being responsible can be dismissed.

Judging from our experience, if any difference occurs, it does so rapidly, so that the situation seen on first complete examination after the operation may usually be regarded as the end-result.

We have also found the best anatomic results to be achieved in patients in whom the obstruction was due entirely or mainly to a vessel. The disappearance or regression of the dilatation in such cases is striking. In patients with stenosis, on the other hand, where the vessel was not responsible for the obstruction and where plastic surgery was performed, regression of dilatation after operation was less conspicuous. This discrepancy in the state of the renal pelvis in the two groups suggests that the congenital inhibitory malformation represented by fixation and stenosis is associated with congenital dilatation of the renal pelvis.

Urography and renal angiography in combination yield the best information on obstructed pelviureteric junction. Only on the actual local narrowing of the junction will pyelography give better information. This information is, however, less valuable than all the important details on morphology, actual and potential function that can be obtained from urography and angiography and direct comparison between the two sides. The supplementary information on the junction sometimes obtainable only by pyelography can only be gained at the price of considerable risk of infection.

3. Vessels and hydronephrosis

The significance of the vessels occupies a central position in the debate on the cause of hydronephrosis. This applies to supplementary arteries or ordinary branches, especially the lower polar artery. The problem can be successfully attacked roentgenologically by means of renal angiography and by comparison between the findings in this examination with those obtained on urography, at operation and on post-operative urography. The discovery that multiple arteries are common in patients with hydronephrosis and demonstrable by renal angiography might lead to an overestimation of the rôle played by the vessels in the causation of hydronephrosis. A comparison between the findings in accordance with the principles set forth above provides a better basis for proper evaluation of the rôle of the various causal factors in a given case of hydronephrosis. Our material, analyzed by BOIJSEN (1959), consists of 39 cases of hydronephrosis in which supplementary arteries were found on renal angiography, in which these supplementary arteries were verified at operation, in which the pelviureteric junction was carefully examined during operation, and in which urography was performed both before and after surgery. The cause of the obstruction was found to be due to the artery alone in 14 cases, artery + adhesions in 2, and artery + adhesion + intracanalicular stenosis in 1 case, adhesions alone in 4 cases, and stenosis alone in 11. In 17 cases out of 39 the supplementary artery was a causal factor and in 14 of them it was the only cause of the obstruction. In all the other cases *i.e.* more than half, the vessel was in no way responsible. In all of the cases in which the vessel was a causal factor it ran ventrally to the renal pelvis. The supplementary artery regularly arose within 40 mm of the origin of the main renal artery from the aorta.

Criteria arguing for a supplementary artery causing hydronephrosis are as follows: the artery runs in caudolateral direction to the lower pole of the kidney and is displaced in a curve with the convexity facing caudally; the artery arises within 40 mm of the main artery. In the absence of any deformity of the contralateral pelviureteric junction, the vessel may be the cause of obstruction. Other-

wise it is probable that the obstruction by the vessel is only secondary to a congenital stenosis or that the vessel has nothing to do with the stenosis. Like other
rules, this rule is not without exception.

On contemplated transposition of a vessel and check examination of the results,
renal angiography is, of course the only acceptable examination method.

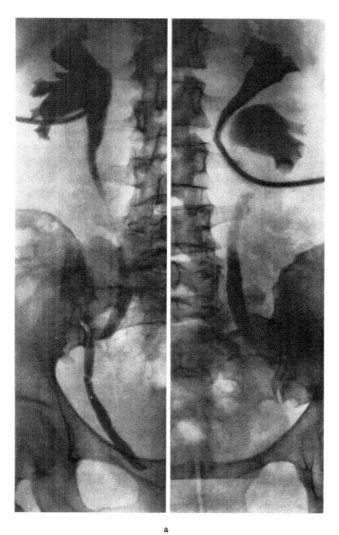

a

Fig. 198a and b. Pyelostomy and antegrade pyelography bilaterally. Amputation of cervix uteri with accidental
bilateral ligation of ureters and consequent anuria. Pyelostomy 2 days later. a Antegrade pyelography: Complete
blocking of caudal end right ureter; somewhat more cranially, also of left ureter. Operation. (See next page)

II. Dilatation of varying origin

As mentioned in the introduction, a variety of urinary diseases, particularly in
childhood, are often associated with dilatation of the urinary pathways. The
roentgen findings are largely the same except for differences due to differences in
the primary disease.

Dilatation of the urinary tract is seen, for example, in the presence of stone in
the ureter, tumour in or encroaching upon the ureter, vesical tumour involving the

ureteric orifice, inflammatory edema or shrinkage as in tuberculosis, in certain vascular anomalies such as anteureteric inferior caval vein, in lesions of the ureter, such as in association with ureterolithotomy and in narrow ureterostomies or uretero-enteroanastomoses, in post-radiotherapeutic edema or cicatricious contraction etc. (Fig. 198). Ureteric dilatation is also apt to occur in a large number of diseases obstructing flow to and emptying of the bladder. In all of these diseases unilateral or bilateral dilatation of varying severity occurs as well as temporary or permanent impairment of renal function.

Broadly speaking, the principal remarks set forth above on the investigation of cases with obstruction of the pelviureteric junction hold also for these types of dilatation. The special investigation of the local obstruction due to the primary disease is added. Renal function should be the centre of interest (Figs. 199, 200).

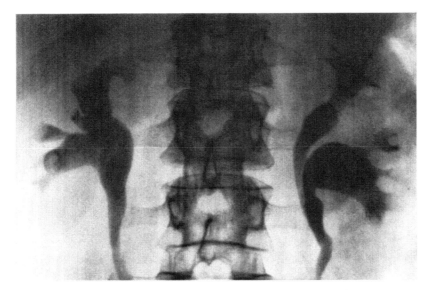

Fig. 198b. Postoperative urography. Good excretion. No dilatation

It might not be out of place again to stress the value of renal angiography in the evaluation of any impairment of renal function due to stasis and for deciding whether conservative or radical methods should be performed if surgery is contemplated.

As to the examination technique, it should be borne in mind that the examiner should try to obtain a complete filling of a dilated renal pelvis and of a dilated ureter on urography. This may be secured by utilizing the high specific gravity of the contrast urine. Thus the patient should be placed in the supine position so that the confluence will be the lowest point in the renal pelvis, and the distal part of the ureter lower than the proximal portion. If the caudal part of the ureter is obstructed, the patient may be allowed to get up and walk about for a while (one minute to an hour depending on the nature and degree of the obstruction) so that the contrast medium may sink to the obstruction (Fig. 201).

A few further details on special conditions are given below.

1. Dilatation of the urinary tract in infants

Dilatation of the urinary pathways in childhood is very often due to diseases in the bladder and/or urethra and are therefore dealt with in greater detail in Part II of this volume.

A large number of diseases in childhood can cause dilatation of the urinary tract. According to CAMPBELL (1951), more than 90% of all serious urologic diseases in childhood are due to urinary stasis in association with infection. This is the case in meningocele, for example, and other innervation disorders. Bladder neck obstruction is another common cause, as is ureterocele and urethra valve

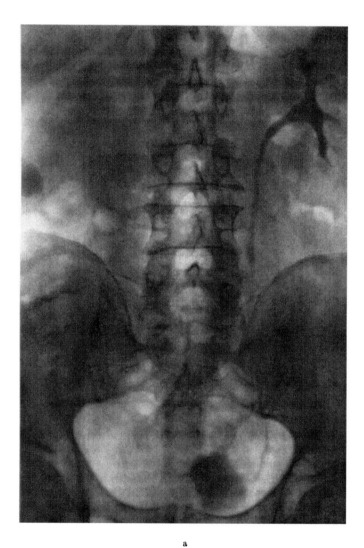

a

Fig. 199a—c. Dilatation because of obstruction of right ureter by bladder carcinoma. a Urography. Very slight excretion on right side. (Continued next page)

(see Fig. 205). In infants with a duplicated renal pelvis, which is more common in girls than in boys, and with symptoms of disease of the urinary tract ureterocele is common (see below).

If urination is difficult, the pressure in the urinary tract will be enhanced by the raised intravesical pressure, partly because the emptying of the ureter into the bladder will be obstructed and partly because an incompetent ureteric orifice does not provide a barrier against the increased intravesical pressure.

The dilatation may affect the urinary pathways on one or both sides. Unilateral dilatation should draw the examiner's attention to the possibility of the obstruction being in the distal part of that ureter, such as a ureterocele. The fact that the dilatation is present only on one side, however, does not necessarily mean that the obstruction must be prevesical. It might simply mean that only one of the ureteric orifices is incompetent.

The severity of the dilatation varies. It is often considerable with marked tortuosity of both ureters. In such cases one may speak of megaloureter. Some authors try to distinguish a type of ureteric dilatation of mainly functional origin and differing in roentgen appearance from other types of dilatation. Such distinction is, as a rule, not possible.

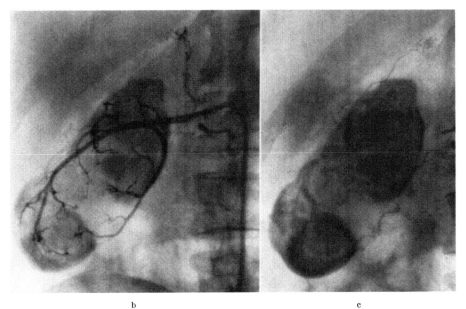

b   c

Fig. 199 b and c. Renal angiography: Marked vascular and parenchymal atrophy. Large sinus caused by dilated kidney pelvis. Irregular accumulation of contrast medium in kidney parenchyma and irregularity of kidney surface because of pyelonephritis

Roentgen examination with contrast medium is often simplest in association with urethrocystography, which should always be performed. It cannot be stressed enough that *investigation of the urinary tract in children should, as a rule, include urethrocystography because the cause of the disease is often found in the bladder and in the urethra.* In other words, the examiner should not rely too much on urography in the examination of children. On urethrocystography reflux of the contrast medium up into the ureters and renal pelves will often occur without special measures. This filling, if desired, can be facilitated by placing the patient with the head-end low. In small infants a filling can be regularly obtained by lifting them up by the feet with the head down.

Instrumental pyelography should only be resorted to in exceptional cases. The diagnostic problems can, as a rule, be solved by urethrocystography and urography, since, as mentioned above, dilatation of the urinary tract in infants is largely due to changes in the bladder and urethra (which are described in part II). Therefore as mentioned, urethrocystography is almost always a necessary supplementary examination in the investigation of urinary tract dilatation in children or at any

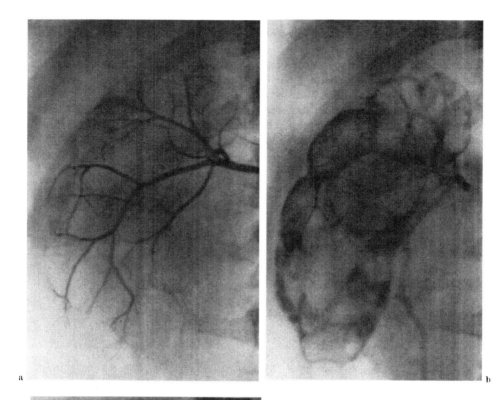

a   b

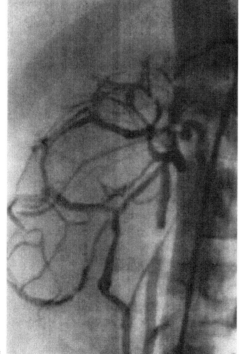

Fig. 200a—c. Hydronephrosis with complete
atrophy and renal vein thrombosis. a Renal angiography, arterial phase. Pronounced atrophy of
main renal artery and intrarenal branches. b Late
nephrographic, early venous phase: Practically
complete atrophy of parenchyma. Main venous
trunk blocked. Intrarenal veins stretched. Filling
of spermatic vein. c Selective phlebography. Main
renal vein thin and markedly irregular—re-cana-
lised thrombosed vein (patho-anatomically
verified). Venous drainage via collaterals

c

rate makes careful examination of the bladder during urography necessary. It must, however, be borne in mind that even primary ureteric changes, *e.g.* ureter valve, unilateral or bilateral, may cause hydronephrosis.

2. Dilatation in prostatic hypertrophy

Micturition difficulties in prostatic hypertrophy impair drainage of the renal pelvis and ureter. Drainage might be impaired still more by the angulation of the distal part of the ureters due to the base of the bladder being lifted by the enlarged prostatic gland. The common involvement of the urinary tract indicates roentgen examination, particularly if operation is contemplated. Experience has shown that, as far as contraindications for prostatectomy are concerned, the abnormal urogram is of direct positive value (TROELL 1935, BRAASCH & EMMETT; V. HERMANN & KRAUS; MINDER 1936, LIEDBERG 1941).

a) Plain radiography

Since most of these patients are fairly old, it may be difficult to delimit the kidneys because of the thinness of the fatty capsule. In addition, the kidneys are often low because of pulmonary emphysema and senile kyphosis and their caudal poles are then projected onto the bony pelvis. The presence of

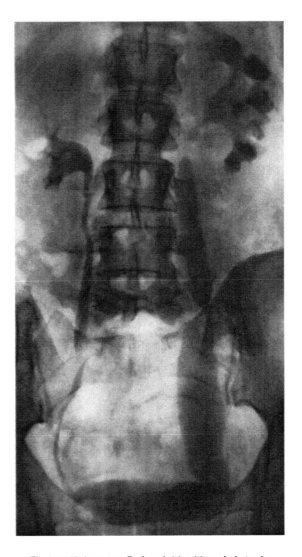

Fig. 201. Hydroureter. Pyelonephritis with marked atrophy of papillae

stone must be excluded and calcifications due to stone be distinguished from vascular calcifications so common in these age classes. If the renal pelvis is markedly dilated, it is often possible to recognize its medial part.

b) Urography

Delayed excretion and dilatation of the renal pelves and ureters are common findings in advanced prostatic hypertrophy. The patient is placed in prone position for a while to secure a filling of the whole renal pelvis and the ureters. The dilated ureters are often very tortuous and dilatation most pronounced in their distal parts. The lower ureter swings more or less sharply medially-cranially before entering the bladder.

After establishment of drainage for a month or so the roentgenographic appearance becomes more normal: dilatation becomes less marked, excretion starts earlier, contrast density increases, and the emptying time of the renal pelvis becomes shorter. The bladder and urethra are, of course, of great diagnostic interest, but changes in these parts of the urinary tract are dealt with in part II.

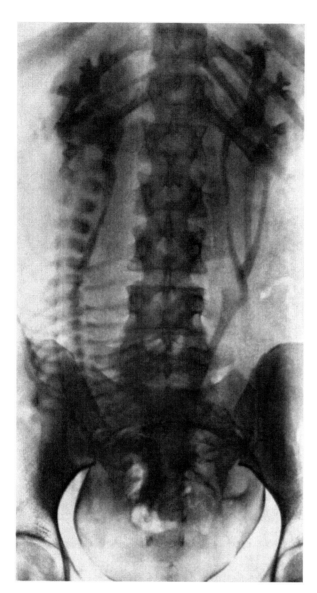

Fig. 202. Dilatation during pregnancy. Urography: Slight bilateral dilatation, somewhat more marked on the right side

3. Dilatation of the urinary tract during pregnancy

Ever since CRUVEIL-HIER (1842) at autopsy demonstrated that severe dilatation of the upper urinary tract occurs during pregnancy the phenomenon has received much attention and prompted much speculation. Pyelographic and particularly urographic investigations have proved such distension to be common. In fact, it occurs in almost every pregnant woman. Dilatation of the renal pelvis and ureter, often in association with tortuosity, thus also increase in length of the ureter, occurs in more than 90% of all cases and is somewhat more common in multiparae than in primigravidae. Dilatation on the right side is more common, where it occurs twice as often as on the left. As a rule, it is also more pronounced on the right side in bilateral cases. Dilatation involves the renal pelvis and ureter, the latter to a much less extent or not at all distally. The dilatation usually ceases at the innominate line or at the level where the ureter crosses the iliac artery. The dilatation commences in the tenth week of pregnancy in primigravidae and in the sixth week in multiparae (SENG 1929) and it is more pronounced and more frequently seen in multiparae. During the first two to four months dilatation is only moderate

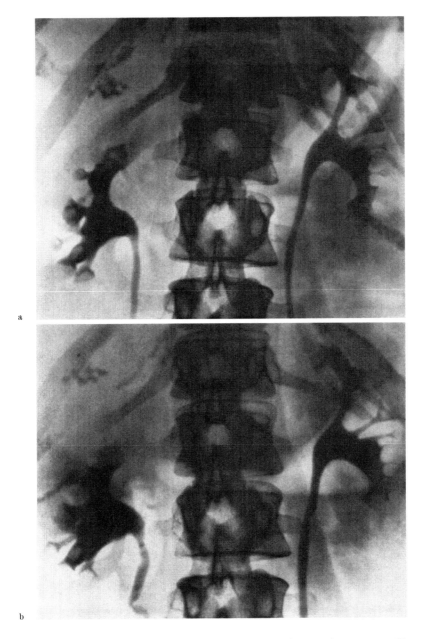

Fig. 203 a and b. Persisting slight dilatation of right kidney pelvis and ureter after pregnancy. Urography: a Before pregnancy. b Three years later, two years after uncomplicated pregnancy

but gradually becomes more pronounced with advancing pregnancy and then the ureters are often pushed laterally, even the segment in the small pelvis.

Already during the last part of pregnancy a certain regression of the dilatation may be seen (Fig. 202), and after parturition the urinary pathways rapidly recover

17*

ordinary width. Thus BRAASCH & EMMETT (1951) stated: ,,In more than half the
cases the urinary tract returns to normal within two weeks after delivary. In
almost all cases it will have returned to normal by the end of 12 weeks.'' However,
slight widening may persist for a long time, and the right renal pelvis will often
be permanently slightly widened and the upper part of the ureter may be dilated

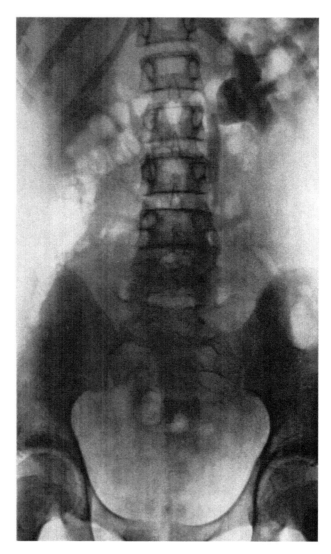

Fig. 204. Dilatation of urinary tract of same type as in pregnancy. Dilatation due to large ovarian dermoid cyst
without hormonal disorder

for the rest of life (OLLE OLSSON 1956) (Fig. 203). This might explain the majority
of cases with slight dilatation in which the right renal pelvis is, as a rule, slightly
wider than the left. Most conspicuous is the frequently persisting slight dilatation
of the right ureter in the part cranial to the crossing of the iliac artery. In cases
with such dilatation fixation to the artery may obviously readily cause dilatation
of a ureter with laxity of its wall. If pregnancy has been complicated by severe
pyelitis, the widening may persist for a long time (CRABTREE, PRATHER & PRIEN

1937, PUHL & JACOBI 1932, CONTIADES 1937). It may also be permanent (BRAASCH & MUSSEY 1945).

Opinions have differed from one period to another on the cause of the dilatation. Thus, in the beginning it was explained on purely mechanical grounds it being supposed that the dilatation was due to pressure of the enlarged uterus against the ureters on their way across the bony pelvis. With increasing knowledge of hormones attempts were made to explain the dilatation on purely hormonal grounds and, on the basis of experiments on mice and monkeys, to ascribe the dilatation entirely to a hormonal effect. It is, however, difficult to explain why the pelvic parts of the ureter are not dilated and why dilatation is more common on the right side. Another point arguing against the hormone theory as the only explanation is that in patients receiving oestrogen therapy—thus not pregnant—the ureter does not become dilated and that no such dilatation is seen in quadrupeds (KEATES 1954). In addition, dilatation of similar type may be seen in tumour of the small pelvis without oestrogen production (Fig. 204). A mechanical factor is undoubtedly mainly responsible. On the other hand I have observed that in low ureteric stone in gravidae a resulting dilatation of the ureter is much more marked also in the distal part of the ureter than in non-pregnant women. A certain laxity of the ureteric wall is undoubtedly present and in fact responsible for the severity of dilatation.

BAKER & LEWIS (1935) offer a simple explanation for the fact that distension is more frequently seen on the right side. In a post mortem study of a pregnant woman they noticed that the sigmoid colon acted as a pressure absorber in that it absorbed most of the pressure that would otherwise be exerted on the left ureter by the enlarged uterus. With this in mind they studied pregnant women with contrast enema, and the findings they made suggested not only that the colon functions as a pressure absorber and thereby protects the left ureter, but that it is also responsible for the so-called physiologic dextroposition of the pregnant uterus, which exerts a strong pressure against the right ureter. If the ureteric dilatation developing during pregnancy with decreased tonus of the ureter does persist to a certain extent for the rest of life, there is reason to give more attention to this problem in view of the risks it might imply.

There is, however, also reason to warn against unnecessary roentgen examination of these factors or complete investigation of other urinary tract disease during pregnancy. This restriction is dictated by the amount of radiation necessary for proper examination of a pregnant woman and the large amount of secondary radiation from the uterus to the ovaries.

4. Local dilatation of the urinary tract

A widening of a single calyx or a group of calyces is called hydrocalicosis. It is due to a process obstructing the lumen of a branch or a stem of a calyx (Fig. 205). Corresponding parts of the renal pelvis are widened and the papillae are flattened. The process is often associated with marked atrophy of the papilla, which enlarges the cavity filled with contrast medium.

Hydrocalicosis is thus always secondary to a pathologic lesion. A stone wedged in a calyceal stem, narrowing of an already narrow part of the renal pelvis by inflammatory edema or contraction such as in tuberculosis etc. is the cause of hydrocalicosis. The roentgen changes in this condition and its differential diagnosis are therefore discussed together with the fundamental diseases.

As described under the sub-heading "calyces" in chapter F hydrocalicosis has been regarded as a disease *sui generis*, an assumption void of supportive evidence.

5. Dilatation of the urinary tract in double renal pelvis

The conditions capable of causing a dilatation of the urinary tract and described above can also cause dilatation of one of the renal pelves of a duplicated kidney.

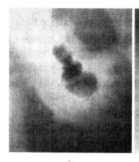
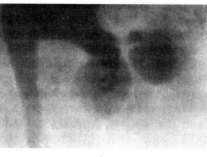
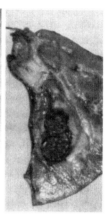

Fig. 205a—c. ¡Plain radiography. a Stones in caudal part of left kidney. b Urography: Stone obstructs flow from caudal calyces, which are severely dilated and corresponding papillae are atrophic. c Operative specimen. Polar nephrectomy

c

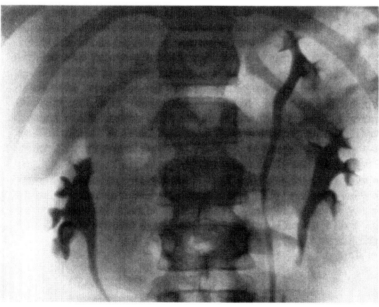
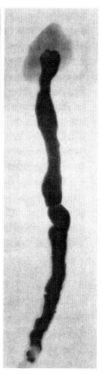

a

Fig. 206a and b. Dilatation of cranial pelvis in double kidney. Ureterocele right. a Urography. Double kidney on left side, single kidney pelvis on right side, but position of pelvis within kidney with large cranial pole definitely argues for presence of another dilated pelvis. Extirpation of cranial pole of kidney and widened ureter. b Pyelogram of specimen

b

The diagnostic problems are the same as those described above for kidneys with a single pelvis. However, this anomaly offers certain diagnostic difficulties. This is the case when the dilatation is due to an ectopic orifice of one of the ureters and in all cases in which a filling is obtained of only one of the pelves on urography.

It is nearly always the renal pelvis belonging to the cranial kidney which is problematic, and the examination is usually indicated by urinary incontinence.

The purpose of the examination is to demonstrate whether a double kidney is present. If excretion of contrast medium can be demonstrated in both pelves in the double kidney, the diagnosis is, of course, simple. As a rule, however, stasis in the upper renal pelvis has existed for such a long time that no excretion will be seen in this part. In some of these cases plain radiography and excretion urography will show the shape of the kidney and of the renal pelvis to be such as to indicate

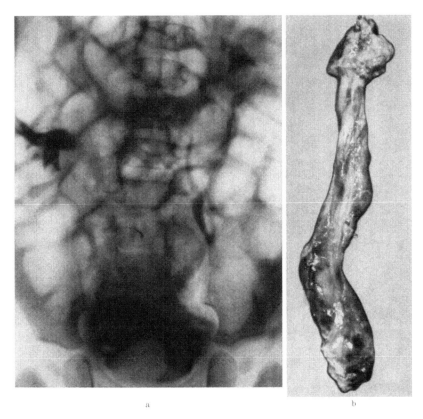

Fig. 207 a and b. Dilatation of cranial kidney pelvis in double kidney due to ureterocele. a Urography: Displacement of contrast filled kidney pelvis in right kidney due to marked dilatation of pelvis to cranial part of kidney in which no excretion takes place. Ureterocele in bladder. b Operative specimen

the existence of a second renal pelvis (Fig. 206). Sometimes the combined findings in plain radiography and urography permit a firm diagnosis, since it may show a large cranial renal pole with a long distance between the outline of the pole and the cranial calyx. The cranial part of the renal pelvis of the lower kidney may then be compressed and flattened.

In some of these cases, especially in adults, differentiation from tumour and cyst may be difficult. Despite dilatation of a cranial renal pelvis, which can originally be very small, the diagnosis may sometimes be difficult if the renal pole is only slightly enlarged and the contrast filled renal pelvis of ordinary shape.

Renal angiography may be valuable. In the nephrogram atrophy of the renal parenchyma will be seen in the area corresponding to the dilated renal pelvis (ECKERBOM & LILJEQUIST 1952, IDBOHRN & SJÖSTEDT 1954) (Fig. 208). In some

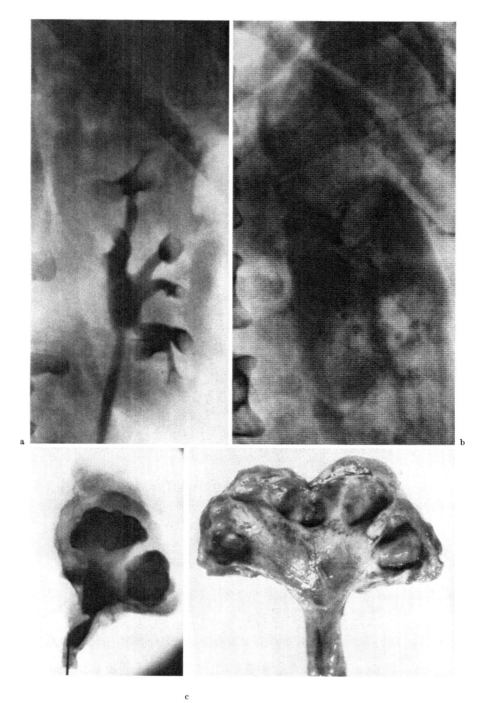

c

Fig. 208a—c. Double kidney pelvis with dilatation of cranial pelvis and atrophy of corresponding parenchyma. Woman, age 36 years, with incontinence after third delivery. a Urography: Slight malrotation of left kidney. Cranial calyces slightly flattened and above them small space-occupying process, probably dilated cranial part of double kidney pelvis. b Renal angiography. Nephrographic phase: Cranial pole has markedly widened sinus surrounded by thin rim of parenchyma—hydronephrosis cranial kidney pelvis with pronounced parenchymal atrophy. The ureter to this kidney pelvis was found to open ectopically in the urethra. Partial nephrectomy. c Specimen (pyelography and photo)

of these cases a ureterocele can be found at urography (Fig. 207). If roentgen examination has given reason to suspect a double renal pelvis with hydronephrosis of the cranial pelvis, a thorough search must be made for a ureter with an ectopic orifice. The ectopic ureter often has a ureterocele extending down into the bladder neck and posterior urethra. In a monograph ERICSSON (1954) described 20 cases of ureterocele. In 14 of them the orifice was ectopic. As to ureterocele, see chapter V. a.

O. Backflow

The backflow or reflux phenomenon has received much space in the literature and has been the subject of experimental, anatomic and clinical investigations. In some of the clinical studies its importance from the points of view discussed has undoubtedly been over-rated. The phenomenon is of particular interest from a purely roentgen-diagnostic point of view and here it will be discussed only from this angle.

The reflux phenomenon is due to leakage of contrast medium in the proximal part of the renal pelvis during pyelography and urography. The refluxes may be tentatively divided into the following groups.

1. Reflux into renal parenchyma, such as tubular reflux and interstitial reflux varying in severity up to subcapsular reflux.

2. Reflux into blood stream, so-called pyelovenous reflux.

3. Reflux into lymphatics.

4. Reflux into sinus with sub-groups fornix reflux, peripelvic reflux, perirenal reflux and reflux further into the retroperitoneal space.

These groups sometimes occur in combination and often represent different stages of one and the same sequence of events.

The reflux phenomenon was first observed by anatomists in association with the production of casts of the renal pelvis. They found that fluid injected into the ureter escaped through the renal vein.

However, the phenomenon did not rouse wide interest until after the advent of pyelography, when these anatomic experiments were reproduced clinically. But many years elapsed after the introduction of pyelography before the phenomenon received systematic attention. HINMAN & LEE-BROWN (1924) and FUCHS (1925) studied the phenomenon anatomically, experimentally, and to a certain extent clinically. In recent years reflux in association with urography (OLLE OLSSON 1948) has received wide attention. Interest has been focused mainly on reflux to the blood stream, *i.e.* pyelovenous backflow.

It is generally agreed that reflux is due to a rupture of the fornix of one or more calyces with overflow of the renal pelvic contents into the sinus and then into the perivascular spaces, which extend from the main part of the sinus into the renal parenchyma. When the extravasate dissects along veins in this stage, ruptures occur in the walls of the veins with passage of contrast medium into their lumina. Such ruptures readily occur when the pressure in the veins is low, while relatively high pressure in the veins tends to prevent reflux (MINDER 1930).

On the basis of autopsy studies and of certain animal experiments far-reaching conclusions have been drawn and accepted as holding for man. It was presumed that experiments on the above mentioned material furnished sufficient evidence to attach clinical significance to backflow with regard to features of the pathophysiology of hydronephrosis, for example, as well as to most accidents in retrograde pyelography. It must be observed that when definite and far-reaching assertions were made in this respect, they were not supported by a single correlated clinical observation. A perusal of the literature shows that the term pyelovenous backflow has been used for practically any extravasation beyound the border of the renal pelvis.

From a roentgen-diagnostic point of view it is important to remember that refluxes can occur in association with both pyelography and urography. The majority of publications on reflux deal with pyelography, and many authors claim that reflux is observed only in association with pyelography. A large monograph on reflux during urography (OLLE OLSSON 1948) has, however, shown that the phenomenon, although frequently in early stages only, is not uncommon even during this type of examination.

The roentgen findings in the various types of reflux are outlined below.

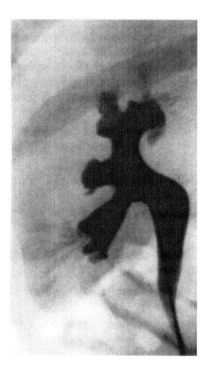

Fig. 209. Tubular and tubulo-interstitial backflow in kidney poles. Small fornical extravasations medial part, cranial calyx and caudal part of middle calyx

I. Tubular backflow

(Fig. 209; see also Fig. 211)

From the middle of a calyx a fairly homogeneous wedge-shaped area of increased density is seen to extend out into the corresponding papilla, widening towards the cortex. Sometimes the increased density is streaky with the streaks converging towards the calyx. This type of backflow is due to contrast medium from the renal pelvis flowing into the collecting tubules, which are thus more or less filled with contrast medium. These changes can be observed as a streaky accumulation of contrast medium in a large portion of the kidney e.g. a renal pole or a single pyramid, and continue right out to the periphery of the kidney, sometimes involving large portions of the kidney (KÖHLER 1953). When it involves an entire pyramid or more than one pyramid, it is, in my opinion, not always due to canalicular backflow but to contrast medium situated interstitially, a tubulo-interstitial backflow. Sometimes the contrast medium in this type of reflux during pyelography is forced through the renal parenchyma out into the subcapsular space, where it spreads to a varying degree in a thin layer.

Tubular backflow can be seen during urography as an increase in density of the papillae (see Fig. 213). It may be considerable and be seen in all or only some of the papillae. In urography it is obviously not a question of backflow but rather of stasis, the increased intrapelvic pressure occurring on ureteric compression making it difficult for the contrast medium excreted by the kidney to flow to the renal pelvis. Tubular backflow occurs readily in patients with particularly wide ducts (HINKEL 1957).

II. Reflux to blood-stream. Pyelovenous backflow

The contrast medium runs as one or several fairly broad bands via the renal hilum towards the spine. Perusal of the literature will show that most cases presented as evidence of pyelovenous backflow are not accompanied by illustrations showing contrast filling of veins. KÖHLER (1953) reported that he had never succeeded in finding a single illustration in the literature of a retrograde pyelography in which it would be possible to identify a contrast-filled renal vein. OLLE OLSSON (1948) has described a case seen during urography, which most probably shows a true contrast filling of a vein, thus an illustration of pyelovenous reflux.

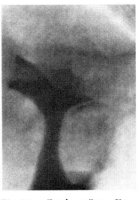

Fig. 210. Fornix reflux. Urography. Small extravasate outside calyx. Calyceal wall appears as filling defect between contrast medium inside and outside calyx

The possibility of pyelo-arterial backflow was suggested by BAUER (1957) on the basis of a very incomplete and inconclusive examination of autopsy specimens.

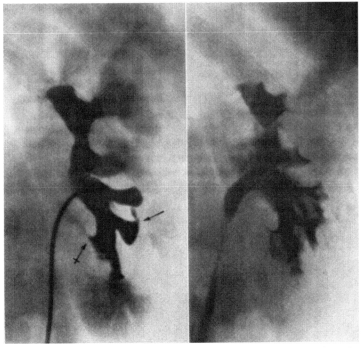

a   b

Fig. 211a and b. Backflow of different types in same patient. Blind pyelography. a Tubular and tubulo-interstitial backflow into several pyramids reaching kidney surface. At ↑ fornix rupture with small extravasate to sinus. At ⇕ fornix rupture with extravasate from sinus into perivascular space. b Later stage of examination. Tubular backflow disappeared. Widespread extravasation into sinus surrounding most calyces and branches and reaching hilum. Catheter withdrawn

III. Reflux to sinus

(Figs. 210, 211, 212, 213; see also Figs. 209, 214, 215, 216)

This is the commonest type of reflux. The extravasate is generally seen in the form of a horn-shaped projection protruding a few millimetres from the boundary of a calyx. The projection may be directed laterally towards the renal parenchyma or substantially medially, towards the sinus. The extravasate is often less

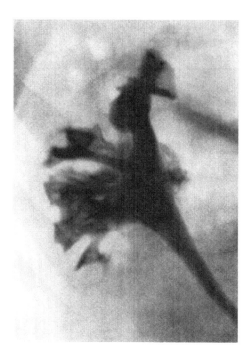

distinctly defined, at least laterally. When the calyx is studied in axial projection, the extravasate can generally be seen surrounding a part of the circumference of the calyx. In the upper or lower portion of the renal pelvis these extravasates often assume a characteristic form resembling an overflow from the boundary of the uppermost or lowermost calyx. In the majority of cases the extravasates—no matter whether they are solitary or multiple—are of this type.

In addition to the small extravasate at the calyceal border, contrast medium is often demonstrable around the stem of that calyx from which the extravasate springs. Medial to the calyx, this medium is well outlined and is separated from the contrast medium in the calyx by a nonopaque zone, about 1 mm wide. This zone corresponds to the thickness of the calyx wall. The lateral outline of the extravasated contrast urine is usually ill-defined. In some cases medium is visible as an irregular

Fig. 212. Large sinus-backflow. Blind pyelography. From ruptures at edge of most calyces contrast medium flows into sinus and out through hilum

accumulation further medially around the confluence of the pelvis or adjacent or surrounding the stem of neighbouring calyces.

In some cases with very extensive extravasation of this type the opaque medium escapes via the hilum along the ureter or around the kidney (Fig. 214).

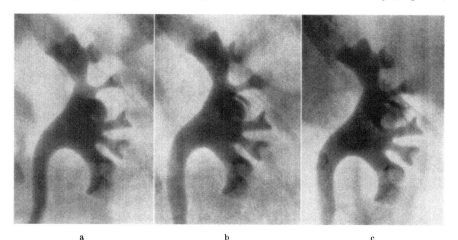

a   b   c

Fig. 213a—c. Development of sinus reflux. Urography. a 10 min. after ureteric compression. No reflux. b 14 min later. Rupture of part of fornix of middle calyx with small extravasate around cranial half of axially projected calyx. c Some minutes later. The extravasate has spread around the stems of the nearby calyces. Note increased contrast density in papillae caused by tubular stasis

It can, particularly in association with renal colic (OLLE OLSSON 1948, 1953), spread out into the retroperitoneal space and far down the ureter (Figs. 215, 216, 217).

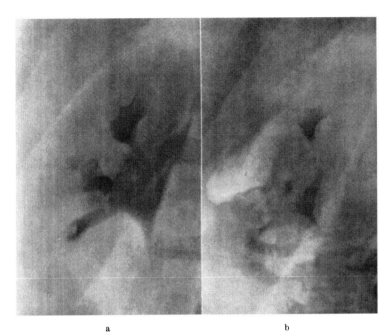

a   b

Fig. 214a and b. Large sinus-perihilar backflow. Urography. After 15 minutes ureteric compression patient felt pain in right side. a Urogram shows sinus extravasate passing through hilum to medial surface of kidney. b Release of compression. Rapid absorption of extravasate

IV. Pyelolymphatic backflow

From one or more fornices, which often show sinus reflux of varying extent spreading along the calyces, well defined, thin, somewhat irregular single or multiple streaks may be seen extending towards the renal hilum, from where they often distinctly bend along the ureter. They may be single or multiple, each appearing as a separate fine line. Their course coincides with that of lymph vessels at the hilum, as seen in anatomic preparations. Their appearance agrees well with lymphangiograms e.g. of the lymphatics of the arms or legs. An illustrative case has been described by ABESHOUSE (1934).

Pyelolymphatic extravasation has been considered a rare phenomenon. Perusal of the literature shows, however, that several of these cases said to illustrate pyelovenous contrast filling undeniably belong to the group of pyelolymphatic backflow. The frequency of these must therefore be considered higher than hitherto generally imagined.

Pyelolymphatic reflux can occur with or without chyluria.

V. Relation of reflux to bloodstream

Above, the reflux phenomenon has been considered only from a roentgendiagnostic point of view. Far-reaching conclusions have been made on observed or assumed signs of backflow in pyelograms without due attention to or proper interpretation of the findings. In addition the clinical and physiologic importance attached to backflow has not always been based on strictly logical grounds.

The changes observed on roentgen examination and described in the literature as pyelovenous reflux are, as a rule, simply signs of sinus extravasation or mostly pyelolymphatic backflow. Illustrations unequivocally showing flow of contrast medium into a vein on clinical examination are, as mentioned, rare.

In an endeavour to find a sound basis for the evaluation of the frequency and significance of the pyelovenous reflux and to elucidate the relation between the

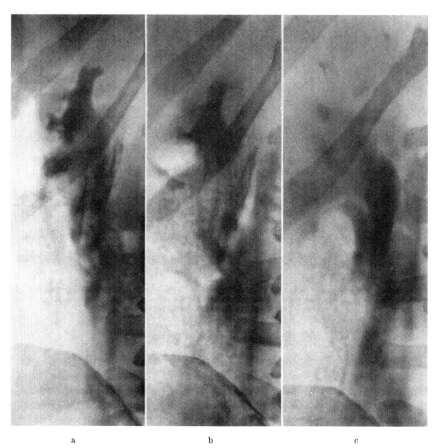

a   b   c

Fig. 215a—c. Backflow to retroperitoneal space in renal colic. Urography, acute examination during pain and 5 hours after onset of pain. No ureteric compression. a 19 minutes after contrast injection. Extravasation from calyces in middle part of kidney into sinus, through hilum and out into retroperitoneal space, along ureter. No contrast filling of dilated ureter which appears as filling defect in extravasate. b 25 minutes later. Extravasate has spread even more. c Another 5 minutes later (prone position). Filling of dilated ureter. Extravasate around ureter has begun to diminish

refluxes and the bloodstream OLLE OLSSON (1948) carried out the following experiments. Fluorescein-sodium was incorporated in the contrast medium for retrograde pyelography. A solution of this substance, when injected intravenously, gives a fluorescence detectable in the skin and mucosae when inspected under long-wave ultra-violet illumination. Thus, if fluorescein-sodium is added to the contrast medium used in association with retrograde pyelography, a fluorescence-phenomenon should be detectable, if the medium finds its way into the circulation via pyelovenous backflow. A fluorescence, easiest to inspect in the conjunctiva bulbi, was seen on intravenous injection of $^{1}/_{2}$—1 cc of 20% fluorescein-sodium solution. Fluorescein-sodium was added to the contrast medium used for instrumental pyelography of 10 patients. Multiple pyelograms were taken under fluoroscopic control with gentle application of only slight pressure. The following

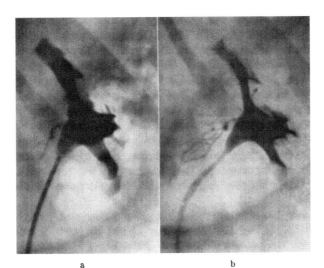

a   b

Fig. 216a and b. Pyelolymphatic backflow. Pyelography. a Rupture of fornices in middle of kidney. b Increasing filling of lymphatics

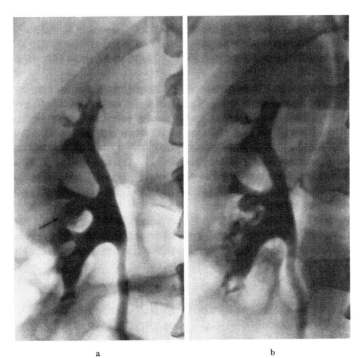

a   b

Fig. 217a and b. Development of reflux. Urography. a After 20 minutes ureteric compression. Slight extravasation at brim of middle calyx (arrow). b A few minutes later: spreading of extravasate in sinus and filling of lymphatic

observations were made: In 6 of the 10 cases no backflow could be observed in the films and no fluorescence was demonstrable. No fluorescence was seen when the films showed small sinus refluxes, 3 cases, which implies that there was no escape of the substance to the veins in this type of reflux. In 2 of these cases fluorescence was seen, but only when, after small sinus extravasations had been demonstrated, the pressure was intentionally raised abruptly. In one case the contrast fluid passed into the vein without such intentional increase in pressure. In none of these cases was contrast medium seen in the vein, but in all 3 of them sinus extravasation was pronounced. Backflow thus occurs readily on retrograde pyelography. Usually it can be avoided by the use of a proper technique. The escape is limited to a sinus reflux, but it can assume the character of a pyelovenous reflux without escape into the vein being demonstrable in the films, probably because the contrast medium is rapidly carried off by the blood. This has long been known. On unilateral pyelography contrast medium has been seen in the contralateral kidney, which must imply that the contrast medium has passed into the bloodstream and that the patient has received an intravenous injection producing excretory urograms with contrast excretion also in the other kidney.

Köhler (1953) has also examined this phenomenon and found that a pressure of 80—100 mm/Hg is, on the average, sufficient to produce reflux in normal human kidneys. Much lower values have been found by Risholm & Öbrink in an investigation in which a very small volume of albumin marked with ^{131}J was injected into the renal pelvis in association with routine cystoscopy. Immediately after the injection the ureter was blocked and the pressure was measured. The radioactivity in the blood was followed by collection of samples at short intervals and preliminary experiments showed that the radioactivity of the blood increased rapidly when the intrapelvic pressure exceeded 15—20 cm water. Since the albumin molecules are too large to pass from the renal pelvis to the bloodstream under normal conditions it is assumed that reflux may occur at this pressure in the renal pelvis.

The final evidence has been produced by anatomic examinations by Staubesand (1956). He has shown good agreement between the anatomic and the roentgen findings described above. In corrosion preparations of normal human kidneys he thus found that the presence of an open communication between the calyx and the renal sinus is always preceded by rupture of the mucosa. Sinus extravasates often flow along the calyceal wall into the sinus. They often also follow the perivascular spaces into the renal parenchyma. Then—though rarely— they enter the venous blood. More frequently the fluid emanating from the renal pelvis hugs the vessel walls.

These observations underline how important it is to use a gentle technique in the performance of pyelography and how necessary it is to perform the examination under fluoroscopic control, as mentioned in the chapter on retrograde pyelography.

VI. Frequency of reflux

The frequency of reflux varies widely with the technique used. Pyelography by the conventional technique should, as stressed above, always be performed under fluoroscopic control, if reflux is to be avoided. If this precaution is not observed, refluxes of various types will be common. In a series of pyelograms of 207 kidneys Köhler (1953) found sinus reflux in 65, pyelolymphatic in 56, pyelovenous in 1 kidney, tubular reflux in 66 and both tubular reflux and sinus reflux in 19.

During urography refluxes occur after application of ureteric compression with the exception of the type that will be described in association with reflux during acute renal colic. But then, compression must have been applied for a while, the renal pelvis must be well filled, and the pressure must have increased so that fornix rupture may occur. As a rule, the refluxes are therefore seen after prolonged compression and at the end of the compression period. During the course of an examination it is possible in very rare cases to follow the development of the reflux from one film to another and its growth from a small contrast extravasate in the edge of a calyx to a large one spreading along a calyceal stem to the adjacent calyx, then along the confluence and occasionally out through the renal hilum.

As to the frequency during urography, LINDBOM (1943) found sinus reflux in 15 cases out of 900 in which ureteric compression had been applied. OLLE OLSSON (1948) found the phenomenon in 37 out of 988 similar cases, and BOYARSKY, TAYLOR & BAYLIN (1955) gave a frequency of 2.9% in association with urography.

VII. Significance of reflux from a roentgen-diagnostic point of view

The refluxes are usually roentgen-diagnostic artefacts caused by the increased pressure in the renal pelvis produced by the method, *i.e.* injection of contrast

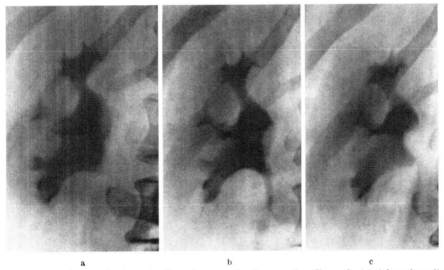

a   b   c

Fig. 218a—c. Peripelvic reflux in renal colic causing expanding tissue reaction. Urography (a) 10 days after colic. Irregular impression from hilum into medial part of confluence. Regression (b) and (c) 1 and 3 weeks later

medium via a catheter for pyelography and application of ureteric compression for urography.

In one situation, however, the roentgenologically demonstrable reflux phenomenon is part of a patho-physiologic sequence of events, namely when reflux is seen in connection with acute renal colic. Small refluxes attributable to renal colic and seen during the actual attack have been described by FUCHS (1931), HENDRIOK (1934) and LINDBOM (1943). During such attacks, however, widespread refluxes can be seen in which contrast medium, via ruptures in the fornix, continues through the sinus and renal hilum out into the retroperitoneal space, often far down along the ureter. A number of such cases have been described by OLLE OLSSON (1948 and 1953) (see Fig. 215). Cases have also been published by PERSKY & JOELSON (1954) and by SENGPIEL (1957). Features of this type of reflux are given in further detail in the chapter on ureterolithiasis.

The pathologist HAMPERL (1949) has shown that gross jelly-like masses may be seen in the fat tissue of the renal hilum and even in retroperitoneal fat tissue

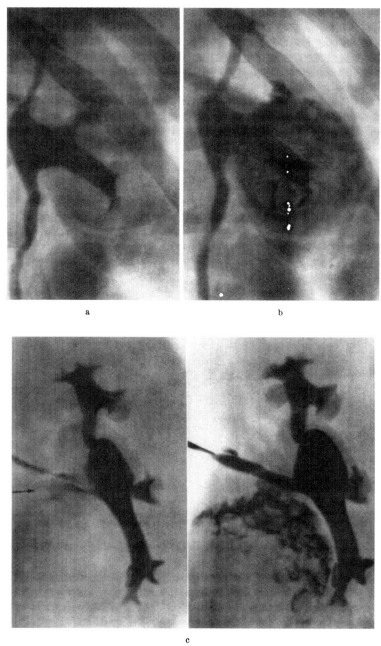

Fig. 219a—c. Backflow into a tumor. Urography. a 10 minutes after application of ureteric compression. Flattening and slight displacement of caudal branch. b 10 minutes later. From edge of cranially displaced calyx backflow into superficial part of tumour. Nephrectomy. Renal carcinoma. c Pyelograms of operative specimen. Note rupture at edge (arrow) of displaced calyx

along the ureters at post-mortem examinations of cases with urinary stasis. The spread of the jellylike mass showed that it was due to some kind of infiltration, as might be expected of a fluid substance that spares the tissue structure; it was definitely related to ruptures of the fornix. It is surprising that such changes should not have been noticed earlier by pathologists, for they are not rare. Even in patho-anatomic material refluxes are thus not uncommon.

The extravasate occurring during such a reflux can result in a tissue reaction of differential roentgen-diagnostic importance. Such a case has been described by FAJERS & IDBOHRN (1957) from our department in which urography 3 days after an attack of renal colic showed changes in the renal pelvis, and in which follow-up showed findings that could be interpreted as renal pelvic tumour but which was considered due to tissue reaction after backflow. Explorative surgery in another hospital revealed that the right kidney was embedded in firm adhesions. The hilum was edematous and was felt to contain an obscure lump the size of a hazelnut. Nephrectomy was done. Histologically wide-spread peripelvic refluxes with old haemorrhages were seen (Fig. 218). We have since seen further cases of this type.

Refluxes are also important from a diagnostic and particularly differential-diagnostic point of view. From a diagnostic point of view, those few cases might be mentioned in which contrast medium had escaped into a tumor in association with retrograde pyelography (BITSCHAI 1927, FUCHS 1930,

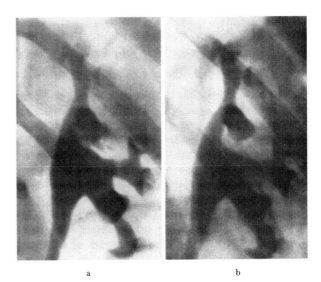

a   b

Fig. 220a and b. Healing of sinus reflux. Urography: Tuberculosis suspected. a Irregular extravasation around calyx cranial to middle of kidney. Probably backflow, but papillary destruction cannot be excluded. b 19 days later. No reflux. No pathologic changes. Edge of calyx sharp

v. ILLYÉS 1932, SCHUBERT 1933, HERRNHEISER & STRNAD 1936, MEUSER 1943) or during urography (OLLE OLSSON 1948) (Fig. 219). In another case the last mentioned author reported reflux around a small calcified space-occupying lesion.

Diagnostically, refluxes are also important, particularly in retrograde pyelography, because, if the reflux is large, small anatomic changes may escape detection. In the event of extensive backflow, pyelography is therefore unreliable.

When pyelography has been performed with thorotrast, contrast medium can have escaped into the renal tissue or renal sinus. Thorotrast residue may then remain in the tissues for the rest of life. On roentgen examination it can be seen as thin linings of single calyces or parts of the renal pelvis, the contrast lying in the sinus along the renal pelvis (SVOBODA 1954). It may also be seen as radial streaks of contrast medium running from one or more papillae out towards the periphery of the kidney.

From a differential-diagnostic point of view, refluxes are important in the presence of papillary destruction, particularly papillary ulceration in renal tuberculosis. The literature contains several reports in which a reflux was obviously interpreted as a destructive process and nephrectomy had been performed unnecessarily (OSSINSKAYA 1937, RENANDER 1939). The importance of considering

18*

fornix reflux in the differential diagnosis of papillary ulceration has been stressed (LINDBOM; OLLE OLSSON; STEINERT 1943). The differential-diagnosis is established by the following procedure: if, during the course of urography, a change is seen that may be a fornix reflux, compression is maintained, and then the reflux will develop and the contrast medium will spread out along the calyceal stem. On occasion this is not possible. The differential-diagnosis can then be established by re-examination a few days later. Experience has shown that ruptures causing refluxes rapidly close (Fig. 220).

Reflux may also be of differential-diagnostic importance in traumatic renal rupture because the roentgen findings in small ruptures are the same as in reflux. This must be kept in mind on retrograde pyelography for suspected renal rupture. Urography in the acute stage of the disease does not give rise to this differential-diagnostic difficulty because urography in the acute stage of suspected renal rupture is performed without the application of ureteric compression.

VIII. Risks associated with reflux

The most important risks from a roentgen-diagnostic point of view are those mentioned above, namely the backflow may mask anatomic changes and, secondly, it may be misinterpreted as some pathologic process. Another risk is that, as mentioned, in retrograde pyelography reflux may occur with "injection" of a large amount of contrast medium into the blood stream and consequent excretion. Retrograde pyelography is sometimes used instead of urography in order to avoid the strain placed on the kidneys by the excretion of contrast medium. In such cases the technique used for pyelography should be so gentle as not to cause reflux. CEDERLUND (1942) stressed that pyelography entails a great risk of large amounts of contrast medium being inadvertently injected into the blood-stream and POLITANO (1957) writes in a discussion of retrograde pyelography: "Obviously any substance unsuitable for intravenous use should not be used or used only with great care."

As to other risks, many authors claim that reflux is important because it favours spread of infection in the kidneys and blood-stream, introduction into the blood-stream of depressants and of other substances secreted with the urine, etc. Much of the discussion is based on more or less unfounded assumptions. It falls beyond the scope of this presentation of the roentgen-diagnosis of reflux.

P. Injury to kidney and ureter

The increasing number of traffic accidents has increased the importance of diagnosing renal injury in association with trauma to the trunk. Roentgen examination not only plays an important rôle in the diagnosis but also acts as a guide when deciding whether treatment should be active or expectant.

Opinions differ on the clinical evaluation of renal damage and particularly whether treatment should be conservative or surgical, the choice of cases for surgery and the time for such operation, some authors adopting a very active attitude, while others prefer to try conservative treatment as long as possible. Without assuming any definite attitude regarding these questions, it may be stated that the opinions of all except adherents of most active surgery base their decision to a large extent on the roentgen findings. In the discussion of roentgen examination there are two points of particular interest, namely the examination method and the time of the examination.

The first point to be decided upon is whether pyelography should be performed or not. Many consider this examination contra-indicated on the grounds that instrumentation can cause a recurrence of haemorrhage by detaching a clot and, secondly, the examination involves a risk of infection. The question then is what information can be obtained by methods not requiring instrumentation.

Concerning the time of roentgen examination, there is wide agreement that the examination should be done as soon as possible in order that the roentgen findings may be included among the data to be considered for deciding whether treatment should be conservative or active. It appears that this opinion is supported by the fact that renal damage often produces few symptoms during the first few hours and that symptoms from the urinary tract may be masked by symptoms from other organs with the result that valuable time is lost before institution of treatment of any renal lesions.

I. Classification of renal ruptures

ADAMS (1943) recognized three groups of renal ruptures: I. Contusions and its subgroups a) Without subcapsular haematoma and b) With subcapsular haematoma. II. Fracture with subgroups a) Incomplete and b) Complete and III. Tears of the renal vessels or ureter. The third type is usually associated with other severe renal injuries but may occur alone. To the last mentioned injuries may be added post-traumatic infarction of the kidney, which may occur because of a secondary thrombosis. This consequence of trauma has received increased theoretic interest since the publication of cases in which vascular spasm was assumed to be the cause of the infarcts, and by the work of TRUETA, BARCLAY, DANIEL, FRANKLIN & PRICHARD (1947), (compilation by LYNCH and LARGE 1951).

This classification is based on clinical pathologic findings. Classifications based partly on roentgen findings are also available. McKAY, BAIRD & LYNCH (1949) thus distinguished three types of renal rupture. Group I. Patients with intact pyelograms and clear renal and psoas shadows and not requiring exploration. Group II. Patients with any rupture of the renal collecting system or loss of renal and psoas shadows, these to be explored in 72 hours. Group III. Those patients in unresponsive or recurring shock due to rupture of the renal vascular pedicle, these to be operated on as an immediate life-saving procedure.

HODGES, GILBERT & SCOTT (1951) recommend the following classification: I. Minor injuries, II. Major injuries, III. Critical injuries. The urographic or pyelographic demonstration that the pelvis and calyceal system are intact is the greatest single criterion for placing injuries in the minor group. To the second group are assigned cases with evidence of urinary extravasation in the retrograde pyelogram. Since perirenal haematoma belongs to this group plain radiography is of importance for classification. In the group "critical injuries" urography is necessary only to check that the kidney on the other side is not damaged. Like all other classifications, this one is incomplete in so far as there may be evidence of extravasation without the injury being classified as major injury.

The renal rupture may vary from a small capsular rupture or a medullary scratch to small or large fractures of the renal parenchyma and further to total contusion of the kidney or laceration of the renal pedicle. In capsular damage, possibly in association with parenchymal damage, a perirenal haematoma will develop and may enclose the entire kidney or it may be localized around the actual rupture of the capsule. If the capsule is intact, the haematoma may be intracapsular.

The changes that can be demonstrated roentgenographically are thus a change in the bed of the kidney and a change in the size, shape and position of the kidney, and pyelography and urography will show any extravasation of contrast medium and patency of ureter and urography also the state of renal function.

II. Plain radiography

The discussion of roentgen examination of patients with renal injury has been centered mainly on the question whether pyelography or urography is preferable, and it appears that the valuable information available from plain radiography has not received the attention it deserves. The examination is usually made in the acute stage with the patient unprepared, so that intestinal contents may make it difficult to judge the anatomy of the retroperitoneal space. Trauma may have caused local or generalized meteorism, which may make the analysis still more difficult.

A reflex skoliosis of the spine with the concavity facing the injured side is sometimes present. This must be remembered in the evaluation of the edge of the psoas muscle. A blurring of the edge of the psoas muscle in a case with trauma to the trunk is frequently referred to as a sign of kidney rupture. Even slight skoliosis, true or due to the position of the patient on the examination table, may, however, cause the sharp outline of the psoas muscle to disappear, and this should then not be interpreted as being due to bleeding or edema.

Injury to the tissue around the kidney causes changes that may be misinterpreted as renal damage. Laceration of muscles can, for example, cause perirenal haematoma and displace the kidney. A perirenal haematoma may be so local as to simulate a local bulge in the outline of the kidney. In the presence of a large perirenal haematoma the retroperitoneal soft tissue anatomy is blurred and an increased density is seen. The kidney can be displaced in different ways depending on the site and longest diameter of the haematoma. The kidney is displaced easiest by a haematoma situated dorsally, where the capsular space is broadest and loosest so that the kidney will be displaced ventrally. This increases the object—film distance and thereby produces an enlargement of the image of the kidney in the film. This should not be interpreted as a true enlargement of the kidney owing to intracapsular haemorrhage.

If the haematoma is intrarenal, the kidney will be enlarged and plump but well defined.

Plain radiography will often also show fractures of one or more of the lower ribs or of the transverse process of one or more lumbar vertebrae. If a transverse process is fractured, a haematoma will often be seen in the psoas muscle. The lateral edge of the muscle is then well defined in its cranial part, for instance, whereas further down a soft tissue density is seen due to haematoma. The lower renal pole may then be displaced laterally by the haematoma, and urography is then usually necessary to demonstrate whether the kidney is intact.

III. Urography and pyelography

If plain radiography is possible, urography is usually also possible. In recent years more and more authors have realized the diagnostic possibilities of urography in renal injury. It is also now widely believed that urography should be given preference and retrograde pyelography should only be resorted to if information obtained by urography is uncertain (LJUNGGREN 1936). Critical voices have, however, also been raised against urography. In 1951 HODGES, GILBERT & SCOTT

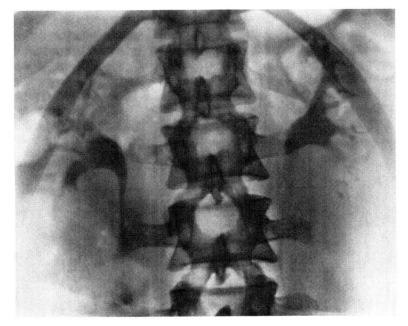

a

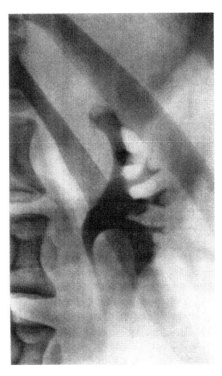

b

Fig. 221a and b. Kidney rupture, caudal pole. Traffic accident. Haematuria. a Urography: Left kidney enlarged; retroperitoneal haematoma; good excretion of contrast medium and ureter filled. Rupture of lower calyces with slight extravasation of contrast urine. Blood clot in caudal branch. Conservative treatment. b Urography 2 years later: Complete recovery

wrote: "Moreover, it has become increasingly apparent in this study that excretory urography, while extremely valuable in demonstrating the presence of a normally functioning kidney on the opposite side, is frequently unsatisfactory in delineating the extent of injury on the affected side." In my opinion, their remarks hold only for exceptional cases. Urography will, as a rule, give sufficient information to judge the situation.

An important advantage of urography is that it shows whether the contra-lateral kidney is functioning. Cases are on record in which nephrectomy for renal rupture has been performed on patients with only one kidney.

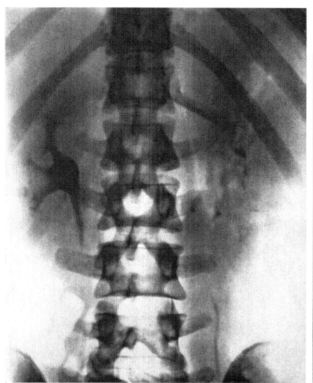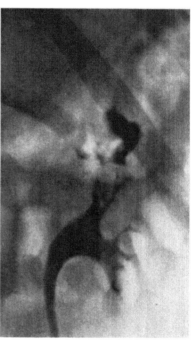

a   b

Fig. 222a and b. Kidney rupture with intra- and extrarenal haematoma. Car accident. Haematuria. a Uro-graphy: Enlargement left kidney; impaired excretion; deformity of kidney pelvis. Ureter normal. Conservative treatment. b 6 weeks later. Marked regression of kidney size. Contrast excretion fairly good. Ruptured cranial branch and contrast-filled irregular cavity in cranial pole

The urographic findings in renal injury may be divided into two groups: 1. excretion is observed, 2. no excretion is observed. In the latter group, which contains few of the cases of renal rupture, a clot may block excretion or the kidney may be so severely damaged as not to function. It must be stressed in this connexion that there is no evidence of the possibility of shock or reflex anuria being responsible for non-functioning of only one of the kidneys. If urography shows absence of function on one side only, pyelography may be resorted to, it being of great importance to check whether the ureter has been torn. Laceration will cause extravasation of contrast medium and the localization and degree of rupture can be estimated. Pyelography in cases with suspected renal damage should always be performed under fluoroscopic control in order to avoid refluxes simulating a traumatic rupture.

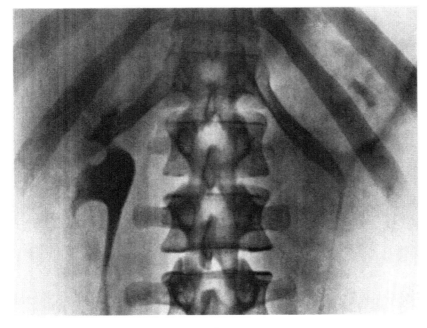

a

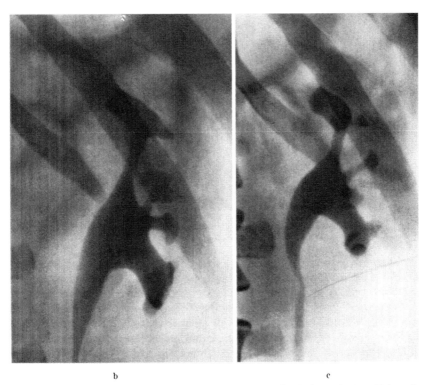

b   c

Fig. 223a—c. Fall from horse. Shock. Haematuria. Roentgen examination during acute stage: Retroperitonea haematoma to the left. a Urography: Contrast excretion on left side. Incomplete filling, compression of kidney pelvis. No extravasation. Ureter normal. b 17 days later: Normal excretion. No rupture. Kidney flattened by retroperitoneal residual haematoma. c 1¹/₂ years later: Normal

In the former group, with excretion during urography, the situation can usually be cleared up without pyelography. Only in those very few cases in which no contrast medium passes into the ureter need pyelography be employed to check the possibility of ureteric rupture. In all other cases urography will show the extent of the damage (Figs. 221, 222, 223). Special attention should be given to those films taken soon after the injection of contrast medium, in order to find out which parts of the kidney are excreting urine. Sometimes excretion will be seen in only one or a few calyces, while the rest of the renal pelvis contains no contrast medium. Gradually a filling

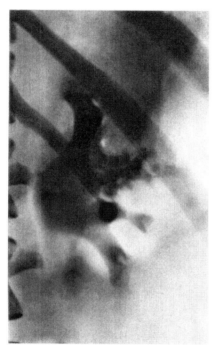 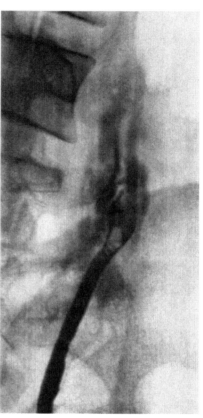

Fig. 224   Fig. 225

Fig. 224. Kidney fracture. Trauma against back (fall from bar during gymnastics). Haematuria. Urograpny: 33 minutes after injection of contrast medium. No ureteric compression. Straight rupture from middle calyx to surface. Perirenal haematoma. Contrast urine escapes through rupture and spreads in sinus along adjacent parts of kidney pelvis as in sinus backflow

Fig. 225. Rupture of ureter by balloon catheter used for study of kidney pelvis in pyelography. Extravasation of contrast medium around ruptured ureter. Blood clots in ureter

will be obtained also of the lacerated parts of the renal pelvis and contrast medium will flow out into the renal tissue or around the kidney. Compression caused by bleeding or edema may also be demonstrated. Calyces into which urine is excreted may be dilated because of compression of the corresponding branch or by blockage of the branch by a blood clot. Small ruptures appear as small extravasates of contrast medium along one or more calyces. They may be of the same appearance as a sinus reflux (Fig. 224). In these cases such an extravasation cannot be due to reflux because urography is, of course, done without ureteric compression being applied.

If the patient is not operated upon, urography may be performed again a few days later and then slight ureteric compression may possibly be applied to obtain a better filling of the renal pelvis for a more detailed study of its morphology. On such check examination it is striking to note how soon a rupture closes.

In children, in whom trauma is common and in whom renal tumours are often symptomless and therefore liable to assume considerable proportions, the injury

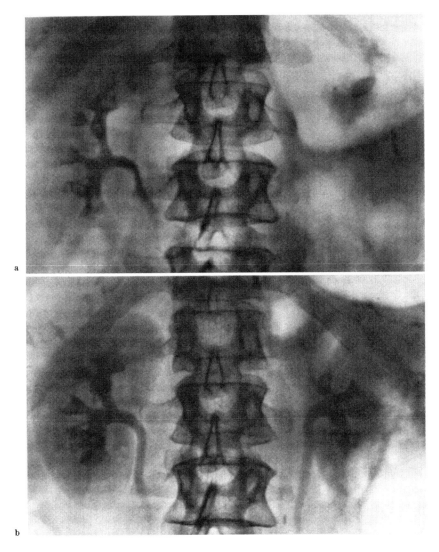

a

b

Fig. 226a and b. Kidney rupture. Fall against hard edge. Haematuria. Roentgen examination during acute stage. Left kidney enlarged, ill defined. Roentgen anatomy of retroperitoneal space deranged. Kidney rupture with perirenal haematoma. a Urography: Large extravasation in cranial part left kidney. Ureter filled (b) 5 months later. Small kidney. Cranial branch changed into a small irregular sprout.—Residuum after kidney rupture

may occur in a kidney with a tumour. LEVANT & FELDMAN (1952) have described two cases of embryoblastoma, which had been symptomless and were discovered on rupture in association with trauma.

The renal pelvis may also be ruptured during instrumental examination. It may be perforated by a catheter. STRNAD (1936) has shown that a simple, ordinary ureteric catheter can perforate the renal pelvis and then usually at the fornix of the cranial calyx (compare Fig. 175 in chapter K). Check examination of such a case with consequent injection of contrast medium subcapsularly showed that the rupture healed very soon (KÖHLER 1953).

Injection of contrast medium can rupture a pathologically changed renal pelvis (BARETZ 1936). The rupture in connexion with the reflux or backflow phenomenon will not be discussed here (see chapter O).

More or less acute perforation may also be produced by decubital lesions caused by stone in the renal pelvis, and spontaneous rupture of the renal pelvis has also been described (RENANDER 1941). Concrements in a calyx can perforate the renal parenchyma and pass directly out into the perirenal space. One case of bilateral perforation has been described by MARQUART (1958).

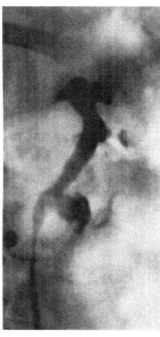

Ureteric injury may occur in association with renal lesion but also alone and then usually following instrumental examination. The diagnosis is based on the disturbed flow through the ureter and on the development of extravasation and offers the same problems as those described above in injury to the renal pelvis and upper ureter. Inflation of the balloon of Dourmashkin's special catheter can rupture the ureter (Fig. 225).

As mentioned, renal ruptures show excellent healing tendencies and check examination of small fresh ruptures of the reflux type will often show that they have closed within a few days. Even severe ruptures show a strong tendency to heal. On review of 54 cases of renal injury several years after the accident STEINBOCK (1948) found that the shape of the renal pelvis was normal in 40; only in 2 was the kidney functionless, one had a hydronephrosis and the other a pyenephrosis with stone. Seven cases showed small changes of the renal pelvis due to scar formation. On the

Fig. 227. Old kidney rupture. Urography. Late result of rupture of caudal pole

other hand, on review of 13 patients a varying interval after trauma to the region of kidney, COLSTON & BAKER (1937) found marked pathologic changes in the kidney or in the perirenal tissue. They claim traumatization of the kidney and haematuria to indicate immediate examination and follow-up at regular intervals to avoid any late complications. Old kidney ruptures may show different degrees of deformation of the kidney pelvis on check examination, mainly depending on extent and localization of the damage (Figs. 226, 227). An uncommon late complication is the development of a large intrarenal cyst. I have seen a case in which a cyst the size of a child's head and containing clear fluid developed within three months of trauma.

During follow-up after renal trauma *renal angiography* may be helpful. We have had a case in our department in which the kidney was fractured and a large fragment of the kidney was separated off but with its vessel of supply intact.

IV. Perirenal haematoma

Haemorrhage around the kidney may develop in association with trauma or it may be spontaneous. A possible cause of retroperitoneal haematoma to be borne in mind is perforation of a vessel by a needle or catheter during the increasingly common arterial and venous puncture and catheterization for different purposes.

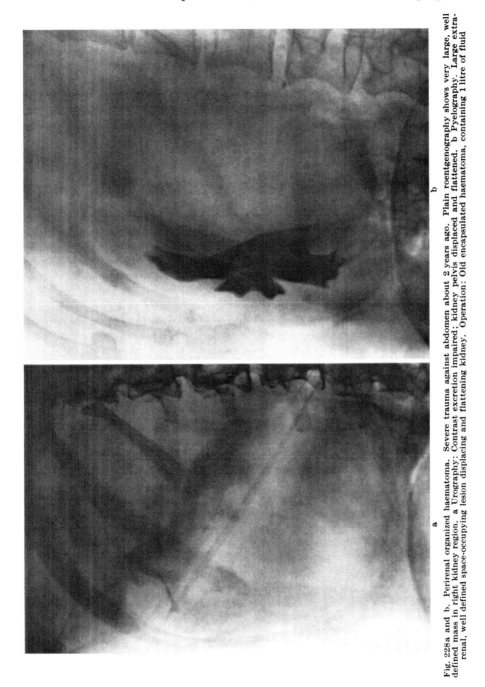

Fig. 228a and b. Perirenal organized haematoma. Severe trauma against abdomen about 2 years ago. Plain roentgenography shows very large, well defined mass in right kidney region. a Urography: Contrast excretion impaired; kidney pelvis displaced and flattened. b Pyelography. Large extrarenal, well defined space-occupying lesion displacing and flattening kidney. Operation: Old encapsulated haematoma, containing 1 litre of fluid

An equally important, if not more important, possibility is bleeding into the perirenal space in association with percutaneous renal biopsy. Haematoma around the right kidney may also be due to liver biopsy with haemorrhage into the right retroperitoneal space.

Spontaneous perirenal haematoma can occur in association with hemophilia (JASIENSKI 1937).

The roentgen findings in these different types of haematoma agree essentially with what is described below in connection with perinephritis of varying extent. However, no signs of edema will be seen.

Old extrarenal haematomas can be well delineated and simulate a well defined space-occupying lesion (Fig. 228). Examination with contrast medium will then often show severe displacement of the kidney and possible impression of the renal pelvis. Such haematomas may also be the cause of large shell-shaped calcifications at the site of the kidney or of irregular perirenal calcifications (MILLER & CORDONNIER 1949, ENGEL & PAGE 1955). Old haematomas can develop into hygromas (KEMM 1923).

Q. Perinephritis, abscess and carbuncle of the kidney

A local inflammatory process in the perirenal tissue is known as perinephritis. Other names used for this condition are perinephritic abscess, paranephritis, epinephritis etc. According to ISRAEL (1901), the two last-mentioned names should be reserved for inflammation of the fatty capsule respectively fibrous capsule of the kidney. But the inflammatory process usually involves all the soft tissues around the kidney and the name perinephritis, which simply indicates the presence of inflammation around the kidney, is therefore satisfactory.

The inflammation may be due to an intrarenal lesion. In renal carbuncle, one or more renal abscesses can perforate the capsule out into the space enclosed by the renal fascia (see chapter E. II. 2. Retroperitoneal pneumography). An inflammatory process may also involve the perirenal tissue via the lymphatics. Particularly the hilum is rich in lymphatics, as is obvious from pyelolymphatic reflux (see chapter O Backflow) and the possibility of spreading through the hilum to the perirenal space is obvious from conditions in association with backflow.

Perinephritis may, however, also be secondary to inflammatory lesions in tissues adjacent the kidney, such as osteitis of the ribs or the spine, pancreatitis, perforated duodenal ulcer, diverticulitis of the colon etc. It may be a metastatic process due to spread of material from a septic process, such as furunculosis, directly to the bed of the kidney.

A perinephritis can break through the renal fascia or can propagate through the open caudal part of the latter. However, it does not usually spread from one side to the other. The spine and the large vessels form a barrier against such spread. The main reason why the condition does not spread in this direction, however, is that the renal fascia is closed medially. This has been shown in autopsy studies. MITCHELL (1939) injected contrast medium post mortem and observed that the passage of the opaque medium from the bed of the kidney on one side to that on the other occurred only via the pelvis. This is also known from wide experience with retroperitoneal pneumography.

Perinephritis may extend around the entire kidney, but, as a rule, it is most pronounced dorsal to the kidney and caudally towards the opening of the renal fascia. This is due to the basic local anatomy e.g. the fatty capsule is thickest dorsally and the infection spreads along the path offering least resistance. It is also in part due to the fact that the patients have usually been lying for a long time on their back. The outline of the lesion may be indistinct, but it may also be sharp like that of a well defined small or large abscess. On examination the disease may be in the acute or chronic stage or it may be healing with fibrosis.

The roentgen findings vary considerably with the patho-anatomic type and stage of the disease. The course of the disease may be followed by repeated examinations at various intervals.

I. Rôle of roentgen examination

Perinephritis does not uncommonly remain concealed until post mortem examination (CAMPBELL 1930, HIGGINS 1932 and others). Roentgen examination is therefore indicated in all cases of obscure fever, and on examination of patients for a dubious abdominal or urinary tract disease the possibility of perinephritis should be considered. It is often to be read in the literature that roentgen examination is of but little value in the diagnosis of perinephritis. As a matter of fact, however, the roentgen findings are abundant. Perinephritis is not infrequently diagnosed as an accidental finding. In our series from 1943 (WELIN) a roentgen diagnosis was made in 9 patients in whom the disease had been clinically suspected and in 8 in whom the disease had not been suspected and who had been examined radiologically for some other urinary tract disease.

RIGLER & MANSON (1931) claimed that the roentgen findings are uncertain within 10 days after onset of symptoms and that the absence of roentgen findings after a period of 14 days should throw grave doubt upon the diagnosis of perinephritic abscess. In view of the varying clinical symptomatology of perinephritis, inclusion of such a time factor in the roentgen examination is fruitless. If the examination is properly performed, the roentgen findings are so valuable that, practically speaking, negative findings exclude the possibility of perinephritis despite the length of the history, provided the examination is performed under favourable conditions. If the history is short and strongly suggestive of perinephritis and roentgenography negative, the examination should, of course, be repeated after a time.

As to the so-called plastic perinephritis or perirenal fascitis see page 325.

II. Roentgen findings

In the discussion of the roentgen findings it should be pointed out that some of them, by themselves or in combination, may be fairly characteristic but that the findings are, as a rule, non-specific since each may be due to some other disease. Yet in combination and together with the clinical findings they usually permit a diagnosis. Therefore roentgen examination is a valuable adjunct in the diagnosis.

The roentgen findings were first exhaustively described by LAURELL in 1921, since when only details have been added.

1. Plain radiography

Sometimes one of the kidneys is enlarged. Edema, however, is often present in the renal capsule or around the kidney which prevents the kidney or part of it from being outlined. Owing to the extent of the pathologic process, which may vary widely, and owing to the degree of edema, which may likewise vary considerably, the anatomy of the retroperitoneal space may be deranged in such a way as to mask the lateral outline of the psoas muscle or part of it. If the process extends far laterally, the anatomy of the soft tissues of the flank may also be changed.

The abscess may vary in size with consequent variation in the roentgen findings. The findings also vary with the severity of the inflammatory edema. If the process is very acute, the edema pronounced, and the outline diffuse, the roentgen findings will be dominated by a blurring of the normal roentgen anatomy of the soft tissues. If the process is long-standing and well defined, the findings may be the same as those produced by a local space-occupying lesion.

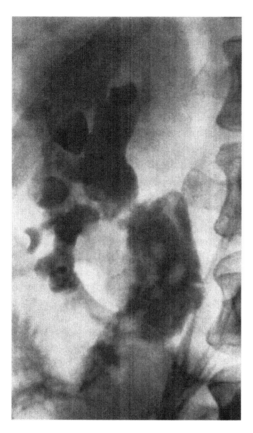

Fig. 229. Perirenal abscess. Pyelolithotomy. Infection and fistulation postoperatively. Antegrade pyelography via fistula. Filling of irregular fistula and large irregular abscess cavity adjacent kidney

The kidney may be displaced, often laterally and caudally, and its mobility may be diminished, as may be seen by the limitation of its movements with the respiratory cycle. The kidney may also be displaced ventrally. Owing to the examination conditions (increased object—film distance on examination in supine position) the kidney may then appear larger than it really is.

The outline of various organs and muscle layers, which is often very distinct owing to the difference between the density of fat and other soft tissues, is blurred by edema because the increased amount of fluid decreases the difference in density of the various tissues. This implies a more or less general increase in the density of the retroperitoneal space, which may be striking.

Meteorism is often generalized, but it may be more or less limited to the local inflammatory process.

Muscle contracture often causes skoliosis with the concavity facing the side involved by the perinephritis. Gas in the colon and stomach often makes it possible to observe displacement, of or impressions in, these organs.

The findings are not pathognomonic. They may be caused by all types of inflammatory processes in the retroperitoneal space. Acute pancreatitis may thus cause roentgen changes of the same nature as unilateral perinephritis.

All of the findings mentioned must be judged with caution and with due allowance for the influence of the examination technique on the results. Thus, in emaciated patients the soft tissue markings may be absent owing to lack of retroperitoneal fat, and thus not to any edema. Skoliosis may be due to the patient not being properly placed on the examination table, or it may be due to spinal deformity. Skoliosis as such can also prevent the lateral border of the psoas muscle from appearing in the usual way (this has been described in detail by SKARBY 1946). In the presence of skoliosis the kidney may be tilted less than otherwise and therefore appear wider. A kidney may also—as mentioned—appear larger than it really is, if it is lifted ventrally by a dorsal abscess. Intestinal contents may also make it difficult to judge the state of the retroperitoneal space. Since these patients have often been bed-ridden for a long time, considerable fecal matter and meteorism are common.

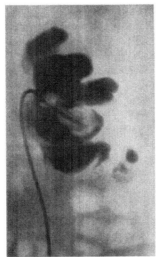 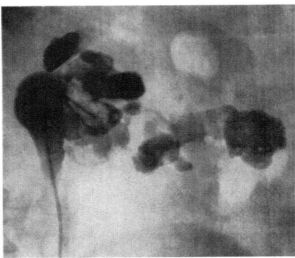

a   b

To the findings described above direct changes may be added. Sometimes gas is seen in the abscess, sometimes it is abundant as in a case in a diabetic described by BRAMAN & CROSS (1956). Otherwise the amount of gas is usually small, and if the pus is thick, the gas will be seen as small bubbles. On examination with the horizontal beam and the patient standing or lying, fluid levels will form against the gas.

An old process may calcify and then be surrounded by an irregular calcium shell or irregular calcium deposits may be seen in the abscess. This is very common in tuberculous perinephritis. Sometimes a stone may be seen in the abscess e.g. a renal or ureteric stone that has perforated and caused the abscess in which it is embedded. If the abscess is due to a projectile, the latter or part of it may be seen in the abscess.

2. Examination with contrast medium

Since the abscess presses against the kidney, pyelography or urography will often show deformation of the renal pelvis and displacement of the ureter. If the abscess is small and

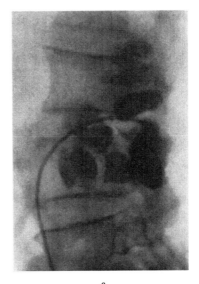

c

Fig. 230a—c. Perinephritic abscess caused by fistulation from chronic pyelonephritis with papillary necrosis and pyonephrosis. Pyelography: Dilated, deformed kidney pelvis with detritus. Contrast agent escapes through fistulae from caudal calyx (a) into irregular space posteriorly—laterally (b and c)

well defined, the deformation of the renal pelvis may resemble that seen in the presence of an intrarenal space-occupying lesion near the surface of the kidney. The abscess and the oedema, however, more often cause a more generalized compression by the pressure to which the kidney is exposed. The pyelographic findings vary with the direction of the pressure and position of the patient and the extent to which the renal pelvis is filled. Therefore, during the examination the technical conditions, *e.g.* the density of the contrast medium, the degree of filling, and the posture of the patient should be varied in order to decide which factors are constant. Since the space-occupying lesion is often situated behind the kidney, lateral projections are usually informative. With due consideration to the pathologic anatomy it is, as a rule, not difficult to decide whether the lesion is extrarenal or intrarenal (DEUTICKE 1940, OVERGAARD 1942). PREHN (1946) reported a case in which rotation of 90° of the upper calyx in a kidney was described by the author as a new sign of perinephritis. In reality the accompanying reproduction of a pyelogram shows a lateral and caudal displacement of the renal pelvis and a large bow-shaped impression in the medial part as well as an impression laterally in the gas-filled stomach, thus a large expanding process which, judging from the pyelogram, was well defined and located mediodorsally. Undoubtedly perirenal abscess has often been mis-diagnosed as an expanding process in the kidney. On the

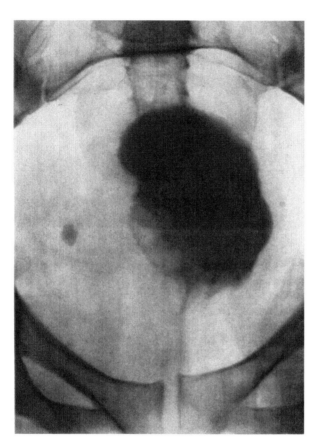

Fig. 231. Abscess around distal part of ureter with fairly large stone. The abscess displaces bladder, impresses its right part and causes inflammatory edema in bladder mucosa

other hand, it must be remembered that renal carbuncle and perinephritis in combination are so common that in the presence of a local expanding process and a perirenal component the possibility of renal carbuncle must always be considered.

If the lesion has perforated into the renal pelvis, contrast medium can flow into the abscess on retrograde pyelography (Figs. 229, 230) (ALKEN 1937, WELIN 1943). If the abscess is due, for example, to a perforated diverticulum of the colon, on examination of the colon with contrast medium the fistula may be filled with the contrast medium which may enter the abscess cavity.

On perforation to the surface of the skin, fistulography may be done. Water soluble contrast medium is injected into the fistula, possibly via a catheter. With suitable injection pressure and suitable posture of the patient contrast medium may fill the entire cavity. The abscess may also be filled by percutaneous puncture of the abscess and injection of gas (LAURELL 1931) or by positive contrast (FECI 1927).

The roentgen-diagnostic signs described above also hold true for abscess formation around the ureter in perforation by stone, for example. An abscess around the distal end of the ureter may impress or encroach upon the bladder (Fig. 231). The bladder mucosa then shows edema of the type not seldom seen in diverticulitis of the colon with abscess formation involving the bladder wall.

3. Indirect roentgen findings

In addition to the signs described above the examination may show a number of indirect signs. The diaphragm on the diseased side is often higher owing to the space-occupying nature of the process or owing to interference with the motility of the diaphragm, the abscess often being situated directly on the dorsal part of the diaphragmatic musculature, which extends far caudally. The diaphragmatic excursions are often limited on the diseased side. Therefore lamellar atelectases are seen in the basal part of the lung of the side involved. The pleural cavity on that side often contains fluid. NESBIT & DICK (1940) stated that of 85 patients with perinephritic abscesses, 14 (16.5%) were found to have supraphrenic complications. The frequency varies of course with the examination technique. If the patient can be examined only at the bed-side, the frequency of pathologic findings will be lower than otherwise. Examination in the lateral position with the beam horizontal—and this is the only way to demonstrate small amounts of pleural effusion—will very often demonstrate pleural involvement. Judging from the above mentioned publication, the examination of the chest was incomplete and included only frontal views, so that the frequency found was undoubtedly low.

An abscess can perforate the diaphragm and cause empyema or it may perforate to the pericardium and cause pyopericarditis.

As mentioned, gas in the intestines and colon is sometimes sufficient to diagnose displacement of these organs. On examination with contrast medium the displacement can, however, often be shown more clearly, and narrowing of the lumen respectively mucosal edema can be demonstrated. If the process is on the left side, the changes are often striking in the descending colon or if it is on the right side in the duodenum, which is close to the right kidney.

An osteitis in the form of spondylitis, for example, or osteomyelitis of the ribs or of one or more transverse processes of the vertebrae can also be diagnosed roentgenologically. Such osteitis may be the primary cause of the abscess formation. It may, however, also be secondary, an erosion of skeletal parts being produced by an abscess lying in direct contact with the skeleton.

It is clear from what has been set forth above that the roentgen findings in perinephritis are abundant and often permit a diagnosis and sometimes also demonstration of the origin of the perinephritic abscess. The frequency of different components given by different authors varies. These frequencies are, however, of less importance. Here, as in all cases, roentgen diagnosis should not consist of a list of various components of very different importance but in integrating the various roentgen-diagnostic observations to a general picture that can be described in terms of clinical pathology.

III. Carbuncle and abscess of the kidney

Carbuncle and renal abscess are local inflammatory processes in the kidney. The former is also called furuncle and anthrax. As to the latter designation it

19*

should be observed that in Romance languages anthrax (French) and antrace (Italian) mean a carbuncle in general, while in English the term anthrax means a carbuncle caused by the Bacillus anthracis. Renal carbuncle should be regarded as the tumor-like multilocular inflammatory process in the parenchyma. The fact that it is multilocular indicates that it is composed of several larger or smaller abscesses. In addition, it consists of more or less firm granulation tissue. The cut surface may resemble that of a well defined renal carcinoma. The renal abscess differs from a carbuncle by being uni-locular.

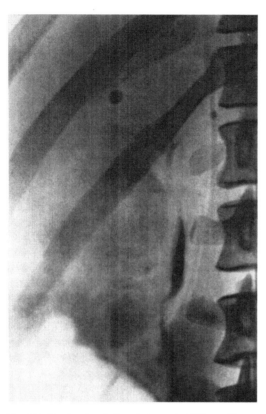

Fig. 232. Renal carbuncle in anterior part of kidney. Elevated temperature. Pain on right side. Tenderness. Right kidney moderately enlarged and plump. Outline sharp cranially but blurred laterally. Urography. Good excretion of contrast medium. Kidney pelvis compressed

Renal infection is often a manifestation of a pyaemia and one may therefore sometimes see a renal carbuncle in one kidney, for example, and a solitary renal abscess or multiple cortical abscesses in the other kidney. The disease may occur in all ages down to childhood. It has always been very rare in our clientele. Renal carbuncle can break through the fibrous capsule of the kidney, or infection may be carried via the lymphatics out into the surroundings. This results in perinephritis. The carbuncle is thus often not diagnosed as such but as perinephritis.

The findings on plain roentgenography are therefore dominated by signs of perinephritis as described above. If the perinephritic changes are mild the carbuncle may be seen as a local, large or small bulge in the outline of the kidney or as a general enlargement of the kidney. In this respect the findings resemble those described for renal tumour.

A bulge in the outline of the kidney due to a carbuncle may be combined with changes in the capsule and the pararenal tissue. The findings on plain radiography may then resemble those seen in tumours infiltrating peri-renally.

Examination with contrast medium

Renal carbuncles and renal abscesses are rare, and experience with pyelography and urography is therefore limited. It was formerly widely believed that pyelography was of little diagnostic help. A case described by LJUNGGREN (1931) showed that both pyelography and urography gave definite information about the expansion which together with the clinical findings gave the pre-operative diagnosis of renal carbuncle. A compilation by SPENCE & JOHNSTON (1939) also shows the value of examination with contrast medium. In 36 cases of renal carbuncle roentgen examination had been performed in 30, and in 26 urography or pyelography had been done. In 4 of these cases pyelography revealed no signs of a pathologic condition, while 22 showed some abnormality or another. In a compilation by GRAVES & PARKINS (1936) of 66 cases, only 15 gave positive find-

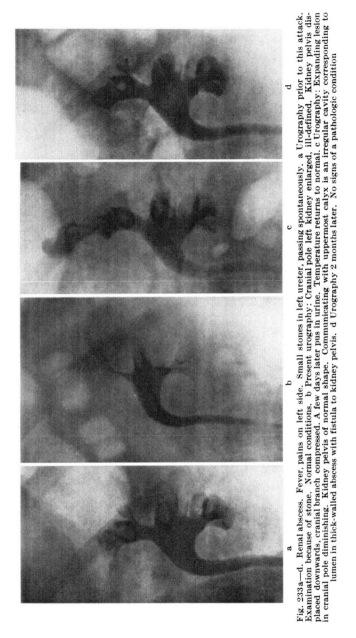

Fig. 233a.—d. Renal abscess. Fever, pains on left side. Small stones in left ureter, passing spontaneously. a Urography prior to this attack. Examination because of stone. Normal conditions. b Present urography: Cranial pole left kidney enlarged, ill-defined. Kidney pelvis displaced downwards, cranial branch compressed. A few days later pus in urine. Temperature returns to normal. c Urography: Expanding lesion in cranial pole diminishing. Kidney pelvis of normal shape. Communicating with uppermost calyx is an irregular cavity corresponding to lumen in thick-walled abscess with fistula to kidney pelvis. d Urography 2 months later. No signs of a pathologic condition

ings on pyelography. It may be presumed that the examination in some of these cases was not complete. Detection of an expanding process by pyelography often requires projections at different angles.

Pyelography and urography will show signs of expansion and the remarks given in association with deformation of the renal pelvis and ureter in the presence of solid tumour or cysts apply here, too (Fig. 232).

A renal carbuncle may fistulate into the renal pelvis and empty via the latter (Fig. 233).

In view of the fact that the patient is often referred for examination because of an acute infection, perinephritis is an important differential diagnosis. On the

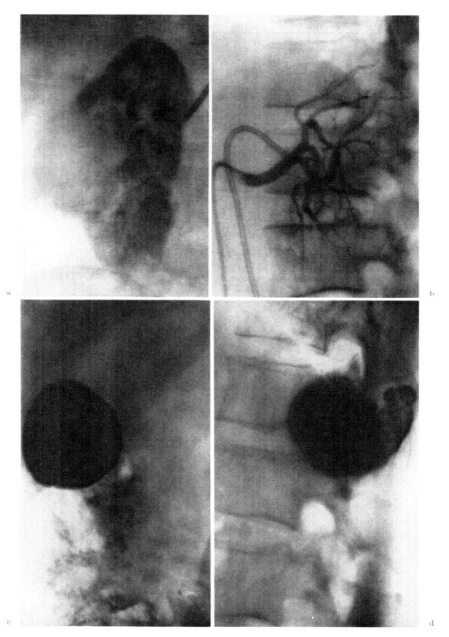

Fig. 234a—c. Renal abscess. Urography showed space-occupying lesion in right kidney. Renal angiography: a Nephrographic phase. Avascular space-occupying lesion, definitely not tumour, but not characteristic of cyst. b Lateral view arterial phase. Displacement of vessels around expanding lesion dorsally. Percutaneous puncture: Thin pus. Contrast medium injected into cavity. c Frontal, d lateral view of cavity

other hand, in perinephritis one must always have in mind the possibility that the process may be of intrarenal origin.

Pyelography will sometimes show not only signs of an expanding process but also severe contractions with rapid filling and emptying of the renal pelvis, which is not seen in non-inflammatory space occupying lesions.

Renal angiography may be helpful. We have seen a case of a large chronic renal abscess in which the angiogram showed displacement of the vessels in the arterial phase and in which the nephrogram showed a filling defect resembling that of a cyst (Fig. 234). In chronic renal abscess renal angiography can be resorted to and the method should be remembered in the differentiation of the lesion from cyst and avascular tumour.

On angiography a renal carbuncle may show a hyper-vascularized region of the type sometimes seen in smaller portions of the kidney in florid pyelonephritis. The hypervascularity may be localized in a large, well defined portion of the kidney. This hypervascularity does not include pathologic vessels of the type occurring in malignant renal tumour. It should, however, be remembered in the differential diagnosis of renal tumour (DE VRIES 1959).

In this connection syphilitic gumma should be mentioned, which, like a chronic renal abscess, roentgenologically resembles a space-occupying lesion (HUNTER 1939).

R. Gas in the urinary tract

A wide variety of conditions are accompanied by gas in varying amount in the urinary tract, particularly in the renal pelvis. The examiner must therefore be familiar with the roentgen findings.

Gas in the urinary tract may be masked by intestinal gas. If the amount of gas in the urinary tract is large, the entire renal pelvis will be filled as in a gas pyelogram. Thanks to the typical form of such an accumulation of gas it is readily recognized as such in the urinary tract. If only a small amount of gas is present in the renal pelvis, projections must be taken at different angles to ascertain that the gas observed really is situated within the kidney. The outline of such gas is then often found to correspond to some part of the renal pelvis, such as a calyx. The gas usually migrates on change of position of the patient, and on examination of the patient in the standing position it will be seen in the cranial group of calyces. It may, however, be entrapped in a cavity formel in a pathologic process.

Gas in the urinary tract may be of intra- or extra-renal origin.

Development of gas in the urinary tract

In the presence of gas-producing bacteria in an inflammatory renal lesion gas may occur in the urinary tract. In urine in diabetics, for example, fermentation can take place with the formation of carbon dioxide. In sugar-free urine, which contains protein, gas may be produced by Bact. coli or Bact. aerogenes. Bact. coli can also produce sulphuric acid from the urinary sulphates.

Gas may be produced in the wall of the urinary tract and bullae can be formed which may rupture with escape of the gas into the lumen of the bladder or kidney pelvis. This is what happens in emphysematous or phlegmonous cystitis.

One case of spontaneous gas pyelogram has been described by NOGUEIRA (1935) in which the cause is not known and one by OLLE OLSSON (1939) in a diabetic with pyelonephritis in whom the urinary sugar had been fermented by Bact. coli. In this case the gas pyelogram demonstrated the occurrence of multiple papillary necroses (Fig. 235). A case of gas formation by the same type of bacteria has been described by BRAMAN & CROSS (1956) in a patient with a coexistent perinephritic abscess, which also contained gas.

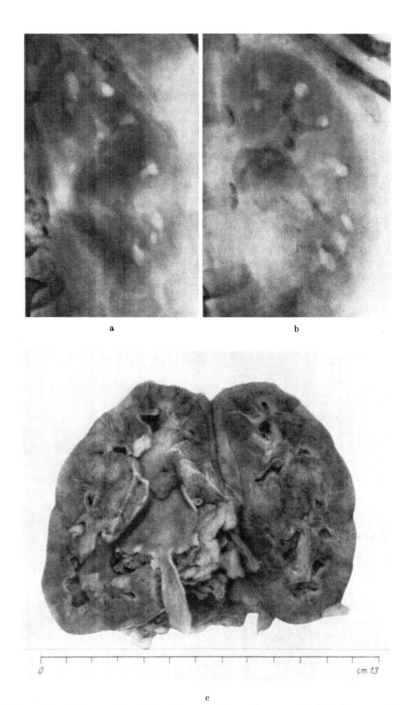

c

Fig. 235a—c. Gas in kidney pelvis and in cavities caused by papillary necrosis. Diabetic woman, 69 years of age, with glucosuria and pyuria. Gas formed by fermentation delineates kidney pelvis and cavities at site of papillae—papillary necrosis. a Plain roentgenogram. b Urogram. c Specimen

Gas may also enter the urinary tract from without. This may occur through direct exposure to the external environments, and is common in association with catheterization of the ureter.

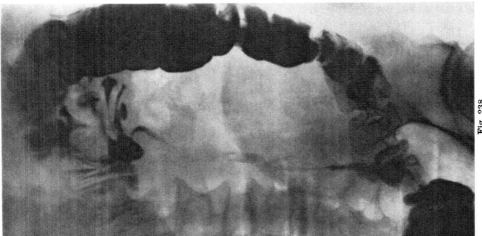

Fig. 238

Fig. 237

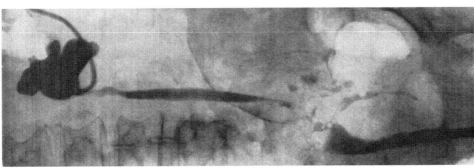

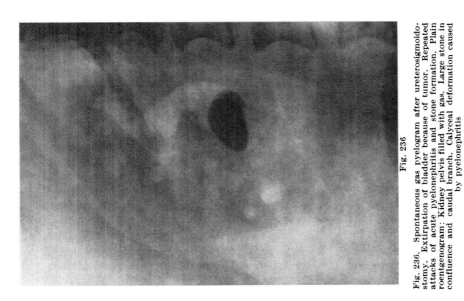

Fig. 236

Fig. 236. Spontaneous gas pyelogram after ureterosigmoidostomy. Extirpation of bladder because of tumor. Repeated attacks of acute pyelonephritis and stone formation. Plain roentgenogram: Kidney pelvis filled with gas. Large stone in confluence and caudal branch. Calyceal deformation caused by pyelonephritis

Fig. 237. Fistula between distal part of ureter and cavity after extirpation of rectum. During operation ureter had to be divided and then sutured. Antegrade pyelography via pyelostomy

Fig. 238. Ureterosigmoidostomy after extirpation of bladder 2 months previously. Passage of barium from rectum to urinary tract during examination of colon

Gas can also enter via a cutaneous ureterostomy and via perforating lesions, either from without, by a weapon for instance, or from within by fistulation caused by a concrement. Gas may, however, also enter via a direct communication between the urinary pathways and a cavity which normally contains gas. This is the case on transplantation of the ureter to the intestine, *e.g.* ureterosigmoideostomy (Fig. 236). A patient with an incompetent ureteroenteroanastomosis may continuously have gas in the renal pelvis. Gas may also enter the urinary tract on spontaneous fistulation with the digestive tract and in inflammatory processes, tumors or necroses. The fistula may communicate with the stomach, small intestine or large intestine. It may be primary in the urinary tract, primary in the gastrointestinal tract, or primary in the tissues outside these organs (Fig. 237). A glandular process, inflammatory or of neoplastic nature, may infiltrate both the urinary tract and the gastrointestinal canal and form a fistula between them. One case has been described by NARINS & SEGAL (1959) in which a large staghorn concrement migrated via a fistula into the intestines and was passed *per rectum*.

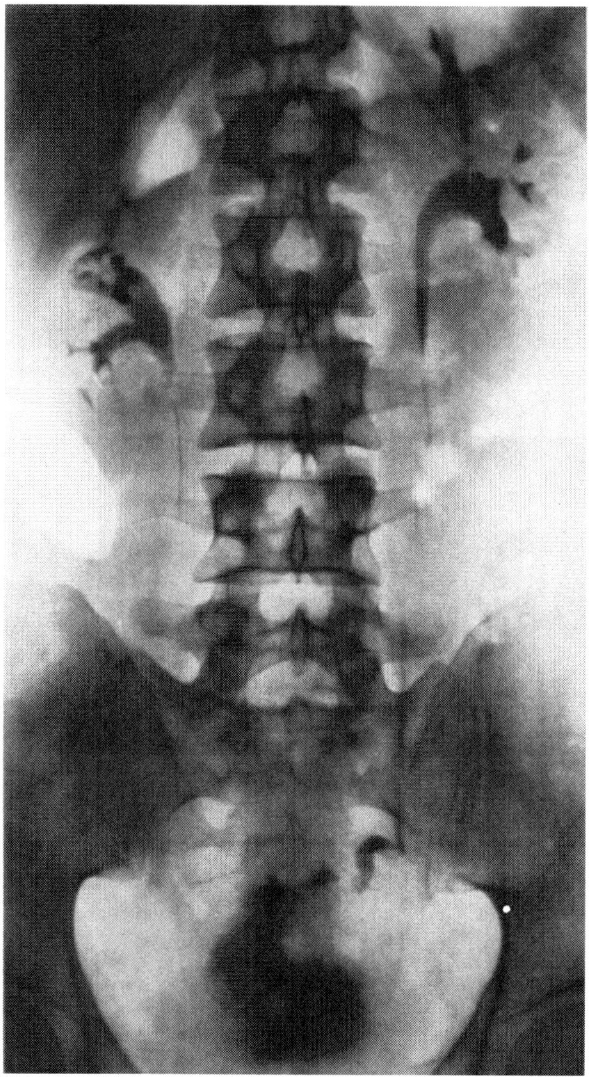

On fistulation between the urinary and the gastrointestinal tract, spontaneous or surgical, infection is liable to occur with

Fig. 239. Ureterosigmoidostomy. Well-functioning anastomosis. No dilatation of urinary tract

concrement formation or renal damage of the type described in the chapter on pyelonephritis. In the presence of such fistulation into the colon, barium contrast can flow into the urinary tract on examination of the colon with a contrast enema (Fig. 238). This can give rise to barium concrements. Contrast medium may also pass in the opposite way, namely in urography, for example, from the ureters over into the large intestine, where the contrast medium may spread over the major part of the latter (Fig. 239). On urography of patients with ureteroenteroanastomosis, I have observed contrast excretion by the kidneys during urography to continue much longer than otherwise. This can hardly imply anything but that the contrast medium excreted and transported to the colon is absorbed to some extent by the intestine and re-excreted.

S. Papillary necrosis

Papillary necrosis was long regarded as rare and the diagnosis as remarkable. Separation of one or more of the renal papillae is, however, not uncommon, as has been shown in recent years. In the literature the disease has been described under the name of papillary necrosis, papillitis necroticans renalis, renal papillary necrosis, necrotizing renal papillitis, renal medullary necrosis etc.

Patho-anatomically the changes are characterized by necrotic destruction of usually several papillae, which are partly or entirely separated. All forms from partial to total demarcation are seen which may affect an entire papilla, only its tip or both the papilla and the pyramid. The disease may be unilateral but it is usually bilateral with affection of several papillae, though the changes may involve only one papilla.

Separated parts of a papilla or entire papillae may be excreted with the urine, often in association with renal colic. They may also persist in the renal pelvis and then have a tendency to collect calcium and form concrements.

The disease is more common in females than in males and shows the highest incidence in age classes above 40 years. It is

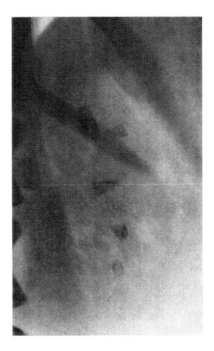

Fig. 240. Calcified necrotic papillae

most common in diabetics (GÜNTHER 1937). At autopsy of 859 diabetics EDMONDSON, MARTIN & EVANS (1947) found 107 (12.4%) with urinary tract infection, and 29 (27.1%) of them had papillary necrosis. Of 31,141 non-diabetic subjects, 1,023 had urinary tract infection and of these, 21 had papillary necrosis. Several other autopsy series and clinical series have shown that the disease is more common among diabetes and in patients with pyelonephritis. Urinary obstruction also favours papillary necrosis.

1. Plain radiography

Plain radiography often shows enlargement of the kidney. Sometimes stone —calcified papillae or fragments—may be seen in the renal pelvis, ureter or bladder. The concrements are often multiple, they increase in density from one examination to the other at intervals of weeks and often have the shape of papillae (Fig. 240; see also Fig. 75). Sometimes a defined papilla-shaped part of a stone may be seen as the nucleus of an irregular concrement. Micro-radiography of a stone removed from such a kidney has also shown such a papilla to be the core of the concrement (ENGFELDT & LAGERGREN 1958). Sometimes parenchymal calcifications corresponding to one or more necrotic papillae that have not been separated are observed. These calcifications are rounded or oval and less radiopaque and resemble a shell owing to collection of calcium on the outer surface of necrotic papillae (LUSTED, STEINBACH & KLATTE 1957). On occasion plain radiography will show the presence of gas in the renal pelvis produced by Bact. coli in the urine in diabetics (see Fig. 235). This gas may fill the entire cavity formed on separation of the papillae. Papillary necrosis can then be diagnosed from such a spontaneous gas pyelogram (OLLE OLSSON 1939).

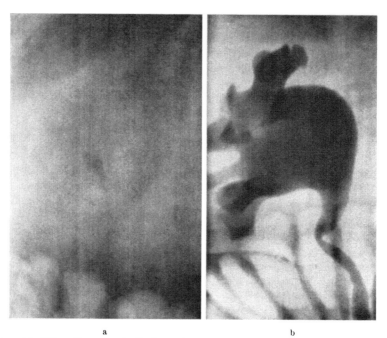

a   b

Fig. 241a and b. Old papillary necrosis. Pyelonephritis. Stones in both kidneys. On right side stone has the form of a papilla (a). b Pyelography: Well defined defect in uppermost papilla corresponding to shed papilla

2. Urography and pyelography

The characteristic pyelographic appearance of papillary necrosis was first described by GÜNTHER (1937) and ALKEN (1938) and the first case diagnosed by urography was described by OLLE OLSSON (1939). We have since diagnosed many cases by urography. Some authors claim that pyelography is the only roentgen method that can be used. The choice of examination method depends in reality on the functional capacity of the kidneys. If function is good, urography is preferable. A case described by ESKELUND (1945) in which he claims pyelography to be responsible for papillary necrosis with a fatal issue can, however, hardly be used as an argument against pyelography. Instrumentation of diabetics must be performed under strictly aseptic conditions in order to prevent the introduction of new bacteria (WALL 1956).

In the contrast-filled renal pelvis papillary necrosis will be manifested by an accumulation of contrast medium at the site of a papilla. The changes may resemble those of papillary destruction in other diseases, e.g. tuberculous papillary ulceration. The appearance varies widely with the extent and stage of the process.

Papillary necrosis cannot be diagnosed until the papilla has changed in such a way as to permit the entrance of contrast medium into a demarcation zone. If the entire papilla is separated or if only a fragment has been shed from the side or middle of a papilla the defect thus produced will be filled with contrast medium (Fig. 241). If the process is florid, the persistent papillary surface may be irregular and, in fact, the earliest finding is an irregularity of a papillary tip. In longstanding processes the surface is smooth and the calyx affected assumes a more or less spherical shape. If the papilla or pyramid is not separated entirely, a varying amount of the contrast medium can enter the demarcation zone (Fig. 242). It may then resemble certain forms of sinus reflux. If the entire pyramid is outlined but not separated, a large irregular ring of contrast medium will be seen around a calyx or a group of calyces, where the separated papilla or pyramid is responsible for the contrast defect in the center of the ring. This type of changes is very characteristic of papillary necrosis (Fig. 243).

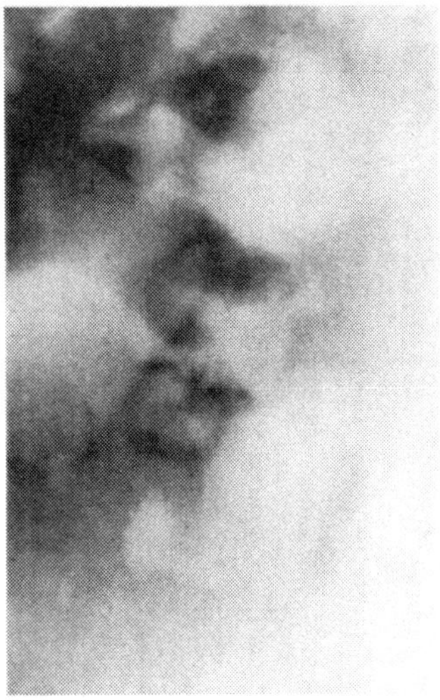

Fig. 242. Papillary necrosis. Chronic pyelonephritis with acute exacerbation. Urography: Delayed excretion. Irregularity of edge of caudal calyces. Contrast urine fills narrow, irregular necrotic zone in papilla

In the renal pelvis, usually in a calyx, one or more filling defects are often seen owing to separation of one or more papillae. The defects may be distinctly papilla-shaped.

Papillary necrosis embraces several problems. The number of cases observed has increased with increasing knowledge of its roentgen appearance. It was

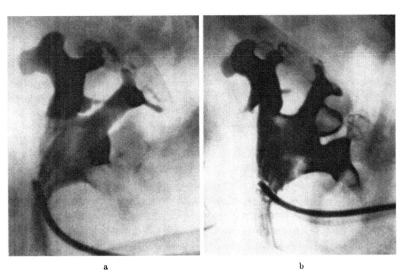

a   b

Fig. 243a and b. Papillary necrosis. Antegrade pyelography in pyelostomy. Shed papillae in calyces and branches in middle and caudal part of kidney pelvis. Contrast urine penetrates into necrotic zones in papillae

formerly believed that papillary necrosis was a dramatic acute disease with a fatal issue. However, not all cases of papillary necrosis run a dramatic course and not all are fatal. THELEN (1947) made a distinction between local and diffuse types, both with an acute, a sub-acute and a chronic course respectively.

It is of importance to bear the diagnostic criteria in mind, since papillary necrosis may represent a very severe acute situation and because energetic therapy can control necrotizing pyelonephritis. It can arrest necrosis and prevent the formation of concrements. The possibility of papillary necrosis must also always be considered in chronic cases with papillary changes of obscure nature.

Papillary necrosis has been regarded as related to and being an accompaniment of pyelonephritis in diabetics as well as in non-diabetics. Renal function studied by EDVALL (1958) in cases of chronic pyelonephritis on one hand and of cases

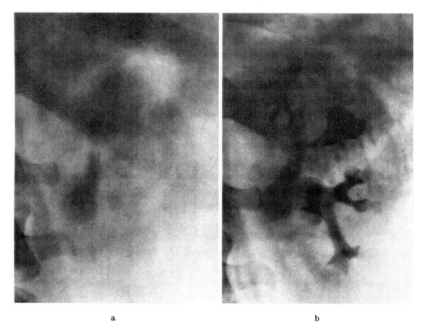

a   b

Fig. 244a and b. Stone causing local stasis of cranial pole, secondary pyelonephritis with papillary necrosis. Stone in confluence and cranial branch. a Plain roentgenogram. b Urography. In cranial pole filling of defects in papillae, displacement of branch to adjacent calyx and narrowing of branch and stems. Partial nephrectomy: Local pyelonephritis with papillary necrosis

with papillary necrosis on the other suggest that it is a question of two independent diseases. This is also supported by the finding of papillary necrosis without infection (HULTENGREN 1958) which thus gives reason to doubt a relation between papillary necrosis and pyelonephritis.

It is of interest to note that of 31 patients with papillary necrosis HULTENGREN found as many as 29 to have a history of severe headache or migraine. This makes the widely supposed relation between the abuse of phenacetin and related substances and renal injury with papillary necrosis spring to mind (SPÜHLER & ZOLLINGER 1953, AXELSSON 1958).

In my experience, however, destruction of one or more papillae is not uncommon in pyelonephritis. The more the examiner is interested in pyelonephritis and the more he performs urography in this disease with ureteric compression for detailed investigation of the morphology of the renal pelvis, particularly of the calyces, the more frequently will changes be found due to destruction of papillae (Fig. 244).

Knowledge of the roentgen changes after recovery from papillary necrosis is still limited. As mentioned, in some cases rounded defects or rounded cavities are seen at the site of an entire papilla or part of it (Fig. 245a, b). Some of the

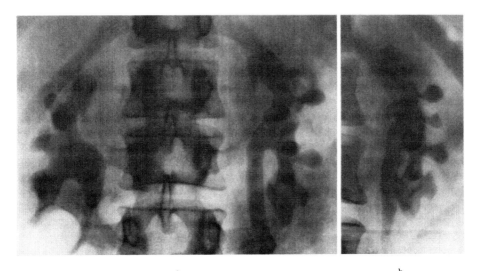

a   b

Fig. 245a and b. Bilateral old papillary necrosis in pyelonephritis. For 5 years repeated attacks of pyelonephritis with passage of papilla fragments. a and b Urography: Defects in most papillae with corresponding widening of calyces. b Oblique view of left kidney

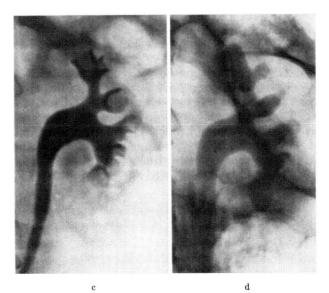

c   d

Fig. 245c and d. Chronic pyelonephritis for at least 5 years. Now acute exacerbation. Urography (c) 8 months previously. No changes. d During acute exacerbation. Slightly decreased density of contrast urine. Calyces plump. Large papillary ulceration in caudal pole and small ulcerations in several papillae, one above middle of kidney resembling a calyceal border evagination

changes known as hypoplasia coincide in appearance with those seen after papillary necrosis. As mentioned, papillary necrosis can also produce some of the changes characteristic of pyelonephritis. Certain so-called calyceal diverticula also fall within this group (Fig. 245c, d).

3. Renal angiography

The changes in the papillae so far have not been diagnosed by renal angiography. This is easily understood since papillary necrosis is thought to occur because normally the arterial supply to the papillae is poor.

T. Medullary sponge kidney

In recent years a peculiar type of kidney disease has been described under the heading of medullary sponge kidney. It has been found incidentally at roentgen examination for a wide variety of clinical symptoms.

Medullary sponge kidney is thus a roentgen diagnostic entity consisting of widening of the collecting tubules in the papillae demonstrable by urography or pyelography. The disease was first described in 1938 by LENARDUZZI; the second case was not reported until 10 years later by DAMMERMANN. Since then a large number of case reports have been published in which the changes have been described under different names such as dilatation of the intrarenal urinary pathways, cystic dilatation of the urinary pathways, cystic disease of the renal pyramids, cystic dilatation of the pelvic urinary pathways, congenital cystic dilatation of the renal collecting tubules etc. The condition is usually named spongy kidney (rene a spugna in Italian, rein à éponge in French, Schwammniere in German). Detailed descriptions have been given by CACCHI & RICCI (1949), GÜNTHER (1950), LHEZ (1954)—12 cases—and LINDVALL (1959), whose 35 cases represent the largest material on record. The epithet "medullary" was suggested by DI SIENO & GUARESCHI (1956) to distinguish this spongy kidney from the completely spongy kidney, i.e. the microcystic degeneration of the entire kidney in newborns.

The diagnosis is based, as mentioned, on the roentgen findings. Neither clinically nor pathologically does it appear to be an entity.

Patho-anatomically it is characterized by changes situated in the pyramids. It is also usually conceived as a congenital malformation consisting of a disturbance at the important border between nephrogenic tissue and derivatives from the Wolffian ducts. The changes are not seen in the cortex. They may be localized to one or more pyramids in one or both kidneys, which may be involved to a varying extent. The pyramids may be enlarged and the collecting tubules are ectatic or cystic. The cysts may be in communication with the tubules or they may end blindly. The cysts and the dilated ducts often contain concrements.

1. Roentgen diagnosis. Plain radiography

The kidneys may be of ordinary size, but they may also be slightly enlarged or diminished and then often have an irregular outline. In many cases, about half, plain roentgenography will show calcifications, often 1—2 mm in diameter, but they may be larger and of irregular shape (Fig. 246a). They are situated close to the renal hilum, while the periphery is free from such calcifications.

The number of calcifications may vary from a single stone to several hundreds. They may occur on one or both sides. They may also be scattered throughout the kidney or localized to a part of it. Sometimes only one papilla or part of it shows calcifications. The changes vary in severity from one part of a kidney to another. If only one papilla or group of papillae is involved, a local accumulation of small calcifications may be seen. These are of fairly characteristic appearance and even when less numerous and small, their appearance in plain roentgenograms will suggest medullary sponge kidney.

2. Urography

The excretion of contrast medium is usually normal. The renal pelvis and the calyces may be of ordinary outline. Papillary hypertrophy, however, is common and occasionally grotesque. One or a pair of papillae may be hypertrophic, while

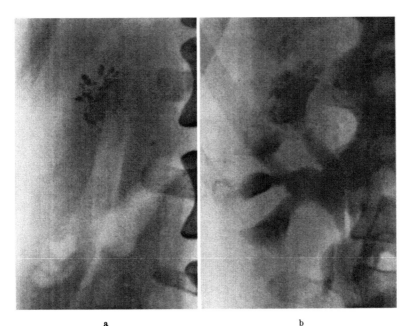

a   b

Fig. 246a and b. Localized medullary sponge kidney—cranial pole right side. a Plain roentgenogram. Characteristic small calculi. b Urography: Calculi in dilated ducts

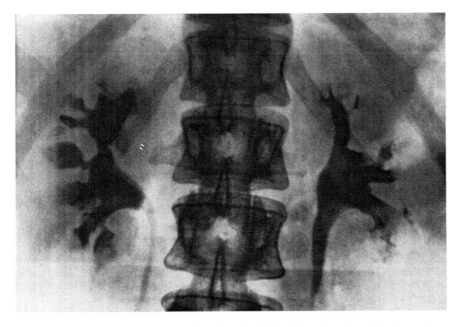

Fig. 247. Medullary sponge kidney bilaterally. Urography: Widened ducts in most papillae at some places looking like ordinary tubular stasis, some with slight cystic dilatation

others also showing changes may be of ordinary size. Papillary hypertrophy is characteristic of the disease but it is not pathognomonic, since it may also occur in other diseases.

At the site of the papillae accumulations of contrast medium may show well defined cavities varying in size from very small to several millimetres in diameter (Fig. 246b, 247, 248). The contrast density in the entire papilla may be irregularly increased or the pyramids may be striated. The calyceal border may be normal and separated by a zone of parenchyma from the cystic dilatated papillary ducts, which are filled with contrast medium. The cavities filled may, however, extend to the calyces and thereby cause small or large irregularities in the calyceal border. Large cystic cavities along a calyceal border may therefore resemble papillary

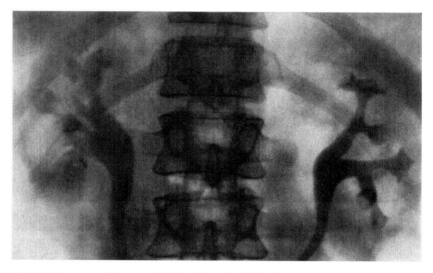

Fig. 248. Medullary sponge kidney on right side. Urography: Delayed excretion on right side, cystic dilatation in most papillae and marked increase in size of some papillae with corresponding flattening of ca yces

destruction. In some cases the changes may be very pronounced in some parts of the kidney and very slight in others. They often affect only one papilla.

The characteristic changes are more readily demonstrable by urography than by pyelography. Only in exceptional cases are they more distinct in pyelograms. This is because on pyelography the contrast medium cannot force its way up through the narrow mouth of the widened ducts. This might help to explain why the condition, though not uncommon, was discovered so late. During urography the contrast filling comes from the parenchyma and thus provides a much better possibility of obtaining a contrast filling of the dilated collecting tubules.

With our present knowledge renal angiography does not contribute to the diagnosis, but shows ordinary vascular anatomy (ALKEN, SOMMER & KLING 1951).

The condition is of differential diagnostic significance, particularly against tuberculosis. This holds both for urography and plain radiography. The disease has undoubtedly occasionally been misinterpreted as tuberculosis and resulted in unnecessary nephrectomy.

The condition must also be distinguished from papillary necrosis as well as from nephrocalcinosis.

U. Generalized diseases of the renal parenchyma

The term generalized diseases of the renal parenchyma embraces such conditions as pyelonephritis, glomerulonephritis and tubular nephritis. Roentgendiagnostically these conditions have much in common, such as the indications for roentgen examination. Most cases with uraemia belong to this group and may therefore be taken together in the discussion of the importance of roentgen examination in the evaluation of the amount of functioning renal parenchyma, in the diagnosis or follow-up of generalized or, for example, pulmonary edema and in its differentiation from other surgical urologic conditions resulting in uraemia. In other words, they occupy a central position in the discussion of acute renal insufficiency.

A firm diagnosis of these conditions is often difficult because patho-anatomic verification is often not available. Operative biopsy and more often percutaneous needle biopsy is resorted to with increasing frequency. The use of percutaneous biopsy is, however, limited by the risk of haemorrhage it involves. Moreover, biopsy specimens removed by this technique or any other are only of value if they are taken from the actual site of any changes. Particularly in pyelonephritis, in which the severity of the changes in one and the same kidney is known to vary widely from one part to another, the percutaneous technique may therefore be of limited diagnostic value. In glomerulonephritis, in which the pathologic process is roughly even in the entire kidney, percutaneous needle biopsy might yield reliable information. As to pyelonephritis, it is often a complication to some other disease such as stone, which dominates both the clinical and roentgenological findings. Roentgenologists interested in the diagnosis of pyelonephritis—and every roentgenologist certainly should have this disease in mind when examining urologic cases—will find that in different diseases the roentgen findings will very often give evidence of additional changes caused by pyelonephritis. However, if it is to be possible to distinguish signs more or less specific of certain diseases and give diagnostic criteria satisfactory definitions, the diseases producing symptoms under investigation must be grouped according to a firm and definite diagnosis excluding other possibilities. This grouping must therefore as a rule be based on patho-anatomic evidence. In generalized parenchymal changes this rule has often not been observed, roentgen-diagnostic signs having been related to diseases diagnosed merely clinically, and sometimes not very strictly, and therefore the roentgen symptomatology is sometimes not satisfactorily described.

The diseases referred to above have a common roentgen-diagnostic baseline, where the differential-diagnosis is of less importance in the acute stage. It is represented by acute renal insufficiency. In this clinical entity roentgen examination is of importance from several points of view, which are discussed below.

I. Acute renal insufficiency

1. General considerations

General considerations on the roentgen examination of patients with acute renal insufficiency, as elaborated in cooperation with the units for internal and surgical renal diseases of our hospital, are set forth below.

Patients with acute renal insufficiency are, as a rule, in a poor general condition, often moribund, which makes roentgen examination difficult and requires well planned, quick and reliable examination with the aid of proficient assistance.

20*

The first point to decide is whether the renal insufficiency is due to changes in the renal parenchyma such as generalized parenchymatous changes, toxic damage, tumour etc. or to obstructed drainage such as by stone, tumour, post-radiotherapeutic edema, periureteritis obliterans etc. It should be observed that a retroperitoneal tumour extending from the intestines or the bladder or from the female

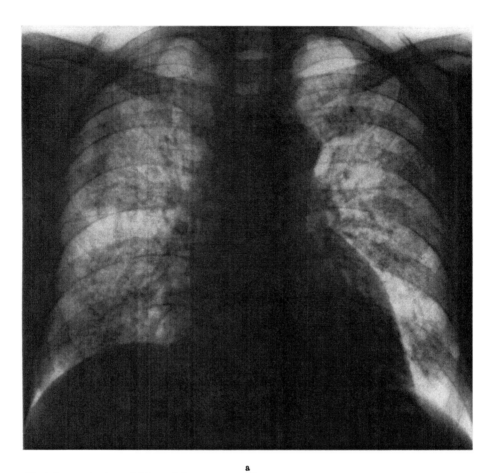

a

Fig. 249a—c. Acute renal failure. Pulmonary edema characteristically localized in central parts of lobe (a)

genital organs may obstruct both ureters. In addition to instrumental examination for checking the patency of the ureters the examiner must be on the watch for any signs suggesting stone or other obstacle obstructing urinary flow. The roentgenologist should therefore pay special attention to the size of the kidneys and the width of the renal pelvis. Dilatation of the renal pelvis can, as mentioned, sometimes be detected in plain roentgenograms. The possibility of the patient having only one kidney should regularly be checked.

The next step is to assess the amount of renal parenchyma. If the kidneys can be outlined, the mass of renal parenchyma can be estimated in plain roentgenograms in accordance with the principles given in chapter E. Such estimation is important not only in the general evaluation, but particularly in the choice of therapy. This is influenced by the type of changes in the kidneys causing the acute renal insufficiency, for example, if any enlargement of the kidneys can be demonstrated and ascribed to an acute disease from which the patient can probably make a complete recovery or if severely contracted kidneys are found to cause the insufficiency.

The size of the kidneys is of prognostic importance. This point will be reverted to later.

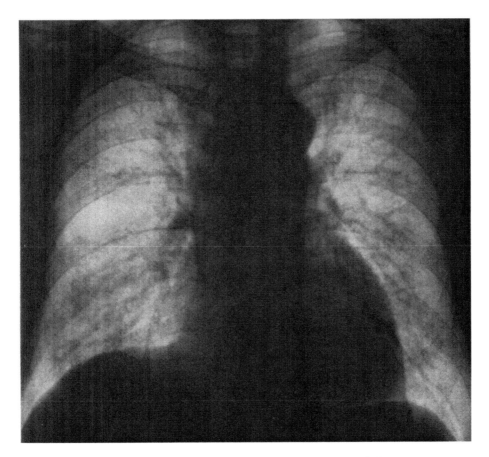

Fig. 249 b. One week later after treatment. Marked regression of edema

2. Edema

The next point to receive attention during the acute stage of the disease is the fluid balance, a factor of decisive importance in acute renal insufficiency. Examinations of patients in a state of acute renal insufficiency bring into sharp focus the importance of roentgen examination for checking edema. Of great value is the examination of the lungs. This is apparent from the fact that, as pointed out by several workers in this field, even in severe pulmonary edema the physical findings are often scanty and contrast sharply with the lung changes seen roentgenologically. This makes the roentgen examination of these patients essential because pulmonary edema is a serious and life-threatening complication. In pulmonary edema of this type the changes are usually bilateral but may differ markedly in extent from side to side, and occasionally they may be unilateral. The changes usually involve the major portion of the lungs. The peripheral parts of the lungs are free as pointed out above all by HERRNHEISER (1958). The changes are thus localized to the central portion of each lung and each lobe (Fig. 249).

A differential diagnosis is naturally of importance in the planning of treatment. It is sometimes difficult to distinguish between this type of pulmonary edema and cardiac edema respectively certain types of pneumonia or atelectases, particularly since a combination of these lesions is not unusual. As mentioned,

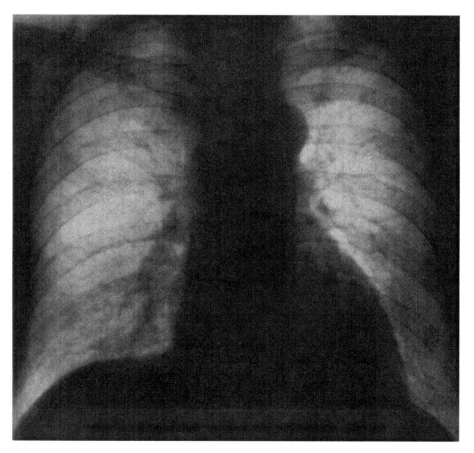

Fig. 249 c. Another 12 days later. Complete disappearance of edema

this pulmonary edema is characterized by the changes being bilateral and localized mainly to the centre of the lung, the margin of the lungs being entirely free from changes. Experimental investigations on dogs at our department with various types of pulmonary edema induced by different methods and in different vascular regions (BORGSTRÖM, ISING, LINDER & LUNDERQUIST 1960) have shown this most distinctly. These investigations—still in progress—have also shown that the characteristic localization of the changes might be due to their relation to the regions of supply of the bronchial arteries. The changes consist essentially of pronounced edema in the wall of the large bronchi in contrast to the cardiac edema and different types of pneumonia in which the filling of the alveoli is the main feature.

The pulmonary changes are reversible. Check-examinations of the chest are therefore of great value in the management of acute renal insufficiency.

The presence of any edema can also usually be detected on plain roentgenography of the urinary tract. In the examination of the patient in the acute stage it is often difficult to recognize the outline of the kidneys, mainly because of the conditions under which the examination is performed. The patient is often unable to co-operate during the examination, he is not prepared for the examination, and uraemia is often accompanied by considerable meteorism. Ascites and retroperitoneal edema also often add to the difficulty in recognizing the outline of the kidneys, but, on the other hand, these conditions add to the diagnostic information of the examination the fact that edema is present. (It is assumed that the reader is familiar with the roentgen diagnosis of ascites.) Retroperitoneal edema has been described in the chapter on perinephritis. In these cases the edema is more generalized with a marked increase in density of the entire retroperitoneal space. This increase abolishes the difference in contrast between organs and tissues in the retroperitoneal space, and it is often not possible to define the psoas muscles, kidneys etc. In the treatment of the fluid retention with regression of the edema as a consequence the kidneys gradually become distinct.

3. Estimation of the size of the kidneys

Estimation of the size of the kidneys during the course of the disease is important. If the kidneys are enlarged, it may be due not only to stasis, which has been dismissed from the differential diagnosis by this stage of the disease, but to generalized parenchymatous changes such as glomerulonephritis, tubular nephritis, pyelonephritis etc. General enlargement of the kidneys might also be due to amyloidosis and other types of nephrosis before the kidney has begun to shrink, infiltration of the kidney by leukaemic tissue (STERNBY 1955) and infarction of the kidney. Extensive granuloma formation in the kidneys in sarcoidosis, for example, also belongs to this group of conditions. These diseases can lead to a considerable enlargement of both kidneys. Another condition to be borne in mind is polycystic kidney described in chapter L. In the stage of acute renal insufficiency polycystic kidneys are usually so large as to offer no diagnostic difficulties.

If the kidneys are small, glomerulonephritis and pyelonephritis are prevalent together with hypoplasia, but many diseases may have a final stage of kidney contraction such as collagenous disease, arthritis urica etc.

Glomerulonephritis and tubular nephritis are of roentgen-diagnostic interest mainly in the investigation of the effect of the disease on the size of the kidney. Pyelonephritis is of greater diagnostic interest because it is the most common renal disease.

On check examination soon after the acute stage the following points should be borne in mind.

a) Enlarged kidneys

In acute and sub-acute glomerulonephritis, in tubular nephritis and acute pyelonephritis, in gross bilateral renal cortical necrosis and in the early stages of some other conditions the kidneys may be enlarged. The enlargement is then sometimes considerable. Both kidneys are enlarged to the same extent except in pyelonephritis, in which only one kidney may be affected or occasionally only part of one kidney. The kidneys are plump but have a smooth surface. Sometimes they cannot be completely outlined because of edema. Oblique views facilitate recognition of their border. Body section radiography may sometimes be useful.

It is important to follow the course of the disease. If there is any doubt about the size of the kidney, check examination should be performed as soon as the edema has abated. Repeated check examinations for any further change in the size of the kidney should preferably be done at intervals of 2 weeks and later at longer intervals. During such roentgen follow-up persistence of the increased size of the kidney shows that the pathologic process is still active. In some cases the kidney may assume and then retain normal size, while in others the kidney may continue to diminish, *i.e.* to develop into a contracted kidney.

b) Kidneys smaller than normal

Chronic glomerulonephritis and pyelonephritis as well as late stages of tubular nephritis, renal cortical necrosis, and some other diseases may be accompanied by pronounced shrinkage of the kidneys. In pyelonephritis the change is usually more severe on one side than on the other. In unilateral small kidney only pyelonephritis (and hypoplasia) need be considered. In patients with a small solitary kidney the question arises whether the smallness is congenital or due to shrinkage. It is, as mentioned, often not possible to answer this question. What is described in the literature as a hypoplastic kidney due to an embryologic disorder may in reality be a contracted kidney due to early pyelonephritis (see chapter Anomalies).

Below the variation in the size of the kidney will be discussed against the background of two diseases, namely glomerulonephritis and tubular nephritis.

4. Glomerulonephritis

On examination of acutely ill patients the examiner must first ascertain the stage of the disease, patients not infrequently having glomerulonephritic shrunken kidneys without any earlier history. In acutely ill patients the kidneys are often normal-sized, but sometimes they are enlarged, occasionally markedly so. On the other hand, the kidneys may be smaller than normal. This means that the uraemia is not due to acute glomerulonephritis and, if the kidneys are very small, the uraemia represents a final stage of renal insufficiency.

In anuria recognition of the stage of the disease is of paramount importance. Extremely active therapy is available and must be applied, especially in cases of acute glomerulonephritis with anuria. It has been demonstrated by RUDEBECK (1946) that the mortality from acute glomerulonephritis (diagnosed clinically), is highest when the clinical picture at the onset of the disease is very intense; on the other hand—if these patients survive this initial stage—the prospects are not worse than for those in whom the clinical picture was moderate in the beginning. Therefore every effort must be taken to try to carry the patient over the acute condition.

The rate at which the disease progresses from an acute to a chronic stage seems to vary widely from one case to another. According to VOLHARD & FAHR (1914), acute nephritis sometimes reaches the stage of a contracted kidney within a few months. On the other hand, one case was reported in which glomerulonephritis was still in the subchronic stage after $3^1/_2$ years. The possibilities for the pathologist to obtain a clear idea of the general course of glomerulonephritis are, of course, limited, because fortunately the percentage of cases coming to post-mortem examination is relatively small. Here roentgen examination can contribute considerably to our knowledge of the patho-anatomic course of the disease, because it is practically always possible, by repeated check examination, to follow the gross anatomic changes, as judged by the size of the kidney.

In a given case the routine roentgen examination plays another rôle; by assessing the size of the kidney in the course of the disease it is often possible to evaluate the actual condition as well as the prognosis, because the size of the kidney reflects the amount of surviving parenchyma. Check-examinations may show how enlarged kidneys reassume a normal size or how enlarged or ordinary-sized kidneys become smaller and continue to do so until the stage of contracted kidney is reached.

5. Tubular nephritis

Patients with tubular nephritis usually come for roentgen examination in the stage of acute renal failure. What is said above about acute renal insufficiency is applicable on this stage.

On roentgen examination of a patient with tubular nephritis it might be well to remember the following and more or less widely accepted stages: the initial stage during which the injury takes place, the anuric-oliguric stage, which is defined as the period during which the daily urinary volume is 400 ml or less and which is said to last about 10—12 days, the diuretic stage, defined as beginning when the daily urinary volume exceeds 400 ml and with still reduced renal function, and the late diuretic stage when the kidney function gradually improves and in most cases becomes normal.

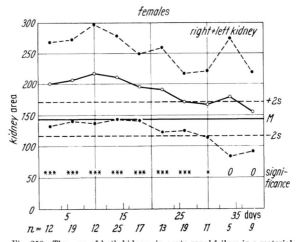

Fig. 250. The area of both kidneys in acute renal failure in a material of 66 cases. The straight lines represent the mean value and the standard deviation in 100 cases with "healthy" kidneys. (After MOËLL)

Roentgenologically, the initial stage is a diagnostic stage in which plain roentgenography of the abdomen can show equal enlargement of both kidneys with an outline varying in distinctness with the severity of retroperitoneal edema.

In the anuric-oliguric stage the purpose of the examination is often to decide whether the patient has edema, especially pulmonary edema and to check the effect of therapeutic procedures. In the diuretic stages the question is mainly to assess the prognosis, as judged by the rate at which the kidney returns to normal size or shrinks still further. As a rule, the kidneys return to normal size within one or a few months, but sometimes a slight enlargement persists for a long time (Fig. 250). Sometimes they shrink. It should be observed that gross bilateral renal cortical necrosis may be the final stage of grave tubular nephritis.

6. Gross bilateral cortical necrosis

Gross bilateral cortical necrosis occurs most frequently in association with concealed accidental haemorrhage (SHEEHAN & MOORE 1952) and since oliguria—anuria is a predominant clinical feature, what was said above about acute renal insufficiency also applies to the disease. Formerly the disease was of less interest from a roentgen-diagnostic point of view because it often runs a rapid and fatal course. By means of rational conservative therapy, and, when indicated, the artificial kidney (dialysis, ultrafiltration), it has, however, become possible to keep patients with renal insufficiency alive for a long time. MOËLL (1957) has described 2 cases of gross bilateral cortical necrosis treated at the department for internal renal diseases and examined in our department, one with 70, the other with 116 days oliguria—anuria. Both patients contracted acute renal failure in connection with delivery. In the early stage of the disease the size of the kidneys was distinctly increased. However, shrinkage was afterwards rapid, the outlines became irregular. Cortical calcifications appeared in one case after two months.

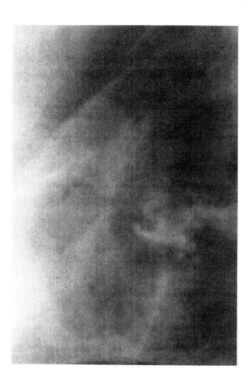

Fig. 251. Chronic pyelonephritis. Scattered calcifications in medullary part of kidney

In the other case cortical calcifications could be seen in post-mortem films of the kidneys.

Judging from observations made by MOËLL, renal cortical necrosis is obviously more common than widely assumed. He has found cortical calcifications in some cases of advanced tubular nephritis.

7. Pyelonephritis

Pyelonephritis will be described in greater detail. The roentgen-diagnosis of pyelonephritis so far is difficult because the disease varies in extent and course from case to case and because many of the roentgen-diagnostic findings are not specific. When collecting diagnostic signs characteristic of a disease, the important search for invariants must be strictly limited to cases with the diagnosis established as firmly as possible, in other words a patho-anatomic diagnosis. The abundant literature on the roentgen findings in pyelonephritis is based mainly on examination of cases with the disease diagnosed on clinical grounds but not confirmed by patho-anatomic examination. In addition, data on the motility, tonus etc. of the urinary tract in pyelonephritis are often founded on less satisfactory examination methods and described in terms for which the examination technique does not furnish complete cover. Nevertheless some publications on the roentgen diagnosis of pyelonephritis deserve due consideration (WULFF 1936, PRÉVÔT & BERNING 1950, BRAASCH & EMMETT 1951, DEJDAR & PRAT 1958, BOIJSEN; DEJDAR 1959 etc.). DEJDAR & PRAT (1958) stressed the importance of roentgen examination in the investigation of pyelonephritis. Though their illustrations are not convincing in all respects and though their material consisted of cases diagnosed only clinically, the results they obtained are interesting.

a) Plain roentgenography

In the acute stage one or both kidneys are enlarged. The enlargement is seldom severe. The kidney increases a centimeter or so in length and breadth and

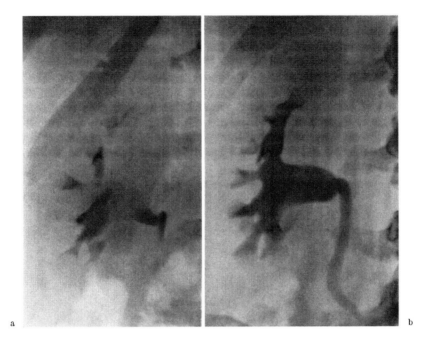

a   b

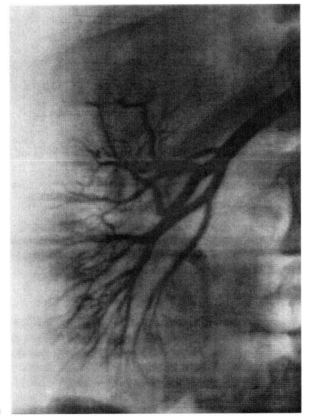

c

Fig. 252a—c. Pyelonephritis. a Urography: Multiple impressions in kidney pelvis because of high plasticity of pelvis wall. b During ureteric compression the impressions diminish and disappear. c Renal angiography—arterial phase. Impressions in kidney pelvis coincides largely with intrarenal arterial branches

appears plump and swollen. As the disease heals the kidney assumes normal size. But the decrease in size may continue and within some months result in unilateral, bilateral or locally contracted kidney. If shrinkage is generalized, the length of the kidney may be reduced to 4—7 cm and the breadth to 3—4 cm. The kidney may then have an irregular surface and it may increase in density owing to deposition of calcium in the renal parenchyma appearing as small, irregular, opaque, multiple, scattered calcifications (Fig. 251). I cannot confirm DEJDAR's (1959) statement that the kidneys decrease in density. Only in the very few cases with severe changes and replacement lipomatosis (see below) in which the paren-

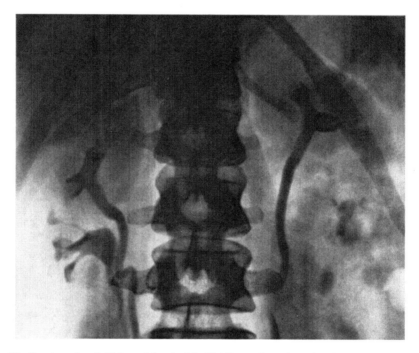

Fig. 253. Chronic pyelonephritis in caudal parts of double kidneys. Operation on left side showed marked pyelonephritic atrophy. Note compensatory hypertrophy of cranial part of both kidneys with marked nephrographic effect during angiography

chyma is replaced to a large extent by fatty connective tissue can the sinus increase in size and the central part of the kidney then appear less dense.

On clinical exacerbation of lesions in a pyelonephritic contracted kidney, the kidney will, even if extremely small, often increase in size.

b) Urography

Excretion urography should be performed when possible. This method is the most gentle and in addition to demonstration of morphologic changes, it yields information on renal function. In the differential diagnosis between acute pyelonephritis, acute abdominal disease or renal and ureteric stone we have found that in most of the patients examined at our department with urography in the acute stage excretion is ordinary (WULFF 1936), *i.e.* time of onset of excretion, density of contrast urine and drainage. Occasionally, however, excretion may be somewhat delayed, the contrast density may be somewhat low and drainage slow because of slight stasis caused by inflammatory edema of the ureteric mucosa.

In more chronic cases the roentgen finding will vary with the extent of the process. Excretion may be ordinary, decreased or absent. As a rule, the density of the contrast urine is somewhat decreased. It should be observed that urography performed for assessing renal function is, as mentioned in chapter E III. 2. b), a crude method. The renal morphology will also vary widely with the severity and extent of the process. In the early stage and in an acute exacerbation of a chronic process the filling of the stems of the calyces is often defective because of a swelling of the mucosa and contraction of the renal pelvis and the pelvis wall is markedly mouldable (Fig. 252). On occasion it may be difficult to obtain sharp films because of marked contractions in rapid succession. These contractions can be demonstrated by cineradiography.

In this connection it should be observed that the motility of the kidney pelvis should not be studied with the aid of retrograde pyelography because it is in-

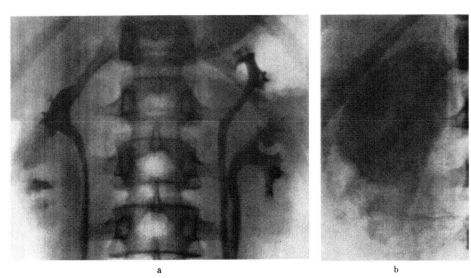

a   b

Fig. 254a and b. Woman, aged 38. Attacks of pyelonephritis since 5 years of age. Urography. a Double kidney bilaterally. Delayed function of caudal part of right kidney. Widened, deformed calyces in this part. Aortic renal angiography. b Nephrographic phase, right kidney: Marked atrophy of caudal part of kidney

fluenced considerably by catheterization and injection of the contrast medium. Investigation of the motility under such conditions will give misleading results.

In more advanced stages other changes appear owing to affection of the parenchyma. Destruction of one or more papillae leads to dilatation of the calyces, which then become more or less spherical. The calyces may extend far out into the renal parenchyma and even reach the surface of the kidney. All transitional forms ranging from normal to pronounced pathologic appearances are seen. Care should, of course, be taken to secure correct projections of the calyces, as stressed by DEJDAR and PRAT (1958). The earliest change consists simply of a flattening of the calyces. In local or generalized hypoplasia, it is often not possible to decide whether anomalies or pyelonephritis or perhaps both are responsible for the changes seen, as mentioned in chapter F. With our present knowledge of the roentgen features of pyelonephritis the scope of the term hypoplasia is in sore need of revision (Figs. 253, 254, 255).

All stages of papillary necrosis are observed with the details described in chapter S (see Fig. 245). Often only the final stages are seen with deformed calyces extending to the surface of the kidney. Judging from even modern text-books, these changes are not widely known.

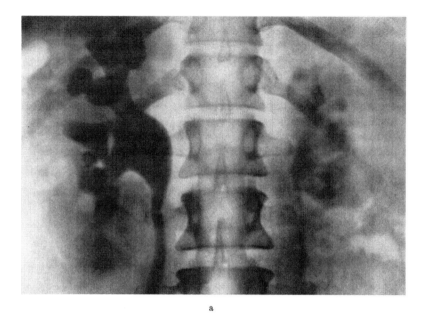

a

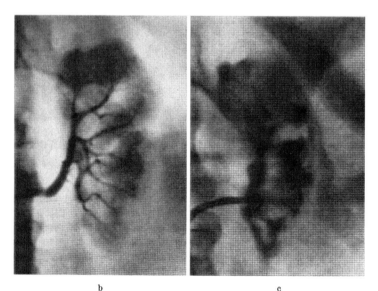

b   c

Fig. 255a—c. Pyelonephritis in hypoplastic kidney. a Urography: Small irregular left kidney with delayed func-tion. Compensatory hypertrophy of right kidney. Renal angiography: b Arterial phase. Irregular kidney with marked atrophy of vessels. c Final stage of renal angiography. Excretion of contrast urine filling irregular, widened calyces

In very advanced stages with pyonephrosis (Fig. 256) the same roentgen findings can be made as in stone pyonephrosis, described in chapter G.

Of greatest interest is, of course, the early diagnosis, particularly since effective therapy is now available for this stage of the disease. Slight changes of the calyces and of the motility and plasticity of the renal pelvis in combination seems to be sufficient to permit a firm diagnosis. Pyelonephritis is often responsible for the changes with distinct indentations in the renal pelvis by vessels and by the

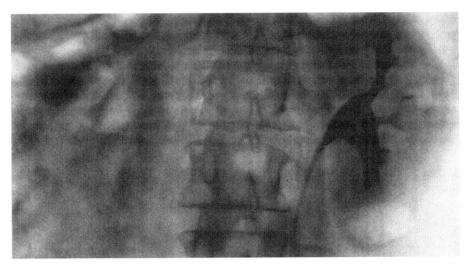

a

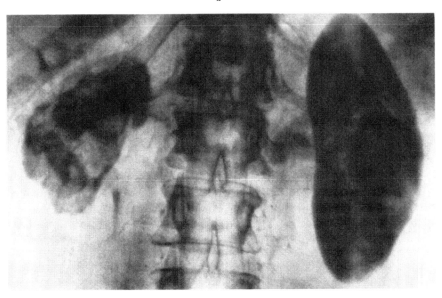

b

Fig. 256a—c. Chronic pyelonephritis. Contracted kidney. a Urography: No excretion on right side. Renal angiography: Marked atrophy of renal artery and branches. b Nephrographic phase. Small irregular kidney with wide sinus, thin cortex and widespread scar formation

edge of the parenchyma, as described in chapter E III. This point, however, requires further research with cineradiography in association with urography of cases in which a patho-anatomic diagnosis can be made.

c) Renal angiography

The angiographic findings vary with the extent of the process. The examination method provides good possibilities of judging the vascularity and amount of functioning parenchyma of the kidney. Of particular interest is the possibility of assessing local changes in the parenchyma. In local florid processes irregular areas may be seen with abundant delicate vessels and a diffuse increase in contrast as a sign of an inflammatory focus. In the cortical part of the parenchyma more or less extensive cicatrization and a varying number of small cysts may be seen. A tendency to spasm can sometimes be noted.

The findings in renal angiography are scanty and have not yet been analysed systematically in large series. Renal angiography will surely prove useful in the diagnosis of the condition, particularly if nephrectomy or partial nephrectomy is contemplated. Investigation of the angiographic changes in pyelonephritis is of importance for assessing the rôle played by pyelonephritis in a pathologic vascular pattern in association with other diseases combined with pyelonephritis.

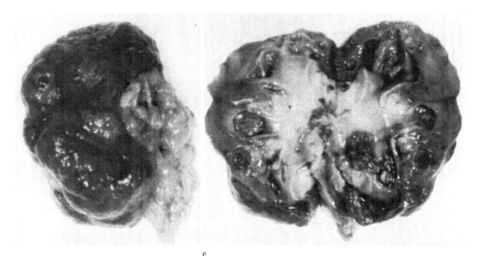

c

Fig. 256c. Operative specimen

8. Replacement lipomatosis

In association with diseases causing destruction of the renal parenchyma and a decrease in the volume of parenchyma fibrosis or fatty replacement of the tissue destroyed is sometimes seen. This condition is called replacement lipomatosis, renal lipomatosis, fibrolipomatosis renis, fibrosis and fatty replacement of destroyed renal cortex, fatty replacement of kidney etc. (Kutzmann 1931, Peacock & Balle 1936, Roth & Davidson; Priestly 1938, Frumkin 1947, Simril & Rose 1950, Hamre 1957). The condition is generally due to pyelonephritis. The accumulation of fat is always intra-capsular and should be distinguished from the rare lipoma in or adjacent a kidney. The fatty connective tissue is most abundant in the renal sinus around the renal pelvis, which may be dilated. Advanced cases are rare. It is of roentgen-diagnostic importance from the following points of view.

Replacement lipomatosis may be extensive and become a source of error to be borne in mind in the evaluation of the amount of renal parenchyma, as judged by the size of the kidney. A kidney may thus appear to be only slightly decreased or even increased in size but nevertheless have only a small amount of parenchyma left, the intracapsular content consisting of fibrous or fatty tissue. While replacement lipomatosis of low grade is common, severe replacement lipomatosis is rare and therefore seldom gives rise to an erroneous diagnosis.

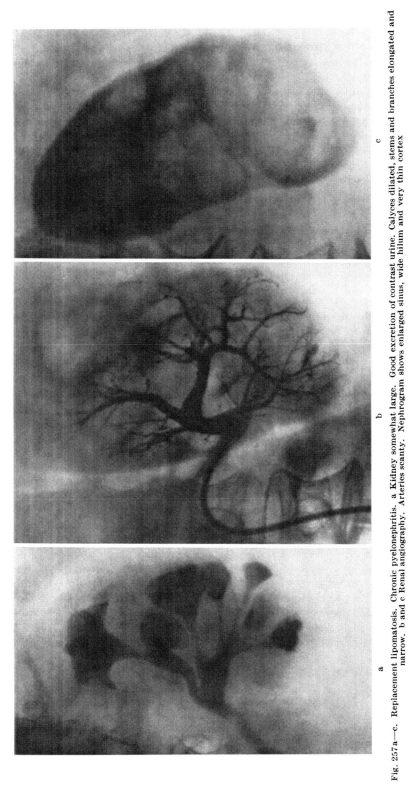

Fig. 257 a—c. Replacement lipomatosis. Chronic pyelonephritis. a Kidney somewhat large. Good excretion of contrast urine. Calyces dilated, stems and branches elongated and narrow. b and c Renal angiography. Arteries scanty. Nephrogram shows enlarged sinus, wide hilum and very thin cortex

Sometimes fat accumulates locally and causes a certain expansion of the kidney. On pyelographic examination it might then be misinterpreted as a tumour, particularly as the condition is usually unilateral. Most cases described in the literature were originally diagnosed as tumour and the diagnosis of replacement lipomatosis was made at operation or patho-anatomic examination.

Careful examinations usually will, however, suggest the diagnosis because the amount of renal parenchyma is reduced and because of the expansiveness with co-existent signs of shrinkage of the renal pelvis. Erroneous diagnoses can be avoided by resorting to renal angiography in the investigation of obscure space-occupying processes. This examination gives the diagnosis because of the absence of any demonstrable pathologic vessels and of any defined defect suggestive of tumour or cyst, while the sinus of the kidney will be widened and the parenchyma thin, and secondly because of the demonstration of generalized or local vascular changes of types that can be seen in pyelonephritis (Fig. 257).

9. Compensatory renal hypertrophy

If one of the kidneys is missing, as in aplasia, or if function is poor, as in severe hypoplasia, or if one of the kidneys has been removed or has ceased to function owing to such conditions as stasis, infections or degeneration, the other kidney will, as a rule, increase in size. This increase is called compensatory hypertrophy for the want of a better name. There is general agreement that this increase in size is due to growth in size of different parts of the nephron, whereas the number of nephrons does not increase, or at most only slightly.

Plain roentgenography of the urinary tract, particularly on comparison with films taken before development of the disease causing hypertrophy of the kidney, will show a marked increase in size of the latter. The increase is as a rule generalized and the kidney becomes plump. If any part of the kidney is the seat of a pathologic process, the rest of the kidney may also show compensatory hypertrophy, while the pathologically changed part will retain its original size. This explains the varying appearance of the kidney in some cases of local hypoplasia of one kidney in which the other kidney shows marked, generalized hypoplasia. Preserved parts of the locally hypoplastic kidney may hypertrophy to such an extent as to suggest the presence of a space-occupying lesion.

The healthy or residual kidney does not always increase in size. In a series of nephrectomized patients examined before and after nephrectomy SCHROEDER (1944) found an increase in the size of the remaining kidney in two thirds. The increase was less marked in the higher age-classes. Hypertrophy can occur in patients somewhat above 50 years, as shown by HANLEY (1940).

The increase in area in SCHROEDER's material was, on the average, 30 per cent, and somewhat larger in females than in males and larger in young patients than in elderly ones. In an experimental investigation on dogs WIDÉN (1958) found that on total obstruction of a ureter for at most 30 days, the other kidney increased in size by 20 per cent. After a ligation period of more than 30 days the kidney showed a statistically probable further increase of 15 per cent.

The kidney usually increases rapidly and then retains a certain size, though a continuous increase for 2—3 years has also been noted (BRAASCH & MERRICKS 1938). These authors pointed out that the large single kidney (in agenesia on the other side) is situated somewhat more caudally than the usual position of a normal kidney.

Urography often shows that in so-called compensatory enlargement of the kidney the width of the renal pelvis is also slightly increased. This is most readily demonstrated in cases in which urograms are available from the time before nephrectomy.

In these cases renal angiography also shows that the renal artery is wider than normally. IDBOHRN (1956) found that on unilateral ligation of the ureter in rabbits the caliber of the renal artery on the other side rapidly increased to a moderate extent and WIDÉN made the same observations in dogs.

V. Miscellaneous changes particularly of ureter

Since the ureter is exposed to essentially the same injurious agents as the kidneys and the renal pelvis, a large number of diseases can occur simultaneously or successively in the kidney pelvis, the ureter, and the bladder with primary or secondary involvement of the ureter. Therefore the normal roentgen anatomy and physiology of the ureter was described in the chapter on Urography and Pyelography. For the same reason the pathology of the ureter has been included in special chapters on tumours, tuberculosis, stone, anomalies, trauma, urinary tract dilatation etc. The ureters can, however, be affected by a wide variety of other pathologic changes calling for supplementary consideration.

Since the ureter is simply a duct for transporting the urine formed in the kidneys and accumulated in the renal pelvis to the bladder, and since this pathway is long and narrow, most of the pathologic changes of the ureter obstruct drainage. Some of these changes have been described in detail in the chapter on Urinary tract dilatation. Others have been mentioned and call for further description, while others being less common were not included in previous chapters.

a) Ureterocele

A ureterocele is a widening of the distal part of the ureter ballooning into the bladder. It is also called ureteric cyst or ureteric phimosis. The nomenclature is not strictly correct. As pointed out by BÉTOULIÈRES, JAUMES & COLIN (1959), the name ureterocele literally means a prolaps of the ureter into the bladder. Ureter cyst or cystic dilatation of the ureter, on the other hand, should mean a closed formation. Therefore in the French literature the term *dilatation pseudo-cystique de l'uretère terminal* has been used. In English the condition is usually referred to as ureterocele.

The distal end of the ureter shows a round or usually oval widening. Since this end bulges into the bladder under the mucosa it will appear in the cystogram as a filling defect at either or both ureteric orifices. On simultaneous filling of the ureter and bladder, as in urography, the dilated end of the ureter will be filled with contrast medium, which is separated from the contrast medium in the bladder by a defect a few millimetres wide. This defect corresponds to the wall of the ureter and the bladder mucosa.

The size of ureterocele varies widely depending in part on whether the ureteric orifice is obstructed or not. It might consist of such a slight widening of the end of the ureter that it may not be demonstrated in the urogram unless films are taken in proper projection with a suitable contrast filling around the ureteric orifice. The filling of a small ureterocele may also be intermittent depending on the flow of urine in the ureter. It may also vary with the extent to which the bladder is filled and disappear on distension of the bladder.

Ureterocele can, however, also assume considerable proportions and fill almost the entire bladder (RUDHE 1948). Then a large round symmetric or asymmetric well-defined formation is seen surrounded by a layer of contrast medium.

In such cases urination is difficult simply because the ureterocele obstructs the internal vesical orifice (GUTIERREZ 1939). When a ureterocele of this type occurs in a man in or above middle age, differentiation from prostatic hypertrophy is important.

As mentioned, in duplication of the ureter dilatation of the ureter draining the upper renal pelvis is common (see chapter Urinary tract dilatation). In such cases urography will show the renal pelvis and the ureter to be widened. In the bladder a ureterocele of varying size will be seen. The ureteric orifice is often ectopic. The ureterocele is then usually situated near the mid-line in the base of the bladder near the neck of the latter. If the ureteric orifice is ectopic, the ureterocele can prolapse out through the urethral orifice in females. A uretero-cele in the bladder at the internal orifice can, on straining, be pressed out into the urethra.

When a ureterocele causes stasis, only one of the ureters may be widened, *i.e.* that which has ureterocele. It may, however, also involve the other ipsilateral ureter, and sometimes the ureters on both sides according to the position and size of the uretero-cele.

If the ureterocele has developed in the poste-rior part of the urethra, ureterocystography will give more detailed infor-mation than urography.

Stasis in the ureter favours stone formation, and the finding of one or more concrements in or above a ureterocele is not uncommon. A concrement situ-ated at the ureteric orifice and seen in the cystogram separated from the contrast filling of the bladder by a contrast-free zone is pathognomonic of concrement in a ureterocele (ÅKERLUND 1935). The finding is thus the same as contrast in the ureterocele with simultaneous filling of the bladder, as described above. Some-times, however, a stone of ordinary appearance may be seen above a ureterocele or several concrements moving freely in the ureter (PETROVČIĆ & DUGAN 1955).

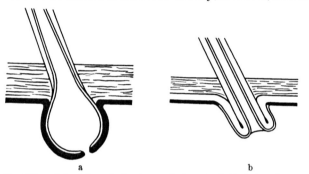

a   b

Fig. 258a and b. Schematic drawing. a Ureterocele. b Ureteric prolapse.
(After STAEHLER 1959)

b) Ureteric prolapse

Ureteric prolapse is rare. It consists of an invagination of the ureter through the ureteric orifice (Fig. 258). The formation bulging into the bladder thus has the ureteric lumen in the middle surrounded by a wall of ureteric mucosa. It appears in the contrast-filled bladder as an oblong filling defect in the direction of the ureter (WEMEAU, LEMAITRE & DEFRANCE 1959).

c) Ureteric endometriosis

In endometriosis of the adnexa and peritoneum the ureters may become involved. Bladder endometriosis can also affect the ureters if it is situated near the ureteric orifice. Endometriosis localized to the ureter is rare. Cases have been described by RANDALL (1941) and the latest by KAIRIS (1958). Most authors have reported only a single case. A narrowing is seen in the distal part of the ureter. Its appearance is not characteristic. Endometriosis should be suspected if urinary symptoms are found to be due to a narrowing of the distal third of the ureter in a women who reports that the symptoms usually increase in severity in association with menstruation.

d) Herniation of the ureter

A case has been described (LINDBOM 1947) in which urography of a patient with repeated left-sided attacks of renal colic for 8 years revealed hydronephrosis on that side, and retrograde ureterography with a bulb catheter showed a loop of the ureter like a hernia protruding in the direction of the sciatic foramen. At the neck the loop was constricted, and above the constriction the ureter was dilated. It was thus diagnosed as ureteric herniation in the sciatic foramen and obstructing flow. Operation verified this finding.

The ureter can also herniate down into a scrotal hernia (JEWETT & HARRIS 1953).

e) Ureteric involvement by aortic aneurysm

Two cases have been described (CRANE 1958) in which an aneurysm in the lumbar aorta caused hydronephrosis by pressing against respectively through extensive collagenous connective tissue formations encasing the ureter.

f) Ureteric diverticula

Small diverticula have been described, but not verified, in the presence of ureteric changes (HOLLY & SUMCAD 1957). Large congenital diverticula have been reported in a few cases. They may calcify (McGRAW & CULP 1952) and become so large as to contain one litre of fluid. As a rule, however, they are smaller and occur anywhere along the ureter. They are usually diagnosed as strictures because the neck of the diverticulum is narrow and it is therefore difficult to obtain a filling of the diverticulum.

g) Regional ureteritis

Ureteritis is common in inflammatory processes of the urinary tract, such as pyelonephritis or secondary to processes above the ureter *e.g.* pyenephrosis, or in processes located immediately outside the ureter such as appendicitis, salpingitis, regional ileitis. It may also be secondary to a condition within the ureter, *e.g.* stones. Such stones can occasionally be difficult to discover. They may be situated in a decubital lesion in the ureteric wall and later cause formation of scars and mucosal hyperplasia with long, severe ureteric stenosis as a result (ELLEGAST & SCHIMATZEK 1957).

Primary inflammatory infiltration along a few centimetres of the ureter has been described as causing moderate dilatation of the urinary tract (DREYFUSS & GOODSITT 1958, NORING 1958). This so-called regional ureteritis has no special characteristics. Ureteric changes with irregular narrowing along fair lengths of the ureter can occur in periarteriitis (polyangiitis) nodosa (FISHER & HOWARD 1948).

h) Peri-ureteritis obliterans

The disease was first described by ORMOND (1948). In recent years various authors have contributed with one or more cases each (HARLIN & HAMM 1952, CHISHOLM, HUTCH & BOLOMEY 1954, RAPER 1955, CIBERT, DURAND & RIVIÈRE 1956, STUEBER 1959 and others). It is usually called peri-ureteritis obliterans, primary retroperitoneal inflammatory process or primitive peri-ureteritis.

The disease usually involves the upper and middle portion of the ureter and the changes consist of a fibrous inflammatory tissue, in which the ureter is embedded. Pronounced edema is often present and microscopically a sclerosing type of inflammatory fibrosis is seen. The ureter is irregularly narrowed and displaced along a fair part of its length, the distal part usually being spared.

Urinary tract dilatation of varying degree occurs. It is often considerable, since the disease runs a slow and initially asymptomatic course with the result that the patient does not seek medical advice until late, by when renal insufficiency has developed.

The disease can probably be of varying origin. The roentgen findings do not differ from those caused by other chronic inflammatory peri-ureteric inflammation of known origin.

Higher up plastic perinephritis may be seen around the entire kidney. It has also been called perirenal fascitis representing a chronic inflammation in Gerotas fascia resulting in a stricture of the ureter with anuria.

It has been discussed whether these two diseases might represent one and the same clinical entity. HUTCH, ATKINSON & LOQUVAM (1959) believed that although these two diseases have some features in common and may ultimately prove to be related, they should be considered separate entities. They claim that the plastic peri-ureteritis may be unilateral and that the ureter can also be changed in its pelvic part which is not the case in plastic peri-nephritis.

I am inclined to believe that at least in some cases the disease may be due to reflux from the renal pelvis, which via the sinus and hilum spreads to the peri-renal tissue. Such refluxes may be unilateral or bilateral. In previous investigations (OLLE OLSSON 1948, 1953, HAMPERL 1949) it has been shown that reflux can cause pronounced fibrosis, and extra-renal fibrosis due to reflux has been described by IDBOHRN & FAJERS (1957) (see chapter Backflow).

i) Bilharziosis

In infection with Bilharzia changes of hyperplastic type can occur in the ureter with abundant small papillomatous formations, which may calcify. The changes may, however, also be of hypoplastic type with mucosal atrophy. In both types the lumen of the ureter is irregularly narrowed and may be obstructed (MAKAR 1948).

k) Amyloidosis

In amyloidosis, primary or secondary, the kidneys and urinary pathways may occasionally be involved. It is usually the bladder that is the seat of amyloidosis. Cases of amyloidosis in the renal pelvis and ureter have, however, also been reported, though mostly in the patho-anatomic literature (AKIMATO 1927 and others). They have also been described from a clinical point of view, and it has been stressed that on involvement of the ureter the lumen may be narrow and the length of the ureter involved may appear rigid (GILBERT & MCDONALD 1952, HIGBEE & MILLETT 1956, ANDREAS & OOSTING 1958). The narrowing has been shown to progress and, in the course of several years, to block the ureter entirely with hydronephrosis as a result (HIGHBEE & MILLETT 1956).

The changes described above have no features that might be described as characteristic of the condition. Amyloidosis should, however, be borne in mind as a possible cause of ureteric stricture and in the differentiation between ureteritis and tumour.

l) Leukoplakia

Leukoplakia means a change of the ordinary epithelium into a squamous epithelium characterized by keratinization. It may occur in any part of the urinary tract, such as in the renal pelvis and/or in the ureter. It is regarded as a pre-cancerous lesion. The disease is rare.

Leukoplakia may be so severe as to cause complete stenosis of the ureter or widespread mural changes with multiple moderately irregular strictures. It may also involve only part of the wall of the ureter or the renal pelvis and cause slight narrowing, or it may cause a slight rigidity of a minor part of the wall of the renal pelvis. It can also manifest itself as filling defects in the renal pelvis or as a high mucosa demonstrable in part of the renal pelvis and then resemble papillomatosis. Neither this type of change nor the total obstruction is characteristic of the disease. Therefore, as a rule, the diagnosis cannot be made roentgenologically. Roentgen examination may give a clue, but the diagnosis must be established by other methods. It has been stressed (FALK 1954) that squamous epithelium in large amounts can be found in the urinary sediment. If cystoscopy has diagnosed leukoplakia in the bladder, any roentgenchanges in the ureter and renal pelvis of the type described above may be diagnosed as leukoplakia.

m) Pyeloureteritis cystica

In pyelitis, ureteritis and cystitis cystica, multiple inflammatory cysts occur in the wall of the urinary tract. They are often seen in the entire urinary pathways, but may be localized only to the renal pelvis or the ureter, or more usually, only to the bladder. The cysts may be single or numerous.

Changes may be bilateral, but they are more frequently unilateral. They vary in size from large cysts obstructing flow in the ureter, to small and single mural excrescenses. They are more common in the proximal part of the ureter in contrast to papilloma, which is usually located in the distal portion of the ureter.

Roentgenologically diagnosed pyeloureteritis cystica was first described in 1929 (JACOBY; JOELSON). In urograms and pyelograms the cysts produce filling defects. If the cysts are numerous, some of them will always be seen along the margin as outgrowths from the ureteric wall. This gives the ureter a very irregular outline. If the cysts are numerous and if some of them are large, the diagnosis is thus easy. On detection of a single cyst, one should try to demonstrate it in suitable projections and show that the defect is projecting from the wall and of fixed localization.

It has been stated that a dilatation of the ends of the major calyces with narrowing of the stems of the calyces and a cystic dilatation at the pelviureteric junction and of the ends of the major calyces are characteristic of the disease (HINMAN, JOHNSON & McCORKLE 1936) which, however, is not obligatory and is not typical of this disease.

Instead of cystic the pelvic and ureteric mucosa may be granular, so-called granular pyelitis, which roentgenologically resembles pyelitis cystica. The defects are smaller than the defects produced by cysts (see Fig. 88).

n) Ureteric stump after nephrectomy

After nephrectomy leaving part of the ureter behind there is a possibility of a pathologic process being maintained or developed in the stump. A tuberculous ureteritis can thus cause persistent pyuria and bacilluria. Even if the ureter is not involved at the time of the operation, infected material can, via reflux from the bladder, be transported and deposited in it. Cases have been described in which at operation for stone pyonephrosis with or without stones being left in the ureter, pyoureter has flared up after several years with normal urinary findings (DAVISON 1942, LIVERMORE 1950, BENNETTS, CRANE, CRANE, GUMMESS & MILES 1955). In shrunken bladder the stump of the ureter may develop into a supplementary bladder and thereby increase the urinary reservoir (see Fig. 128).

It is also known that carcinoma can develop in the ureteric stump, even in patients in whom nephrectomy was done but not because of tumor (LOEF & CASELLA 1952).

The question whether primary ureterectomy is indicated or not is debatable and indications vary. RIESER (1950) recommends that retrograde pyelography should regularly be done with contrast filling of the ureter, whose drainage should be followed. A film taken about 1 or 2 hours after the retrograde injection of the contrast medium will indicate whether or not the contents of the ureter will be voided after nephrectomy. The information thus obtained would prove crucial and of material assistance in arriving at a definite decision concerning the indication for ureterectomy. Such a procedure may be of importance in some cases, but it cannot be accepted as a regular routine measure.

References

Acute urography

DITTMAR, F.: Reflektorische Skoliosen bei Erkrankungen der Harnwege. Dtsch. Arch. klin. Med. 184, 249 (1939). — HELLMER, H.: On the technique in urography and the roentgen picture in acute renal and ureteral statis. Acta radiol. (Stockh.) 16, 51 (1935). — HICKEL, R., et P. CORNET: Essai sur la signification et la valeur des images et des signes urographiques fonctionnels. J. Radiol. Électrol. 29 (1948). — WALLDÉN, L.: Administration of contrast medium in urography via the bone marrow. Acta radiol. (Stockh.) 25, 213 (1944).

Amyloidosis

GILBERT, L. W., and J. R. McDONALD: Primary amyloidosis of the renal pelvis and ureter: report of case. J. Urol. (Baltimore) 68, 137 (1952).

Anatomy

ANSON, B. J., E. W. CAULDWELL, J. W. PICK and L. E. BEATON: The blood supply of the kidney, suprarenal gland, and associated structures. Surg. Gynec. Obstet. 84, 313—320 (1947). — GARBSCH, H.: Zum Röntgenbild paraduodenal raumfordernder Prozesse. Radiol. Austr. 10, 71 (1958). — GONDOS, B.: Rotation of the kidney around its transverse axis. Radiology 74, 19—25 (1960). — HESS, E.: Renal mobility. J. Amer. med. Ass. 110, 1818 (1938). — LEMBKE, J.: Flächenkymographische Beobachtung an der pulsatorischen Mitbewegung an den Nieren. Fortschr. Röntgenstr. 85, 42—46 (1956). — MOËLL, H.: Kidney size and its deviation from normal in acute renal failure. Acta radiol. (Stockh.) Suppl. 206 (1961). — Size of normal kidneys. Acta radiol. (Stockh.) 46, 640—645 (1956). — RÖHRIG, H.: Kongenitale thorakale Ektopie der rechten Niere. Fortschr. Röntgenstr. 89, 371 (1958). — SANDERS jr., P. W.: Medial renal ptosis. J. Urol. (Baltimore) 77, 24—26 (1957).

Aneurysm

ABESHOUSE, B. S.: Aneurysm of the renal artery: report of two cases and review of the literature. Urol. cutan. Rev. 55, 451 (1951). — ATKINSON, R. L.: Aneurysm of the renal artery. J. Urol. (Baltimore) 72, 117 (1954). — BEGNER, J. A.: Aortography in renal artery aneurysm. J. Urol. (Baltimore) 73, 720 (1955). — BOIJSEN, E., and G. JÖNSSON: Renal arteriovenous aneurysm. To be published in Acta radiol. — GARRITANO, A. P., G. T. WOHL, C. K. KIRBY and A. L. PIETROLUONGO: The roentgenographic demonstration of an arteriovenous fistula of renal vessels. Amer. J. Roentgenol. 75, 905 (1956). — KEY, E., and Å. ÅKERLUND: Fall von verkalktem Aneurysma in der Arteria renalis. Fortschr. Röntgenstr. 25

(1917—1918). — LJUNGGREN, E., et G. EDSMAN: Remarques sur l'arteriographie rénale. Dixième Congrès de la Soc. Int. d'Urol. Athènes 10.—18. Avril 1955. Vol. II, p. 140. Athènes 1956. — RENCK, G.: Über das Renalisaneurysma, besonders vom röntgenologischen Gesichtspunkt. Acta radiol. (Stockh.) 7, 309 (1926). — SCHULZE-BERGMANN, G.: Über das arteriovenöse Aneurysma der Niere. Z. Urol. 47, 661 (1954). — SCHWARTZ, J. W., A. A. BORSKI and E. J. JAHNKE: Renal arteriovenous fistula. Surgery 37, 951 (1955). — SLOMINSKI-LAWS, M. D., J. H. KIEFER and C. W. VERMEULEN: Arteriovenous aneurysm of the kidney: case report. J. Urol. (Baltimore) 75, 586 (1956). — SPROUL, R. D., R. G. FRASER and K. J. MACKINNON: Aneurysm of the renal artery. J. Canad. Ass. Radiol. 9, 45 (1958).

Angiography

ABESHOUSE, B. S.: Thrombosis and thrombophlebitis of the renal veins. Urol. cutan. Rev. 49, 661—675 (1945). — ABESHOUSE, B. S., and A. T. TIONGSON: Paraplegia, a rare complication of translumbar aortography. J. Urol. (Baltimore) 75, 348—355 (1956). — AGUZZI, A., A. MARLEY e S. CHIUPPA: Valutazione critica delle technice di aortografia addominale. Boll. Soc. med.-chir. Pavia 68, 1153 (1954). — AHLBÄCK, S.: The suprarenal glands in aortography. Acta radiol. (Stockh.) 50, 341 (1958). — AJELLO, L., M. MELIS, G. BALDUZZI e G. BENEDETTI: L'arteriografia renale in condizioni normali e patologiche. Minerva chir. (Torino) 13, 1000—1014 (1958). — ALKEN, C. E.: La rénovasographie peropératoire. J. Urol. méd. chir. 57, 623 (1951). — Renovasographie bei Teilresektionen der Niere und ihre Bedeutung für die Diagnostik isolierter Prozesse am Nierenparenchym. Z. Urol. Sonderh. 1952, 121. — ALKEN, C. E., u. F. SOMMER: Die Renovasographie. Z. Urol. 43, 420—423 (1950). — ALLEN, C. D.: Urological symptoms produced by abdominal aneurysms. Urol. cutan. Rev. 44, 462 (1940). — AMBROSETTI, A., u. R. SESENNA: Arteriographische Untersuchungen an der tuberkulösen Niere. Urol. int. (Basel) 1, 153 (1955). — ANTHONY jr., J. E.: Complications of aortography. Arch. Surg. (Chicago) 76, 28 (1958). — ANTONI, N., and E. LINDGREN: Steno's experiment in man as complication in lumbar aortography. Acta chir. scand. 98, 230—247 (1949). — Aortography. J. Amer. med. Ass. 148, 652 (1952). — ARNOLD, M. W., W. E. GOODWIN and J. A. C. COLSTON: Renal infarction and its relation to hypertension. Urol. Surv. 1, 191 (1951). — BARNES, B. A., R. S. SHAW, A. LEAF and R. R. LINTON: Oliguria following diagnostic translumbar aortography: report of a case. New Engl. J. Med. 252, 1113 (1955). — BARON, G. J., and R. H. KOENEMANN: Arteriovenous fistula of the renal vessels. A case report. Radiology 64, 85 (1955). — BAURYS, W.: Serious complications associated with the newer diagnostic methods in urology. J. Urol. (Baltimore) 75, 846 (1956). — BAZY, L., J. HUGUIER, H. REBOUL, P. LAUBRY et J. AUBERT: Sur quelques aspects technique de l'artériographie. Arch. Mal. Coeur 41, 97 (1948). — BECKMANN, G. F.: Translumbar aortography. Transactions of southeastern section of the A.U.A. p. 144, apr. 1954. — BEGNER, J. A.: Aortography in renal artery aneurysm. J. Urol. (Baltimore) 73, 720 (1955). — BERG, O. C.: Acute renal failure following translumbar aortography. Sth. med. J. (Bgham, Ala.) 49, 494—496 (1956). — BERGENDAL, S.: Zur Frage der Hydronephrose bei Nierengefäßvarianten. Acta chir. scand. Suppl. 45 (1936). — BERRY, J. F., J. J. ROBBINS and E. L. PIRKEY: Abdominal aortography. Arch. Surg. (Chicago) 70, 173 (1955). — BERRY, N. E., E. P. WHITE and J. O. METCALFE: Abdominal aortography in urology. Canad. med. Ass. J. 66, 215 (1952). — BIERMAN, H. R., E. R. MILLER, R. L. BYRON, K. S. DOD, K. H. KELLY and D. H. BLACK: Intra-arterial catheterization of viscera in man. Amer. J. Roentgenol. 66, 555 (1951). — BOBLITT, D. E., M. M. FIGLEY and E. F. WOLFMAN jr.: Roentgen signs of contrast material dissection of aortic wall in direct aortography. Amer. J. Roentgenol. 81, 826 (1959). — BOHNE, A. W., and G. L. HENDERSON: Intrarenal arteriovenous aneurysm: case report. J. Urol. (Baltimore) 77, 818—820 (1957). — BOIJSEN, E.: Angiographic studies of the anatomy of single and multiple renal arteries. Acta radiol. (Stockh.) Suppl. 183 (1959). — CHAUVIN, E.: Sull'arteriografia renale. Minerva chir. (Torino) 13, 1134—1135 (1958). — CHIAUDANO, C.: Arteriografia renale. Torino 1955. — CHIAUDANO, M.: Aspetti arteriografici dei reni in condizioni patologiche. Minerva chir. (Torino) 13, 1074—1082 (1958). — Comportamento arteriografico del rene normale. Minerva chir. (Torino) 13, 1082—1090 (1958). — CHRISTOPHE, L., et D. HONORÉ: L'artériographie par injection et prises de clichés automatiques. J. Chir. (Paris) 63, 5 (1947). CLARK, C. G.: Unilateral renal injury due to translumbar aortography. Lancet 1958 I, 769. — CONGER, K. B., H. REARDON and J. AREY: Translumbar aortography followed by fatal renal failure and severe hemorrhagic diathesis. Arch. Surg. (Chicago) 74, 287 (1957). — CREEVY, C. D., and W. E. PRICE: Differentiation of renal cysts from neoplasms by abdominal aortography: Pitfalls. Radiology 64, 831—839 (1955). — CUÉLLAR, J.: New technique of translumbar aortic catheterization. J. Urol. (Baltimore) 75, 169 (1956). — DANIEL, P. M., M. M. L. PRICHARD and J. N. WARD-MCQUAID: The renal circulation after temporary occlusion of the renal artery. Brit. J. Urol. 26, 118 (1954). — DETAR, J. H., and J. A.

HARRIS: Venous pooled nephrograms: technique and results. J. Urol. (Baltimore) **72**, 979 (1954). — DETERLING jr., R. A.: Direct and retrograde aortography. Surgery **31**, 88—114 (1952). — DOSS, A. K.: Translumbar aortography: its diagnostic value in urology. J. Urol. (Baltimore) **55**, 594 (1946). — DOSS, A. K., H. C. THOMAS and T. B. BOND: Renal arteriography, its clinical value. Tex. St. J. Med. **38**, 277 (1953). — DOS SANTOS, R., A. LAMAS et J. P. CALDAS: L'artériographie des membres, de l'aorte et de ses branches abdominales. Bull. Soc. nat. Chir. **55**, 587 (1929). — DUNN, J., and H. BROWN: Unilateral renal disease and hypertension. J. Amer. med. Ass. **166**, 18 (1958). — EDHOLM, P., and S. I. SELDINGER: Percutaneous catheterization of the renal artery. Acta radiol. (Stockh.) **45**, 15 (1956). — EDLING, N. P. G., and C. G. HELANDER: On renal damage due to aortography and its prevention by renal tests. Acta radiol. (Stockh.) **47**, 473 (1957). — Nephrographic effect in renal angiography. Acta radiol. (Stockh.) **51**, 17 (1959). — Angionephrographic effect in renal damage. Acta radiol. (Stockh.) **51**, 241 (1959). — EDLING, N. P. G., C. G. HELANDER, F. PERSSON and Å. ÅSHEIM: Renal function after selective renal angiography. Acta radiol. (Stockh.) **51**, 161—169 (1959). — EDLING, N. P. G., C. G. HELANDER and S. I. SELDINGER: The nephrographic effect in depressed tubular excretion of umbradil. Acta radiol. (Stockh.) **48**, 1 (1957). — EDSMAN, G.: Accessory vessels of the kidney and their diagnosis in hydronephrosis. Acta radiol. (Stockh.) **42**, 26 (1954). — Angionephrography and suprarenal angiography. Acta radiol. (Stockh.) Suppl. **155** (1958). — Angionephrography in malignant renal tumours. Urol. int. (Basel) **6**, 117 (1958). — EIKNER, W. C., and CH. BOBECK: Renal vein thrombosis. J. Urol. (Baltimore) **75**, 780 (1956). — EVANS, A. T.: Renal arteriography. Amer. J. Roentgenol. **72**, 574 (1954). — EVANS, J. A., e A. F. GOVONI: Angionefrografia associata a stratigrafia. Radiol. med. (Torino) **41**, 1120 (1955). — FABRE, P.: L'angiographie rénale. X. congrès de la soc. int. d'urol. Aten 1955, p. 345. — FARIÑAS, P. L.: A new technique for the arteriographic examination of the abdominal aorta and its branches. Amer. J. Roentgenol. **46**, 641 (1941). — FERNSTRÖM, I., and K. LINDBLOM: Simultaneous stereoangiography. Acta radiol. (Stockh.) **44**, 230 (1955). — FONTAINE, R., P. WARTER, F. BILGER, M. KIM et R. KIENY: De l'intérêt de l'aortographie pour le diagnostic des affections rénales. J. Radiol. Électrol. **37**, 733—737 (1956). — FORST, H.: Der aortographische Nachweis der einseitigen Nierenaplasie. Z. Urol. **50**, 366 (1957). — GANSAU, H.: Cavographie. Fortschr. Röntgenstr. **84**, 575—580 (1956). — GARRITANO, A. P., G. T. WOHL, C. K. KIRBY and A. L. PIETROLUONGO: The roentgenographic demonstration of an arteriovenous fistula of renal vessels. Amer. J. Roentgenol. **75**, 905 (1956). — GASPAR, M. R., and P. G. SECREST: Chylothorax as a complication of translumbar aortography. Arch. Surg. (Chicago) **75**, 193—196 (1957). — GAYLIS, H., and J. W. LAWS: Dissection of aorta as complication of translumbar aortography. Brit. med. J. **1956**, 1141. — GESENIUS, H.: Die abdominale Aortographie. Fortschr. Röntgenstr. **76**, 24 (1952). — GOLLMAN, G.: Die gezielte Angiographie und ihre diagnostischen Möglichkeiten (Kathetermethode). Radiol. austr. **9**, 117—123 (1956). — Eine Modifizierung der Seldingerschen Kathetermethode zur isolierten Kontrastfüllung der Aortenäste. Fortschr. Röntgenstr. **87**, 211 (1957). — Zur Technik der Angiographie mittels Katheter. Fortschr. Röntgenstr. **89**, 281 (1958). — Die isolierte Angiographie der Aortenäste mit perkutan eingeführtem Katheter, ihre Indikation und Ergebnisse. Fortschr. Röntgenstr. **89**, 383 (1958). — GOODWIN, W. E., P. L. SCARDINO and W. W. SCOTT: Translumbar aortic puncture and retrograde catheterization of the aorta in aortography and renal arteriography. Ann. Surg. **132**, 944 (1950). — GOSPODINOW, G. I., u. J. B. TOPALOW: Phlebographie der Nierenvene auf dem Wege der Vena spermatica sinistra. Fortschr. Röntgenstr. **91**, 664—669 (1959). — GOTTLOB, R., G. ZINNER u. F. GOLDSCHMIDT: Über die Testmethoden zur Feststellung der lokalen schädlichen Wirkung von Röntgenkontrastmitteln bei der Angiographie. Langenbecks Arch. klin. Chir. **285**, 591 (1957). — GRAVES, F. T.: The anatomy of the intrarenal arteries in health and disease. Brit. J. Surg. **43**, 605—616 (1956). — GREGG, D. McC., J. M. ALLCOCK and F. R. BERRIDGE: Percutaneous transfemoral selective renal arteriography (including cineradiology). Brit. J. Radiol. **30**, 423—435 (1957). — GROSSMAN, L. A., and J. A. KIRTLEY: Paraplegia after translumbar aortography. J. Amer. med. Ass. **166**, 1035 (1958). — HANLEY, H. G.: Cineradiography of the urinary tract. Brit. med. J. **1955** II, 22—23. — HARE, W. S. C.: Damage to the spinal cord during translumbar aortography. J. Fac. Radiol. (Lond.) **8**, 258 (1957). — HARRISON, C. V., M. D. MILNE and R. E. STEINER: Clinical aspects of renal vein thrombosis. Quart. J. Med. **25**, 285—298 (1956). — HARVARD, M.: Renal angiography. J. Urol. (Baltimore) **70**, 15 (1953). — HAUSCHILD, W.: Peridurale Kontrastmittelinjektion bei der Aortographie. Fortschr. Röntgenstr. **88**, 154 (1958). — HELANDER, C. G.: Nephrographic effect and renal arteriographic damage. Acta radiol. (Stockh.) Suppl. **163** (1958). — HELANDER, C. G., and Å. LINDBOM: Roentgen examination of the inferior vena cava in retroperitoneal expanding process. Acta radiol. (Stockh.) **45**, 287 (1956). — HELLSTRÖM, J.: Über die Varianten der Nierengefäße. Z. urol. Chir. **24**, 253 (1928). — HOL, R., and O. SKJERVEN: Spinal cord damage in abdominal aortography. Acta radiol. (Stockh.) **42**, 276 (1954). — HOLM, O. F.: Registrering genom aortografi av lokala recidiv efter nefrectomi för hypernefrom (renalt adenocarcinom). Svenska Läk.-Tidn. **54**, 3388 (1957). — Hou-Jensen, H. M.: Die Verästelung der Arteria renalis in der Niere des Menschen. Berlin: Springer 1929. — Hughes, F., A. Barcia, O. Fiandra y J. Viola: Angiografia renal por via femoral. An. Hosp. S. Cruz (Barcelona) **17**, 1—8 (1957). Aneurysm of the renal artery. Acta radiol. (Stockh.) **49**, 117 (1958). — Idbohrn, H.: Angiographical diagnosis of carotid body tumours. Acta radiol. (Stockh.) **35**, 115—123 (1951). — Renal angiography in cases of delayed excretion in intravenous urography. Acta radiol. (Stockh.) **42**, 333—352 (1954). — Indovina, I.: La circolazione renale studiata mediante isotopi radioattivi. Minerva chir. (Torino) **13**, 1090—1096 (1958). — Isaac, F., T. H. Brem, E. Temkin and H. J. Movius: Congenital malformation of the renal artery, a cause of hypertension. Radiology **68**, 679 (1957). — Isaac, F., I. Schoen and P. Walker: An unusual case of Lindau's disease. Cystic disease of the kidneys and pancreas with renal and cerebellar tumors. Amer. J. Roentgenol. **75**, 912 (1956). — Jones, R. N., and F. G. Wood: Renal arteriography. Practitioner **175**, (1047) 293—299 (1955). — Kaufman, J. J., D. E. Burke and W. E. Goodwin: Abdominal venography in urological diagnosis. J. Urol. (Baltimore) **75**, 160—168 (1956). — Landelius, E.: Death following renal arteriography in a child. Acta chir. scand. **109**, 469—472 (1955). — Lasio, E., G. Arrigoni e A. Civino: L'aortografia addominale in chirurgia urologica. Arch. ital. Urol. **27**, 424 (1954). — Indicazioni e limiti dell'aortografia addominale in urologia. Minerva chir. (Torino) **13**, 1096—1100 (1958). — Leger, L., C. Proux et M. Duranteau: Phlébographie rénale et cave inférieure par injection intra-parenchymateuse. Presse méd. **65**, 141 (1957). — Leriche, R., P. Beaconsfield and C. Boely: Aortography: its interpretation and value. A report of 200 cases. Surg. Gynec. Obstet. **94**, 83—90 (1952). — Liese, G. J.: Angiotomography: a preliminary report. Radiology **75**, 272—275 (1960). — Lindblom, K., and S. I. Seldinger: Renal angiography as compared with renal puncture in the diagnosis of cysts and tumours. X. congrès de la soc. int. d'urol. Aten 1955, p. 331. — Lindgren, E.: Technique of abdominal aortography. Acta radiol. (Stockh.) **39**, 205 (1953). — Ljunggren, E., et G. Edsman: Remarques sur l'arteriographie rénale. X. congrès de la soc. int. d'urol. Aten 1955 II, pp. 140—147. — Lockhart, J., A. Pollero, A. Corlere y J. Héctor: La cavografia de los tumores del testiculo. Arch. esp. Urol. **12** (1956). — Lodin, H., and L. Thorén: Renal function following aortography carried out under ganglionic block. Acta radiol. (Stockh.) **43**, 345—354 (1955). — Löfgren, F.: Das topographische System der Malpighischen Pyramiden der Menschenniere. Lund: A. B. Gleerupska Univ.-bokhandeln 1949. — Löfgren, F. O.: Renal tumour not demonstrable by urography but shown by renal angiography. Acta radiol. (Stockh.) **42**, 300 (1954). — Loose, K. E.: The importance of serial aortography for demonstration of blood vessels in pelvis and kidney. Radiol. clin. (Basel) **23**, 325 (1954). — Lopatkin, N. A.: Renal angiography and its diagnostic significance (Russian text). Vestn. Hir. **78**, 74 (1957). — Malisoff, S. and M. Cerruti: Aneurysm of the renal artery. J. Urol. (Baltimore) **76**, 542—549 (1956). — Maluf, N. S. R.: Internal diameter of renal artery and renal function. Surg. Gynec. Obstet. **107**, 415 (1958). — Maluf, N. S. R., and C. B. McCoy: Translumbar aortography as a diagnostic procedure in urology. Amer. J. Roentgenol. **73**, 533 (1955). — Manfredi, D., R. Begani e L. G. Frezza: La roentgencineangiografia renale selettiva. Minerva chir. (Torino) **13**, 1100—1103 (1958). — Margolis, G., A. K. Tarazi and K. S. Grimson: Contrast medium injury to the spinal cord produced by aortography. J. Neurosurg. **13**, 349 (1956). — McAfee, J. G.: A survey of complications of abdominal aortography. Radiology **68**, 825—838 (1957). — McAfee, J. G., and J. K. V. Willson: A review of the complications of translumbar aortography. Amer. J. Roentgenol. **75**, 956 (1956). — McCormack, J. G.: Paraplegia secondary to abdominal aortography. J. Amer. med. Ass. **161**, 860 (1956). — McDonald, D. F., and J. M. Kennelly jr.: Intrarenal distribution of multiple renal arteries. J. Urol. (Baltimore) **81**, 25 (1959). — McDowell, R. F. C., and I. D. Thompson: Inferior mesenteric artery occlusion following lumbar aortography. Brit. J. Radiol. **32**, 344 (1959). — McLelland, R.: Renal artery aneurysms. Amer. J. Roentgenol. **78**, 256—265 (1957). — Meldolesi, G.: Il quadro angiografico renale nel blocco degli ureteri. Minerva chir. (Torino) **13**, 1104—1109 (1958). — Migliardi, L.: Sull'angiografia renale. Minerva chir. (Torino) **13**, 1135 (1958). — Miller, A. L., A. W. Brown and G. C. Tomskey: Pelvic fused kidney. J. Urol. (Baltimore) **75**, 17 (1956). — Morino, F., e A. Tarquini: Il contributo dell'arteriografia selettiva allo studio della patologia renale. Minerva chir. (Torino) **13**, 1018—1041 (1958). — Mulholland, S. W.: Abdominal crises with urologic implications. J. Amer. med. Ass. **166**, 455 (1958). — Muller, H.: Arteriography by retrograde catheterization of the aorta in renal pathology. Arch. chir. neerl. **5**, 108 (1953). — Murray, R. S., and G. C. Tresidder: Renal angiography. Brit. med. Bull. **13**, 61—63 (1957). — Myhre, J. R.: Arteriovenous fistula of the renal vessels. A case report. Circulation **14**, 185—187 (1956). — Nesbitt, T. E.: A criticism of renal angiography. Amer. J. Roentgenol. **73**, 574 (1955). — Nicolich, G., e G. B. Cerruti: La nostra esperienza in angiografia renale e vescicale. Minerva chir. (Torino) **13**, 1109—1111

(1958). — NORDMARK, B.: Double formations of the pelves of the kidneys and the ureters. Embryology, occurrence and clinical significance. Acta radiol. (Stockh.) **30**, 267 (1948). — NOTTER, G., u. C. G. HELANDER: Über den Wert der Cavographie bei Diagnose und Behandlung retroperitonealer Testistumormetastasen. Fortschr. Röntgenstr. **89**, 409 (1958). — NUNNO jr., R. DE: L'arteriografia strumentale selettiva del rene. Arch. ital. Urol. **29**, 159—168 (1956). — Technique, indications et limites de l'artériographie sélective instrumentale du rein. Presse méd. **65**, 792 (1957). — L'arteriografia selettiva strumentala del rene. Minerva chir. (Torino) **13**, 1014—1018 (1958). — ÖDMAN, P.: Percutaneous selective angiography of the main branches of the aorta. Acta radiol. (Stockh.) **45**, 1 (1956). — OLHAGEN, B.: Hypernefromdiagnos vid negativ urografi. Svenska Läk.-Tidn. **51**, 7 (1954). — OLIVERO, S., F. MORINO e F. MARGAGLIA: Comportamento delle curve glicemiche a seguito dell'arteriografia addominale selettiva. Minerva chir. (Torino) **13**, 1111—1117 (1958). — OLSSON, OLLE: Renal angiography. X. congrès de la soc. int. d'urol. Aten 1955 I, p. 298. — Arteriografia renale per via transfemorale. Minerva chir. (Torino) **13**, 1041—1044 (1958). — Renal angiography in the pre-diagnostic phase. IX. I. C. R. München 1959. — PEIRCE, C.: Arteriografia renale transfemorale. Minerva chir. (Torino) **13**, 1045—1048 (1958). — PEIRCE, E. C. II: Percutaneous femoral artery aortography: Its use in the evaluation of retroperitoneal masses. J. int. Coll. Surg. **20**, 16—28 (1953). — PEIRCE, E. C. II, and W. P. RAMEY: Renal arteriography: report of a percutaneous method using the femoral artery approach and a disposable catheter. J. Urol. (Baltimore) **69**, 578—585 (1953). — PETTINARI, V., e M. SERVELLO: L'indagine arteriografica e flebografica del rene. Minerva chir. **13**, 1117—1122 (1958). — PIRONTI, L., e A. TARQUINI: Alcuni casi di tumore primitivo del rene studiati con l'arteriografia renale selettiva. Minerva chir. **13**, 1122—1131 (1958). — POIRIER, P., et A. CHARPY: Traité d'anatomie humaine. Paris: Masson & Cie. 1923. — POST, H. W.A., and W. F. W. SOUTHWOOD: The technique and interpretation of nephrotomograms. Brit. J. Radiol. **32**, 734—738 (1959). — POTTS, I. F.: Translumbar aortography. Med. J. Austr. **1**, 173 (1954). — Further experiences in aortography. Med. J. Austr. **1955** I, 232. — POUTASSE, E. F.: Occlusion of renal artery as cause of hypertension. Circulation **13**, 37—48 (1956). — Renal artery aneurysm: report of 12 cases, two treated by excision of the aneurysm and repair of renal artery. J. Urol. (Baltimore) **77**, 697—708 (1957). — POUTASSE, E. F., and H. P. DUSTAN: Arteriosclerosis and renal hypertension. J. Amer. med. Ass. **165**, 1521 (1957). — POUTASSE, E. F., A. W. HUMPHRIES, L. J. MCCORMACK and A. C. CORCORAN: Bilateral stenosis of renal arteries and hypertension: Treatment by arterial homografts. J. Amer. med. Ass. **161**, 419—423 (1956). — PROVET, H., J. W. LORD and J. R. LISA: Aneurysm of the renal artery. Amer. J. Roentgenol. **78**, 266—269 (1957). — PYRAH, L. N., and J. W. COWIE: Two unusual aortograms. J. Fac. Radiol. (Lond.) **8**, 416 (1957). — RADNER, S.: Subclavian angiography by arterial catheterization. Acta radiol. (Stockh.) **23**, 359—364 (1949). — RANDALL, A., and E. W. CAMPBELL: Anomalous relationship of the right ureter to the vena cava. J. Urol. (Baltimore) **34**, 565 (1935). — REAGAN jr., G. W., and G. CARROLL: Arteriography as observed in 80 patients at St. Louis city hospital. J. Urol. (Baltimore) **66**, 467 (1951). — RICHES, E. W.: The present status of renal angiography. Brit. J. Surg. **42**, 462 (1955). — RICHES, E. W., and I. H. GRIFFITHS: Renal angiography. X. congrès de la soc. int. d'urol. Aten 1955, p. 271. — RITTER, J. S.: Aortography. J. Urol. (Baltimore) **73**, 155 (1955). — ROBECCHI, M., F. MORINO e A. TARQUINI: L'arteriografia renale selettiva per via omerale nella pratica urologica. Minerva med. (Torino) **47**, 1639 (1956). — ROBINSON, ALAN S.: Acute pancreatitis following translumbar aortography: case report with autopsy findings seven weeks following aortogram. A.M.A. Arch. Surg. **72**, 290—294 (1956). — ROSSI, A.: Aortografia addominale translombare, o arteriografia renale selettiva? Minerva chir. (Torino) **13**, 1131—1134 (1958). — ROUX-BERGER, J. L., J. NAULLEAU et X. J. CONTIADÈS: Cortico-surrénalome malin. Aortographie. Exérèse. Guérison opératoire. Bull. Soc. nat. Chir. **60**, 791—802 (1934). — SAMUEL, E., and M. DENNY: An evaluation of the hazards of aortography. Arch. Surg. (Chicago) **76**, 542 (1958). — SANTE, L. R.: Evaluation of aortography in abdominal diagnosis. Radiology **56**, 183 (1951). — SANTOS, J. C. DOS: L'angiographie rénale. X. congrès de la soc. int. d'urol. Aten 1955, p. 229. — Phlébographie d'une veine cave inférieure suturée. J. Urol. méd. chir. **39**, 586 (1935). — Technique de l'Aortographie. J. int. Chir. **2**, 609 (1937). — SCHIMATZEK, A.: Aortographie. Verh.ber. der Dtsch. Ges. für Urologie, Leipzig 1958, S. 257. — SCHWARTZ, J. W., A.A. BORSKI and E. J. JAHNKE: Renal arteriovenous fistula. Surgery **37**, 951—954 (1955). — SELDINGER, S. I.: Catheter replacement of the needle in percutaneous arteriography. Acta radiol. (Stockh.) **39**, 368 (1953). — SILVIS, R. S., W. F. HUGHES and F. H. HOLMES: Aneurysm of the renal artery. Amer. J. Surg. **91**, 339—343 (1956). — SKOP, V., and V. TEICHMANN: The aortographic picture in Grawitz tumours of the kidney. Čsl. Roentgenol. **9**, 148 (1955). — SLOMINSKI-LAWS, M. D., J. H. KIEFER and C. W. VERMEULEN: Arteriovenous aneurysm of the kidney: case report. J. Urol. (Baltimore) **75**, 586 (1956). — SMITH, G. I., and V. ERICKSON: Intrarenal aneurysm of the renal artery: case report.

J. Urol. (Baltimore) **77**, 814—817 (1957). — SMITH, P. G.: A résumé of the experience of the making of 1500 renal angiograms. J. Urol. (Baltimore) **70**, 328 (1953). — SMITH, P. G., T. W. RUSH and A. T. EVANS: An evaluation of translumbar arteriography. J. Urol. (Baltimore) **65**, 911 (1951). — The technique of translumbar arteriography. J. Amer. med. Ass. **148**, 255 (1952). — SMITHUIS, T.: The problem of renal segmentation in connection with the modes of ramification of the renal artery and the renal vein. Acta chir. neerl. **8**, 227 (1956). — SOMMER, F., u. P. SCHÖLZEL: Beobachtung einer aszendierenden Aortenthrombose nach Aortographie. Fortschr. Röntgenstr. **86**, 609—613 (1957). — STEINER, R. E.: Venography in relation to the kidney. Brit. med. Bull. **13**, 64—66 (1957). — STIRLING, W. B.: Aortography. Its application in urological and some other conditions. Edinburgh and London: E. & S. Livingstone Ltd. 1957. — TARAZI, A. K., G. MARGOLIS and K. S. GRIMSON: Spinal cord lesions produced by aortography in dogs. Arch. Surg. (Chicago) **72**, 38 (1956). — THOMSON, H. S., G. MARGOLIS, K. S. GRIMSON and H. M. TAYLOR: Effects of intra-arterial injection of iodine contrast media on the kidney of the dog. Arch. Surg. (Chicago) **74**, 39 (1957). — TILLANDER, H.: Magnetic guidance of a catheter with articulated steel tip. Acta radiol. (Stockh.) **35**, 62—64 (1951). — TILLE, D.: Zur Technik und Indikation der Aortographie insbesondere der Renovasographie. Z. Urol. **52**, 121 (1959). — TRUC, E. e R. PALEIRAC: I difetti di diffusione gassosa retro-peritoneale fisiologici. Minerva chir. (Torino) **13**, 1135—1137 (1958). — UNGEHEUER, E.: Indikationen zur Aortographie. Med. Klin. **52**, 16 (1957). — VELZER, D. A. VAN, and R. R. LANIER: A simplified technic for nephrotomography. Radiology **70**, 77 (1958). — VOGLER, E.: Die Aortographie in ihrer Anwendung zur Darstellung der Durchblutung innerer Organe. Radiol. austr. **9**, 13 (1956). — VOGLER, E., u. R. HERBST: Angiographie der Nieren. Stuttgart: Georg Thieme 1958. — VOTH, H., u. H. FINKE: Zum Röntgenbild der Nierennekrose. Fortschr. Röntgenstr. **87**, 266—267 (1957). — WAGNER jr., F. B.: Arteriography in renal diagnosis: Preliminary report and critical evaluation. J. Urol. (Baltimore) **56**, 625 (1946). — WALTER, R. C., and W. E. GOODWIN: Aortography and pneumography in children. J. Urol. (Baltimore) **77**, 323 (1957). — WEYDE, R.: Die abdominale Aortographie, insbesondere bei Nierenkrankheiten. Radiol. clin. (Basel) **23**, 313 (1954). — WIDÉN, T.: Renal angiography during and after unilateral ureteric occlusion. Acta radiol. (Stockh.) Suppl. **162** (1958). — WINTER, C. C.: Unilateral renal disease and hypertension: Use of the radioactive diodrast renogram as a screening test. J. Urol. (Baltimore) **78**, 107—116 (1957). — WOHL, G. T.: Use of contrast media in the recognition of hypertension of renal origin. Radiology **69**, 672 (1957). — WOODRUFF jr., J. H., and R. E. OTTOMAN: Radiologic diagnosis of renal tumours by renal angiography. J. Canad. Ass. Radiol. **7**, 54—58 (1956). — WYATT, G. M., and B. FELSON: Aortic thrombosis as a cause of hypertension: an arteriographic study. Radiology **69**, 676 (1957). — ZHEUTLIN, N., D. HUGHES and B. J. O'LOUGHLIN: Radiographic findings in renal vein thrombosis. Radiology **73**, 884—890 (1959).

[Anomalies

ABOULKER, P., et C. MOTZ: Un cas d'uretère rétro-cave. J. Urol. méd. chir. **59**, 391 (1953). — ABRAMS, A., L. and A. L. FINKLE: Reversible suppressed function in unilateral renal malrotation. J. Amer. med. Ass. **163**, 641 (1957). — ALLANSMITH, R.: Ectopic ureter termination in seminal vesicle; unilateral polycystic kidney: report of a case and review of the literature. J. Urol. (Baltimore) **80**, 425 (1958). — ANDERSON, G. W., G. G. RICE and B. A. HARRIS jr.: Pregnancy and labor complicated by pelvic ectopic kidney. J. Urol. (Baltimore) **65**, 760 (1951). — ANDERSSON, J. C., and A. S. C. ROBERTSON: Solitary ectopic pelvis kidney. Brit. J. Urol. **24**, 207 (1952). — ANSON, B. J., and L. E. KURTH: Common variations in the renal blood supply. Surg. Gynec. Obstet. **100**, 157 (1955). — ASK-UPMARK, E.: Über juvenile maligne Nephrosklerose und ihr Verhältnis zu Störungen in der Nierenentwicklung. Acta path. microbiol. scand. **6**, 383—442 (1929). — AXILROD, H. D.: Triplicate ureter. J. Urol. (Baltimore) **72**, 799 (1954). — BAGGENSTOSS, A. H.: Congenital anomalies of the kidney. Med. Clin. N. Amer. **35**, 987 (1951). — BANKER, R. J., and W. H. CARD: Calyceal diverticula. J. Urol. (Baltimore) **72**, 773 (1954). — BARLOON, J. W., W. E. GOODWIN and V. VERMOOTEN: Thoracic kidney. J. Urol. (Baltimore) **78**, 356—358 (1957). — BEGG, R. C.: Sextuplicitas renum: a case of six functioning kidneys and ureters in an adult female. J. Urol. (Baltimore) **70**, 686 (1953). — BENNETT, J. P.: Renal cysts communicating with the pelvis. Illinois med. **79**, 232 (1941). — BIBUS, B.: Ein seltener Fall von Nierenmißbildung. Z. Urol. **47**, 28 (1954). — BIE, K.: Ureteral duplications, ectopic ureter and ureterocele. J. Oslo Cy Hosp. **8**, 201 (1958). — BOLADO, J. L. I.: Rinon en herradura. Arch. esp. Urol. **13**, 220 (1957). — BORELL, U., and I. FERNSTRÖM: Congenital solitary pelvic kidney. A study of its blood supply by aortography. J. Urol. (Baltimore) **72**, 618 (1954). — BRAASCH, W. F.: Anomalous renal rotation and associated anomalies. Trans. Amer. Ass. gen.-urin. Surg. **23**, 1 (1930). — BRAIBANTI, T.: Considerazioni su un caso di dispasia cistica del rene. Ann. Radiol. diagn. (Bologna) **21**, 412 (1949). —

BROOMÉ, A.: Komplex urogenital missbildning. Nord. Med. **59**, 51 (1958). — BRUNELLI, B., e M. DARDARI: Raro aspetto di cisti pielogenica. Nunt. radiol. (Firenze) **21**, 33—39 (1955). — BULGRIN, J. G., and F. H. HOLMES: Eventration of the diaphragm with high renal ectopia. Radiology **64**, 249 (1955). — BURKLAND, C. E.: Clinical considerations in aplasia, hypoplasia and atrophy of the kidney. J. Urol. (Baltimore) **71**, 1 (1954). — BUTLER, T. J.: Solitary ectopic pelvic kidney. Brit. J. Surg. **38**, 522 (1951). — CAMPBELL, M. F.: Urology. I. Philadelphia and London: W. B. Saunders Company 1954. — Renal ectopy. J. Urol. (Baltimore) **24**, 187 (1930). — CAMPOS FREIRE, G.: Uretère rétrocave et rein hypoplasique. J. Urol. méd. chir. **59**, 868 (1953). — CATHRO, A. J. McG.: Section of the inferior vena cava for retrocaval ureter: A new method of treatment. J. Urol. (Baltimore) **67**, 464 (1952). — CHALKLEY, T. S., and L. E. SUTTON: Infected solitary cyst of the kidney in a child, with a review of the literature. J. Urol. (Baltimore) **50**, 414 (1943). — CHAUVIN, H. F.: Sur les images radiologiques d'uretère rétro-cave. J. Urol. méd. chir. **60**, 266 (1954). — CHWALLA (1935) cit. GILL (1952). — COPPRIDGE, W. M.: Bilateral pelvic kidneys. J. Urol. (Baltimore) **32**, 231 (1934). — COUVELAIRE, R.: Autre exemple d'uretère rétro-cave. J. Urol. méd. chir. **59**, 65 (1953). — CULVER, H.: Extravesical ureteral opening into the genital tract in a male. Trans. Amer. Ass. gen.-urin. Surg. **30**, 295 (1937). — DALLA BERNARDINA, L., and E. RIGOLI: La cisti pielogenica. Quad. radiol. **23**, 109 (1958). — DAMM, E.: Solitärcysten der Niere. Z. urol. Chir. **35**, 102 (1932). — DAVIDSON, B.: Renal ectopia with abdominal and pelvic symptomatology. Urol. cutan. Rev. **42**, 334 (1938). — DAY, R. V.: Ectopic opening of the ureter in the male with report of a case. J. Urol. (Baltimore) **11**, 239 (1924). — DEÁK, J.: Eine seltene Nierenentwicklungsanomalie. Fortschr. Röntgenstr. **85**, 250—252 (1956). — DEMOULIN, M., u. L. NICKELS: Kelchzysten der Niere. Fortschr. Röntgenstr. **83**, 208 (1955). — DERBES, V. J., and W. A. DIAL: Postcaval ureter. J. Urol. (Baltimore) **36**, 226 (1936). — DORSEY, J. W.: Solitary hydrocalyx secondary to a dumbbell calculus. J. Urol. (Baltimore) **62**, 742 (1949). — DREYFUSS, W.: Anomaly simulating a retrocaval ureter. J. Urol. (Baltimore) **82**, 630—632 (1959). — DUFF, P. A.: Retrocaval ureter: Case report. J. Urol. (Baltimore) **63**, 496 (1950). — DUFOUR, A., et P. SESBOÜÉ: L'uretère rétro-cave. J. Urol. méd. chir. **58**, 433 (1952). — Uretère rétrocave diagnostiqué avant l'opération et guéri par urétéroplastie. J. Urol. méd. chir. **58**, 390 (1952). — ECKERBOM, H., and B. LILIEQUIST: Ectopic ureter. Acta radiol. (Stockh.) **38**, 420 (1952). — EKSTRÖM, T.: Renal hypoplasia. A clinical study of 179 cases. Acta chir. scand. Suppl. **203** (1955). — EKSTRÖM, T., and A. E. NILSON: Retrocaval ureter. Acta chir. scand. **118**, 53—59 (1959). — EMMETT, J. L., J. J. ALVAREZ-IERENA and J. R. McDONALD: Atrophic pyelonephritis versus congenital renal hypoplasia. J. Amer. med. Ass. **148**, 1470 (1952). — ENGEL, W. J.: Aberrant ureters ending blindly. J. Urol. (Baltimore) **42**, 674 (1939). — The late results of partial nephrectomy for calyectasis with stone. J. Urol. (Baltimore) **57**, 619 (1947). — Ureteral ectopia opening into the seminal vesicle. J. Urol. (Baltimore) **60**, 46 (1948). — ERICKSEN, L. G.: Rupture of congenital solitary kidney. Report of a case in which the diagnosis was made during life. Amer. J. Roentgenol. **39**, 731 (1938). — ESCH, W., u. K. HALBEIS: Zu den Kelchzysten der Niere. Radiol. Austr. **10**, 65 (1958). — EVERS, E.: Zwei Fälle mit seltener Ureteranomalie (akzessorische Blindureter). Acta radiol. (Stockh.) **25**, 121 (1944). — FALLENIUS, GÖSTA: Beitrag zur Röntgendiagnostik der Nierenektopie. Acta radiol. (Stockh.) **23**, 455 (1942). — FELTON, L. M.: Should intravenous pyelography be a routine procedure for children with chryptorchism or hypospadias? J. Urol. (Baltimore) **81**, 335 (1959). — FERGUSON, G., and J. N. WARD-McQUAID: Stones in pyelogenic cysts. Brit. J. Surg. **42**, 595 (1955). — FEY, B., GOUYGOU et TEINTURIER: Diverticules kystiques des calcies. J. Urol. méd. chir. **57**, 1 (1951). — GILL, R. D.: Triplication of the ureter and renal pelvis. J. Urol. (Baltimore) **68**, 140 (1952). — GLENN, J. F.: Fused pelvic kidney. J. Urol. (Baltimore) **80**, 7 (1958). — GOLDSTEIN, A. E., and E. HELLER: Ectopic ureter opening into a seminal vesicle. J. Urol. (Baltimore) **75**, 57 (1956). — GONDOS, B.: High ectopy of the left kidney. Amer. J. Roentgenol. **74**, 295 (1955). — GRAVES, F. T.: The anatomy of the intrarenal arteries in health and disease. Brit. J. Surg. **43**, 605 (1956). — GRAVES, R. C., and L. M. DAVIDOFF: Anomalous relationship of the right ureter to the inferior vena cava. J. Urol. (Baltimore) **8**, 75 (1922). — GRUBER, G.: Entwicklungsstörungen der Nieren und Harnleiter. In HENKE-LUBARSCH' Handbuch der speziellen pathologischen Anatomie und Histologie, Teil 4. Berlin 1925. — HAMILTON, G. R., and A. B. PEYTON: Ureter opening into seminal vesicle complicated by traumatic rupture of only functioning kidney. J. Urol. (Baltimore) **64**, 731 (1950). — HARRIS, A.: Renal ectopia — special reference to crossed ectopia without fusion. J. Urol. (Baltimore) **42**, 1051 (1939). — HARRISON, J. H., and T. W. BOTSFORD: Experiences in the management of congenital anomaly of the kidney in the army. J. Urol. (Baltimore) **55**, 309 (1946). — HEIDENBLUT, A.: Das Kelchdivertikel der Niere. Fortschr. Röntgenstr. **84**, 230 (1956). — HELLMER, H.: Nephrography. Acta radiol. (Stockh.) **23**, 233—254 (1942). — HELLSTRÖM, J.: Über die Varianten der Nierengefäße. Z. urol. Chir. **24**, 253 (1928). — HENNIG, O.: Überbleibsel von Urnierenanlagen. Z. Urol. **47**, 493 (1954). — HESLIN, J. E., and C. MAMONAS:

Retrocaval ureter; report of four cases and review of literature. J. Urol. (Baltimore) **65**, 212 (1951). — HOLM, H.: On pyelogenic renal cysts. Acta radiol. (Stockh.) **29**, 87 (1948). — HOU-JENSEN, H.: Die Verästelung der Arteria renalis in der Niere des Menschen. Z. Anat. Entwickl.-Gesch. **91**, 1 (1930). — IDBOHRN, H., and S. SJÖSTEDT: Ectopic ureter not causing incontinence until adult life. Acta obstet. gynec. scand. **33**, 457 (1954). — ITIKAWA, T., u. H. TANIO: Über den Ureterprolapsus und das angeborene Divertikel des Nierenkelchs. Z. Urol. **33**, 395—398 (1939). — KATZEN, P., and B. TRACHTMAN: Diagnosis of vaginal ectopic ureter by vaginogram. J. Urol. (Baltimore) **72**, 808 (1954). — KRETSCHMER, H. L.: Hernia of the kidney. J. Urol. (Baltimore) **65**, 944 (1951). — LAIDIG, C. E., and J. M. PIERCE jr.: Retrocaval ureter — unusual cause of ureteral obstruction. J. Amer. med. Ass. **171**, 2312 to 2314 (1959). — LAU, F. T., and R. B. HENLINE: Ureteral anomalies. J. Amer. med. Ass. **96**, 587 (1931). — LAUGHLIN, V. C.: Retrocaval (circumcaval) ureter associated with solitary kidney. J. Urol. (Baltimore) **71**, 195 (1954). — LJUNGGREN, E.: Beitrag zur Röntgendiagnostik der Nierentuberkulose. Z. Urol. **36**, 155 (1942). — MAYER, R. F., and G. L. MATHES: Retrocaval ureter. Sth. med. J. (Bgham, Ala) **51**, 945 (1958). — McDONALD, D. F., and J. M. KENNELLY jr.: Intrarenal distribution of multiple renal arteries. J. Urol. (Baltimore) **81**, 25—26 (1959). — MEISEL, H. J.: Ectopic ureter opening into a seminal vesicle. J. Urol. (Baltimore) **68**, 579 (1952). — MESSERSCHMIDT, O.: Beitrag zur Röntgendiagnose der „Cystome des nephrogenen Gewebes". Fortschr. Röntgenstr. **79**, 529 (1953). — MILLER jr., A. L., A.W. BROWN and G. C. TOMSKEY: Pelvic fused kidney. J. Urol. (Baltimore) **75**, 17 (1956). — MOLINA, L. F. R., and R. M. SABUCEDO: The retrocaval ureter. Radiologia (Panama) **7**, 115 (1957). — MOORE, G. W., and W. I. BUCHERT: Unilateral multicystic kidney in an infant. J. Urol. (Baltimore) **78**, 721 (1957). — MULLEN jr., W. H., and W. J. ENGEL: Circumcaval ureter. Radiology **59**, 528 (1952). — NATVIG, P.: Two cases of solitary renal cyst with communication to the renal pelvis. Acta radiol. (Stockh.) **22**, 732 (1941). — NORDMARK, B.: Double formations of the pelves of the kidneys and the ureters. Embryology, occurrence and clinical significance. Acta radiol. (Stockh.) **30**, 267—278 (1948). — OCHSNER, H. C.: Cysts of the kidney. Amer. J. Roentgenol. **65**, 185 (1951). — ØDEGAARD, H.: Crossed renal ectopia. Acta radiol. (Stockh.) **27**, 543 (1946). — ÖSTLING, K.: Röntgenologische und pathologisch-anatomische Veränderungen bei Erweiterungen einzelner Nierenkelche. Acta radiol. (Stockh.) **15**, 28 (1934). — PASQUIER, C. M., and R. K. WOMACK: Ectopic opening of ureter into seminal vesicle. J. Urol. (Baltimore) **70**, 164 (1953). — PERRIN (1927) cit. GILL (1952). — PETROVČIĆ, F., and O. KRIVEC: Triple ureter: with report of a case. Brit. J. Radiol. **28**, 627 (1955). — PETROVČIĆ, F., and N. MILIĆ: „Horseshoe" kidney with crossed ureter condition after right nephrectomy. Brit. J. Radiol. **29**, 114 (1956). — PICK, J .W., and B. J. ANSON: Retrocaval ureter; report of a case, with discussion of its clinical significance. J. Urol. (Baltimore) **43**, 672 (1940). — PONTHUS, P., et F. N. BOUSTANY: Sur le diagnostic radiologique du rein en fer à cheval. Rev. méd. Moy. Or. **13**, 93—98 (1956). — POTTS, I. F.: Solitary ectopic pelvic kidney. Med. J. Aust. **2**, 498 (1953). — PRATHER, G. C.: Calyceal diverticulum. J. Urol. (Baltimore) **45**, 55 (1941). — PRESMAN, D., and RAYMOND F.: A diagnostic method for retrocaval ureter. Amer. J. Surg. **92**, 628—631 (1956). — RANDALL, A., and E. W. CAMPBELL: Anomalous relationship of the right ureter to the vena cava. J. Urol. (Baltimore) **34**, 565 (1935). — RAYER, P. F. O.: Traité des maladies des reins. Paris **3**, 507 (1841). — RIBA, L.W., C. J. SCHMIDLAPP and N. L. BOSWORTH: Ectopic ureter draining into the seminal vesicle. J. Urol. (Baltimore) **56**, 332 (1946). — ROBERTS, R. R.: Complete valve of the ureter: Congenital urethral valves. J. Urol. (Baltimore) **76**, 62 (1956). — RÖHRIG, H.: Kongenitale thorakale Ektopie der rechten Niere. Fortschr. Röntgenstr. **89**, 371 (1958). — RUDSTRÖM, P.: Ein Fall von Nierenzyste mit eigenartiger Konkrementbildung. Acta chir. scand. **85**, 501—510 (1941). — SANDEGÅRD, E.: The treatment of ureteral ectopia. Acta chir. scand. **115**, 149 (1958). — SCHORR, S., and D. BIRNBAUM: Raised position of the right kidney. Radiol. clin. (Basel) **28**, 102—110 (1959). — SCHWARTZ, A., and M. FRÄNKEL: High renal ectopia, detected on routine chest examination. Acta radiol. (Stockh.) **37**, 583 (1952). — SCHWARTZ, J.: An unusual unilateral multicystic kidney in infant. J. Urol. (Baltimore) **35**, 259—263 (1936). — SELDOWITSCH, J. B.: Über die Multiplicität der Nierenarterie und deren chirurgische Bedeutung. Langenbecks Arch. klin. Chir. **89**, 1071 (1909). — SERVANTIE, G.: Un cas d'uretère rétro-cave. J. Radiol. Électrol. **37**, 935—937 (1956). — SESBOÜÉ, P.: L'uretère retro-cave. Thèse, Paris 1952. — SHIH, H. E.: Postcaval ureter. J. Urol. (Baltimore) **38**, 61 (1937). — SPENCE, H. M.: Congenital unilateral multicystic kidney: an entity to be distinguished from polycystic kidney disease and other cystic disorders. J. Urol. (Baltimore) **74**, 693 (1955). — SPILLANE, R. J., and G. C. PRATHER: High renal ectopy: a case report. J. Urol. (Baltimore) **62**, 441 (1949). — STEVENS, A. R.: Pelvic single kidneys. J. Urol. (Baltimore) **37**, 610 (1937). — STITES, J. R., and J. A. BOWEN: Crossed ectopia of the kidney. J. Urol. (Baltimore) **42**, 9 (1939). — TEICHERT, G.: Kelchdivertikel der Niere mit Konkrement. Fortschr. Röntgenstr. **84**, 761—762 (1956). — THOMAS, G. J., and J. C. BARTON: Ectopic pelvic kidney. J. Amer. med. Ass. **106**, 197 (1936). —

THOMPSON, G. J., and J. M. PACE: Ectopic kidney. Surg. Gynec. Obstet. **64**, 935 (1937). — THORSÉN, G.: Pyelorenal cysts. Acta chir. scand. **98**, 476 (1949). — VELZER, D. A. VAN, C. W. BARRICK and E. L. JENKINSON: Postcaval ureter. A case report. Amer. J. Roengenol. **74**, 490 (1955). — WALL, B., and H. E. WACHTER: Congenital ureteral valve: its role as a primary obstructive lesion: classification of the literature and report of an authentic case. J. Urol. (Baltimore) **68**, 684 (1952). — WATKINS, K. H.: Cysts of kidney due to hydrocalycosis. Brit. J. Urol. **11**, 207 (1939). — WILLIAMS, J. I., R. B. CARSON and W. D. WELLS: Renal aplasia: a report of two cases. J. Urol. (Baltimore) **79**, 6 (1958). — WYRENS, R. G.: Calyceal diverticula or pyelogenic cysts. J. Urol. (Baltimore) **70**, 358 (1953). — YOUNG, J. N.: Ureteral opening into the seminal vesicle: report on a case. Brit. J. Urol. **27**, 57 (1955). — YOW, R. M., and R. C. BUNTS: Calyceal diverticulum. J. Urol. (Baltimore) **73**, 663 (1955).

Backflow

ABESHOUSE, B. S.: Pyelographic injection of perirenal lymphatics. Amer. J. Surg. **25**, 427 (1934). — AHLSTRÖM, C. G.: Experimentelle Untersuchung über die pyelovenöse Refluxe. Acta chir. scand. **75**, 162 (1934). — AUVERT, J. (Rapporteur): Les reflux à partir du bassinet. (Refluxt pyélo-rénal.) Ass. Française d'Urologie 51. session Paris, 7 au 12 octobre 1957. Rapp or et informations. — BAUER, D.: Pyelorenal backflow. Amer. J. Roentgenol. **78**, 296—316 (1957). — BITSCHAI, J.: Demonstrationen zum Kapitel der Nierenchirurgie. Z. Urol. **21**, 891 (1927). — BOYARSKY, S., A. TAYLOR and G. BAYLIN: Extravasation in excretory urography. Urol. int. (Basel) **1**, 191 (1955). — CEDERLUND, H.: Beitrag zur Frage des pyelovenösen Rückflusses. Acta radiol. (Stockh.) **23**, 34 (1942). — FAJERS, C. M., and H. IDBOHRN: Peripelvic reflux simulating a tumour of the renal pelvis. Urologia int. (Basel) **5**, 197 (1957). — FUCHS, F.: Untersuchungen über die innere Topographie der Niere. Z. urol. Chir. **18**, 164 (1925). — Pyelovenous backflow in the human kidney. J. Urol. (Baltimore) **23**, 181—216 (1930). — Zur Frage der pyelographisch sichtbaren Nierenbeckenextravasate. Z. urol. Chir. **30**, 392—403 (1930). — Die Hydromechanik der Niere. Z. urol. Chir. **33**, 1—144 (1931). — Die physiologische Rolle des Fornixapparates. Z. urol. Chir. **42**, 80—100 (1936). — HAMPERL, H.: Vävnadsreaktion („främmandekroppsreaktion") mot slem och urin. Nord. Med. **41**, 66 (1949). — HENDRIOCK, A.: Intravenöse Urographie und pelvirenaler Übertritt. Zbl. Chir. **61**, 1822—1827 (1934). — HERRNHEISER, G., u. F. STRNAD: Die Perforationen des Nierenbeckens und des Harnleiters im Pyelogramm. Erg. Med. Strf. **7**, 259—297 (1936). — HINKEL, C. L.: Opacification of the renal pyramids in intravenous urography. Amer. J. Roentgenol. **78**, 317—322 (1957). — HINMAN, F., and R. K. LEE-BROWN: Pyelovenous back flow. J. Amer. med. Ass. **82**, 607 (1924). — ILLYÉS, G. v.: Frühzeitige Feststellung einer kleinen Nierengeschwulst mittels pyelovenösen Refluxes. Z. urol. Chir. **34**, 186 (1932). — KÖHLER, R.: Investigations on backflow in retrograde pyelography. Acta radiol. (Stockh.) Suppl. **99** (1953). — LAMMERS, H. J., TH. SMITHUIS et Å. LOHMAN: De pyelo-veneuze reflux. Ned. T. Geneesk **99**, 3237 (1955). — LINDBOM, Å.: Fornix backflow in excretion urography. Acta radiol. (Stockh.) **24**, 411 (1943). — Miliary tuberculosis after retrograde pyelography. Acta radiol. (Stockh.) **25**, 219 (1944). — MEUSER, H.: Über Hypernephrome. Z. Urol. **37**, 251—261 (1943). — MINDER, J.: Experimentelle und klinische Beiträge zur Frage des pyelovenösen Refluxes und seine klinische Bedeutung. Z. urol. Chir. **30**, 404 (1930). — OLIVIER, A.: Les aspects radiologiques des hémato-lymphochyluries filariennes. J. Radiol. Électrol. **38**, 286—288 (1957). — OLSSON, OLLE: Studies on backflow in excretion urography. Acta radiol. (Stockh.) Suppl. **70** (1948). — ORKIN, L. A.: Spontaneous or nontraumatic extravasation from the ureter. J. Urol. (Baltimore) **67**, 272 (1952). — OSSINSKAYA, V. V.: Refluxes. Vestn. Rentgenol. Radiol. **16**, 25 (1936). — PERSKY, L., and J. J. JOELSON: Spontaneous rupture of renal pelvis secondary to a small ureteral calculus. J. Urol. (Baltimore) **72**, 141 (1954). — PERSKY, L., J. P. STORAASLI an.d G. AUSTEN: Mechanisms of hydronephrosis: Newer investigative techniques. J. Urol. (Baltimore) **73**, 740 (1955). — POLITANO, V. A.: Pyelorenal backflow. J. Urol. (Baltimore) **78**, 1—8 (1957). — PYTEL, A.: A propos de la pathogénèse et du traitement des soi-disant hémorragies rénales essentielles. Acta urol. belg. **24**, 211—244 (1956). — Über den Fornix-Venenkanal als Ursache gewisser Nierenblutungen. Urologia (Treviso) **25** (1958). — QUACK, G.: Pyelorenaler Reflux bei der Ausscheidungsurographie. Fortschr. Röntgenstr. **91**, 411—412 (1959). — RENANDER, A.: Röntgenbefunde bei Nierentuberkulose. Acta radiol. (Stockh.) **20**, 341 (1939). — ROLNICK, H. C., and P. L. SINGER: Effects of overdistention of the renal pelvis and ureter: A study on pyelovenous backflow. J. Urol. (Baltimore) **57**, 834 (1947). — SCHUBERTH, O.: Eine Komplikation bei Pyelographierung. Zbl. ges. Chir. Grenzgeb. **60**, 1825 (1933). — SENGPIEL, G. W.: Renal backflow in excretory urography. Amer. J. Roentgenol. **78**, 289—295 (1957). — SOARES DE GOUVÊA, G.: Spontaneous reflux during excretory urography. Rev. bras. Cir. **22**, 307 (1951). — STAUBESAND, J.: Beobachtungen an Korrosionspräparaten menschlicher Nierenbecken. Fortschr. Röntgenstr. **85**, 33—41 (1956). — STEINERT, R.: Renal tuberculosis and roentgenologic examination. Acta radiol. (Stockh.) Suppl. **53** (1943). — SVOBODA, M.: Thorotrast residue in the kidneys thirteen years after retrograde pyelography. Zbl. Chir. **79**, 1930 (1954). — WEINER, M. E., F. S. ALCORN and E. L. JENKINSON: Subcapsular rupture of the kidney during intravenous urography. Radiology **69**, 853 (1957).

Cyst

ANDRESEN, K.: Beitrag zur Röntgenologie der solitären Nierenzysten. Röntgenpraxis 8, 505 (1936). — BARNETT, L. E.: Hydatid disease. Aust. N.Z. J. Surg. **12**, 240 (1943). — BAURYS, W.: Echinococcus disease of the kidney. J. Urol. (Baltimore) **68**, 411 (1952). — BELTRAN, J. C.: Congenital unilateral multicystic kidney in infancy. J. Urol. (Baltimore) **81**, 602 (1959). — BERGER, I. R., and G. T. COWART: Renal echinococcus disease. Radiology **62**, 852 (1954). — CLAESSEN, G.: The roentgen diagnosis of echinococcus tumors. Acta radiol. (Stockh.) Suppl. **6** (1928). — CLARKE, B. G., W. J. GOADE jr., H. L. RUDY and L. ROCKWOOD: Differential diagnosis between cancer and solitary serous cyst of the kidney. J. Urol. (Baltimore) **75**, 922 (1956). — COPPRIDGE, A. J., and R. K. RATLIFF: Unilateral multicystic disease. J. Pediat. **53**, 330 (1958). — DEAN, A. L.: Treatment of solitary cyst of the kidney by aspiration. Trans. Amer. Ass. gen.-urin. Surg. **32**, 91 (1939). — DEW, H. R.: Hydatid disease. Sidney: Australian medical publishing co. 1928. — DEWEERD, J. H., and H. B. SIMON: Simple renal cysts in children: review of the literature and report of five cases. J. Urol. (Baltimore) **75**, 912 (1956). — DUBILIER, W., and J. A. EVANS: Peripelvic cysts of the kidney. Radiology **71**, 404 (1958). — FINE, M. G., and E. BURNS: Unilateral multicystic kidney: report of six cases and discussion of the literature. J. Urol. (Baltimore) **81**, 42 (1959). — FISH, G. W.: Large solitary serous cysts of the kidney. J. Amer. med. Ass. **112**, 514 (1939). — FRAZIER, T. H.: Multilocular cysts of the kidney. J. Urol. (Baltimore) **65**, 351 (1951). — GOLDSTEIN, H. H., M. L. LIEBERMAN and G. E. OBESTER: Echinococcic disease of the kidney: report of a case of unusual size. J. Urol. (Baltimore) **81**, 596 (1959). — GORDON, I. R. S.: Renal puncture. J. Fac. Radiol. (Lond.) **9**, 108 (1958). — GRABSTALD, H.: Catherization of renal cyst for diagnostic and therapeutic purposes. J. Urol. (Baltimore) **71**, 28 (1954). — HUDSON, P. L.: Echinococcus disease. Sth. med. J. (Bgham, Ala.) **38**, 584 (1945). — HUFFMAN, W. L.: Echinococcus disease of kidney: report of a case. J. Urol. (Baltimore) **78**, 17 (1957). — ISAAC, F., I. SCHOEN and P. WALKER: An unusual case of Lindau's disease. Cystic disease of the kidneys and pancreas with renal and cerebellar tumors. Amer. J. Roentgenol. **75**, 912—920 (1956). — IVEMARK, B. I., and K. LINDBLOM: Arterial ruptures in the adult polycystic kidney. Acta chir. scand. **115**, 100 (1958). — KRETSCHMER, H. L.: Echinococcus disease of kidney. Surg. Gynec. Obstet. **36**, 196 (1923). — LATHAM, W. J.: Hydatid disease. J. Fac. Radiol. (Lond.) **5**, 65 (1953). — LINDBLOM, K.: Diagnostic kidney puncture in cysts and tumors. Amer. J. Roentgenol. **68**, 209 (1952). — LOWSLEY, O. S., and M. S. CURTIS: The surgical aspects of cystic disease of the kidney. J. Amer. med. Ass. **127**, 112 (1945). — MISHALANY, H. G., and D. R. GILBERT: Benign ossified lesion of the kidney — report of a case resembling a hydatid cyst. J. Urol. (Baltimore) **78**, 330 (1957). — MOORE, G. W., and W. I. BUCHERT: Unilateral multicystic kidney in an infant. J. Urol. (Baltimore) **78**, 721 (1957). — MUIR, J. B. G.: Hydatid cyst of kidney. Aust. N.Z. J. Surg. **17**, 305 (1948). — NATVIG, P.: Two cases of solitary renal cyst with communication to the renal pelvis. Acta radiol. (Stockh.) **22**, 732 (1941). — OLIVERO, S.: Il problema diagnostico dei reni cistici con particolare riguardo alla semeiologia arteriografica. Minerva urol. (Torino) **11**, 31—43 (1959). — PISANO, D. J., R. H. ROSEN, B. M. RUBINSTEIN and H. G. JACOBSON: The roentgen manifestations of carcinoma and cyst in the same kidney. Amer. J. Roentgenol. **80**, 603 (1958). — REAY, E. R., and G. L. ROLLESTON: Diagnosis of hydatid cyst of the kidney. J. Urol. (Baltimore) **64**, 26 (1950). — SALANO, P. B. E.: Consideraciones sobre 452 casos de quistes renales, revisados en el „Armed forces institute ot pathology". Arch. esp. Urol. **13**, 299 (1957). — SHIVERS, C. H. DE T., and H. D. AXILROD: Solitary renal cysts. J. Urol. (Baltimore) **69**, 193 (1953). — SNOW, W. T.: Urachal cyst with calculi. Amer. J. Roentgenol. **78**, 323—327 (1957). — SPENCE, H. M.: Congenital unilateral multicystic kidney: an entity to be distinguished from polycystic kidney disease and other cystic disorders. J. Urol. (Baltimore) **74**, 693—706 (1955). — TEPLICK, J. G., M. LABESS and S. STEINBERG: Echinococcosis of the kidney. J. Urol. (Baltimore) **78**, 323 (1957). — WHEELER, B. C.: Use of the aspirating needle in the diagnosis of solitary renal cyst. New Engl. J. Med. **226**, 55 (1952). — WHITE, E. W., and L. BRAUNSTEIN: Renal cystic disease. J. Urol. (Baltimore) **71**, 17 (1954).

Dilatation of the urinary tract

ANDERSON, J. C.: Hydronephrosis and hydrocalycosis, in E. W. RICHES, Modern Trends in urology, Chap. 10, p. 96. London: Butterworth & Co. 1953. — BAKER, E. C., and J. S.

LEWIS jr.: Comparison of the urinary tract in pregnancy and pelvic tumors. J. Amer. med. Ass. **104**, 812 (1935). — BAUER, K. M.: Das Rücklaufzystogramm. Medizinische **1**, 47 (1957). — BENJAMIN, J. A., J. J. BETHEIL, V. M. EMMEL, G. H. RAMSEY and J. S. WATSON: Observations on ureteral obstruction and contractility in man and dog. J. Urol. (Baltimore) **75**, 25 (1956). — BERGENDAL, S.: Zur Frage der Hydronephrose bei Nierengefäßvarianten. Acta chir. scand. Suppl. **45** (1936). — BISCHOFF, P.: Mißbildungen und Entleerungsstörungen der oberen Harnwege im Kindesalter. Verhandlungsber. der Dtsch. Ges. für Urologie, S. 29. Leipzig 1958. — BLIGH, A. S.: Pyelographic changes in pregnancy. Brit. J. Radiol. **30**, 489 (1957). — BRAASCH, W. F., and R. D. MUSSEY: Complications in the urinary tract during pregnancy. Minn. Med. **28**, 543 (1945). — BUCHMANN, E.: Ureterstenosierung und Hydronephrosenbildung durch Krebsinfiltration und Strahleninduration des Parametriums beim Collumcarcinom. Strahlentherapie **99**, 20 (1956). — CASEY, W. C., and W. E. GOODWIN: Percutaneous antegrade pyelography and hydronephrosis. J. Urol. (Baltimore) **74**, 164 (1955). — CONTIADES, X.-J.: A propos de l'origine hormonale de la stase urinaire gravidique. 37. Congr. franc. d'Urol. Paris 1937, p. 473. — COVINGTON jr., T., and W. REESER: Hydronephrosis associated with overhydration. J. Urol. (Baltimore) **63**, 438 (1950). — CRABTREE, E. G., G. C. PRATHER and E. L. PRIEN: End-results of urinary tract infections associated with pregnancy. Amer. J. Obstet. Gynec. **34**, 405 (1937). — CRUVEILHIER: Zit. F. HOFF, Der Schwangerschaftsureter. Beilageheft zu Z. Geburtsh. Gynäk. **125** (1945). — ECKERBOM, H., and B. LILIEQUIST: Ectopic ureter. Acta radiol. (Stockh.) **38**, 420 (1952). — EDELBROCK, H. H.: Ureterovesical obstruction in children. J. Urol. (Baltimore) **74**, 492 (1955). — EDSMAN, G.: Accessory vessels of the kidney and their diagnosis in hydronephrosis. Acta radiol. (Stockh.) **42**, 26 (1954). — FALK, D.: Intermittent obstruction at the ureteropelvic juncture. J. Urol. (Baltimore) **79**, 16 (1958). — FETTER, T. R., and K. C. WARREN: Congenital urinary tract obstructions in children. J. Urol. (Baltimore) **75**, 173 (1956). — FINLAY jr., A. M.: Importance of the postvoiding film in pediatric excretory urography. Tex. St. J. Med. **53**, 781 (1957). — GIBSON, TH. E.: Hydronephrosis: diagnosis and treatment of ureteropelvic obstructions. J. Urol. (Baltimore) **75**, 1 (1956). — GREENE, L. F., J. T. PRIESTLEY, H. B. SIMON and R. H. HEMPSTEAD: Obstruction of the lower third of the ureter by anomalous blood vessels. J. Urol. (Baltimore) **71**, 544 (1954). — HANDEL, J., and S. SCHWARTZ: Value of the prone position for filling the obstructed ureter in the presence of hydronephrosis. Radiology **71**, 102 (1958). — HERMANN, J. v., u. A. F. KRAUS: Zur Indikationsstellung der Prostatektomie auf Grund der Ausscheidungsurographie. Z. urol. Chir. **41**, 441—460 (1936). — HOFF, F.: Der Schwangerschaftsureter. Ein experimenteller Beitrag zum Nachweis seiner Entstehung. Beilageheft Z. Geburtsh. **125** (1943). — HOLDER, E.: Die mechanische Hydronephrose und ihre Fähigkeit zur Rückbildung im Experiment. Ergebn. Chir. Orthop. **40**, 266 (1956). — IDBOHRN, H., and A. MUREN: Renal blood flow in experimental hydronephrosis. Acta physiol. scand. **38**, 200—206 (1956). — IDBOHRN, H., and S. SJÖSTEDT: Ectopic ureter not causing incontinence until adult life. Acta obstet. gynec. scand. **33**, 457 (1954). — KEATES, P. G.: Physical, physiological and hormonal aspects of hydronephrosis. J. Fac. Radiol. (Lond.) **6**, 123 (1954). — KJELLBERG, S. R., N. O. ERICSSON and U. RUDHE: The lower urinary tract in childhood. Stockholm: Almqvist & Wiksell 1957. — KRETSCHMER, H. L., and F. H. SQUIRE: The incidence and extent of hydronephrosis in prostatic obstruction. J. Urol. (Baltimore) **60**, 1 (1948). — LICH jr., R.: The obstructed ureteropelvic junction. Radiology **68**, 337—344 (1957). — LICH jr., R., and M. L. BARNES: A clinicopathologic study of ureteropelvic obstructions. J. Urol. (Baltimore) **77**, 382—387 (1957). — LICH, R., J. E. MAURER and M. L. BARNES: Pyelectasis. J. Urol. (Baltimore) **75**, 12 (1956). — LIEDBERG, N.: Die Urographie als Untersuchungsmethode vor der Prostatektomie. Lund: Håkan Ohlssons förlag 1941. — LINDBLOM, K.: Roentgenographic studies of hydronephrosis due to obstruction at the ureteropelvic junction. Acta radiol. (Stockh.) **32**, 113 (1949). — MALUF, N. S. R.: A method for relief of upper ureteral obstruction within bifurcation of renal artery. J. Urol. (Baltimore) **75**, 229 (1956). — MARCEL, J.-E., et G. MONIN: Complications urinaires hautes aprés curie et roentgenthérapie pour cancer du col utérin. J. Urol. méd. chir. **61**, 249 (1955). — MINDER, J.: Über den diagnostischen und klinischen Wert der Ausscheidungspyelographie. Z. ur. Chir. Gynäk. **42**, 312—363 (1936). — MOORE, T.: Hydrocalicosis. Brit. J. Urol. **22**, 304 (1950). — NESBIT, R. M.: Diagnosis of intermittent hydronephrosis: importance of pyelography during episodes of pain. J. Urol. (Baltimore) **75**, 767 (1956). — O'CONOR, V. J.: Diagnosis and treatment of hydronephrosis. Trans. Amer. Ass. gen.-urin. Surg. **46**, 103 (1954). — ÖSTLING, K.: Röntgenologische und pathologisch-anatomische Veränderungen bei Erweiterungen einzelner Nierenkelche. Acta radiol. (Stockh.) **15**, 28 (1934). — The genesis of hydronephrosis. Acta chir. scand. Suppl. **72** (1942). — PELLEGRINO, A., et P. GIUDICELLI: L'urographie intra-veineuse dans la bilharziose urinaire. J. Radiol. Électrol. **39**, 599 (1958). — PERSKY, L., F. J. BONTE and G. AUSTEN: Mechanisms of hydronephrosis: radioautographic backflow patterns. J. Urol. (Baltimore) **75**, 190 (1956). — PETKOVIĆ, S.:

Versuche zur Behandlung des Megaureters. Verhandlungsber. der Dtsch. Ges. für Urologie, S. 69, Leipzig 1958. — PONTI, C. DE, and U. POGGI: Rilievi clinico-radiologici sui vasi anomali renali. Nunt. radiol. (Firenze) 23, 702 (1957). — PUHL, H., u. H. JACOBI: Über „fixierte" Schwangerschaftsatonie des Ureters. Z. urol. Chir. 35, 384 (1932). — ROBERTSON, H. E.: Hydronephrosis and pyelitis of pregnancy. Philadelphia and London: W. B. Saunders Company 1944. — ROLLESTON, G. L., and E. R. REAY: The pelvi-ureteric junction. Brit. J. Radiol. 30, 617 (1957). — SCHEWE, E. J., and J. M. SALA: Bilateral ureteral obstruction complicating the treatment of carcinoma of the cervix. Amer. J. Roentgenol. 81, 125 (1959). — SENG, M. I.: Dilatation of the ureters and renal pelvis in pregnancy. J. Urol. (Baltimore) 21, 475 (1929). — STIRLING, W. C.: Massive hydronephrosis complicated by hydro-ureter. J. Urol. (Baltimore) 42, 520 (1939). — SWYNGEDAUW, J., L. WEMEAU, M. FLEURY et J. HÉRENT: Les complications urinaires du traitement radiothérapique du cancer du col utérin. J. Radiol. Electrol. 39, 618 (1958). — TRAUT, H. F., C. M. MCLANE and A. KUDER: Physiologic changes in the ureter associated with pregnancy. Surg. Gynec. Obstet. 64, 51—58 (1937). — TROELL, A.: Intravenöse Pyelographie zur Prüfung der Nierenfunktion bei Prostatikern. Chirurg 7, 513—517 (1935). — USON, A. C., D. W. JOHNSON, J. K. LATTIMER and M. M. MELICOW: A classification of the urographic patterns in children with congenital bladder neck obstruction. Amer. J. Roentgenol. 80, 590 (1958). — WAGENEN, G. VAN, and R. H. JENKINS: An experimental examination of factors causing ureteral dilatation of pregnancy. J. Urol. (Baltimore) 42, 1010 (1939). — WALL, B., and H. E. WACHTER: Congenital ureteral valve: its role as a primary obstructive lesion: classification of the literature and report of an authentic case. J. Urol. (Baltimore) 68, 684 (1952). — WILHELM, G.: Beitrag zur Röntgendiagnostik der Hydronephrose durch Lagewechsel beim i.v. Pyelogramm. Fortschr. Röntgenstr. 84, 628—630 (1956). — X-rays during pregnancy. J. Amer. med. Ass. 153, 218 (1953).

Examination methods

ÅKERLUND, Å.: Über die Technik bei Röntgenuntersuchung der freigelegten Niere. Acta chir. scand. 79, 553—565 (1937). — ARENDT, J., and A. ZGODA: The heterotropic excretion of intravenously injected contrast media. Radiology 68, 238—241 (1957). — ASTRALDI, A., y J. V. URIBURU jr.: Radiologia del rinón durante el acto operatorio. Rév. méd. lat.-amer. 21, 891—907 (1936). — BACON, R. D.: Respiration pyelography. Amer. J. Roentgenol. 44, 71 (1940). — BASKIN, A. M., B. M. HARVARD and A. H. JANZEN: Sterile fluoroscopy: preliminary report of a new technique for localization of renal calculi. J. Urol. (Baltimore) 78, 821 (1957). — BECKER, R.: Beitrag zur Verbesserung der röntgenologischen Nierendiagnostik. Münch. med. Wschr. 97, 1104—1105 (1955). — BEER, E.: Roentgenological control of exposed kidneys in operations for nephrolithiasis, with the use of special intensifying casette. J. Urol. (Baltimore) 25, 159—164 (1931). — BENJAMIN, E. W.: Notes on the technique of X-ray control in the operating room. J. Urol. (Baltimore) 25, 165—171 (1931). — BERG, O. C., and D. H. ALLEN: Use of carbonated beverage as an aid in pediatric excretory urography. J. Urol. (Baltimore) 67, 393 (1952). — BERGER, H., u. O. KARGL: Beitrag zur Ureterenkompression bei der Urographie. Bruns' Beitr. klin. Chir. 190, 13 (1955). — BERRY, C. D., and R. R. CROSS: Use of bag ureteral catheters for nephrograms: obstructive nephrograms. J. Urol. (Baltimore) 74, 683 (1955). — BEZOLD, K., H. R. FEINDT u. K. PRESSLER: Der Röntgenbildverstärker im Routinebetrieb. Fortschr. Röntgenstr. 85, 447 (1956). — BODNER, H., A. H. HOWARD and J. H. KAPLAN: Cinefluorography for the urologist. J. Urol. (Baltimore) 79, 356 (1958). — BØGGILD, D.: Some experiences with intravenous pyelography by means of uroselectan. Acta radiol. (Stockh.) 12, 41 (1931). — BOEMINGHAUS, H., u. L. ZEISS: Die Erkrankung der Harnorgane im Röntgenbild. Leipzig: Johann Ambrosius Barth 1933. — BORGARD, W.: Beobachtungen und Untersuchungen bei Pyelitis. Z. Urol. 41, 217—236 (1948). — BUSCHER, A. K.: Beitrag zur Röntgendiagnostik an der freigelegten Niere. Urologia (Treviso) 22, 217 (1955). — CATEL, W., u. R. GARSCHE: Studien bei Kindern mit dem Bildwandler. Fortschr. Röntgenstr. 86, 66 (1957). — CHRISTIANSEN, H.: Some practical hints on the performance of urography on infants. Acta radiol. (Stockh.) 26, 46 (1945). — Clark's applied pharmacology, VIIIth edit. Revised by A. WILSON and H. O. SCHILD. London: Churchill Ltd. 1952. — DENNEHY, P. J.: A method of excretory urography in children. S. Afr. med. J. 28, 949 (1954). — DICK, D. R., R. W. HERRMANN, CH. FERUGSON and C. L. HEBERT: The use of short acting, muscle relaxant drug in diagnostic urography. A preliminary report. J. Urol. (Baltimore) 72, 1260 (1954). — DIHLMANN, W.: Vergleichende Untersuchungen über den Wert der intravenösen Kompressionsurographie. Fortschr. Röntgenstr. 89, 104 (1958). — DURIO, A., A. GRIO N. MASTROBUONO e G. SCAGLIONE: Osservazioni sull'impiego della jaluronidase nella tecnica urografica dell'infanzia. Aggiorn. pediat. 6, 191 (1955). — EBBINGHAUS, K. D.: Die technische Durchführung der intravenösen Pyelographie. Ärztl. Wschr. 1955, 97. — ENGELKAMP, H.: Anwendung der Hartstrahltechnik (200 kV) bei Untersuchungen mit negativen Kontrastmitteln. Fortschr. Röntgenstr. **93**, 230—237 (1960). — EPSTEIN, B. S.: Subcutaneous urography in infants. J. Amer. med. Ass. **164**, 39—41 (1957). — EUPHRAT, E. J.: Polaroid photography as a practical method of providing illustrations of radiographs for clinical records. New Engl. J. med. **252**, 628 (1955). — EVANS, J. A., W. DUBILIER jr. and J. C. MONTEITH: Nephrotomography. Amer. J. Roentgenol. **71**, 213 (1954). — EVANS, J. A., J. C. MONTEITH and W. DUBILIER jr.: Nephrotomography. Radiology **64**, 655—663 (1955). — EVANS, J. A., and N. POKER: Newer roentgenographic techniques in the diagnosis of retroperitoneal tumors. J. Amer. med. Ass. **161**, 1128—1132 (1956). — FRANÇOIS, J.: Technique et valeur du controle radiologique pendant les opérations pour calculs du rein. Proc.-Verb. L'Ass. Fr. d'Urol., Paris 1932, pp. 616—627. — FRIESE-CHRISTIANSEN, A.: Urography on children after administration of the contrast substance by mouth. Acta radiol. (Stockh.) **27**, 197 (1946). — GABRIEL, G.: Experimentelle Untersuchungen über die intravenöse Pyelographie bei pathologischen Zuständen der Niere. Acta radiol. (Stockh.) **11**, 500 (1930). — GETZOFF, P. L.: Use of antihistamine drug prophylaxis against diodrast reactions. J. Urol. (Baltimore) **65**, 1139 (1951). — GIDLUND, Å.: Development of apparatus and methods for roentgen studies in haemodynamics. Acta radiol. (Stockh.) Suppl. **130** (1956). — GILLESPIE, J. B., G. A. MILLER and J. SCHLERETH: Water intoxication following enemas for roentgenographic preparation. Amer. J. Roentgenol. **82**, 1067—1069 (1959). — GREENWOOD, F. G.: Cineradiography in urinary tuberculosis. Brit. J. Radiol. **30**, 493—496 (1957). — GROSSE-BROCKHOFF, F., H. H. LÖHR, F. LOOGEN u. H. VIETEN: Die Punktion des linken Ventrikels zur Kontrastmitteldarstellung seiner Abflußbahn. Fortschr. Röntgenstr. **90**, 300—308 (1959). — GÜNTHER, G. W.: Pyelitische Hämaturie und Nephrektomie. Z. Urol. **43**, 21—28 (1950). — GYLLENSWÄRD, Å., H. LODIN and O. MYKLAND: Prevention of undue intestinal gas in abdominal radiography in infants. Acta radiol. (Stockh.) **39**, 6—16 (1953). — HANLEY, H. G.: Cineradiography of the urinary tract. Brit. med. J. **1955** II, 22—23. — HAJÓS, E.: Methodik des Röntgenschichtverfahrens in der Urologie. Fortschr. Röntgenstr. **91**, 366 (1959). — HEINECKE, H.: Diskussionsäußerung zu PERTHES, Die chirurgische Behandlung der Nephrolithiasis mit besonderer Rücksicht auf die Indiaktionsstellung. Münch. med. Wschr. **54**, 1753 (1907). — HELLMER, H.: On the technique in urography and the roentgen picture in acute renal and ureteral stasis. Acta radiol. (Stockh.) **16**, 51—55 (1935). — HELWIG, F. C., C. B. SCHUTZ and O. E. CURRY: Water intoxication: report of fatal human case, with clinical, pathologic and experimental studies. J. Amer. med. Ass. **104**, 1569—1575 (1935). — HENDRIOCK, A.: Intravenöse Urographie und pelvirenaler Übertritt. Zbl. Chir. **61**, 1822 (1934). — HEUSSER, H.: Die Röntgenuntersuchung der operativ freigelegten Niere. Schweiz. med. Wschr. **18**, 630 (1937). — HILGENFELDT, O.: Das Veratmungspyelogram. Dtsch. Z. Chir. **247**, 411 (1936). — Zbl. Chir. **65**, 1538 (1938). — HOPE, J. W., and F. CAMPOY: The use of carbonated beverages in pediatric excretory urography. Radiology **64**, 66 (1955). — HULTBORN, K. A.: Allergische Reaktionen bei Kontrastinjektionen für die Urographie. Acta radiol. (Stockh.) **20**, 263 (1939). — HUTTER, K.: Zur Röntgendarstellung von Beckengefäßen bei urologischen Fällen. Acta radiol. (Stockh.) **16**, 94 (1935). — JACHES: cit. BENJAMIN, J. Urol. (Baltimore) **25**, 165 (1931). — JENSEN, F.: Ny kompressionsmetode ved intravenøs urografi. Nord. Med. **58**, 1771 (1957). — JOHNSSON, S.: A contribution to the diagnostics of nephromata. Acta radiol. (Stockh.) Suppl. **60**, (1946). — JOSEPHSON, B.: The mechanism of the excretion of renal contrast substances. Acta radiol. (Stockh.) **38**, 299 (1952). — JUTRAS, A.: Roentgen diagnosis by remote control. Telefluoroscopy and cineradiography. Medica Mundi **4**, 77—82 (1958). — KEATES, P. G.: Physical, physiological and hormonal aspects of hydronephrosis. J. Fac. Radiol. (Lond.) **6**, 123 (1954). — An assessment of sodium acetrizoate and an experimental basis for its use in intravenous pyelography. J. Fac. Radiol. (Lond.) **7**, 139 (1955). — KIRSH, I. E.: Is a fluoroscope useful to the general practitioner? J. Amer. med. Ass. **170**, 1141—1142 (1959). — KJELLBERG, S. R., and U. RUDHE: The fetal renal secretion and its significance in congenital deformities of the ureters and urethra. Acta radiol. (Stockh.) **31**, 243 (1949). — KNEISE, O., u. K. L. SCHOBER: Die Röntgenuntersuchung der Harnorgane. Leipzig 1941. — KOCH, C. C., and B. G. NØRGÅRD: Intravenous pyelography. An examination of certain technical problems and a new radiopaque substance. Nord. Med. **54**, 1351 (1955). KOCKUM, J., K. LIDÉN and O. NORMAN: Radiation hazards attending use of transportable image intensifier. Acta radiol. (Stockh.) **49**, 369—376 (1958). — KRETSCHMER, H. L.: Intravenous urography. Surg. Gynec. Obstet. **51**, 404 (1930). — LENTINO, W., E. z. BERTRAM, H. G. JACOBSON and M. H. POPPEL: Intravenously given urographic mediums. Comparative study of eight hundred cases. J. Amer. med. Ass. **161**, 606 (1956). — LILJA, B., and H. WAHREN: On meteorism in pyelography. Acta radiol. (Stockh.) **15**, 41 (1934). — LOWMAN, R. M., H. SHAPIRO, A. LIN, L. DAVIS, F. E. KORN and H. R. NEWMAN: Preliminary clinical evaluation of hypaque in excretory urography. Surg. Gynec. Obstet. **101**, 1 (1955). — MAGNUSSON, W.: On meteorism in pyelography and on the passage of gas through the small intestine. Acta radiol. (Stockh.) **12**, 552 (1931). — MARQUARDT, C. R., J. W. PICK, A. MELA-

MED, A. MARCK and A. H. HOLT: The use of miniature film (renogram) for kidney stone surgery. J. Urol. (Baltimore) 80, 388 (1958). — MAY, F.: Ein Beitrag zur Röntgenphotographie der freigelegten Niere. Z. Urol. (Baltimore) 36, 89—93 (1942). — Meßergebnisse des osmotischen Druckes der zur Zeit gebräuchlichsten Kontrastmittel. Schering AG, Berlin-West, den 16. 1. 1957. — MOORE, TH. D., and R. F. MAYER: Hypaque: an improved medium for excretory urography. Sth. med. J. (Bgham, Ala.) 48, 135 (1955). — NESBIT, R. M., and D. B. DOUGLAS: The subcutaneous administration of diodrast for pyelograms in infants. J. Urol. (Baltimore) 42, 709 (1939). — OLSSON, OLLE, and O. LÖFGREN: Hyaluronidase as a factor hastening the spread and absorption of water-soluble radiopaque substances deposited intracutaneously, subcutaneously or itramuscularly. Acta radiol. (Stockh.) 31, 250—256 (1949). — OPPENHEIMER, G. D.: Evaluation of roentgenography of surgically exposed kidney in treatment of renal calculi. J. Urol. (Baltimore) 43, 253—264 (1940). — PAUL, L. E., and J. H. JUHL: The essentials of roentgen interpretation. New York: Paul B. Hoeber 1959, p. 489. — PENDERGRASS, E. P., J. P. HODES, R. L. TONDREAU, C. C. POWELL and E. D. BURDICK: Further consideration of deaths and unfavorable sequelae following administration of contrast mediums in urography in United States. Amer. J. Roentgenol. 74, 262—287 (1955). — PETRÉN, G.: Ein Fall von Nephrolithiasis mit Röntgenphotographie während der Operation. Acta chir. scand. 77, 338—340 (1936). — PFLAUMER, E.: Die Röntgenphotographie der freigelegten Niere bei der Steinoperation. Z. Urol. 29, 225 (1935). — PFLAUMER, E., and H. FRIEDRICH: Gang und Technik der Röntgenuntersuchung auf Harnsteine. Leipzig 1940. — POST, H. W. A., and W. F. W. SOUTHWOOD: The technique and interpretation of nephrotomograms. Brit. J. Radiol. 32, 734—738 (1959). — PRIESTLEY, J. T.: Surgical considerations in removal of stones from the kidney. Surg. Gynec. Obstet. 67, 798—803 (1938). — PUHL, H.: Röntgenuntersuchung freigelegter Nieren. Zbl. Chir. 63, 1035 (1936). — PUIGVERT GORRO, A.: Die Röntgenuntersuchung der Niere während der Operation. Z. urol. Chir. 47, 32—45 (1943). — QUINBY, W.: Remarks on the operation localization of urinary calculi. Boston med. surg. J. 91, 194 (1924). — RIBBING, S.: Une source d'erreurs négligée dans l'interprétation des pyélographies. Acta radiol. (Stockh.) 14, 545 (1933). — RIBBING, S.: La stratification des liquides opaques dans l'urographie. Acta radiol. (Stockh.) 16, 716 (1935). — ROTH, M., and T. A. NICHOLSON: Comparative study of five urographic contrast media. J. Urol. (Baltimore) 77, 670—681 (1957). — SIMONE F. DE, A. FIUMICELLI e E. DI LEVA: Variazioni dell'effetto urografico sotto l'azione della 1,4-idrazinoftalazina. Progr. med. (Napoli) 12, 135—138 (1956). — SINGLETON, E. B., and G. H. HARRISON: Excretory pyelography in infants. Technique for intravenous injection. Amer. J. Roentgenol. 75, 896—899 (1956). — SOUTHWOOD, W. F. W., and V. F. MARSHALL: A clinical evaluation of nephrotomography. Brit. J. Urol. 30, 127 (1958). — STAUFFER, H. M., M. J. OPPENHEIMER, L.A. SOLOFF and G. H. STEWART: Cardiac physiology revealed by the roentgen ray. Amer. J. Roentgenol. 77, 195—206 (1957). — STEINERT, R.: Effect of enemata on contrast excretion in urography. Acta radiol. (Stockh.) 38, 30 (1952). — A compression apparatus for urography. Acta radiol. (Stockh.) 38, 212 (1952). — SUTHERLAND, C. G.: Renal roentgenoscopy and roentgenography at the operating table. J. Urol. (Baltimore) 33, 1—11 (1935). — SZÉKELY, J.: Intravenás urographia okozta acut veseelégtelenség. Orv. Hetil. 99, 176 (1958). — THESTRUP ANDERSEN, P.: On tomography as an adjunct to urography. Acta radiol. (Stockh.) 30, 225 (1948). — TRUCHOT, P., M. NOIX et R. FABRE: Valeur diagnostique des modifications morphologiques de l'image rénale au cours des examens radiologiques. J. Radiol. Électrol. 38, 1141 (1957). — TUDDENHAM, W. J.: The visual physiology of roentgen diagnosis. Amer. J. Roentgenol. 78, 116—123 (1957). — UEBELHÖR, R.: Die Röntgenaufnahme der freigelegten Niere. Z. urol. Chir. 41, 275—279 (1936). — VAN VELZER, D. A., and R. R. LANIER: A simplified technic for nephrotomography. Radiology 70, 77 (1958). — WALD, A. M.: Nephrography during routine excretory urography. J. Urol. (Baltimore) 75, 572—577 (1956). — WALLDÉN, L.: Administration of contrast medium in urography via the bone marrow. Acta radiol. (Stockh.) 25, 213 (1944). — WARRES, H. L., and A. C. KING: Hyaluronidase in intramuscular excretory urography. Radiology 63, 730 (1955). — WICKBOM, I.: The influence of the blood pressure in urographic examination. Acta radiol. (Stockh.) 34, 1 (1950). — WINTER, C. C.: The value of chlor-trimeton in the prevention of immediate reactions to 70 per cent urokon. J. Urol. (Baltimore) 74, 416 (1955). — WOLKE, K.: Some experiments in rectal pyelography. Acta radiol. (Stockh.) 12, 497 (1931). — Pyelogramm mit einem durch einen Nierenarterienzweig verursachten Füllungsdefekt (Pseudodefekt). Acta radiol. (Stockh.) 17, 566—568 (1936). — YOUNGBLOOD, V. H., J. O. WILLIAMS and A. TUGGLE: Reactions due to intravenous urokon. J. Urol. (Baltimore) 75, 1011—1015 (1956).

Fistula

BLOOM, B.: Spontaneous renoduodenal fistulas. J. Urol. (Baltimore) 72, 1153 (1954).

Foreign body

GONDOS, B.: Foreign body in the left kidney and ureter. J. Urol. (Baltimore) **73**, 35 (1955).

Gas in the urinary tract

BLOOM, B.: Spontaneous renoduodenal fistulas. J. Urol. (Baltimore) **72**, 1153 (1954). — BOIJSEN, E., and J. LEWIS-JONSSON: Emphysematous cystitis. Acta radiol. (Stockh.) **41**, 269 (1954). — BRAMAN, R., and R. R. CROSS jr.: Perinephric abscess producing a pneumonephrogram. J. Urol. (Baltimore) **75**, 194 (1956). — KENT, H. P.: Gas in the urinary tract. J. Fac. Radiol. (Lond.) **7**, 57 (1955). — NARINS, L., and H. SEGAL: Spontaneous passage of a dendritic renal calculus by rectum. J. Urol. (Baltimore) **82**, 274 (1959). — NORTH, J. P., S. O. LIVINGSTON and B. K. LOVELL: Spontaneous renoduodenal fistula. Surgery **39**, 683—687 (1956). — RATLIFF, R. K., and A. C. BARNES: Acquired renocolic fistula: report of two cases. J. Urol. (Baltimore) **42**, 311 (1939). — ROST, G. S., D. COOPER, C. E. KNOUF, P. FERGUSON and A. McCRARY: Acquired renocolic fistula in remaining functioning kidney with recovery: case report. J. Urol. (Baltimore) **75**, 787 (1956). — WEISER, A.: Über einen Fall von Gasgangrän der Harnblase. Z. urol. Chir. Gynäk. **28**, 113 (1929).

Generalized kidney disease

ALEXANDER, J. C.: Pneumopyonephrosis in diabetes mellitus. J. Urol. (Baltimore) **45**, 570 (1941). — BECK, R. E., and R. C. HAMMOND: Renal and osseous manifestation of tuberous sclerosis: case report. J. Urol. (Baltimore) **77**, 578—582 (1957). — BORGSTRÖM, K.-E., U. ISING, E. LINDER and A. LUNDERQUIST: Experimental pulmonary edema. Acta radiol. (Stockh.) **54**, 97—119 (1960). — BRAASCH, W. F., and J. W. MERRICKS: Clinical and radiological data associated with congenital and acquired single kidney. Surg. Gynec. Obstet. **67**, 281 (1938). — BROOKFIELD, R. W., E. L. RUBIN and M. K. ALEXANDER: Osteosclerosis in renal failure. J. Fac. Radiol. (Lond.) **7**, 102 (1955). — BRUN, C.: Acute anuria. Diss. Copenhagen: Ejnar Munksgaard 1954. — CRAWFORD, T., C. E. DENT, P. LUCAS, N. H. MARTIN and J. R. NASSIM: Osteosclerosis associated with chronic renal failure. Lancet **1954II**, 981. — DEJDAR, R.: Die chronische Pyelonephritis in röntgenographischer Darstellung. Fortschr. Röntgenstr. **90**, 196—220 (1959). — DEJDAR, R., u. V. PRAT: Das Röntgenbild der Nieren und der Harnwege bei der chronischen Pyelonephritis. Z. Urol. **51**, 1—25 (1958). — DE PASS, S. W., J. STEIN, M. H. POPPEL and H. G. JACOBSON: Pulmonary congestion and edema in uremia. J. Amer. med. Ass. **162**, 5—9 (1956). — DIAZ-RIVERA, R. S., and A. J. MILLER: Periarteritis nodosa: a clinico-pathological analysis of seven cases. Ann. intern. Med. **24**, 420 (1946). — DOW, J. D.: Radiological findings in Bright's disease. Guy's Hosp. Rep. **107**, 454—474 (1958). — ELLEGAST, H., u. H. JESSERER: Der röntgenologische Aspekt der renalen Osteopathie. Fortschr. Röntgenstr. **89**, 450 (1958). — FREI, A.: Zur Röntgendiagnose der chronischen Pyelonephritis, S. 201. Verhandlungsber. der Dtsch. Ges. für Urologie. Leipzig 1958. — FRUMKIN, J.: Replacement lipomatosis of the kidney. J. Urol. (Baltimore) **58**, 100 (1947). — HAARSTAD, J.: Papillitis necroticans renalis. Nord. Med. **58**, 1759 (1957). — HAMRE, L.: Fibrolipomatosis renis. Nord. Med. **58**, 1769 (1957). — HANLEY, H. G.: The post-operative results of nephrectomy. Brit. J. Surg. **27**, 553 (1940). — HERRNHEISER, G.: Zur Röntgendiagnostik des Lungenödems. Fortschr. Röntgenstr. **89**, 125—135 (1958). — HILLENBRAND, H., and FORST: Renovasographie der chronischen Pyelonephritis. S. 207. Verhandlungsber. der Dtsch. Ges. für Urologie. Leipzig 1958. — HUGHES, B., and G. J. GISLASON: Osteonephropathy: a report of two cases. J. Urol. (Baltimore) **55**, 330 (1946). — JAMES, J. A.: Renal tubular disease with nephrocalcinosis. Report of two unusual cases. J. Dis. Child. **91**, 601—605 (1956). — JESSERER, H.: Röntgenveränderungen am Skelett als Folge von Nierenerkrankungen. Fortschr. Röntgenstr. **84**, 452 (1956). — KNUTSSEN, A., E. R. JENNINGS, O. A. BRINES and A. AXELROD: Renal papillary necrosis. Amer. J. clin. Path. **22**, 327 (1952). — KUTZMANN, A. A.: Replacement lipomatosis of the kidney. Surg. Gynec. Obstet. **52**, 690 (1931). — MACGIBBON, B. H., L. W. LOUGHRIDGE, D. O'B. HOURIHANE and D. W. BOYD: Autoimmune haemolytic anaemia with acute renal failure due to phenacetin and p-aminosalicylic acid. Lancet **1960I**, 7—10. — MARTINI, F.: Malattia di Besnier-Boeck-Schaumann in rene anomalo. Nunt. Radiol. **21**, 461—469 (1955). — MITCHELL jr., R. E., C. R. TITTLE and H. L. BOCKUS: Nephrocalcinosis in patient with duodenal ulcer disease. Report of a case associated with parathyroid adenoma. Gastroenterology **30**, 943 to 949 (1956). — MOËLL, H.: Gross bilateral renal cortical necrosis during long periods of oliguria-anuria. Acta radiol. (Stockh.) **48**, 355 (1957). — Kidney size and its deviation from normal in acute renal failure. Acta radiol. (Stockh.) Suppl. 206 (1961). — MOOLTEN, S. E., and I. B. SMITH: Fatal nephritis in chronic phenacetin poisoning. Amer. J. Med. **28**, 127—134 (1960). — PAPILLON, J., F. PINET, R. BOUVET, A. PINET et J. L. CHASSARD: A propos de deux cas de manifestations urinaires de la maladie de Hodgkin. J. Radiol. Électrol. **38**, 974 (1957). — PEACOCK, A. H., and A. BALLE: Renal lipomatosis. Ann. Surg. **103**, 395 (1936). — PRIESTLEY,

J. B.: Renal lipomatosis or fatty replacement of destroyed renal cortex. J. Urol. (Baltimore) **40**, 269 (1938). — RAKOVEC, S.: Hypertension due to vascular changes in chronic unilateral pyelonephritis. Urol. int. (Basel) **6**, 127 (1958). — ROTH, L. J., and H. B. DAVIDSON: Fibrous and fatty replacement of renal parenchyma. J. Amer. med. Ass. **111**, 233 (1938). — RUDEBECK, J.: Clinical and prognostic aspects of acute glomerulonephritis. Acta med. scand. Suppl. **173** (1946). — SARRUBI, Z.: Radiologie des pyélites et pyélonéphritis. J. Urol. méd. chir. **62**, 372—378 (1956). — SCHROEDER, E.: Kliniske studier over nyrefunktionen hos nephrectomerede. Diss. København: Einar Munksgaard 1944. — SHEEHAN, H. L., and H. C. MOORE: Renal cortical necrosis of the kidney of concealed accidental haemorrhage. Oxford: Blackwell Scientific Publ. 1952. — SIMRIL, W. A., and D. K. ROSE: Replacement lipomatosis and its simulation of renal tumors: a report of two cases. J. Urol. (Baltimore) **63**, 588 (1950). — SPÜHLER, O., u. H. U. ZOLLINGER: Die chronisch-interstitielle Nephritis. Z. klin. Med. **151**, 1 (1953). — STANBURY, S. W.: Azotaemic renal osteodystrophy. Brit. med. Bull. **13**, 57—60 (1957). — STERNBY, N. H.: Studies in enlargement of leukaemic kidneys. Acta haemat. (Basel) **14**, 354—362 (1955). — VOLHARD, F., u. T. FAHR: Die Brightsche Nierenkrankheit. Klinik, Pathologie und Atlas. Berlin: Springer 1914. — ZETTERGREN, L.: Uremic lung. Acta Soc. Med. upsalien. **60**, 161 (1955). — ZOLLINGER, H. U.: Chronische interstitielle Nephritis bei Abusus von phenacetinhaltigen Analgetica (Saridon usw.). Schweiz. med. Wschr. **85**, 746 (1955). — Die Pathologie der chronischen Pyelonephritis. Verhandlungsber. der Dtsch. Ges. für Urologie, S. 165. Leipzig 1958.

Generalized parenchymal changes

GORMSEN, H., T. HILDEN, P. IVERSEN og F. RAASCHOU: Nyrebiopsi ved glomerulonefritis og nefrotisk syndrom. Nord. Med. **54**, 1341 (1955). — REFVEM, O.: Lower nephron nephrosis—akutt nyresvikt. Nord. Med. **54**, 1337 (1955).

Injury

ADAMS, P.: Traumatic rupture of the kidney. Amer. J. Surg. **61**, 316—323 (1943). — ANZILOTTI, A.: Late results of a severe injury of the kidney. Radiol. med. (Torino) **26**, 144 (1939). — BAIRD, H. H., and H. R. JUSTIS: Surgical injuries of the ureter and bladder. J. Amer. med. Ass. **162**, 1357 (1956). — BARETZ, L. H.: Rupture of the kidney following pyelography. J. Amer. med. Ass. **106**, 980 (1936). — CIBERT, J. A. V., et H. CAVAILHER: Hématomes spontanés périrénaux. J. Urol. méd. chir. **50**, 65 (1942). — COLSTON, J. A. C., and W. W. BAKER: Late effects of various types of trauma to the kidney. Arch. Surg. (Chicago) **34**, 99 (1937). — DENIS et PLANCHAIS cit. M. F. LEGUEU: Rupture traumatique d'une hydronéphrose. Bull. Soc. Chir. Paris **35**, 382 (1909). — DRUCKMANN, A., and S. SCHORR: Roentgenographic observation of perforation of the kidney following retrograde pyelography. J. Urol. (Baltimore) **61**, 1028 (1949). — EKMAN, H.: Displacement of the kidney consequent upon spontaneous perirenal hematoma. Acta chir. scand. **93**, 531—551 (1946). — ENGEL, W. J., and I. H. PAGE: Hypertension due to renal compression resulting from subcapsular hematoma. J. Urol. (Baltimore) **73**, 735 (1955). — HAMMEL, H.: Subcutane Nierenverletzung und Ausscheidungsurographie. Z. urol. Chir. **41**, 502 (1936). — HAREIDE, I.: Über die Röntgenuntersuchung bei Nierenverletzungen unter besonderer Berücksichtigung der intravenösen Urographie. Acta radiol. (Stockh.) **21**, 292 (1940). — HERMAN, J., és B. MELLY: Abrodillel végzett intravenás pyelographiáról. Orv. Hétil. **75**, 1—5 (1931). Ref. Z. Urol. **27**, 510 (1933). — HODGES, C. V., D. R. GILBERT and W. W. SCOTT: Renal trauma; study of 71 cases. J. Urol. (Baltimore) **66**, 627—637 (1951). — INCLÁN BOLADO, J. L., y J. CORRAL CASTANEDO: Fracturas de riñon. Estudio clinico. Arch. esp. Urol. **13**, 135 (1957). — JASIENSKI, G.: Sur un cas d'hématimie périrénal spontané chez un hémophile. J. Urol. méd. chir. **44**, 487 (1937). — JONES, R. F.: Surgical management of transcapsular rupture of the kidney: 24 cases. J. Urol. (Baltimore) **74**, 721 (1955). — KAIJSER, R.: Über das sog. spontane perirenale Hämatom. Upsala Läk.-Fören. Förh. **44**, 283 (1938/39). — KEMM, N.: Rupture of the kidney: delayed symptoms; operation; recovery. Brit. med. J. **1923 II**, 1218. — KITTREDGE, W. E., and J. R. CRAWLEY: Surgical renal lesions associated with pregnancy. J. Amer. med. Ass. **162**, 1353 (1956). — LARSEN, K. A., and A. PEDERSEN: Spontaneous rupture of the kidney pelvis. J. Oslo Cy Hosp. **5**, 121—128 (1955). — LEFKOVITS, A. M.: Fatal air embolism during presacral insufflation of air. J. Urol. (Baltimore) **77**, 112—115 (1957). — LEVANT, B., and B. J. FELDMAN: Traumatic rupture of Wilms' tumor. J. Urol. (Baltimore) **67**, 629 (1952). — LISKA, J. R.: Recognition and management of trauma to kidney. J. Urol. (Baltimore) **78**, 525—531 (1957). — LJUNGGREN, E.: Die Bedeutung der Pyelographie bei subkutanen Nierenverletzungen. Z. Urol. **30**, 650 (1936). — LOCKARD, V. M.: Lesions of the upper gastro-intestinal tract in infants and children. Radiology **58**, 696 (1952). — LYNCH jr., K. M.: Management of the injured kidney: Preliminary report. J. Urol. (Baltimore) **60**, 371—380 (1948). — Traumatic urinary injuries: Pitfalls in diagnosis and treatment.

J. Urol. (Baltimore) **77**, 90—95 (1957). — LYNCH jr., K. M., and H. L. LARGE jr.: Posttraumatic ischemic infarction of the kidney due to arteriospasm. Sth. med. J. (Bgham, Ala.) **44**, 600 (1951). — MARQUARDT, H. D.: Zur Methodik der Röntgenuntersuchung der Harnorgane. Medizinische **8**, 316 (1958). — McKAY, H. W., H. H. BAIRD and K. M. LYNCH jr.: Management of the injured kidney. J. Amer. med. Ass. **141**, 575 (1949). — MERTZ, H. O.: Injury of the kidney in children. J. Urol. (Baltimore) **69**, 39 (1953). — MILLER, J. A., and J. J. CORDONNIER: Spontaneous perirenal hematoma associated with hypertension. J. Urol. (Baltimore) **62**, 13—17 (1949). — NAVAS, J.: Contusion renal y litiasis. Arch. esp. Urol. **12**, 96—99 (1956). — O'CONOR, V. J.: Immediate management of the injured ureter. J. Amer. med. Ass. **162**, 1201 (1956). — ORKIN, L. A.: Evaluation of the merits of cystoscopy and retrograde pyelography in the management of renal trauma. J. Urol. (Baltimore) **63**, 9 (1950). — OVERGAARD, K.: A case of internal uroplania. Acta radiol. (Stockh.) **17**, 542 (1936). PRIESTLEY, J. T., and F. PILCHER: Traumatic lesions of the kidney. Amer. J. Surg. **40**, 357 (1938). — RENANDER, A.: Another case of spontaneous rupture of the renal pelvis. Acta radiol. (Stockh.) **22**, 422 (1941). — RITVO, M., and D. B. STEARNS: Roentgendiagnosis of contusions of the kidney. J. Amer. med. Ass. **109**, 1101 (1937). — SARGENT, J. C., and C. R. MARQUARDT: Renal injuries. J. Urol. (Baltimore) **63**, 1 (1950). — SIMON, O.: Das Hämatom des Nierenlagers im Röntgenbild. Fortschr. Röntgenstr. **59**, 178 (1939). — STRNAD, F.: Nierenperforation und pyelovenöser Reflux. Fortschr. Röntgenstr. **53**, 175 (1936). — TRUETA, J., A. E. BARCLAY, P. M. DANIEL, K. J. FRANKLIN and M. M. L. PRICHARD: Studies of the renal circulation. Oxford: Blackwell scientific publications 1947. — USON, A. C., S. T. KNAPPENBERGER and M. M. MELICOW: Nontraumatic perirenal hematomas: a report based on 7 cases. J. Urol. (Baltimore) **81**, 388 (1959). — WOODRUFF jr., J. H., R. E. OTTOMAN, J. H. SIMONTON and B. D. AVERBROOK: The radiologic differential diagnosis of abdominal trauma. Radiology **72**, 641 (1959). — YDÉN, S.: Cyst rupture in 6 cases of polycystic renal disease. Acta radiol. (Stockh.) **42**, 17 (1954).

Nephro- and ureterolithiasis

ÅKERLUND, Å.: Ein typisches Röntgenbild bei Konkrementbildung in einer Ureterozele. Acta radiol. (Stockh.) **16**, 39 (1935). — ALBRIGHT, F., W. V. CONSOLAZIO, F. S. COOMBS, H. W. SULKOWITCH and J. H. TALBOTT: Metabolic studies and therapy in a case of nephrocalcinosis with rickets and dwarfism. Bull. Johns Hopk. Hosp. **66**, 7 (1940). — ALBRIGHT, F., L. DIENES and H. W. SULKOWITCH: Pyelonephritis with nephrocalcinosis. J. Amer. med. Ass. **110**, 357 (1938). — ALLYN, R. E.: Uric acid calculi. J. Urol. (Baltimore) **78**, 314—317 (1957).— ANTHONSEN, W., and C. J. CHRISTOFFERSEN: Nephrolithiasis. Nord. Med. **8**, 1943 (1940). — ARNESEN, A.: Der akute Nierensteinanfall. Z. urol. Chir. Gynäk. **45**, 94 (1939). — ASK-UPMARK, E.: Über Röntgenuntersuchung der Nieren bei gewissen diagnostisch schwer zu deutenden Krankheitsfällen in der inneren Medizin. Acta med. scand. **96**, 390 (1938). — BAINES, G. H., J. A. BARCLAY and W. T. COOKE: Nephrocalcinosis associated with hyperchloraemia and low plasma-bicarbonate. Quart. J. Med. **14**, 113 (1945). — BAKER, R., and J. P. CONELLY: Bilateral and recurrent renal calculi. J. Amer. med. Ass. **160**, 1106 (1956). — BEARD, D. E., and W. E. GOODYEAR: Hyperparathyroidism and urolithiasis. J. Urol. (Baltimore) **65**, 638 (1950). — BIE, K., and Y. KJELSTRUP: Urinveiskonkrementer hos småbarn. Nord. Med. **58**, 1777 (1957). — BIRDSALL, J. C.: The incidence of urinary tract obstruction in renal calculus formation. J. Urol. (Baltimore) **42**, 917 (1939). — BOEMINGHAUS, H.: Über die Funktion der Niere bei akutem komplettem Ureterverschluß. Langenbecks Arch. klin. Chir. **171**, 109—115 (1932). — BOEMINGHAUS, H., u. L. ZEISS: Zur Erholungsfähigkeit mechanisch bedinter Stauungszustände im Nierenbecken-Harnleitersystem. Z. Urol. **29**, 83 (1935). — BOYCE, W. H., and F. K. GARVEY: The amount and nature of the organic matrix in urinary calculi: a review. J. Urol. (Baltimore) **76**, 213 (1956). — BURKLAND, C. E.: Fracture of giant ureteral calculus. J. Urol. (Baltimore) **69**, 366 (1953). — BURNETT, C. H., R. R. COMMONS, F. ALBRIGHT and J. E. HOWARD: Hypercalcemia without hypercalcuria. New Engl. J. Med. **240**, 787—794 (1949). — BUTLER, A. M., J. L. WILSON and S. FARBER: Dehydration and acidosis with calcification at renal tubules. J. Pediat. **8**, 489 (1936). — CANTAROW, A., and B. SCHEPARTZ: Biochemistry, 2nd edit., p. 779. Philadelphia: W. B. Saunders Company 1957. — CARR, R. J.: A new theory on the formation of renal calculi. Brit. J. Urol. **26**, 105 (1954). — CLAESSON, U.: Nephrolithiasis hos barn efter immobilisering för fraktur. Nord. Med. **58**, 1772 (1957). — COLIEZ, R.: La stase pyélo-calicienne artificielle dans le diagnostic radiologique des affections des reins. Gaz. méd. Fr. **50**, 189 (1943). — Les signes radiologiques de stase et de surpression urétéro-rénale au cours de l'urographie intra-veineuse. J. Radiol. Électrol. **28**, 311 (1947). — COMARR, A. E.: A long-term survey of the incidence of renal calculosis in paraplegia. J. Urol. (Baltimore) **74**, 447 (1955). — CONWELL, cit. E. J. McCAGUE (1937). — COUNCILL, W. A., and W. A. COUNCILL jr.: Spontaneous rupture of the renal parenchyma associated with renal lithiasis. J. Urol. (Baltimore) **63**, 441 (1950). — COWIE,

T.: Nephrocalcinosis and renal calculi. Radiological studies in calculus formation. Brit. J. Radiol. **27**, 210—218 (1954). — DAVIS, H.: Metabolic causes of renal stones in children. J. Amer. med. Ass. **171**, 2199—2202 (1959). — DODSON, A. I.: Urological surgery. London 1956. — DUNN, H. G.: Oxalosis. Report of a case with review of the literature. Amer. J. Dis. Child. **90**, 58 (1955). — DWORETZKY, M.: Reversible metastatic calcification (milkdrinker's syndrome). J. Amer. med. Ass. **155**, 830—832 (1954). — EBSTEIN, W., u. A. NICOLAIER: Über die Wirkung der Oxalsäure und einiger ihrer Derivate auf die Nieren. Virchows Arch. path. Anat. **148**, 366 (1897). — ELLIOT, J. S.: Spontaneous dissolution of renal calculi. J. Urol. (Baltimore) **72**, 331 (1954). — ENFEDJIEFF, M.: Detrusorspasmus bei tiefsitzenden Uretersteinen im Röntgenbild. Verhandlungsber. der Dtsch. Ges. für Urologie, S. 276, Leipzig 1958. — ENGEL, W. J.: Nephrocalcinosis. J. Amer. med. Ass. **145**, 288—294 (1951). — Urinary calculi associated with nephrocalcinosis. J. Urol. (Baltimore) **68**, 105—116 (1952). — ENGFELDT, B., and C. LAGERGREN: Nephrocalcinosis. Acta chir. scand. **115**, 46—57 (1958). — EZICKSON, W. J., and J. B. FELDMAN: Signs of vitamin A deficiency in the eye correlated with urinary lithiasis. J. Amer. med. Ass. **109**, 1706 (1937). — FASSBENDER, C. W.: Über Nieren- und Harnleiterkonkremente bei Kleinstkindern. Fortschr. Röntgenstr. **85**, 451—453 (1956). — FEINDT, W.: Röntgenologischer Nachweis eines partiellen Sekretionsausfalles der Niere bei Harnleiterkonkrement und gedoppelter Ureteranlage. Fortschr. Röntgenstr. **73**, 62 (1950). — FRITJOFSSON, A.: Njurstenar och deras behandling. Nord. Med. **59**, 733 (1958). — GAUJOUX, J.: Four cases of urolithiasis impossible to see on the X-ray picture. Écho méd. Cevennes **55**, 1 (1954). — GOLDSTEIN, A. E., and B. S. ABESHOUSE: Calcification and ossification of the kidney. Radiology **30**, 544, 667 (1937). — GRANOFF, M. A.: Migration of renal stones associated with pyonephrosis and perinephric abscess into lung. J. Urol. (Baltimore) **42**, 302 (1939). — GREENSPAN, E. M.: Hyperchloremic acidosis and nephrocalcinosis. Arch. intern. Med. **83**, 271 (1949). — GÜRSEL, A. E.: Renal lithiasis invisible without opaque medium. J. Radiol. Électrol. **36**, 360—361 (1955). — HAMMARSTEN, G.: Terapi-inducerade urinvägsstenar. Opusc. med. (Stockh.) **3**, 19 (1958). — HAMRE, L.: Bilaterale ureterstener med uremi. Nord. Med. **58**, 1775 (1957). — HELLMER, H.: Nephrography. Acta radiol. (Stockh.) **23**, 233 (1942). — HELLSTRÖM, J.: Röntgendiagnostikens begränsning och möjligheter vid njur- och uretärstenar. Nord. Med. **8**, 1725 (1934). — Njur- och uretärsten. Inledn. föredrag vid Nord. Kir. för. 20: e möte i Köpenhamm 1935. — HERZAN, F. A., and F. W. O'BRIEN: Acceleration of delayed excretory urograms. Influence of ingested ice water on the kidney function. Amer. J. Roentgenol. **68**, 104 (1952). — HICKEL, R.: Figures urographiques particulières: les ombres précapillaires (ou images dites „en boules") et la néphrographie. J. Radiol. Électrol. **27**, 509 (1946). — HIGGINS, C. C., and E. E. MENDENHALL: Factors associated with recurrent formation of renal lithiasis with report of new method for qualitative analysis of urinary calculi. J. Urol. (Baltimore) **42**, 436 (1939). — HOLST, S.: Silikatsten i urinveiene. Nord. Med. **60**, 1169 (1958). — HOWELL, R. D.: Milk of calcium renal stone. J. Urol. (Baltimore) **82**, 197—199 (1959). — KAUFMANN, S. A.: The acceleration of delayed excretory urograms with ingested ice water. J. Urol. (Baltimore) **74**, 243 (1955). — KEATING jr., F. R.: Some metabolic aspects of urinary calculi. J. Urol. (Baltimore) **79**, 663 (1958). — KEYSER, L. D.: Newer concepts of stone in the urinary tract. J. Urol. (Baltimore) **42**, 420 (1939). — KIMBROUGH, J. C., and J. C. DENSLOW: Urinary tract calculi in recumbent patients. J. Urol. (Baltimore) **61**, 837—845 (1949). — KIRSNER, J. B., W. L. PALMER and E. HUMPHREYS: Morphologic changes in the human kidney following prolonged administration of alkali. Arch. Path. (Chicago) **35**, 207—225 (1943). — KJELLBERG, S. R.: Fälle mit geschichteten und facettierten Nierensteinen. Acta radiol. (Stockh.) **16**, 571 (1935). — KNEISE, O., u. K. L. SCHOBER: Die Röntgenuntersuchung der Harnorgane. Leipzig: Georg Thieme 1941. — KNUTH, D.: Die seitliche Röntgenaufnahme in der Nierensteindiagnostik und ihre Fehlerquellen. Röntgenpraxis **11**, 679 (1939). — LAGERGREN, C.: Biophysical investigations of urinary calculi. Acta radiol. (Stockh.) Suppl. **133** (1956). — LAGERGREN, C., and H. ÖHRLING: Urinary calculi composed of pure calcium phosphate. Acta chir. scand. **117**, 335—341 (1959). — McCAGUE, E. J.: The incidence and prevention of renal and vesical calculi in the fracture and traumatic group. Amer. J. Surg. **38**, 85—88 (1937). — MEADS, A. M.: Fibrin calculi of the kidney. J. Urol. (Baltimore) **42**, 1157 (1939). — MELDOLESI, G.: Il quadro angiografico renale nel blocco degli ureteri. Minerva chir. (Torino) **13**, 1104 (1958). — MILLER, J. M., I. FREEMAN and W. H. HEATH: Calcinosis due to treatment of duodenal ulcer. J. Amer. med. Ass. **148**, 198—199 (1952). — MOORE, C. A., and C. C. DODSON: Urinary tract calculi in children, renal and vesical calculi in an 8-month-old child. Amer. J. Dis. Child. **88**, 743 (1954). — MORTENSEN, J. D., A. H. BAGGENSTOSS, M. H. POWER and D. G. PUGH: Roentgenographic demonstration of histologically identifiable renal calcification. Radiology **62**, 703—712 (1954). — MORTENSEN, J. D., and J. L. EMMETT: Nephrocalcinosis: a collective and clinicopathologic study. J. Urol. (Baltimore) **71**, 398—406 (1954). — MORTENSEN, J. D., J. L. EMMETT and A. H. BAGGENSTOSS: Clinical aspects of nephrocalcinosis. Proc. Mayo Clin. **28**,

305—312 (1953). — MUSCETTOLA, G.: Raro caso di pseudocalcolo transparente intraureteropelvico in uretero-pielografia. Radiol. med. (Torino) **26**, 767 (1939). — NEUSTEIN, H. B., S. S. STEVENSON and L. KRAINER: Oxalis with renal calcinosis due to calcium oxalate. J. Pediat. **47**, 624—633 (1955). — NICE, C. M., A. R. MARGULIS and L. G. RIGLER: Roentgen diagnosis of abdominal tumors in childhood. Springfield, Ill.: Ch. C. Thomas 1957. — OLSSON, OLLE: Renal colic in cases of tumor and tuberculosis of the kidney: roentgenologic views. J. Urol. (Baltimore) **63**, 118—127 (1949). — Backflow in excretion urography during renal colic. Modern trends in diagnostic radiology (1953), chap. 13. — OSTRY, H.: Nephrocalcinosis. Canad. med. Ass. J. **65**, 465 (1951). — PARSONS, J.: Magnesium dibasic phosphate identified as a crystalline component of a urinary calculus. J. Urol. (Baltimore) **76**, 228 (1956). — PERSKY, L., D. CHAMBERS and A. POTTS: Calculus formation and ureteral colic following acetazolamide (diamox) therapy. J. Amer. med. Ass. **161**, 1625 (1956). — PHEMISTER, D. B.: Ossification in kidney stones attached to the renal pelvis. Ann. Surg. **78**, 239 (1923). — PITTS jr., H. H., J. W. SCHULTE and D. R. SMITH: Nephrocalcinosis in a father and three children. J. Urol. (Baltimore) **73**, 208 (1955). — PRIEN, E. L.: Studies in urolithiasis. II. Relationships between pathogenesis, structure and composition of calculi. J. Urol. (Baltimore) **61**, 821 (1949). — Studies in urolithiasis. III. Physicochemical principles in stone formation and prevention. J. Urol. (Baltimore) **73**, 627 (1955). — PRIEN, E. L., and C. FRONDEL: Crystallography of the urinary sediments with clinical and pathological observations in sulfonamide drug therapy. J. Urol. (Baltimore) **46**, 748 (1941). — Studies in urolithiasis. I. The composition of urinary calculi. J. Urol. (Baltimore) **57**, 949—991 (1947). — RANDALL, A.: The initiating lesions of renal calculus. Surg. Gynec. Obstet. **64**, 201 (1937). — RENANDER, A.: Spontane konkrementäre Nierenbeckenperforation. Acta radiol. (Stockh.) **21**, 343 (1940). — The roentgen density of the cystine calculus. Diss. Stockholm 1941. — RICKER, W., and M. CLARK: Sarcoidosis. Amer. J. clin. Path. **19**, 725 (1949). — RISHOLM, L.: Studies on renal colic and its treatment by posterior splanchnic block. Acta chir. scand. Suppl. **184** (1954). — ROSENBAUM, D., W. COGGESHALL and R. T. LEVIN: Chronic glomerulonephritis with severe renal tubular calcification. Amer. J. med. Sci. **221**, 319 (1951). — ROSENOW, E. C.: Renal calculi: a study of papillary calcification. J. Urol. (Baltimore) **44**, 19 (1940). — SANDEGÅRD, E.: Prognosis of stone in the ureter. Acta chir. scand. Suppl. **219** (1956). — SAUPE, E.: Röntgendiagramme von menschlichen Körpergeweben und Konkrementen. Fortschr. Röntgenstr. **44**, 204 (1931). — SCHIFFER, E.: Füllungsdefekt bei retrograder Pyelographie, vorgetäuscht durch einen Nierenkelchkrampf. Acta radiol. (Stockh.) **17**, 93 (1936). — SCHNEIDER, P. W.: Beitrag zur Nephrokalzinose. Radiol. clin. (Basel) **28**, 34 (1959). — SCHÜPBACH, A., u. M. WERNLY: Hyperkalzaemie und Organverkalkungen bei Boeckscher Krankheit. Acta med. scand. **115**, 401 (1943). — SEIFTER, J., and H. R. TRATTNER: Simplified qualitative analysis of urinary calculi by spot tests. J. Urol. (Baltimore) **42**, 452 (1939). — SGALITZER, M.: Röntgenuntersuchung im Krankenzimmer. Wien. med. Wschr. **86**, 864 (1936). — SMITH, D. R., F. O. KOLB and H. A. HARPER: The management of cystinuria and cystine-stone disease. J. Urol. (Baltimore) **81**, 61—71 (1959). — STÅHL, F.: Urolithiasis als Komplikation bei orthopädischen Erkrankungen. Acta chir. scand. **87**, 342 (1942). — STENSTRÖM, R.: Nefrokalcinos vid poliomyelit med adningsförlamning. Nord. Med. **55**, 647 (1956). — STOUT, H. A., R. H. AKIN and E. MORTON: Nephrocalcinosis in routine necropsies; its relationship to stone formation. J. Urol. (Baltimore) **74**, 8 (1955). — TOVBORG JENSEN, A., u. J. E. THYGESEN: Über die Phosphatkremente der Harnwege. Z. Urol. **32**, 659 (1938). — TWINEM, F. P.: The relation of renal stone formation and recurrence to calyceal pathology. J. Urol. (Baltimore) **44**, 596 (1940). — VERMOOTEN, V.: The incidence and significance of the deposition of calcium plaques in the renal papilla. J. Urol. (Baltimore) **46**, 193 (1941). — WIESER, C., u. U. M. ISLER: Viszerale Röntgenbefunde bei Osteomyelosklerose. Radiol. clin. (Basel) **26**, 329 (1957). — WILDBOLZ, E.: Klinik der Pyurie im Kindesalter. Schweiz. med. Wschr. **89**, 665 (1959). — WINER, J. H.: Practical value of analysis of urinary calculi. J. Amer. med. Ass. **169**, 1715 (1959). — WULFF, H. B.: Om värdet av urografi vid diagnostiken av njur- och uretärstensanfallet. Nord. Kir. För. Förhandl. Kbh. 1935. — Urography in 125 cases of acute renal and abdominal conditions. Acta radiol. (Stockh.) **16**, 77 (1935). — Die Zuverlässigkeit der Röntgendiagnostik — besonders hinsichtlich des Wertes der Urographie — und die Prognose bei Nieren- und Harnleitersteinen. Acta radiol. (Stockh.) Suppl. **32** (1936). — Über die sog. reflektorische Steinanurie. Lund 1941. — Urinary excretion in acute unilateral renal and ureteral blocking. Lund: Håkan Ohlssons boktryckeri 1948. — ZOLLINGER, H. U., u. H. ROSENMUND: Urämie bei endogen bedingter subakuter und chronischer Calciumoxalatniere. Schweiz. med. Wschr. **82**, 1261 (1952).

Papillary necrosis

ABESHOUSE, B. S., and J. O. SALIK: Pyelographic diagnosis of lesions of the renal papillae and calyces in cases of hematuria. Amer. J. Roentgenol. **80**, 569 (1958). — ALKEN, C. E.: Die

Papillennekrose. Z. Urol. **32**, 433 (1938). — AXELSSON, U.: Papillitis necroticans renalis och hemolytisk anemi hos fenazonmissbrukare. Nord. Med. **59**, 903 (1958). — CHRISTOFFERSEN, J. C., and K. ANDERSEN: Renal papillary necrosis. Acta radiol. (Stockh.) **45**, 27 (1956). — EDMONDSON, H. A., H. E. MARTIN and E. EVANS: Necrosis of renal papillae and acute pyelonephritis in diabetes mellitus. A.M.A. Arch. intern. Med. **79**, 148 (1947). — EDVALL, C. A.: Unilateral renal function in chronic pyelonephritis and renal papillary necrosis. Acta chir. scand. **115**, 11 (1958). — ESKELUND, V.: Necrosis of the renal papillae following retrograde pyelography. Acta radiol. (Stockh.) **26**, 548 (1945). — EVANS, J. A., and W. D. ROSS: Renal papillary necrosis. Radiology **66**, 502—508 (1956). — FOORD, R. D., J. D. N. NABORRO and E. W. RICHES: Diabetic pneumaturia. Brit. med. J. **1956**I, 433. — GARRETT, R. A., M. S. NORRIS and F. VELLIOS: Renal papillary necrosis: a clinicopathologic study. J. Urol. (Baltimore) **72**, 609 (1954). — GAUSTAD, V., and J. HERTZBERG: Acute necrosis of the renal papillae in pyelonephritis, particularly diabetes. Acta med. scand. **136**, 331 (1950). — GÜNTHER, G. W.: Die Papillennekrosen der Niere bei Diabetes. Münch. med. Wschr. **84**, 1695 (1937). — Die Mark- und Papillennekrosen der Niere, Pyelonephritis und Diabetes. Z. Urol. **41**, 310 (1948). — HARRISON, J. H., and O. T. BAILEY: The significance of necrotizing pyelonephritis in diabetes mellitus. J. Amer. med. Ass. **118**, 15 (1942). — HULTENGREN, N.: Renal papillary necrosis. Acta chir. scand. **115**, 89 (1958). — HYAMS, J. A., and H. R. KENYON: Localized obliterating pyelonephritis. J. Urol. (Baltimore) **46**, 380 (1941). — JOHNSTON, D. H.: Repeated bouts of renal papillary necrosis diagnosed by examination of voided tissue. Arch. intern. Med. **90**, 711 (1952). — KNUTSEN, A., E. R. JENNINGS, O. A. BRINES and A. AXELROD: Renal papillary necrosis. Amer. J. clin. Path. **22**, 327—336 (1952). — LUSTED, L. B., H. L. STEINBACH and E. KLATTE: Papillary calcification in necrotizing renal papillities. Amer. J. Roentgenol. **78**, 1049 (1957). — MANDEL, E. E.: Renal medullary necrosis. Amer. J. Med. **13**, 322 (1952). — MANDEL, E. E., and H. POPPER: Experimental medullary necrosis of the kidney. A.M.A. Arch. Path. **52**, 1 (1951). — MELLGREN, J., u. G. REDELL: Zur Pathologie und Klinik der Papillitis necroticans renalis. Acta chir. scand. **84**, 439 (1941). — MOREAU, R., R. DEUIL, J. CROSNIER, C. BIATRIX et P. THIBAULT: Nécrose papillaire rénale au cours du diabète. Presse méd. **62**, 599—600 (1954). — MUIRHEAD, E. E., J. VANATTA and A. GROLLMAN: Papillary necrosis of the kidney. J. Amer. med. Ass. **142**, 627 (1950). — OLSSON, OLLE: Spontanes Gaspyelogramm. Acta radiol. (Stockh.) **20**, 578 (1939). — OTTOMAN, R. E., J. H. WOODRUFF, S. WILK and F. ISAAC: The roentgen aspects of necrotizing renal papillitis. Radiology **67**, 157 (1956). — PRAETORIUS, G.: Papillitis necroticans bei schwerer chronischer Pyelonephritis. Z. Urol. **31**, 298 (1937). — PRÉVOT, R., u. H. BERNING: Zur Röntgendiagnostik der Pyelonephritis. Fortschr. Röntgenstr. **73**, 482 (1950). — ROBBINS, E. D., and A. ANGRIST: Necrosis of renal papillae. Ann. intern. Med. **31**, 773 (1949). — ROBBINS, S. L., G. K. MALLORY and T. D. KINNEY: Necrotizing renal papillitis: a form of acute pyelonephritis. New Engl. J. Med. **235**, 885 (1946). — SARGENT, J. C., and J. W. SARGENT: Unilateral renal papillary necrosis. J. Urol. (Baltimore) **73**, 757 (1955). — SHEEHAN, H. L.: Medullary necrosis of the kidneys. Lancet **1937**II, 187. — SIMON, H. B., W. A. BENNETT and J. L. EMMETT: Renal papillary necrosis: a clinicopathologic study of 42 cases. J. Urol. (Baltimore) **77**, 557—567 (1957). — SLIPYAN, A., and S. BARLAND: Renal papillary necrosis: case report. J. Urol. (Baltimore) **68**, 430 (1952). — SPÜHLER, O.: Probleme der interstitiellen Nephritis. Schweiz. med. Wschr. **83**, 145 (1953). — SPÜHLER, O., u. H. U. ZOLLINGER: Die chronisch-interstitielle Nephritis. Z. klin. Med. **151**, 1 (1953). — SWARTZ, D.: Renal papillary necrosis. J. Urol. (Baltimore) **71**, 385 (1954). — THELEN, A.: Papillitis necroticans bei chronischer Pyelonephritis. Z. Urol. **40**, 67 (1947). — THORSÉN, G.: Pyelorenal cysts. Acta chir. scand. **98**, 476 (1949). — WALL, B.: Pyelographic changes in necrotizing renal papillitis. J. Urol. (Baltimore) **72**, 1 (1954). — WELCH, N. M., and G. C. PRATHER: Pneumonephrosis. A complication of necrotizing pyelonephritis. J. Urol. (Baltimore) **61**, 712 (1949). — WHITEHOUSE, F. W., and H. F. ROOT: Necrotizing renal papillitis and diabetes mellitus. J. Amer. med. Ass. **162**, 444 (1956). — WIESEL, B. H., and J. F. A. McMANUS: Necrotizing renal papillitis. Sth. med. J. (Bgham, Ala.) **43**, 403 (1950). — ZOLLINGER, H. U.: Problèmes des néphritis et néphroses. J. Urol. méd. chir. **61**, 581 (1955).

Perinephritis

ALKEN, C. E.: Perinephritische Eiterungen mit seltenem Verlauf. Z. Urol. **31**, 773 (1937). — ATCHESON, D. W.: Perinephric abscess with a review of 117 cases. J. Urol. (Baltimore) **46**, 201 (1941). — BALL, W. G.: Renal carbuncle. Brit. J. Urol. **6**, 248 (1934). — BANGERTER, J.: Über einen Fall von Nierenkarbunkel mit multiplen Rindabszessen in der anderen Niere. Schweiz. med. Wschr. **67**, 310 (1937). — BARON, E., and L. J. ARDUINO: Primary renal actinomycosis. J. Urol. (Baltimore) **62**, 410 (1949). — BEER, E.: Roentgenographic evidence of perinephritic abscess. J. Amer. med. Ass. **90**, 1375 (1928). — BERGSTRAND, H.: Über die Nierenveränderungen bei tödlicher Sulfathiazolschädigung. Acta med.

scand. **118**, 97 (1944). — BRAMAN, R-, and R. R. CROSS jr.: Perinephric abscess producing a pneumonephrogram. J. Urol. (Baltimore) **75**, 194—197 (1956). — DAVIDSON, B.: Solitary cortical abscess (carbuncle) of the kidney in a child simulating tumor. Urol. cutan. Rev. **40**, 260 (1936). — DEUTICKE, P.: Die Bedeutung der Pyelographie für die Diagnose des paranephritischen Abszesses. Zbl. Chir. **67**, 2214 (1940). — Über pyelographische Befunde bei Entzündungen des Nierenlagers. Z. Urol. **34**, 89 (1940). — DROSCHL, H.: Klinischer Beitrag zur Diagnose des Nierenkarbunkels. Zbl. Chir. **64**, 1209 (1937). — EMMETT, J. L., and J. T. PRIESTLEY: Solitary renal abscess (carbuncle): report of case. Proc. Mayo Clin. **11**, 764 (1936). — FECI, L.: Contributo radiologico alla diagnosi degli ascessi perirenali. Arch. ital. Urol. **4**, 503 (1927). — FOULDS, G. S.: Diagnosis of perinephric abscess. J. Urol. (Baltimore) **42**, 1 (1939). — FRIEDMAN, L. J.: Roentgen signs of perinephritic abscess. Med. J. Rec. **127**, 648 (1928). — FRIMANN-DAHL, J.: Røntgenundersøkelser ved akutte abdominalsykdommer. Oslo: Johan Grundt Tanum 1942. — GARDINI, G. F.: Contributo allo studio del foruncolo renale. Arch. ital. Urol. **11**, 504 (1934). — GOLDSTEIN, A. E., and O. MARCUS: Roentgenological diagnosis of perinephritic abscess and perinephritis. Amer. J. Roentgenol. **40**, 371 (1938). — GRAVES, C. G., and L. E. PARKINS: Carbuncle of the kidney. J. Urol. (Baltimore) **35**, 1 (1936). — GUSZICH, A.: Zur Frage der Diagnostik des Nierenkarbunkels. Z. urol. Chir. **40**, 449 (1935). — HENCZ, L.: Späteres Schicksal eines Patienten mit operiertem Nierenkarbunkel. Z. urol. Chir. Gynäk. **43**, 186 (1937). — HJORT, E.: Om nyreabscess og nyrekarbunkel. Med. rev. Bergen **54**, 376 (1937). — HUNTER, A. W.: Gumma of kidney. J. Urol. (Baltimore) **42**, 1176 (1939). — ILLYÉS, G. DE: Suppurations of the renal parenchyma. Brit. J. Urol. **9**, 101 (1937). — INGRISH, G. A.: Carbuncle of the kidney: report of ten cases. J. Urol. (Baltimore) **42**, 326 (1939). — JAMES, T. G. I.: A case of carbuncle of the kidney. Brit. J. Urol. **6**, 156 (1934). — KICKHAM, C. J. E., and F. L. COLPOYS jr.: Periureteral fascitis. J. Amer. med. Ass. **171**, 2202—2204 (1959). — LAURELL, H.: Ein Beitrag zur Röntgendiagnostik der Peri- bzw. der Paranephritis. Upsala Läk.-Fören. Förh. **26**, XXXVIII (1920/21). — LAZARUS, J. A.: Carbuncle of the kidney. Amer. J. Surg. **25**, 155 (1934). — LEAKE, R., and T. B. WAYMAN: Retroperitoneal encysted hematomas. J. Urol. (Baltimore) **68**, 69 (1952). — LIPSETT, PH.: Roentgenray observations in acute perinephritic abscess. J. Amer. med. Ass. **90**, 1374 (1928). — LJUNGGREN, E.: Beitrag zur Röntgendiagnostik der Nierenkarbunkel. Z. urol. Chir. **31**, 258 (1931). — McNULTY, P. H.: Carbuncle of the kidney: review of the literature, discussion of unilateral localized lesions of the kidney and report of a case. J. Urol. (Baltimore) **35**, 15 (1936). — MENVILLE, J. G.: The lateral pyelogram as a diagnostic aid in perinephritic abscess. J. Amer. med. Ass. **111**, 231 (1938). — MILLER, R. H.: Diagnosis of peripephric abscess. Ann. Surg. **106**, 756 (1937). — MITCHELL, G. A. G.: The spread of retroperitoneal effusions arising in the renal regions. Brit. med. J. **1939**, 1134. — MOORE, T. D.: Renal carbuncle. J. Amer. med. Ass. **96**, 754 (1931). — MORALES, O.: A case of roentgenologically observed perirenal oedema after therapy with sulphanilamide preparations. Acta radiol. (Stockh.) **26**, 334 (1945). — NESBIT, R. M., and V. S. DICK: Pulmonary complications of acute renal and perirenal suppuration. Amer. J. Roentgenol. **44**, 161 (1940). — O'CONOR, V.: Carbuncle of the kidney. J. Urol. (Baltimore) **30**, 1 (1933). — OVERGAARD, K.: A case of paranephritic abscess with characteristic pyelogram. Acta radiol. (Stockh.) **23**, 180 (1942). — PARKS, R. E.: The radiographic diagnosis of perinephric abscess. J. Urol. (Baltimore) **64**, 555 (1950). — PREHN, D. T.: A pyelographic sign in the diagnosis of perinephric abscess. J. Urol. (Baltimore) **55**, 8 (1946). — RÉVÉSZ, V.: Die direkte Röntgendiagnostik der peri- und paranephritischen Eiterungen und die Röntgenuntersuchung der chronischen Perinephritis. Fortschr. Röntgenstr. **34**, 48 (1926). — RIGLER, L. G., and M. H. MANSON: Perinephritic abscess. Amer. J. Surg. **13**, 459 (1931). — RIPPY, E. L.: Review of local cases of perinephritic abscess. Year book of urol., p. 208, 1938. — SHANE, J. H., and M. HARRIS: Roentgenologic diagnosis of perinephritic abscess. J. Urol. (Baltimore) **32**, 19 (1934). — SKARBY, H.-G.: Beiträge zur Diagnostik der Paranephritiden. Acta radiol. (Stockh.) Suppl. **62** (1946). — SPENCE, H. M., and L. W. JOHNSTON: Renal carbuncle; case report and comparative review. Ann. Surg. **109**, 99—108 (1939). — STITES, J. R., and J. A. BOWEN: Diagnostic difficulties in perinephritic abscess. Sth. med. J. (Bgham, Ala.) **30**, 1062 (1937). — SZACSVAY, S. v.: Ein Beitrag zur Diagnose und Therapie des Nierenkarbunkels. Z. urol. Chir. **40**, 70 (1935). — TAYLOR, W. N.: Carbuncle of the kidney. Amer. J. Surg. **22**, 550 (1933). — VRIES, G. H. DE: Angiogramm eines Nierenkarbunkels. Fortschr. Röntgenstr. **90**, 640—641 (1959). — WELIN, S.: Über die Röntgendiagnostik der Paranephritis. Fortschr. Röntgenstr. **67**, 162 (1943). — WOODRUFF, S. R., and S. L. GROSSMAN: Renal carbuncle. Urol. cutan. Rev. **40**, 240 (1936).

Plain radiography

ALBRIGHT, F., P. C. BAIRD, O. COPE and E. BLOOMBERG: Studies on the physiology of the parathyroid glands. Amer. J. Med. Sci. **187**, 49 (1934). — ALBRIGHT, F., and E. C. REIFENSTEIN jr.: The parathyroid glands and metabolic bone disease. Baltimore 1948. —

ARONS, W. L., W. R. CHRISTENSEN and M. C. SOSMAN: Nephrocalcinosis visible by x-ray associated with chronic glomerulonephritis. Ann. intern. Med. 42, 260 (1955). — ASK-UPMARK, E.: Über Röntgenuntersuchung der Nieren bei gewissen diagnostisch schwer zu deutenden Krankheitsfällen in der inneren Medizin. Acta med. scand. 96, 390 (1938). — BAUER, H.: Beitrag zu den Nierenverkalkungen. Dtsch. Z. Chir. 254, 1 (1940). — BURNETT, C. H., R. R. COMMONS, F. ALBRIGHT and J. E. HOWARD: Hypercalcemia without hypercalcuria or hypophosphatemia, calcinosis and renal insufficiency. New Engl. J. Med. 240, 787 (1949). — FUSI, G.: Considerazioni sull'iperparatiroidismo in nefropatie. Radiol. med. (Torino) 40, 551—574 (1954). — HAMRE, L.: Fibrolipomatosis renis. Nord. Med. 58, 1769 (1957). — HEIDENBLUT, A.: Röntgendiagnostik des verkalkten Renalisaneurysmas. Fortschr. Röngenstr. 83, 868—871 (1955). — HELLSTRÖM, J.: Clinical experiences of twenty one cases of hyperparathyroidism with special reference to the prognosis following parathyroidectomy. Acta chir. scand. 100, 391 (1950). — Further observations regarding the prognosis and diagnosis in hyperparathyroidism. Acta chir. scand. 105, 122 (1953). — Primary hyperparathyroidism. Observations in a series of 50 cases. Acta endocr. (Kbh.) 16, 30 (1954). — Calcification and calculus formation in a series of seventy cases of primary hyperparathyroidism. Brit. J. Urol. 27, 387 (1955). — KESHIN, J. G., and A. JOFFE: Varices of the upper urinary tract and their relationship to portal hypertension. J. Urol. (Baltimore) 76, 350 (1956). — LEWIS, S., and R. D. DOSS: Calcified hydropyonephrosis. Radiology 70, 866 (1958). — LILJA, B., and H. WAHREN: On meteorism in pyelography. Acta radiol. (Stockh.) 15, 41 (1934). — MARTZ, H.: Renal calcification accompanying pyloric and high intestinal obstruction. Arch. intern. Med. 65, 375—389 (1940). — MISHALANY, H. G., and D. R. GILBERT: Benign ossified lesion of kidney. J. Urol. (Baltimore) 78, 330—336 (1957). — MUSCHAT, M., and L. KOOLPE: Parenchymal calculosis of the kidneys. J. Urol. (Baltimore) 42, 293 (1939). — NESBIT, R. M., and W. B. CRENSHAW: Aneurysm of the renal artery. J. Urol. (Baltimore) 75, 380 (1956). — NUGENT, C. A., and W. STOWELL: Localization of the kidney for renal biopsy. J. Urol. (Baltimore) 82, 193 (1959). — PACCIARDI, A., and P. L. MICHELASSI: Diagnostic criteria for the evaluation of renal calcifications on routine roentgenograms. Ann. Radiol. diagn. (Bologna) 31, 30 (1958). — PANICHI, S., e I. BONECHI: Determinazione radiologica delle dimensioni del rene. Valori normali. Minerva med. (Torino) 49, 3261 (1958). — PETRÉN, T.: La situation des reins en hauteur chez l'enfant. Stockholm: Iduns Tryckeri A.-B. 1934. — RIEMENSCHNEIDER, P. A.: Multiple large aneurysms of the splenic artery. Amer. J. Roentgenol. 74, 872 (1955). — RONNEN, J. R. v.: The roentgen diagnosis of calcified aneurysms of the splenic and renal arteries. Acta radiol. (Stockh.) 39, 385 (1953). — ROSENBERG, M. L.: Hypercalcuria and metabolic bone disease. Calif. Med. 81, 382 (1954). — SCHORR, S., and D. BIRNBAUM: Raised position of the right kidney. Radiol. clin. (Basel) 28, 102 (1959). — WOLKE, K.: Pyelogramm mit einem durch einen Nierenarterienzweig verursachten Füllungsdefekt (Pseudodefekt). Acta radiol. (Stockh.) 17, 566 (1936).

Polycystic disease

BILLING, L.: The roentgen diagnosis of polycystic kidneys. Acta radiol. (Stockh.) 41, 305—315 (1954). — BORSKI, A. A., and J. C. KIMBROUGH: Bilateral carcinoma in polycystic renal disease — an unique case. J. Urol. (Baltimore) 71, 677—681 (1954). — CLARKE, B. G., I. S. HURWITZ and E. DUBINSKY: Solitary serous cysts of kidney. J. Urol. (Baltimore) 75, 772 (1956). — HOOPER, J. W.: Cystic disease of the kidney in infants. J. Urol. (Baltimore) 79, 917—924 (1958). — IVEMARK, B., och K. LINDBLOM: Förkalkningar i adulta polycystnjurar. Nord. Med. 59, 882 (1958). — MENASHE, V., and D. R. SMITH: Apparently unilateral polycystic kidney. A cause for abdominal calcific shadows. Amer. J. Dis. Child. 94, 313 (1957). — RALL, J. E., and H. M. ODEL: Congenital polycystic disease of the kidney: review of the literature and data on 207 cases. Amer. J. med. Sci. 218, 399—407 (1949). — SPRING, M., and S. W. GROSS: Ruptured aneurysm of the circle of Willis associated with polycystic kidneys. A.M.A. Arch. intern. Med. 102, 806 (1958). — VIDAL, B., e G. ENGLARO: Sulla semeiologia radiologica del rene policistico. Radiol. med. (Torino) 43, 647 (1957).

Preparation of the patient

GYLLENSWÄRD, Å., H. LODIN and O. MYKLAND: Prevention of undue intestinal gas in abdominal radiography in infants. Acta radiol. (Stockh.) 39, 6 (1953). — KOSENOW, W.: Verbesserung der Säuglings- und Kleinkinder-Urographie durch gleichzeitige Flüssigkeits- und Luftfüllung des Magens. Fortschr. Röntgenstr. 83, 396 (1955). — Einfache Methode zur Verbesserung der Ausscheidungsurogramme bei Säuglingen und Kleinkindern. Mschr. Kinderheilk. 103, 407 (1955). — SLANINA, J.: The value of hydrogen peroxide and tannic acid in cleansing enema. Radiol. clin. (Basel) 27, 197 (1958).

Pyelography

ALFERMANN, F.: Die Anwendung des Bewegungspyelogramms zur Differentialdiagnostik von Bauchtumoren. Bruns' Beitr. klin. Chir. 180, 199 (1950). — BAURYS, W.: Serious complications associated with the newer diagnostic methods in urology. J. Urol. (Baltimore) 75, 846 (1956). — BLOOM, J., and J. F. RICHARDSON: The usefulness of a contrast medium containing an antibacterial agent (retrografin) for retrograde pyelography. J. Urol. (Baltimore) 81, 332 (1959). — BOWEN, J. A., and E. L. SHIFLETT: Intravenous urography in the upright position. Radiology 36, 672 (1941). — BREUER, F.: Zur Bedeutung des Veratmungspyelogramms für die Erkennung paranephritischer Abszesse. Zbl. Chir. 64, 683 (1937). — BURROS, H. M., V. H. J. BORROMEO and D. SELIGSON: Anuria following retrograde pyelography. Ann. intern. Med. 48, 674 (1958). — CASEY, W. C., and W. E. GOODWIN: Percutaneous antegrade pyelography and hydronephrosis. J. Urol. (Baltimore) 74, 164 (1955). CHAMBERLIN, G. W., and I. IMBER: Pyelography for the diagnosis of lesions of the body and tail of the pancreas. Radiology 63, 722 (1954). — EBERL, J.: Die Urinschichtung bei der intravenösen Pyelographie. Fortschr. Röntgenstr. 86, 74 (1957). — EISLER, F.: Neueste Fortschritte der röntgenologischen Steindiagnose. Referat 5. Tagg der Dtsch. Ges. für Urologie, 29. 9.—1. 10. 1921, Wien. Dtsch. med. Wschr. 1921, 1380. — ETTINGER, A.: Layer formation in pyelography. Amer. J. Roentgenol. 49, 783—794 (1943). — FEY, B., P. TRUCHOT et M. NOIX: Étude radiocinématographique de l'uretère normal et pathologique. J. Radiol. Électrol. 39, 328 (1958). — FLOYD, E., and J. C. GUY: Translumbar percutaneous antegrade pyelography as an adjunct to urologic diagnosis. J. med. Ass. Ga 45, 13 (1956). — GEREMIA, B., e A. GAMBA: Urografia discendente destra da pielografia ascendente sinistra. Acta chir. ital. 14, 141 (1958). — GOLLMANN, G.: Zur Vermeidung störender Luftblasen bei der retrograden Pyelographie. Fortschr. Röntgenstr. 84, 487 (1956). — GRIEVE, J., and K. G. LOWE: Anuria following retrograde pyelography. Brit. J. Urol. 27, 63 (1955). — HESS, E.: Respiration pyelography as an aid in diagnosis. J. Urol. (Baltimore) 42, 4, 381 (1939). — JUNKER, H.: Durchleuchtung und Momentaufnahme von Nierenbecken und Ureter. Z. Urol. 30, 231 (1936). — KLAMI, P.: Retrograde pyelography with hydrogen peroxide in the contrast medium. Acta radiol. (Stockh.) 42, 181 (1954). — LAURELL, H.: On the differential-diagnosis: pyonephrosis or retroperitoneal tumour. Acta radiol. (Stockh.) 3, 226—227 (1924). — LICHTENBERG, A. v.: Grundsätzliches zur Ausscheidungsurographie auf Grundlage von 2000 Untersuchungen mit sieben Nierenkontrastmitteln. Verh. III. Internat. Radiologenkongr. Paris 1931, S. 931. — Principles and new advances in excretion urography. Brit. J. Urol. 3, 119 (1931). — The principles of intravenous urography. J. Urol. (Baltimore) 25, 249 (1931). — Grundlagen und Fortschritte der Ausscheidungsurographie. Langenbecks Arch. klin. Chir. 171, 1, 3 (1932). — LINDBOM, Å.: Miliary tuberculosis after retrograde pyelography. Acta radiol. (Stockh.) 25, 219 (1944). — MANGELSDORFF, B.: Die Veratmungspyelographie und ihre Verwertbarkeit in der urologischen Diagnostik. Fortschr. Röntgenstr. 74, 416 (1951). — MEYER, E.: Kritische Besprechung der direkten Kontrastfüllung der Harnwege und Erfahrungen mit dem neuen Kontrastmittel Thorotrast. Z. Urol. 26, 157 (1932). — PIERSON, L. E., and E. M. HONKE: Respiration pyelography in the diagnosis of perinephric abscess. J. Urol. (Baltimore) 47, 580 (1942). — PRÉVÔT, R.: Intravenöse gezielte Pyelographie. Fortschr. Röntgenstr. 59, 52 (1939). — PRÉVÔT, R., u. H. BERNING: Zur Röntgendiagnostik der Pyelonephritis. Fortschr. Röntgenstr. 73, 482 (1950). — PYTEL, A.: Percutaneous antegrade pyelography (Russian text). Vestn. Rentgenol. Radiol. 33, 15 (1958). — ROTH, R. B., A. F. KAMINSKY and E. HESS: Bactericidal additive for pyelographic mediums. J. Urol. (Baltimore) 74, 563—566 (1955). — SALINGER, H., and F. SAALBERG: Pyeloscopy. Acta radiol. (Stockh.) 27, 617 (1946). — SARRUBI ZALDIVAR, D.: Radiologie des pyelites et pyelonephrites. J. Urol. méd. chir. 62, 372—378 (1956). — SAVINO, F. M.: A pyelographic test for renal fixity during respiration. Brit. J. Urol. 19, 29 (1947). — SCHEELE, K.: Die Radiographie der oberen Harnwege als diagnostisches Mittel bei Tumoren des Bauches. Ergebn. med. Strahlenforsch. 4, 41 (1930). — SCHIFFER, E.: Füllungsdefekt bei retrograder Pyelographie, vorgetäuscht durch einen Nierenkelchkrampf. Acta radiol. (Stockh.) 17, 93 (1936). — WADSWORTH, G. E., and E. UHLENHUTH: The pelvic ureter in the male and female. J. Urol. (Baltimore) 76, 244 (1956). — WEENS, H. S., and T. J. FLORENCE: The diagnosis of hydronephrosis by percutaneous renal puncture. J. Urol. (Baltimore) 72, 589 (1954). — WEISER, M.: Strahlentod durch Thorotrast. Röntgenblätter 10, 270—276 (1957). — WICKBOM, I.: Pyelography after direct puncture of the renal pelvis. Acta radiol. (Stockh.) 41, 505 (1954). — WOLKE, K.: Pyelogramm mit einem durch einen Nierenarterienzweig verursachten Füllungsdefekt (Pseudodefekt). Acta radiol. (Stockh.) 17, 566 (1936). — ZIEGLER, J.: Bedeutung und Technik der Ureterkompression bei der Ausscheidungspyelographie. Dtsch. med. Wschr. 56, 1772 (1930).

Radiation protection

ARDRAN, G. M., H. E. CROOKS, F. H. KEMP and R. OLIVER: Radiation dose to staff in medical x-ray departments. Brit. J. Radiol. 30, 600 (1957). — ARDRAN, G. M., and F. H.

KEMP: Protection of the male gonads in diagnostic procedures. Brit. J. Radiol. **30**, 280 (1957). — Reduction of radiation doses administered during chest radiography. Tubercle (Lond.) **38**, 403 (1957). — BAKER, W. J., F. R. PORTNEY and R. FIRFER: A study of x-ray hazards. Urol. int. (Basel) **1**, 135 (1955). — A study of x-ray hazards of retrograde urography. J. Urol. (Baltimore) **74**, 174 (1955). — BÖÖK, Jan A.: Joniserande strålning och genetisk morbiditet. Sv. Läk.-Tidn. **54**, 517—530 (1957). — BRAESTRUP, C. B.: Past and present radiation exposure to radiologists from the point of view of life expectancy. Amer. J. Roentgenol. **78**, 988 (1957). — CHAMBERLAIN, R. H.: Radiation protection comes of age. J. Amer. med. Ass. **153**, 488—491 (1953). — A summary: today's problems in radiation hazards and what is being done to control them. Amer. J. Roentgenol. **78**, 1000 (1957). — DEUEL, H. J. jr., A. L. S. CHENG, G. D. KRYDER and M. E. BINGEMANN: Protective effect against X-irradiation of methyl linoleate in the rat. Science **117**, 254—255 (1953). — *Exposure of man to ionizing radiation arising from medical procedures.* Phys. in Med. Biol. **2**, 107—151 (1957). — FAILLA, G., and P. McCLEMENT: The shortening of life by chronic whole-body irradiation. Amer. J. Roentgenol. **78**, 946 (1957). — GLASS, B.: The genetic basis for the limitation of radiation exposure. Amer. J. Roentgenol. **78**, 955 (1957). — KAPLAN, H. S.: An evaluation of the somatic and genetic hazards of the medical uses of radiation. Amer. J. Roentgenol. **80**, 696 (1958). — KOCKUM, J., K. LIDÉN and O. NORMAN: Radiation hazards attending use of transportable image intensifier. Acta radiol. (Stockh.) **49**, 369 (1958). — LARSSON, L.-E.: Radiation doses to patients and personnel in modern roentgen diagnostic work. Acta radiol. (Stockh.) **46**, 680—689 (1956). — Radiation doses to the gonads of patients in Swedish roentgen diagnostics. Acta radiol. (Stockh.) Suppl. **157** (1958). — LAUGHLIN, J. S., M. L. MEURK, I. PULLMAN and R. S. SHERMAN: Bone, skin, and gonadal doses in routine diagnostic procedures. Amer. J. Roentgenol. **78**, 961 (1957). — NORWOOD, W. D.: Common sense approach to the problem of genetic hazard due to diagnostic radiology. J. Amer. med. Ass. **167**, 1928 (1958). — The determination of injury from the internally deposited radioisotope plutonium. J. occupat. Med. **1**, 269—276 (1959). — NORWOOD, W. D., J. W. HEALY, E. E. DONALDSON, W. C. ROESCH and C. W. KIRKLIN: The gonadal radiation dose received by the people of a small american city due to the diagnostic use of roentgen rays. Amer. J. Roentgenol. **82**, 1081—1097 (1959). — RUSSELL, L. B., and W. L. RUSSELL: Radiation hazards to embryo and fetus. Radiology **58**, 369 (1952). — SPIEGLER, G., and B. E. KEANE: Scatter doses received on the lower extremities of the diagnostic radiologist. Brit. J. Radiol. **28**, 140 (1955). — STANFORD, R. W., and J. VANCE: Quantity of radiation received by reproductive organs of patients during routine diagnostic X-ray examinations. Brit. J. Radiol. **28**, 266 (1955). — STIEVE, F. E.: Untersuchungen über Maßnahmen zur Reduzierung der Strahlenbelastung der männlichen Keimdrüsen bei röntgendiagnostischen Maßnahmen in deren Umgebung. Fortschr. Röntgenstr. **90**, 373 (1959). — STONE, R. S.: Common sense in radiation protection applied to clinical practice. Amer. J. Roentgenol. **78**, 993 (1957). — SWENSON, P. C.: The radiation hazards of diagnostic procedures. Radiology **63**, 876 (1954). — TAYLOR, L. S.: Practical suggestions for reducing radiation exposure in diagnostic examinations. Amer. J. Roentgenol. **78**, 983 (1957). — WARREN, S.: Longevity and causes of death from irradiation in physicians. J. Amer. med. Ass. **162**, 464 (1956). — WOERT jr., I. VAN, P. I. KEARNEY, I. KILICOZLU and J. F. ROACH: Radiation hazards of intravenous pyelography. J. Amer. med. Ass. **166**, 1826 (1958).

Retroperitoneal pneumography

ANDERSEN, P. E.: Pneumoretroperitoneum in suprarenal disease. Acta radiol. (Stockh.) **43**, 289 (1955). — BERNARDINI e R. SALVATI: Retropneumoperitoneo, nuovo mezzo di indagine radiologica. Gaz. int. Med. Chir. **44**, 301 (1950). — BIBUS, B.: Die Pneumoradiographie des Nierenlagers. Wien. klin. Wschr. **52**, 256 (1939). — BLAND, A. B.: A simplified apparatus for presacral carbon dioxide injection. J. Urol. (Baltimore) **79**, 171 (1958). — BONOMINI e BACCAGLINI: Pneumoretroperitoneo e pneumomediastino. L'enfisema diagnostico dei tessuti areolari profondi del tronco. Bologna: Cappelli 1953. — BRODNY, M. L., and H. A. CHAMBERLIN: A simple apparatus for pneumoadrenalography. J. Urol. (Baltimore) **42**, 211 (1939). — CAHILL, G. F.: Air injections to demonstrate the adrenals by X-ray. J. Urol. (Baltimore) **34**, 238—243 (1935). — CARELLI, M. H.: Sur le pneumopéritoine et sur une méthode personelle pour voir le rein sans pneumopéritoine. Bull. Soc. méd. Hôp. Paris **45**, 1409 (1921). — COCCHI, U.: Retropneumoperitoneum und Pneumomediastinum. Stuttgart: Georg Thieme 1957. — Fortschr. Röntgenstr. Erg.-Bd. **79**. — COONEY, J. D., R. D. AMELAR and A. ORRON: Renal displacement and rotation during retroperitoneal pneumography. Arch. Surg. (Chicago) **70**, 405 (1955). — COPE, O., and R. SCHATZKI: Tumors of the adrenal glands. Arch. intern. Med. **64**, 1222 (1939). — DODSON, A. I.: Urological surgery. London 1956. — DURANT, E. M., J. LONG and M. J. OPPENHEIMER: Pulmonary (venous) air embolism. Amer. Heart J. **33**, 269—281 (1947). — EVANS, A. T.: Combined use of contrast media in retroperitoneal tumors. Critical evaluation. Arch.

Surg. (Chicago) **70**, 191 (1955). — Evans, J. A., and N. Poker: Newer roentgenographic techniques in the diagnosis of retroperitoneal tumors. J. Amer. med. Ass. **161**, 1128—1132 (1956). — Fagerberg, S.: Pneumoretroperitoneum. Acta radiol. (Stockh.) **37**, 519 (1952). — Fontaine, R., P. Warter, P. Frank, G. Stoll et R. Raber: De l'intérêt du rétropneumopéritoine pour le diagnostic des malformations et néoplasmes du rein. J. Radiol. Électrol. **36**, 708 (1955). — Franciosi, A. U., A. F. Govoni and C. G. Pasquinelli: Retroperitoneum associated with laminagraphy. Amer. J. Roentgenol. **72**, 1034 (1954). — Gandini, D., and A. Gibba: Present trends in the diagnoses of surgical renal diseases by means of pneumoretroperitoneum combined with the usual radio-urological technique. Nunt. Radiol. **20**, 707 (1954). — Gennes, L. de, J. P. May et G. Simon: Le rétropneumoperitoine (nouveau procedé d'exploration radiologique de l'abdomen). Presse méd. **21**, 351—352 (1950). — Giraud, G., P. Betoulieres, H. Latour y M. Pelissier: La neumostratigrafia. Arch. esp. Med. interna **2**, 79—103 (1956). — Giraud, M., P. Bret, M. Kuentz et A. Anjou: Bilan de cent examens après pneumorétropéritoine. J. Radiol. Électrol. **35**, 838—846 (1954). — Glassman, I., R. Shapiro and F. Robinson: Air embolism during presacral pneumography: a case report. J. Urol. (Baltimore) **75**, 569 (1956). — Iavazyan, A. V.: Visualization of kidney anomalies by the aid of presacral pneumoretroperitoneum (Russian text). Vestn. Rentgenol. Radiol. **32**, 60—62 (1957). — Köhler, H.: Indikationsgebiet der Pneumoradiographie. Dtsch. Ges. Urol. 1926, S. 119. — Landes, R. R., and C. L. Ransom: Presacral retroperitoneal pneumography utilizing carbon dioxide: further experiences and improved technique. J. Urol. (Baltimore) **82**, 670—673 (1959). — Levine, B.: Use of helium in perirenal insufflation: preliminary reports. J. Urol. (Baltimore) **67**, 390 (1952). — Macarini, N., et L. Oliva: Sur l'insufflation rétropéritonéale associée à la stratigraphie tridimensionell. J. belge Radiol. **34**, 281—297 (1951). — Majela de Abreu Guedes, G.: Nossa experiencia com o retro-pneumoperitoneo. Rev. bras. Cir. **32**, 193—198 (1956). — Mencher, W. H.: Perirenal insufflation. J. Amer. med. Ass. **109**, 1338—1341 (1937). — Meneghini, C., u. G. Dell'Adami: Die Insufflation des extraperitonealen Bindegewebes in der Röntgendiagnostik der oberen Harnorgane mit besonderer Berücksichtigung der Möglichkeiten der Stratigraphie. Fortschr. Röntgenstr. **76**, 181—190 (1952). — Montero, J. J.: Aplasia renal y retropneumoperitoneo. Arch. esp. Urol. 14, 26 (1958). — Moos, F. von: Die Tomographie beim Pneumoretroperitoneum. Schweiz. med. Wschr. **82**, 629—632 (1952). — Mosca, L. G.: El enfisema retroperitoneal: Su técnica, sus indicaciones y resultados. Pren. méd. argent. **38**, 1025—1035 (1951). — Mosenthal, A.: Unsere Erfahrungen mit der „Pneumoradiographie des Nierenlagers" nach P. Rosenstein. Z. urol. Chir. **12**, 303 (1923). — Palubinskas, A. J., and C. J. Hodson: Transintervertebral retroperitoneal gas insufflation. Radiology **70**, 851—854 (1958). — Polvar, G., et P. Braggion: Mobilità renale e pneumoaddome extraperitoneale. Minerva urol. (Torino) **4**, 221—227 (1952). — Porcher, Bonomini e Oliva: L'insufflazione retroperitoneale in radiodiagnostica. Torino: Minerva Medica 1954. — Puigvert-Gorro, A., et Moya-Prats: Les infiltrations periviscerales en radiologie urinaire. J. Urol. méd. chir. **55**, 63—67 (1949). — Ransom, C. L., R. R. Landes and R. McLelland: Air embolism following retroperitoneal pneumography: a nation-wide survey. J. Urol. (Baltimore) **76**, 664 (1956). — Reinhardt, K.: Zur Technik des Retropneumoperitoneums. Dtsch. med. Wschr. **77**, 804—806 (1952). — Ritter, A., u. R. Allemann: Diagnostische Ergebnisse der Pyelographie und Pneumoradiographie. Schweiz. med. Wschr. **53**, 927—932, 955—961 (1923). — Rosenstein, P.: Die Pneumoradiographie des Nierenlagers. Z. Urol. **15**, 447 (1921). — Rossi, L.: Il retropneumoperitoneo. Ann. Radiol. diagn. (Bologna) **23**, 340 (1951). — Ruiz Rivas, M.: Nueva tecnica de diagnostico radiografico aplicable a organos y estructuras retroperitoneales, mediastinicas y cervicales. Rev. clín. esp. **25**, 206 (1947). — Diagnostico radiologico. El neumorriñon. Tecnica original. Arch. esp. Urol. **4**, 228—233 (1948). — Roentgenological diagnosis. Generalized subserous emphysema through a single puncture. Amer. J. Roentgenol. **64**, 723—734 (1950). — Russ, F. H., D. L. Glenn and C. Gianturco: Gas embolism during extraperitoneal insufflation. Radiology **61**, 637—638 (1953). — Salvati, R.: Utilità e indicazioni della insufflazione retroperitoneale nella pratica e nella radiodiagnostica urologica. Minerva urol. (Torino) **8**, 201—203 (1956). — Schulte, E.: Gasembolie bei der extraperitonealen Pneumoradiographie. Fortschr. Röntgenstr. **91**, 87 (1959). — Senger, F. L., G. R. Horton, J. J. Bottone, H. Y. H. Chin and M. C. Wilson: Perirenal air insufflation by the paracoccygeal retro rectal route. N. Y. St. J. Med. **53**, 2823 (1953). — Sinner, W.: Die Bedeutung des Retropneumoperitoneums in der Nierendiagnostik. Z. Urol. **48**, 564 (1955). — Sövényi, E.: Unsere Erfahrungen mit der retroperitonealen Luftinsufflation (Retropneumoperitoneum). Radiol. clin. (Basel) **28**, 198 (1959). — Steinbach, H. L., R. P. Lyon, E. R. Miller and D. R. Smith: Extraperitoneal pneumography. Calif. Med. **75**, 202 (1951). — Steinbach, H. L., and D. R. Smith: Extraperitoneal pneumography in diagnosis of retroperitoneal tumours. Arch. Surg. (Chicago) **70**, 161—172 (1955). — Vespignani, L.: The roentgen reticular appearance of the perirenal fat tissue in extraperitoneal pneumoabdomen (retropneumo, peritoneum) and tomography. Acta radiol. (Stockh.) **36**,

509 (1951). — VESPIGNANI, L., et R. ZENNARO: La stratigraphie en projection latérale du rein normal et pathologique avec le „pneumo-abdomen extra-péritoneál". J. Radiol. Électrol. **32**, 720—726 (1951). — WALTER, R. C., and W. E. GOODWIN: Aortography and retroperitoneal oxygen in urologic diagnosis: a comparison of translumbar and percutaneous femoral methods of aortography. J. Urol. (Baltimore) **70**, 526 (1953). — Aortography and pneumography in children. J. Urol. (Baltimore) **77**, 323—328 (1957). — WILHELM, S. F.: Gas insufflation through the lumbar and presacral routes. Surg. Gynec. Obstet. **99**, 319 (1954).

Sponge kidney

ALKEN, C. E., F. SOMMER and F. KLING: Renovasographie vor Teilresektion der Niere bei Markcystensteinbildung im oberen Pol. Z. Urol. **44**, 569—576 (1951). — ARDUINO, L. J.: A case of pyelitis and cystitis cystica. J. Urol. (Baltimore) **55**, 149 (1946). — BALESTRA, G., e B. DELPINO: In tema di rene a spugna e di nefrocalcinosi. Radiol. med. (Torino) **42**, 745—764 (1956). — BARATA, L. S.: Um caso de rim esponja. Urologia (P. Alegre) **1**, 40—45 (1951). — BEITZKE, H.: Über Zysten im Nierenmark. Charité-Ann. **32**, 285—293 (1908). — BRAIBANTI, T.: Considerazioni au di un caso di displasia cistica del rene. Ann. Radiol. diagn. (Bologna) **21**, 412 (1949). — BRUNI, P.: Rene a spugna associato a cistopatia cistica. Urologia (Treviso) **21**, 148—153 (1954). — BUTLER, A. M., J. L. WILSON and S. FARBER: Dehydration and acidosis with calcification at renal tubules. J. Pediat. **8**, 489—499 (1936). — CACCHI, R.: La malattia cistica delle piramidi renali o „Rene a spugna". Relazione ufficiale al XXX. Congr. della Soc. Italiana di Urologia, Napoli 19.—20.—21. ottobre 1957. Cremona 1957. — CACCHI, R., et V. RICCI: Sur une rare maladie kystique multiple des pyramides rénales le „rein en éponge". J. Urol. méd. chir. **55**, 497—519 (1949). — CARINATI, A.: In tema di displasie cictiche renali con particolare riguardo ad un caso di „rene a spugna". Radiol. **12**, 79 (1956). — CETNAROWICZ, H., Z. CZECHOWSKA, M. KOPEĆ and J. ZABO-KRZYCKI: Cystic disease of renal pyramids. Pol. Przegl. radiol. **22**, 233 (1958). — CIRLA, A., e S. GALDINI: Contributo allo studio del rene a spugna. Radiol. med. (Torino) **42**, 605—610 (1956). — DAMMERMANN, H. J.: Urologentreffen Düsseldorf 1948. Zit. GÜNTHER 1950. — Markcystenniere unter dem Bild einer Solitärcyste. Z. Urol. **44**, 230—232 (1951). — DARGET, R., et R. BALLANGER: Sur un cas de rein „en éponge". J. Urol. méd. chir. **60**, 713—715 (1954). — DELMAS, J., RACHOU, J. PHILIPPON et BENEJAM: Reins „en éponge". J. Radiol. Électrol. **39**, 844 (1958). — DELZOTTO, L., e P. TURCHETTO: Il rene a spugna; contributo casistico. Urologia (Treviso) **22**, 240—244 (1955). — DI SIENO, A., e B. GUARESCHI: Il quadro radiologico del rene a spugna midollare. Radiol. clin. (Basel) **25**, 80—103 (1956). — Il rene a spugna midollare con calcolosi multipla endocavitaria ed i suoi possibili rapporti con la nefrocalcinosi. Radiol. med. (Torino) **42**, 167—183 (1956). — EKSTRÖM, T., B. ENG-FELDT, C. LAGERGREN and N. LINDVALL: Medullary sponge kidney. Stockholm: Almqvist & Wiksell 1959. — FIUMICELLI, A., G. SAMMARCO e G. C. VERDECCHIA: Rena a spugna midollare e nefrocalcinosi: diagnosi differenziale. Radiol. med. (Torino) **42**, 1018 (1956). — FONTOURA MADUREIRA, H.: Doenca quistica das piramides renais (Rim em esponja). J. Soc. Ci. Med. Lisboa **117**, 6 (1943). — GAYET, R.: Deux cas de maladie kystique des pyramides rénales un rein en éponge. Actes du 44. Congr. Francais d'urologie, p. 473—477. Paris: G. Doin & Cie. 1950. — Discussion to HICKEL: Un cas de „rein en éponge". J. Urol. méd. chir. **59**, 409 (1953). — GIANNONI, R., B. VIDAL e L. ENGLARO: Contributo alla casistica del rene a spugna. Urologia (Treviso) **23**, 625—633 (1956). — GIBBA, A., e D. GANDINI: Contributo casistico alla studio del rene a spugna. Urologia (Treviso) **21**, 596—606 (1954). — GIORDANO, G.: Rene a spugna (caso con ipertensione a crisi). Nunt. Radiol. **22**, 380—388 (1956). — GÜNTHER, G. W.: Die Markcysten der Niere. Z. Urol. **43**, 29—46 (1950). — HICKEL, R.: Un cas de „rein en éponge". J. Urol. méd. chir. **59**, 408—409 (1953). — HOGNESS, J. R., and J. M. BURNELL: Medullary cysts of kidneys. Arch. intern. Med. **93**, 355—366 (1954). — JOSSERAND, P., R. ANNINO, L. MUGNIERY, L. ROUVÉS et H. MERLE: Le rein en éponge. Pédiatrie **7**, 31—42 (1952). — LENARDUZZI, G.: Reperto pielografico poco commune (dilatazione delle vie urinarie intrarenali). Radiol. med. (Torino) **26**, 346 (1939). — Sul rene a spugna. Radiol. med. (Torino) **35**, 992 (1949). — La forma circoscritta di rene a spugna. Radiol. med. (Torino) **37**, 776 (1951). — Evoluzione del rene a spugna. Radiol. med. (Torino) **38**, 57 (1952). — Rene a spugna parcellare. Radiol. med. (Torino) **38**, 1084 (1952). — LHEZ, A.: Le rein en éponge. J. Urol. méd. chir. **60**, 575—588 (1954). — LINDVALL, N.: Roentgenologic diagnosis of medullary sponge kidney. Acta radiol. (Stockh.) **51**, 193—206 (1959). — MARINI, A.: Il rene a spugna. Boll. Soc. med.-chir. Cremona **11**, 65—78 (1957). — MASETTO, I., e P. BRAGGION: Rene a spugna. Nunt. Radiol. **22**, 47—69 (1956). — MATHIS, R. I., y G. BERRI: Rinen en esponja. Rev. argent. Urol. **24**, 383—388 (1955). — MULVANEY, W. P., and W. T. COLLINS: Cystic disease of the renal pyramids. J. Urol. (Baltimore) **75**, 776—779 (1956). — NEUHAUS, W.: Multiple Zysten der Tubuli recti. Fortschr. Röntgenstr. **84**, 108 (1956). — NEVEU, J.: Un cas de „maladie kystique multiple des pyramides rénales". J. Urol. méd.

chir. **56**, 564—565 (1950). — PANSADORO, V.: Su un caso di malattia cistica multipla delle piramidi renali o rene a spugna. Quad. Urol. **1**, 125 (1952). — PELOT, G.: Discussione a HICKEL: un cas de „rein en éponge". J. Urol. méd. chir. **59**, 410 (1953). — Discussione a LHEZ: Le rein en éponge. J. Urol. méd. chir. **60**, 587 (1954). — PETKOVIC, S.: Contribution à l'étude de la maladie kystique des pyramides rénales. J. Urol. méd. chir. **58**, 425—432 (1952). — POLITANO, V.A.: Pyelorenal backflow: clinical significance and interpretation. J. Urol. (Baltimore) **78**, 1 (1957). — POWELL, R. E.: An unusual congenital deformity of the kidney. Canad. med. Ass. J. **60**, 48—50 (1949). — REBOUL, G., M. PÉLISSIER et L. BELTRANDO: A propos d'un cas de rein en éponge. J. Radiol. Électrol. **39**, 795—796 (1958). — RONCORONI, L.: Le calcificazioni della loggia renale nelle formazioni cistiche e nei tumori. Radiol. med. (Torino) **42**, 953 (1956). — RUBIN, E. L., J. C. ROSS and D. P. B. TURNER: Cystic disease of the renal pyramids („sponge kidney"). J. Fac. Radiol. (Lond.) **10**, 134—137 (1959). — SMITH, C. H., and J. B. GRAHAM: Congenital medullary cysts of the kidneys with severe refractory anemia. Amer. J. Dis. Child. **69**, 369—377 (1945). — TOTI, A., e G. DELL' ADAMI: Contributo alla conoscenza della dilatazione cistica delle vie urinarie prepelviche (rene a spugna). Atti Accad. Sci. Ferrara **27**, 2 (1948/49). — VERMOOTEN, V.: Congenital cystic dilatation of renal collecting tubules: New disease entity. Yale J. Biol. Med. **23**, 450—453 (1950/51). — VESPIGNANI, L.: Sull'associazione delle varie forme della malattia cistica renale Radioter. Radiobiol. Fis. med. **5**, 483—498 (1951). — Rene a spugna. Ann. Radiol. diagn. (Bologná) **31**, 276—302 (1958). — ZAFFAGNINI, B., e A. MACCHITELLA: Rene a spugna. Acta chir. ital. **10**, 513—516 (1954).

Tuberculosis

AMBROSETTI, A., u. R. SESENNA: Arteriographische Untersuchungen an der tuberkulösen Niere. Urol. int. (Basel) **1**, 153—171 (1955). — BIONDETTI, P., e F. MARANI: Diagnosi differenziale arteriografica della tubercolosi renale. Minerva chir. (Torino) **13**, 1049—1073 (1958). — CAVAZZANA, P., e C. MENEGHINI: Considerazioni sull'evoluzione radiologica e clinica della tubercolosi urinaria in soggetti trattati con streptomicina e chemioterapici antitubercolari. Radiol. med. (Torino) **42**, 977 (1956). — CHIAUDANO, C., e V. GIONGO: Trattamento chirurgico conservativo della tubercolosi urinaria. Minerva med. Saluzzo 1958. — CIBERT, J.: La tuberculose rénale. Paris 1946. — COOK, E. N., and L. F. GREENE: The use of streptomycin in the treatment of tuberculosis of the urinary tract. J. Urol. (Baltimore) **60**, 187 (1948). — EITZEN, A. C.: Tuberculous contracted kidney: case report. J. Urol. (Baltimore) **42**, 288 (1939). — ERICSSON, N. O., and Å. LINDBOM: Intravenous urography in renal tuberculosis. Brit. J. Urol. **22**, 201 (1950). — FRANZAS, F.: Clarification of radiograms in renal tuberculosis. Acta chir. scand. **106**, 429 (1954). — FRIMANN-DAHL, J.: The radiological investigation of renal tuberculosis. The XXVII Meeting of the scand. surg. soc. in Oslo 1955, p. 22. — Radiological investigations of urogenital tbc. Urol. intern. (Basel) **1**, 396 (1955). — Selective angiography in renal tuberculosis. Acta radiol. (Stockh.) **49**, 31 (1958). — GAY, R.: Focal exclusions in renal tuberculosis. Acta radiol. (Stockh.) **32**, 129 (1949). — GREENWOOD, F. G.: Cineradiography in urinary tuberculosis. Brit. J. Radiol. **30**, 493 (1957). — HALKIER, E.: Behandling af nyretuberkulose med kemoterapeutica. Köpenhamn: Arnold Busck 1956. — HALKIER, E., and J. MEYER: Chemotherapy of renal tuberculosis. Dan. med. Bull. **6**, 97 (1959). — JACOBS, L. G.: Total tuberculosis calcification of a kidney and ureter. Amer. Rev. Tuberc. **71**, 437 (1955). — LANE, T. J. D.: Some observations on renal tuberculosis. Brit. J. Urol. **27**, 27 (1955). — LINDBOM, Å.: Miliary tuberculosis after retrograde pyelografi. Acta radiol. (Stockh.) **25**, 219 (1944). — LINDÉN, K.: Prognostic and therapeutic aspects of urogenital tuberculosis. Acta chir. scand. Suppl. **153** (1950). — LJUNGGREN, E.: Zur Röntgendiagnostik der Nierentuberkulose. Z. Urol. **32**, 40 (1938). — Beitrag zur Röntgendiagnostik der Nierentuberkulose. Z. Urol. **36**, 155 (1942). — Le diagnostic précoce de la tuberculose rénale. Presse méd. **91**, 2089 (1956). — MAY, F.: Zur Behandlung der Urogenitaltuberkulose. Wschr. Klinik u. Praxis **35**, 1525—1527, 1563—1567 (1959). — NESBIT, R. M., and A. W. BOHNE: A present day rationale for the treatment of urinary tuberculosis. J. Amer. med. Ass. **138**, 937 (1948). — OBRANT, K. O. F.: Studier över urogenitaltuberkulosens behandling. Diss. Göteborg 1953. — OLSSON, OLLE: Die Urographie bei der Nierentuberkulose. Acta radiol. (Stockh.) Suppl. **47** (1943). — PUIGVERT, A.: La néphrectomie partielle pour tuberculose. Urol. int. (Basel) **1**, 199 (1955). — RENANDER, A.: Röntgenbefunde bei Nierentuberkulose. Acta radiol. (Stockh.) **20**, 341 (1939). — RODRIGUEZ-LUCCA, B.: Renal tuberculosis simulating hypernephroma. J. Urol. (Baltimore) **77**, 589—592 (1957). — ROSENDAL, T.: Renal tuberculosis. Urol. cutan. Rev. **52**, 340—351 (1948). — STEINERT, R.: Renal tuberculosis and roentgenologic examination. Acta radiol. (Stockh.) Suppl. **53**. — WEYDE, R.: Abdominal aortography in renal diseases. Brit. J. Radiol. **25**, 353 (1952).

Tumour

ABOULKER, P., J. CHOMÉ et P. CORNET: Documents pour l'étude de l'artériographie rénale. J. Urol. méd. chir. **61**, 218 (1955). — ACKERMAN, L. V.: Mucinous adenocarcinoma of the pelvis of the kidney. J. Urol. (Baltimore) 55, 36 (1946). — ADAMS, P. S., and H. B. HUNT: Differential diagnosis of Wilms' tumour assisted by intramuscular urography. J. Urol. (Baltimore) 42, 688 (1939). — AGERHOLM-CHRISTENSEN, J.: A case of adenosarcoma of the kidney (Wilms's mixed tumor). Acta radiol. (Stockh.) 20, 69 (1939). — AGNEW, C. H.: Metastatic malignant melanoma of the kidney simulating a primary neoplasm. A case report. Amer. J. Roentgenol. 80, 813—816 (1958). — AHLBÄCK, S.: The suprarenal glands in aortography. Acta radiol. (Stockh.) 50, 341 (1958). — AHLSTRÖM, C. G., u. S. WELIN: Zur Differentialdiagnostik der Ewingschen Sarkome. Acta radiol. (Stockh.) 24, 67—81 (1943). — AINSWORTH, W. L., and S. A. VEST: The differential diagnosis between renal tumors and cysts. J. Urol. (Baltimore) 66, 740 (1951). — ALBERS, D. D., E. H. KALMON and K. C. BACK: Pheochromocytoma: Report of five cases, one a spontaneous cure. J. Urol. (Baltimore) 78, 301—308 (1957). — ANGULO, R.: Recurrent, nonfunctioning tumor of adrenal capsule. J. Urol. (Baltimore) 78, 309—313 (1957). — ANNAMUNTHODO, H., and R. F. HUTCHINGS: Nephroblastoma (Wilms' Tumor): Case report. J. Urol. (Baltimore) 78, 197 (1957). — ARCADI, J. A.: Mucus-producing cystadenocarcinoma of renal pelvis and ureter: fourth reported case. A.M.A. Arch. Path. 61, 264—268 (1956). — ARCOMANO, J. P., J. C. BARNETT and J. J. BOTTONE: Spontaneous disappearance of pulmonary metastases following nephrectomy for hypernephroma. Amer. J. Surg. 96, 703 (1958). — AUSTEN jr., G.: Calcification of renal tumors. Amer. J. Roentgenol. 49, 580 (1943). — BAILEY, M. K., and V. H. YOUNGBLOOD: Bilateral renal hypernephroma: report of a case. J. Urol. (Baltimore) 63, 593 (1950). — BAKER, W. J., and A. B. RAGINS: Pararenal teratoma: case report. J. Urol. (Baltimore) 63, 982 (1950). — BARTLEY, O., and G. T. HULTQUIST: Spontaneous regression of hypernephromas. Acta path. microbiol. scand. 27, 448 (1950). — BAUER jr., F. C., D. E. MURRAY and E. F. HIRSCH: Solitary adenoma of the kidney. J. Urol. (Baltimore) 79, 377 (1958). — BEATTIE, J. W.: Hypernephroma in seven-year-old white girl. J. Urol. (Baltimore) 72, 625 (1954). — BECK, R. E., and R. C. HAMMOND: Renal and osseous manifestation of tuberous sclerosis: case report. J. Urol. (Baltimore) 77, 578 (1957). — BEER, E.: Some aspects of malignant tumors of the kidney. Surg. Gynec. Obstet. 65, 433 (1937). — BELL, E. T.: A classification of renal tumors with observations on the frequency of the various types. J. Urol. (Baltimore) 39, 238—243 (1938). — BESSE jr., B. E., J. E. LIEBERMAN and L. B. LUSTED: Kidney size in acute leukemia. Amer. J. Roentgenol. 80, 611—617 (1958). — BILLING, L., u. Å. G. H. LINDGREN: Die pathologisch-anatomische Unterlage der Geschwulstarteriographie. Acta radiol. (Stockh.) 25, 625 (1944). — BOHNE, A. W., and W. W. CHRISTESON: Clinical evaluation of a concentrated iodine preparation. Radiology 60, 401 (1953). — BOSHAMMER: Das Pyelogramm bei Nierentumoren. Langenbecks Arch. klin. Chir. 175, 238 (1933). — BRAASCH, W. F., and J. A. HENDRICK: Renal cysts, simple and otherwise. J. Urol. (Baltimore) 51, 1 (1944). — BRODY, H., and H. LIPSHUTZ: Concomitant intrarenal and pararenal angiomyolipomas. J. Urol. (Baltimore) 74, 741 (1955). — BRØNDUM NIELSEN, J.: Sjaelden nyrebaekkentumor. Nord. Med. 58, 1774 (1957). — BULKLEY, G., J., and H. R. DRINKER: Malignant mesenchymoma of the kidney: case report. J. Urol. (Baltimore) 77, 583—588 (1957). — BUMPUS, H. C.: The apparent disappearance of pulmonary metastasis in a case of hypernephroma following nephrectomy. J. Urol. (Baltimore) 20, 185 (1928). — BURKLAND, C. E., and W. F. LEADBETTER: Pyelitis cystica associated with an hemophilus influenzae infection in the urine. J. Urol. (Baltimore) 42, 14 (1939). — CAMPBELL, J. H., C. M. PASQUIER, E. C. ST. MARTIN and P. C. WORLEY: Hypernephroma associated with polycythemia and eczematoid dermatitis. J. Urol. (Baltimore) 79, 12 (1958). — CAMPBELL, M. F.: Bilateral embryonal adenomyosarcoma of the kidney (Wilms tumor). J. Urol. (Baltimore) 59, 567 (1948). — CARNEVALI, G., V. C. CATANIA e S. DI PIETRO: Contributo radio-chirurgico allo studio dei surreni mediante pneumoretroperitoneo. Ann. Radiol. diag. (Bologna) 30, 466 (1958). — CHIAUDANO, M.: Aspetti arteriografici dei reni in condizioni patologiche. Minerva chir. (Torino) 13, 1074 (1958). — CHIDEKEL, N., and O. OBRANT: Hypernephroma metastases demonstrated by pelvic angiography. Acta chir. scand. 114, 46 (1957). — CHYNN, K. Y., and J. A. EVANS: Nephrotomography in the differentiation of renal cyst from neoplasm: a review of 500 cases. J. Urol. (Baltimore) 83, 21—24 (1960). — CLARKE, B. G., W. J. GOADE jr., H. L. RUDY and L. ROCKWOOD: Differential diagnosis between cancer and solitary serous cyst of the kidney. J. Urol. (Baltimore) 75, 922 (1956). — COUVELAIRE, R., et J. AUVERT: La phlébographie cave inférieure dans l'exploration des tumeurs du rein droit. J. Urol. méd. chir. 62, 21—40 (1956). — DEES, J. E.: Prognosis of primary tumors of renal pelvis and ureter. J. Urol. (Baltimore) 75, 419 (1956). — DEUTICKE, P.: Nierentumoren. Dtsch. Z. Chir. 231, 767—797 (1931). — DeWEERD, J. H.: Lipomatous retroperitoneal tumors: urographic findings. J. Urol. (Baltimore) 71, 421 (1954). — DeWEERD, J. H., and A. B. HAGEDORN: Hypernephroma associated with polycythemia. J. Urol. (Baltimore) 82, 29 (1959). — DUFF, P. A., and W. H. GRANGER: Diagnosis of involvement of inferior vena cava in renal neoplasms. J. Urol. (Baltimore) 65, 368 (1951). — EARLY, R., B. BROWN and K. TERPLAN: Fibroblastoma of renal parenchyma. J. Urol. (Baltimore) 80, 417 (1958). — EDELSTEIN, J. M., and S. M. MARCUS: Primary benign neoplasm of the ureter. J. Urol. (Baltimore) 60, 409 (1948). —

ENGEL, W. J.: The significance of renal displacement. J. Urol. (Baltimore) 76, 478—487 (1956). — ERIKSON, S.: Ein Fall von Nierenbeckentumor mit ungewöhnlichem Röntgenbild. Radiol. clin. (Basel) 11, 173 (1942). — ESCOVITZ, W., and S. G. WHITE: Extensive metastatic calcification in a case of malignant melanoma. Ann. West. Med. Surg. 4, 339—342 (1950). — ETTINGER, A., and M. ELKIN: Value of plain film in renal mass lesions (tumors and cysts). Radiology 62, 372 (1954). — EVANS, A. T.: Combined use of contrast media in retroperitoneal tumors. Critical evaluation. Arch. Surg. (Chicago) 70, 191 (1955). — Renal cancer: translumbar arteriography for its recognition. Radiology 69, 657 (1957). — EVANS, J. A.: Nephrotomography in the investigation of renal masses. Radiology 69, 684 (1957). — EVANS, J. A., W. DUBLIER and J. C. MONTEITH: Nephrotomography. Amer. J. Roentgenol. 71, 213—223 (1954). — EVANS, J. A., and N. POKER: Newer roentgenographic technique in the diagnosis of retroperitoneal tumors. J. Amer. med. Ass. 161, 1128 (1956). — FELBER, E.: Asynchronous bilateral benign papilloma of the ureter with subsequent cancer of ureteral stump, bladder, and vagina. J. med. Ass. Ga. 42, 198 (1953). — FERGUSON, CH., G. CAMERON and J. CARRON: Hemangioma of the kidney: report of two cases. J. Urol. (Baltimore) 74, 591 (1955). — FOSTER, D. G.: Large benign renal tumors. J. Urol. (Baltimore) 76, 231 (1956). — GEBAUER, A., and J. LISSNER: Differentialdiagnose retroperitonealer Tumoren. Fortschr. Röntgenstr. 88, 200 (1958). — GIBSON, T. E.: Lymphosarcoma of the kidney. J. Urol. (Baltimore) 60, 838 (1948). — Interrelationship of renal cysts and tumors: report of three cases. J. Urol. (Baltimore) 71, 241 (1954). — GIRAUD, M., P. BRET, M. KUENTZ, A. ANJOU, G. COSTAZ et L. CHOLLAT: Étude radiologique et stratigraphique des tumeurs surrénaliennes. J. Radiol. Électrol. 38, 893 (1957). — GLENN, J. F.: Primary ureteral carcinoma eight years in duration. J. Urol. (Baltimore) 81, 649 (1959). — GLOOR, H. U.: Über Verdrängungen der Niere bei Milztumor. Acta radiol. (Stockh.) 15, 467 (1934). — GOODWIN, W. E., E. V. MOORE and E. C. PEIRCE: Roentgenographic visualization of adrenal glands: use of aortography and/or retroperitoneal pneumography to visualize adrenal glands: combined adrenalography. J. Urol. (Baltimore) 74, 231 (1955). — GRACIA, V., and E. O. BRADFIELD: Simultaneous bilateral transitional cell carcinoma of the ureter: a case report. J. Urol. (Baltimore) 79, 925 (1958). — GRAUHAN: Die Tumorniere im Röntgenbild. Z. urol. Chir. 17, 1—26 (1925). — GREENBERG, A. L.: Right solitary renal cyst, left renal calculus. J. Urol. (Baltimore) 42, 87 (1939). — GREENE, L. B., B. L. HAYLLAR and M. BOGASCH: Epithelial tumors of the renal pelvis and ureter. J. Urol. (Baltimore) 79, 697 (1958). — HALLAHAN, J. D.: Spontaneous remission of metastatic renal cell adenocarcinoma: a case report. J. Urol. (Baltimore) 81, 522 (1959). — HAMER, H. G., and WM. NILES WISHARD jr.: Osteogenic sarcoma involving the right kidney. J. Urol. (Baltimore) 60, 10 (1948). — HAMM, F. C., and L. L. LAVALLE: Tumors of the ureter. J. Urol. (Baltimore) 61, 493 (1949). — HAMM, F. C., and L. J. SCORDAMAGLIA: A diagnostic aid for visualization of the left suprarenal space. J. Urol. (Baltimore) 73, 885 (1955). — HARRISON, F. G., H. L. WARRES and J. A. FUST: Neuroblastoma involving the urinary tract. J. Urol. (Baltimore) 63, 598 (1950). — HARRISON III, R. H., and L. C. DOUBLEDAY: Roentgenological appearance of normal adrenal glands. J. Urol. (Baltimore) 76, 16—22 (1956). — HAUGE, B. N.: Pheochromocytoma. J. Oslo Cy Hosp. 6, 135 (1956). — HEIDENBLUT, A.: Plattenepithelkarzinom des Nierenbeckens. Fortschr. Röntgenstr. 83, 95 (1955). — HEMPSTEAD, R. H., M. B. DOCKERTY, J. T. PRIESTLEY and G. B. LOGAN: Hypernephroma in children: report of two cases. J. Urol. (Baltimore) 70, 152 (1953). — HOLM, O. F.: Nachweis über die Ausbreitung von Rezidiven und lokalen Metastasen durch Aortographie bei einem Falle von operiertem Hypernephrom. Fortschr. Röntgenstr. 86, 399 (1957). — Registrering genom aortografi av lokala recidiv efter nefrectomi för hypernofrom (renalt adenocarcinom). Svenska Läk.-Tidn. 54, 3388 (1957). — HUFFMAN, W. L.: Echinococcus disease of kidney: report of a case. J. Urol. (Baltimore) 78, 17 (1957). — HULSE, C. A., and E. E. PALIK: Renal hamartoma. J. Urol. (Baltimore) 66, 506 (1951). — IMMERGUT, S., and Z. R. COTTLER: Peripelvic lipoma. J. Urol. (Baltimore) 67, 50 (1952). — ISRAEL, J.: Über Fieber bei malignen Nieren- und Nebennierengeschwülsten. Dtsch. med. Wschr. 37, 57—62 (1911). — JANSSON, G.: Die Röntgendiagnose bei Nierenbeckenpapillom. Acta radiol. (Stockh.) 16, 354 (1935). — JOHNSSON, S.: A contribution to the diagnostics of nephromata. Acta radiol. (Stockh.) Suppl. 60 (1946). — JOHNSSON, S. H., and M. MARSHALL jr.: Primary kidney tumors of childhood. J. Urol. (Baltimore) 74, 707 (1955). — KEEN, M. R.: Primary ureteral tumors. J. Urol. (Baltimore) 69, 231 (1953). — KESSEL, L.: Spontaneous disappearance of bilateral pulmonary metastases. J. Amer. med. Ass. 169, 1737 (1959). — KNOX, J., and A. SLESSOR: Phaechromocytoma and neurofibromatosis. Lancet 1955 I, 790—793. — KUCERA, J., and C. DVORACEK: A contribution to the diagnosis of renal adenoma. Acta radiol. bohemosl. 8, 163 (1954). — LASSER, E. C., and W. J. STAUBITZ: Translumbar aortography in urologic diagnosis. J. Amer. med. Ass. 163, 1325—1329 (1957). — LATTIMER, J. K., M. M. MELICOW and A. C. USON: Wilms tumor: a report of 71 cases. J. Urol. (Baltimore) 80, 401 (1958). — LAWS, J. W.: Radiology of the suprarenal glands. Brit. J. Radiol. 31, 352 (1958). — LIEBERTHAL, F.: Multi-locular solitary cyst of the renal hilus. J. Urol. (Baltimore) 42, 321 (1939). — LINDBLOM, K.: Percutaneous puncture of renal cysts and tumors. Acta radiol. (Stockh.) 27, 66 (1946). — LINKE, C. A., I. ROSENTHAL and J. H. KIEFER: Bilateral pheochromocytoma in a 12-year-old boy. J. Urol. (Baltimore) 79, 781 (1958). — LJUNGGREN, E.: Partial nephrectomy in renal tumour. Acta chir. scand. Suppl. 253 (1960). — LJUNGGREN, E., S. HOLM, B. KARTH and R. POMPEIUS: Some aspects of renal tumors with special reference to spontaneous regression. J. Urol. (Baltimore) 82, 553—557 (1959). — LOEB, M. J.: Solitary cysts of the kidney. An hypothesis of common pathogenesis of cysts. Report of three unusual cases. Urol. cutan. Rev. 48, 105 (1944). — LOWMAN, R. M., and L. DAVIS: The role of barium contrast studies in the diagnosis of retroperitoneal tumors. Radiology 69, 641 (1957). — LOWSLEY, O.: Malignant cyst of the kidney. J. Urol. (Baltimore) 74, 586 (1955). — LUSTED, L. B., B. E. BESSE jr. and R. FRITZ: The intravenous urogram in acute leukemia. Amer. J. Roentgenol. 80, 608—610 (1958). — MacLEAN, J. T., and V. B. FOWLER: Pathology of tumors of the renal pelvis and ureter. J. Urol. (Baltimore) 75, 384 (1956). — MACQUET, P., F. VANDENDORP, G. LEMAITRE et R. DU BOIS: L'aortographie dans le diagnostic des tumeurs rénales. J. Radiol. Électrol. 38, 221—224 (1957). — MANN, L. T.: Spontaneous disappearance of pulmonary metastases after nephrectomy for hypernephroma. J. Urol. (Baltimore) 59, 564 (1948). — MASSON, G. M. C., A. C. CORCORAN and D. C. HUMPHREY: Diagnostic procedures for pheochromocytoma. J. Amer. med. Ass. 165, 1555 (1957). — McAFEE, J. G., and C. E. BALLI: Radiological diagnosis of diseases of adrenal origin. Amer. J. med. Sci. 232, 572—599 (1956). — MEISEL, H. J.: Bilateral polyadenomatous kidneys; adenomatosis of the kidneys simulating polycystic disease. J. Urol. (Baltimore) 72, 1140 (1954). — MOONEY, K.: Hamartoma of kidney. J. Urol. (Baltimore) 73, 951 (1955). — NAUMANN, H. N., and S. A. SABATINI: Cholesteatoma of kidney simulating squamous cell carcinoma. J. Urol. (Baltimore) 69, 467 (1953). — NICOL, M., CH. STABERT et G. GUERIN: Néphro-épithélioma calcifié. J. Radiol. Électrol. 39, 64 (1958). — OCKULY, E. A., and F. M. DOUGLASS: Retroperitoneal perirenal lipomata. J. Urol. (Baltimore) 37, 619 (1937). — O'CONOR, V. J.: The diagnosis of tumors of the renal pelvis and ureter. J. Urol. (Baltimore) 75, 416 (1956). — O'CONOR, V. J., A. H. CANNON, TH. C. LAIPPLY, K. SOKOL and E. BARTH: Renal tumors, a round table discussion. Radiology 58, 830 (1952). — PENNISI, S. A., S. RUSSI and R. C. BUNTS: Multiple dissimilar tumors in one kidney. J. Urol. (Baltimore) 78, 205—211 (1957). — PFEIFFER, G. E., and M. M. GANDIN: Massive perirenal lipoma with report of a case. J. Urol. (Baltimore) 56, 12 (1946). — PHILLIPS, C. A. S., and G. BAUMRUCKER: Neurilemmoma (arising in the hilus of left kidney). J. Urol. (Baltimore) 73, 671 (1955). — PIRONTI, L., e A. TARQUINI: Alcuni casi di tumore primitivo del rene studiati con l'arteriografia renale selettiva. Minerva chir. (Torino) 13, 1122 (1958). — PISANO, D. J., R. H. ROSEN, B. M. RUBINSTEIN and H. G. JACOBSON: The roentgen manifestations of carcinoma and cyst in the same kidney. Amer. J. Roentgenol. 80, 603 (1958). — PLAUT, A.: Diffuses dickdarmähnliches Adenom des Nierenbeckens mit geschwulstartiger Wucherung von Gefäßmuskulatur. Z. urol. Chir. 26, 562 (1929). — POUTASSE, E. F.: Value and limitation of roentgenographic diagnosis of adrenal disease. J. Urol. (Baltimore) 73, 891 (1955). — PRATHER, G. C.: Differential diagnosis between renal tumor and renal cyst. J. Urol. (Baltimore) 64, 193 (1950). — PROVET, H., J. R. LISA and S. TRINIDAD: Tubular carcinoma of the kidney within a solitary cyst. J. Urol. (Baltimore) 75, 627 (1956). — PUIGVERT, A.: Polykystose rénale et cancer bilatéral. J. Urol. méd. chir. 64, 30 (1958). — RAGINS, A. B., and H. C. ROLNICK: Mucus producing adenocarcinoma of the renal pelvis. J. Urol. (Baltimore) 63, 66 (1950). — RATLIFF, R. K., W. C. BAUM and W. J. BUTLER: Bilateral primary carcinoma of the ureter, a case report. Cancer (Philad.) 2, 815 (1949). — RICHES, E. W., I. H. GRIFFITHS and A. C. THACKRAY: New growths of the kidney and ureter. Brit. J. Urol. 23, 297 (1951). — ROBECCHI, M., e G. CHIAUDANO: Diagnosi differenziale arteriografica fra cisti e tumori renali. Boll. soc. piemont. chir. 26, 275—281 (1956). — RUDSTRÖM, P.: Ein Fall von Nierenzyste mit eigenartiger Konkrementbildung. Acta chir. scand. 85, 501 (1941). — RUSCHE, C.: Renal hamartoma (angiomyolipoma): report of three cases. J. Urol. (Baltimore) 67, 823 (1952). — SALTZ, N. J., E. M. LUTTWAK, A. SCHWARTZ and G. M. GOLDBERG: Danger of aortography in the localization of pheochromocytoma. Ann. Surg. 144, 118—123 (1956). — SALVIN, B. L., and W. A. SCHLOSS: Papillary adenocarcinoma of the kidney, with aortography resembling huge renal cyst. J. Urol. (Baltimore) 72, 135 (1954). — SANDOMENICO, C., and M. MANSI: Contributo clinico-radiologico alla diagnosi dell'echinococcosi renale. Nunt. Radiol. 22, 270—287 (1956). — SANTOS, R. DOS: L'aortographie dans les tumeurs rénales et pararénales. Arch. Mal. Reins 8, 313 (1934). — SAVIGNAC, E. M.: Primary carcinoma of the ureter. Amer. J. Roentgenol. 74, 628 (1955). — SCHOLL, A. J.: Peripelvic lymphatic cysts of the kidney. Report of two cases. J. Amer. med. 136, 4 (1948). — SCHULTE, T. L., and J. L. EMMETT: Urography in the differential diagnosis of retroperitoneal tumors. J. Urol. (Baltimore) 42, 215 (1939). — SCHWIEBINGER, G. W., and C. V. HODGES: Coexistence of renal tumor and solitary cyst of the kidney. A.M.A. Arch. Surg. 71, 115 (1955). — SHELLEY, H. S.: Renal adenoma. Pyelograms showing the growth over a five year period. J. Urol. (Baltimore) 69, 480 (1953). — SHIVERS, T. C. H. DE, et H. D.

AXILROD: Solitary renal cysts. J. Urol. (Baltimore) **69**, 193 (1953). — A clinical comparison between benign solitary cysts and malignant lesions of the renal parenchyma. J. Urol. (Baltimore) **79**, 363 (1958). — SIMRIL, W. A., and D. K. ROSE: Replacement lipomatosis and its simulation of renal tumours: A report of two cases. J. Urol. (Baltimore) **63**, 588 (1950). — SOUTHWOOD, W. F. W., and V. F. MARSHALL: A clinical evaluation of nephrotomography. Brit. J. Urol. **30**, 127 (1958). — SPENCE, H. M., S. S. BAIRD and E. W. WARE jr.: Cystic disorders of the kidney — Classification, diagnosis, treatment. J. Amer. med. Ass. **163**, 1466—1472 (1957). — SPILLANE, R. J., J. A. SINGISER and G. C. PRATHER: Fibromyxolipoma of the kidney. J. Urol. (Baltimore) **68**, 811 (1952). — STAHL, D. M.: Unusual primary hypernephroma (renal cell carcinoma) of the ureter in a child. J. Urol. (Baltimore) **80**, 176 (1958). — STEARNS, D. B., M. W. SHAPIRO and S. K. GORDON: Reticulum cell sarcoma of the kidney. J. Urol. (Baltimore) **81**, 395 (1959). — STEINBACH, H. L., F. HINMAN jr. and P. H. FORSHAM: The diagnosis of adrenal neoplasms by contrast media. Radiology **69**, 664 (1957). — SÜSSE, H. J., u. H. RADKE: Nachweis und Lokalisierung von Nebennierentumoren mittels Aortographie. Fortschr. Röntgenstr. **86**, 599—604 (1957). — TAYLOR, J. N., and K. GENTERS: Renal angiomyolipoma and tuberous sclerosis. J. Urol. (Baltimore) **79**, 685 (1958). — TAYLOR, W. N.: Tumors of the kidney pelvis. J. Urol. (Baltimore) **82**, 452—458 (1959). — TEPLICK, J. G., M. LABESS and S. STEINBERG: Echinococcosis of the kidney. J. Urol. (Baltimore) **78**, 323 (1957). — THOMPSON, I. M.: Peripelvic lymphatic renal cysts. J. Urol. (Baltimore) **78**, 343—350 (1957). — TWISS, A. C.: Cortical adenomas of arteriosclerotic kidneys. Illinois med. J. **95**, 311 (1949). — VILLAUME, C.: Diffuse papillomatosis of the urinary tract. Acta radiol. (Stockh.) **37**, 401 (1952). — WALLACH, J. B., A. P. SUTTON and M. CLAMAN: Hemangioma of the kidney. J. Urol. (Baltimore) **81**, 515 (1959). — WATKINS, J. P.: Wilms' tumor with ureteral metastases extending into the bladder. J. Urol. (Baltimore) **77**, 593—596 (1957). — WEAVER, R. G., and J. H. CARLQUIST: Two rare tumors of the renal parenchyma. J. Urol. (Baltimore) **77**, 351—357 (1957). — WESOLOWSKI, S.: Primary tumors of the ureter. J. Urol. (Baltimore) **82**, 212 (1959). — WEYDE, R.: Abdominal aortography in renal diseases. Brit. J. Radiol. **25**, 353 (1952). — WHARTON, L. R.: Hypernephromas that are too early to diagnose. J. Urol. (Baltimore) **42**, 713 (1939). — WHITLOCK, G. F., J. R. McDONALD and E. N. COOK: Primary carcinoma of the ureter: a pathologic and prognostic study. J. Urol. (Baltimore) **73**, 245 (1955). — WOODRUFF, J. H., C. C. CHALEK, R. E. OTTOMAN and S. P. WILK: The roentgen diagnosis of renal neoplasms. J. Urol. (Baltimore) **75**, 615 (1956). — WOODRUFF jr., J. H., and R. E. OTTOMAN: Radiologic diagnosis of renal tumours by renal angiography. J. Canad. Ass. Radiol. **7**, 54—58 (1956).

Ureter

ABESHOUSE, B. S.: Primary benign and malignant tumors of the ureter. A review of the literature and report of one benign and twelve malignant tumors. Amer. J. Surg. **91**, 237 to 271 (1956). — ABESHOUSE, B. S., and L. H. TANKIN: Leukoplakia of the renal pelvis and the bladder. J. Urol. (Baltimore) **76**, 330 (1956). — ÅKERLUND, Å.: Ein typisches Röntgenbild bei Konkrementbildung in einer Ureterozele. Acta radiol. (Stockh.) **16**, 39 (1935). — AKIMOTO, K.: Über amyloidartige Eiweißniederschläge im Nierenbecken. Beitr. path. Anat. **78**, 239—242 (1927). — ALTVATER, G.: Primäres Harnleiterkarzinom. Z. Urol. **49**, 121—122 (1956). — AMSELEM, A.: Hidronefrosis bilateral gigante sin obstaculo organico aparente. Med. esp. **23**, 230 (1950). — ANDREAS, B. F., and M. OOSTING: Primary amyloidosis of the ureter. J. Urol. (Baltimore) **79**, 929 (1958). — ARMSTRONG jr., C. P., H. C. HARLIN and C. A. FORT: Leukoplakia of the renal pelvis. J. Urol. (Baltimore) **63**, 208 (1950). — ARNHOLDT, F.: Zur Diagnose der Leukoplakie des Nierenbeckens. Z. urol. Chir. **44**, 292 (1939). — BARON, C.: Leukoplakia of the renal pelvis. J. Urol. (Baltimore) **73**, 941 (1955). — BATES, B. C.: Periureteritis obliterans: a case report with a review of the literature. J. Urol. (Baltimore) **82**, 58 (1959). — BENNETTS, F. A., J. F. CRANE, J. J. Crane, G. H. GUMMESS and H. B. MILES: Diseases of ureteral stump. J. Urol. (Baltimore) **73**, 238 (1955). — BERMAN, M. H., and H. COPELAND: Filling defects of ureterogram caused by a varicose ureteral vein. J. Urol. (Baltimore) **70**, 168 (1953). — BÉTOULIÈRES, P., F. JAUMES et R. COLIN: Dilatation pseudokystique de l'uretère terminal. J. Radiol. Électrol. **40**, 582—586 (1959). — BIANCHI, E.: Roentgenologic findings in uretero-appendicular fistula. Radiol. med. (Milan) **42**, 286—290 (1956). — BORCH-MADSEN, P.: Primary benign tumour of the ureter. Nord. Med. **53**, 956 (1955). — BRADFIELD, E. O.: Bilateral ureteral obstruction due to envelopment and compression by an inflammatory retroperitoneal process. J. Urol. (Baltimore) **69**, 769 (1953). — BRODNY, M. L., and H. HERSHMAN: Pedunculated hemangioma of the ureter. J. Urol. (Baltimore) **71**, 539 (1954). — BURKLAND, C. E., and W. F. LEADBETTER: Pyelitis cystica associated with an hemophilus influenzae infection in the urine. J. Urol. (Baltimore) **42**, 14 (1939). — CANIGIANI, T.: Ein Fall von cystischer Dilatation des vesicalen Ureterendes. Z. urol. Chir. **36**, 172 (1933). — CHINN, J., R. K. HORTON and C. RUSCHE: Unilateral ureteral obstruction as sole manifestation of endometriosis. J. Urol. (Baltimore) **77**, 144—150 (1957). —

CHISHOLM, E. R., J. A. HUTCH and A. A. BOLOMEY: Bilateral ureteral obstruction due to chronic inflammation of the fascia around the ureters. J. Urol. (Baltimore) 72, 812 (1954). — CIBERT, J., L. DURAND et C. RIVIÈRE: Les compressions ureterales par sclerose du tissu cellulo-adipeux peri-ureteral „peri-ureteritis primitives". J. Urol. méd. chir. 62, 705 (1956). — COMPERE, D. E., G. F. BEGLEY, H. E. ISAACKS, T. H. FRAZIER and C. B. DRYDEN: Ureteral polyps. J. Urol. (Baltimore) 79, 209 (1958). — CRANE, J. F.: Ureteral involvement by aortic aneurysm. J. Urol. (Baltimore) 79, 403 (1958). — DAVIS, D. M., and TH. F. NEALON jr.: Complete replacement of both ureters by an ileal loop. J. Urol. (Baltimore) 78, 748 (1957). — DAVISON, S.: Pyoureter seventeen years after nephrectomy. J. Amer. med. Ass. 118, 137 (1942). — DORST, J. D., G. H. CUSSEN and F. N. SILVERMAN: Ureteroceles in children, with emphasis on the frequency of ectopic ureteroceles. Radiology 74, 88—89 (1960). — DREY-FUSS, W.: Anomaly simulating a retrocaval ureter. J. Urol. (Baltimore) 82, 630—632 (1959). — DREYFUSS, W., and E. GOODSITT: Acute regional ureteritis. J. Urol. (Baltimore) 79, 202 (1958). — ELLEGAST, H., u. A. SCHIMATZEK: Zur Differentialdiagnose der Ureterstenosen. Radiol. austr. 9, 209—215 (1957). — ERICSSON, N. O.: Ectopic ureterocele in infants and children. Acta chir. scand. Suppl. 197 (1954). — EVERS, E.: Zwei Fälle mit seltener Ureter-anomalie („Akzessorischer Blindureter"). Acta radiol. (Stockh.) 25, 121 (1944). — EWELL, G. H., and H. W. BRUSKEWITZ: Bilateral ureteral obstruction due to envelopment and compression by an inflammatory retroperitoneal process. Urol. cutan. Rev. 56, 3 (1952). — FALK, C. C.: Leukoplakia of renal pelvis and ureter. J. Urol. (Baltimore) 72, 310 (1954). — FEY, B., P. TRUCHOT et M. NOIX: Étude radiocinématographique de l'uretère normal et pathologique. J. Radiol. Électrol. 39, 328 (1958). — FISHER, R. S., and H. H. HOWARD: Unusual ureterograms in a case of periarteritis nodosa. J. Urol. (Baltimore) 60, 398 (1948). — FRISCHKORN jr., H. B.: Roentgenographic behavior of the ureter. Amer. J. Roentgenol. 75, 877—883 (1956). — GILBERT, L. W., and J. R. MCDONALD: Primary amyloidosis of the renal pelvis and ureter: report of a case. J. Urol. (Baltimore) 68, 137 (1952). — GREENFIELD, M.: True prolapse of the ureter: case report and review of the literature. J. Urol. (Baltimore) 75, 223 (1956). — GUMMESS, G. H., D. A. CHARNOCK, H. I. RIDDELL and C. M. STEWART: Ureteroceles in children. J. Urol. (Baltimore) 74, 331 (1955). — GUTIERREZ, R.: The modern surgical treatment of ureterocele. Surg. Gynec. Obstet. 68, 611 (1939). — HARLIN, H. C., and F. C. HAMM: Urologic disease resulting from nonspecific inflammatory conditions of the bowel. J. Urol. (Baltimore) 68, 383—392 (1952). — HEJTMANCIK, J. H., and M. A. MAGID: Bilateral periureteritis plastica. J. Urol. (Baltimore) 76, 57 (1956). — HELLSTRÖM, J.: Zur Kenntnis der isolierten Dilatation des pelvinen oder juxtavesikalen Harnleiterabschnittes. Acta radiol. (Stockh.) 18, 141 (1937). — HIGBEE, D. R., and W. D. MILLETT: Localized amyloidosis of the ureter: report of a case. J. Urol. (Baltimore) 75, 424 (1956). — HINKEL, C. L., and G. A. MOLLER: Multiple giant ureteral calculi. Amer. J. Roentgenol. 75, 900 (1956). — HINMAN, F., C. M. JOHNSON and J. H. MCCORKLE: Pyelitis and ureteritis cystica. J. Urol. (Baltimore) 35, 174—189 (1936). — HOLLY, L. E., and B. SUMCAD: Diverticular ureteral changes. Amer. J. Roentgenol. 78, 1053 (1957). — HOWARD, T. L.: Giant polyp of ureter. J. Urol. (Baltimore) 79, 397 (1958). — HUNNER, G. L.: Intussusception of the ureter due to a large papillomalike polypus. J. Urol. (Baltimore) 40, 752 (1938). — HUTCH, J. A., R. C. ATKINSON and G. S. LOQUVAM: Perirenal (Gerota's) fascitis. J. Urol. (Baltimore) 81, 76—95 (1959). — IANNACCONE, G., and A. MARSELLA: Dilatations of the ureter: A casuistic contribution and critical review with particular regard to the problem of megaureter. Radiol. med. (Milan) 41, 759 (1955). — IANNACCONE, G., and P. E. PANZIRONI: Ureteral reflux in normal infants. Acta radiol. (Stockh.) 44, 451—456 (1955). — IOZZI, L., and J. J. MURPHY: Bilateral ureteral obstruction by retroperitoneal inflammation. J. Urol. (Baltimore) 77, 402—406 (1957). — IRELAND jr., E. F., and R. CHUTE: A case of triplicate-duplicate ureters. J. Urol. (Baltimore) 74, 342 (1955). — JACOBY, M.: Ureteritis cystica. Z. Urol. 23, 722—723 (1929). — JEWETT, H. J., and A. P. HARRIS: Scrotal ureter: report of a case. J. Urol. (Baltimore) 69, 184 (1953). — JOELSON, J. J.: Pyelitis, ureteritis and cystitis cystica. Arch. Surg. (Chicago) 18, 1570—1583 (1929). — JULIANI, G., and A. GIBBA: Pyelo-ureteral roentgenkymography. Radiol. med. (Milan) 43, 209 (1957). — KAIRIS, Z.: Endometriose des Ureters. Verhandlungs-ber. der Dtsch. Ges. für Urologie, S. 271. Leipzig 1958. — KICKHAM, C. J. E., and H. L. JAFFE: The upper urinary tract in bladder tumors. J. Urol. (Baltimore) 42, 131 (1939). — KINDALL, L.: Pyelitis cystica and ureteritis cystica. J. Urol. (Baltimore) 29, 645—659 (1933). — KLINGER, M. E.: Bone formation in the ureter: a case report. J. Urol. (Baltimore) 75, 793 (1956). — KNUTSSON, F.: The roentgen appearance in ureteritis cystica. Acta radiol. (Stockh.) 16, 43 (1935). — LANDES, R. R., and J. W. HOOKER: Sclerosing lipogranuloma and peri-ureteral fibrosis following extravasation of urographic contrast media. J. Urol. (Baltimore) 68, 403 (1952). — LEWIS, E. L., and R. W. CLETSOWAY: Megaloureter. J. Urol. (Baltimore) 75, 643 (1956). — LINDBOM, Å.: Unusual ureteral obstruction by herniation of ureter into sciatic foramen. Acta radiol. (Stockh.) 28, 225 (1947). — LIVERMORE, G. R.: Stone in the ureteral stump left when nephrectomy is done. J. Urol. (Baltimore) 63, 786 (1950). — LOEF,

J. A., and P. A. Casella: Squamous cell carcinoma occurring in the stump of a chronically infected ureter many years after nephrectomy. J. Urol. (Baltimore) 67, 159 (1952). — Loitman, B. S., and H. Chiat: Ureteritis cystica and pyelitis cystica. A review of cases and roentgenologic criteria. Radiology 68, 345—351 (1957). — Low, H. T., and H. E. Coakley: Leukoplakia of the renal pelvis. J. Urol. (Baltimore) 60, 712 (1948). — Makar, N.: The bilharzial ureter. Brit. J. Surg. 36, 148 (1948/49). — Mayers, M. M.: Diverticulum of the ureter. J. Urol. (Baltimore) 61, 344 (1949). — McGraw, A. B., and O. S. Culp: Diverticulum of the ureter: report of another authentic case. J. Urol. (Baltimore) 67, 262 (1952). — McNulty, M.: Pyelo-ureteritis cystica. Brit. J. Radiol. 30, 648—652 (1957). — Millard, D. G., and S. M. Wyman: Periureteric fibrosis: radiographic diagnosis. Radiology 72, 191—196 (1959). — Miller, J. M., R. J. Lipin, H. J. Meisel and P. H. Long: Bilateral ureteral obstruction due to compression by chronic retroperitoneal inflammation. J. Urol. (Baltimore) 68, 447 (1952). — Mirabile, C. S., and R. J. Spillane: Bilateral ureteral compression with obstruction from a nonspecific retroperitoneal inflammatory process: case report. J. Urol. (Baltimore) 73, 783 (1953). — Morley, H. V., E. J. Shumaker and L. W. Gardner: Intussusception of the ureter associated with a benign polyp. J. Urol. (Baltimore) 67, 266 (1952). — Mulvaney, W. P.: Periureteritis obliterans: a retroperitoneal inflammatory disease. J. Urol. (Baltimore) 79, 410 (1958). — Nilson, A. E.: Roentgen diagnosis of ureterocele and some impeding factors. Acta radiol. (Stockh.) 52, 365—368 (1959). — Noring, O.: Nonspecific ureteritis elucidated by a case of primary ureteritis. J. Urol. (Baltimore) 79, 701 (1958). — Ormond, J. K.: Bilateral ureteral obstruction due to envelopment and compression by an inflammatory retroperitoneal process. J. Urol. (Baltimore) 59, 1072 (1948). — Paull, D. P., J. C. Causey and C. V. Hodges: Perinephritis plastica. J. Urol. (Baltimore) 73, 212 (1955). — Petrovčić, F., and C. Dugan: Ureterocele. Report of an unusual case. Brit. J. Radiol. 28, 374 (1955). — Politano, V. A.: Leukoplakia of the renal pelvis and ureter. J. Urol. (Baltimore) 75, 633 (1956). — Prévôt, R., u. H. Berning: Zur Röntgendiagnostik der Pyelonephritis. Fortschr. Röntgenstr. 73, 482—488 (1950). — Rae, L. J.: Ectopic ureter in childhood. J. Fac. Radiol. (Lond.) 8, 402 (1957). — Randall, A.: Endometrioma of the ureter. J. Urol. (Baltimore) 46, 419 (1941). — Raper, F. P.: Bilateral, symmetrical, periureteric fibrosis. Proc. roy. Soc. Med. 48, 736—740 (1955). — Ratliff, R. K., and W. B. Crenshaw: Ureteral obstruction from endometriosis. Surg. Gynec. Obstet. 100, 414 (1955). — Rennaes, S.: On double renal pelvis and ureteral calculus. Acta radiol. (Stockh.) 31, 37 (1949). — Rieser, C.: A consideration of the ureteral stump subsequent to nephrectomy. J. Urol. (Baltimore) 64, 275 (1950). — Rimondini, C.: Un caso di tumore primitivo dell'uretere destro. Considerazioni radiodiagnostiche e radioterapeutiche. Nunt. Radiol. 23, 596 (1957). — Ríos, P.: Periureteritis primitiva unilateral. Arch. esp. Urol. 14, 97 (1958). — Robbins, J. J., and R. Lich jr.: Metastatic carcinoma of the ureter. J. Urol. (Baltimore) 75, 242 (1956). — Roberts, R. R.: Complete valve of the ureter: congenital urethral valves. J. Urol. (Baltimore) 76, 62 (1956). — Romani, S., e A. Ambrosetti: Le neoplasie dell'uretere. Riv. ital. Radiol. clin. 5, 121 (1955). — Ronnen, J. R. v., and H. Dormaar: A case of pyelo-ureteritis cystica diagnosed by pyelography. Acta radiol. (Stockh.) 34, 96 (1950). — Ross, J. A.: Peri-ureteritis fibrosa, with notes on three cases. J. Fac. Radiol. (Lond.) 9, 142 (1958). — Rudhe, U.: A typical roentgen picture of very large ureteroceles. Acta radiol. (Stockh.) 29, 396 (1948). — Ruiu, A.: La pieloureterite cistica. Quad. Radiol. 23, 263 (1958). — Selman, J.: Ureterocele: roentgenologic diagnosis with report of an unusual case. Amer. J. Roentgenol. 80, 620 (1958). — Senger, F. L., A. L. L. Bell, H. L. Warres and W. S. Tirman: Fate of the ureteral stump after nephrectomy. Amer. J. Surg. 73, 69 (1947). — Senger, F. L., J. J. Bottone and J. H. Kelleher: Bilateral leukoplakia of the renal pelvis. J. Urol. (Baltimore) 65, 528 (1951). — Shaheen, D. J., and A. Johnston: Bilateral ureteral obstruction due to envelopment and compression by an inflammatory retroperitoneal process: report of two cases. J. Urol. (Baltimore) 82, 51—57 (1959). — Stueber jr., P. J.: Primary retroperitoneal inflammatory process with ureteral obstruction. J. Urol. (Baltimore) 82, 41 (1959). — Talbot, H. S., and E. M. Mahoney: Obstruction of both ureters by retroperitoneal inflammation. J. Urol. (Baltimore) 78, 738 (1957). — Taylor, J. A.: Primary carcinoma of the ureter. J. Urol. (Baltimore) 65, 797 (1951). — Twinem, F. P.: Primary tumors of the ureter. J. Amer. med. Ass. 163, 808—813 (1957). — Velzer, D. A. van, C. W. Barrick and E. L. Jenkinson: Postcaval ureter. Amer. J. Roentgenol. 74, 490 (1955). — Vest, S. A., and B. Barelare jr.: Peri-ureteritis plastica: a report of four cases. J. Urol. (Baltimore) 70, 38 (1953). — Wadsworth, G. E., and E. Uhlenhuth: The pelvic ureter in the male and female. J. Urol. (Baltimore) 76, 244 (1956). — Weaver, R. G.: Ureteral regeneration: experimental and clinical, part III. J. Urol. (Baltimore) 79, 31 (1958). — Wellens, P.: La pyélo-urétérite (-cystite) kystique. J. belge Radiol. 41, 465 (1958). — Wemeau, L., G. Lemaitre et G. Defrance: Urétérocèle et prolapsus de l'urètre. J. Radiol. Électrol. 40, 275 (1959). — Williams, J. I., R. B. Carson and W. D. Wells: Reflux ureteropyelograms in children. Sth. med. J. (Bgham, Ala.) 50, 845 (1957). — Willich, E.: Ureterostiumstenose-Ureterocele. Mschr.

Kinderheilk. **105**, 377 (1957). — Wood, L. G., and G. E. Howe: Primary tumors of the ureter: case reports. J. Urol. (Baltimore) **79**, 418 (1958). — Zerbini, E.: Su di un caso di frattura dell'uretere. Nunt. Radiol. **22**, 825 (1956).

Urography

Allen, R. P.: Neuromuscular disorders of the urinary tract in children. Radiology **65**, 325 (1955). — Alwall, N.: Aspiration biopsy of the kidney. Acta med. scand. **143**, 430—435 (1952). — Alwall, N., P. Erlanson and A. Tornberg: The clinical course of renal failure occurring after intravenous urography and/or retrograde pyelography. Acta med. scand. **152**, 163—173 (1955). — Alyea, E. P., and C. E. Haines: Intradermal test for sensitivity to iodopyracet injection, or „diodrast". J. Amer. med. Ass. **135**, 25 (1947). — Arnell, S., and F. Lidström: Myelography with skiodan (abrodil). Acta radiol. (Stockh.) **12**, 287—288 (1931). — Arner, B.: Personal communications 1959. — Astraldi, A., y J. V. Uriburu jr.: Radiologia del rinon durante el acto operatorio. Rév. méd. lat.-amer. **21**, 891—907 (1936). — Babaiantz, L., et C. Wieser: Un nouveau produit de contraste triiodé pour l'urographie intraveineuse. Praxis **44**, 454—456 (1955). — Backlund, V.: Über die Technik der simultanen Telefilmplanigraphie. Acta radiol. (Stockh.) Suppl. **137** (1956). — Bartels, E. D., G. C. Brun, A. Gammeltoft and P. A. Gjørup: Acute anuria following intravenous pyelography in patient with myelomatosis. Acta med. scand. **150**, 297—302 (1954). — Bell, E. T.: Renal diseases. London: Henry Kimpton 1950. — Bell, J. C.: Intravenous urography. Urol. cutan. Rev. **44**, 460 (1940). — Berg, N. O., H. Idbohrn and B. Wendeberg: Investigation of the tolerance of the rabbit's kidney to newer contrast media in renal angiography. Acta radiol. (Stockh.) **50**, 285 (1958). — Berg, V., and M. Dufresne: Excretory urography in the pediatric patient with the aid of carbonated beverage. Harper Hosp. Bull. **14**, 122 (1956). — Bezold, K., H. R. Feindt u. K. Pressler: Der Röntgenbildverstärker im Routinebetrieb. Fortschr. Röntgenstr. **85**, 447 (1956). — Blommert, G., J. Gerbrandy, J. A. Molhuysen, L. A. de Vries and J. G. G. Borst: Diuretic effect of isotonic saline solution compared with that of water. Lancet **1951**, 1011. — Bloom, J., and J. F. Richardson: The usefulness of a contrast medium containing an antibacterial agent (retrografin) for retrograde pyelography. J. Urol. (Baltimore) **81**, 332—334 (1959). — Braasch, W. F., and J. L. Emmett: Excretory urography as a test of renal function. J. Urol. (Baltimore) **35**, 630 (1936). — Clinical urography. Philadelphia and London: W. B. Saunders Company 1951. — Bradley, S. E., and G. P. Bradley: The effect of increased intra-abdominal pressure of renal function in man. J. clin. Invest. **26**, 1010 (1947). — Braun, J. P., et L. Schneider: L'opacification corollaire de la vésicule biliaire après injection intra-veineuse d'une substance de contraste urinaire. J. Radiol. Electrol. **40**, 481 (1959). — Campbell, M.: Clinical pediatric urology. Philadelphia and London: W. B. Saunders Company 1951. — Carlson, H. E.: The proven ineffectiveness of the compression bag in intravenous pyelography. J. Urol. (Baltimore) **56**, 609 (1946). — Catel, W., u. R. Garsche: Studien bei Kindern mit dem Bildwandler. 2. Bewegungs- und Entleerungsvorgänge im Bereich von Nierenkelchen und Nierenbecken. Fortschr. Röntgenstr. **86**, 66 (1957). — Chesney, W. McEvan and James O. Hope: Studies of the tissue distribution and excretion of sodium diatrizoate in laboratory animals. Amer. J. Roentgenol. **78**, No 1, 137—144 (1957). — Chiaudano, M.: Comportamento arteriografico del rene normale. Minerva chir. (Torino) **13**, 1082 (1958). — Counts, R. W., G. B. Magill and R. S. Sherman: Death from intra-abdominal hemorrhage simulating reaction to contrast medium. J. Amer. med. Ass. **165**, 1134 (1957). — Crane, J. J.: Sudden death following intravenous administration of diodrast for intravenous urography. J. Urol. (Baltimore) **42**, 745 (1939). — Crepea, S. B., J. C. Allanson and L. DeLambre: Failure of antihistaminic drugs to inhibit diodrast reactions. N.Y. St. J. Med. **49**, 2556—2558 (1949). — Dargent, M., J. Papillos, J. F. Montbarbon et G. Costaz: Etude systématique de l'urographie pré- et post-opératoire chez des malades traitées par association radium-chirurgie pour cancer du col de l'utérus au stade de début. Lyon chir. **51**, 711—724 (1956). — Etude urographique du cancer du col utérin traité par l'association radium-lymphadénectomie. J. Radiol. Electrol. **39**, 109 (1958). — Davis, D. M.: The hydrodynamics of the upper urinary tract (urodynamics). Ann. Surg. **140**, 839 (1950). — Davis, L. A.: Reactions following excretory pyelography in infants and children. Radiology **71**, 19 (1958). — Davis, L. A., Kee-Chang Huang and E. L. Pirkey: Water-soluble, non-absorbable radiopaque mediums in gastrointestinal examination. J. Amer. med. Ass. **160**, 373—375 (1956). — Detar, J. A., and J. A. Harris: Venous pooled nephrograms: technique and results. J. Urol. (Baltimore) **72**, 979 (1954). — Doll, E.: Ausscheidungsurographie mit Urografin in der Kinderheilkunde. Medizinische **38**, 1384 (1957). — Doyle, O. W.: The use of chlor-trimeton with miokon in intravenous urography. J. Urol. (Baltimore) **81**, 573—574 (1959). — Ebbinghaus, K. D.: Ist die intravenöse Pyelographie bei Nierenschäden kontraindiziert? Ärztl. Wschr. **10**, 736 (1955). — Eberl, J.: Die Urinschichtung bei der i.v. Pyelographie. Fortschr. Röntgenstr. **86**, 74 (1957). — Edling, N. P. G., C. G. Helander and L. Renck: The correlation between contrast excretion and arterial and intrapelvis pressures in urography. Acta radiol. (Stockh.) **42**, 442—450 (1954). — EDLING, N. P. G., C. G. HELANDER and S. I. SELDINGER: The nephrographic effect in depressed tubular excretion of umbradil. Acta radiol. (Stockh.) **48**, 1 (1957). — FEY, B., et P. TRUCHOT: L'urographie intra-veineuse. Paris: Masson & Cie. 1944. — FIGDOR, P. P.: Akute Nierenschäden nach Pyelographien. Z. Urol. **49**, 133—147 (1956). — FINBY, N., J. A. EVANS and I. STEINBERG: Reactions from intravenous organic iodide compounds: Pretesting and prophylaxis. Radiology **71**, 15 (1958). — FINBY, N., N. POKER and J. A. EVANS: Ninety per cent hypaque for rapid intravenous roentgenography; preliminary report. Radiology **67**, 244—246 (1956). — FREI, A.: Ein neues Kontrastmittel zur intravenösen Urographie. Dtsch. med. Wschr. **79**, 1636—1637 (1954). — FROMMHOLD, W., u. H. BRABAND: Zwischenfälle bei Gallenblasenuntersuchungen mit Biligrafin und ihre Behandlung. Fortschr. Röntgenstr. **92**, 47—59 (1960). — GARRITANO, A. P., G. T. WOHL, CH. K. KIRBY and A. L. PIETROLUONGO: The roentgenographic demonstration of an arteriovenous fistula of renal vessels. Amer. J. Roentgenol. **75**, 905 (1956). — GILG, E.: The influence of diphenhydramine (Benadryl) on the side-effects of diodone in urography. Acta radiol. (Stockh.) **39**, 299 (1953). — GÜNTHER, G. W.: Röntgenuroskopie. Stuttgart: Georg Thieme 1952. — HAENISCH, F.: Die Röntgenuntersuchung des uropoetischen Systems. GROEDELS Lehrbuch und Atlas der Röntgendiagnostik. München 1938. — HANLEY, H. G.: Cineradiography of the urinary tract. Brit. med. J. **1955**II, 22—23. — HARROW, B. R.: Intravenous urography using mixtures of radiopaque agents. Radiologie **65**, 265 (1955). — Experiences in intravenous urography using hypaque. Amer. J. Roentgenol. **75**, 870—876 (1956). — HELLMER, H.: Nephrography. Acta radiol. (Stockh.) **23**, 233 (1942). — HERSKOVITS, E.: Mit Perabrodil gefüllte Gallenblase während einer Ausscheidungspyelographie. Röntgenpraxis **10**, 261 (1938). — HERZAN, F. A., and F. W. O'BRIEN: Acceleration of delayed excretory urograms. Amer. J. Roentgenol. **68**, 104 (1952). — HOGEMAN, O.: Elevated nonprotein nitrogen and urography. Upsala Läk.-Fören. Förh. **57**, 161 (1952). — HOL, R., and O. SKJERVEN: Spinal cord damage in abdominal aortography. Acta radiol. (Stockh.) **42**, 276—284 (1954). — HOLLANDER jr., W., and T. F. WILLIAMS: A comparison of the water diuresis produced by oral and by intravenous water loading in normal human subjects. J. Lab. clin. Med. **49**, 182 (1957). — HOLMAN, R. L.: Complete anuria due to blockage of renal tubules by protein casts in a case of multiple myeloma. Arch. Path. (Chicago) **27**, 748—752 (1939). — HOPPE, J. O.: Some pharmacological aspects of radiopaque compounds. Ann. N.Y. Acad. Sci. **78**, 727—739 (1959). — HUGER, W. E., G. MARGOLIS and K. S. GRIMSON: Protective effect of intra-aortic injection of procaine against renal injuries produced in experimental aortography. Surgery **43**, 52—62 (1958). — HULTBORN, K. A.: Allergische Reaktionen bei Kontrastinjektionen für die Urographie. Acta radiol. (Stockh.) **20**, 263 (1949). — HUNNER, G. L.: The fallacy of depending on X-rays in the diagnosis of certain important urological conditions. J. Urol. (Baltimore) **42**, 720 (1939). — HUTTER, K.: Zur Röntgendarstellung der Nierenhohlräume nebst Bemerkungen über die Lagebeziehung des Nierenbeckens zum Musculus psoas. Z. urol. Chir. **30**, 256 (1930). — IDBOHRN, H., and N. BERG: On the tolerance of the rabbit's kidney to contrast media in renal angiography. Acta radiol. (Stockh.) **42**, 121 (1954). — INMAN, G. K. E.: A comparison of urographic contrast media, with particular reference to the aetiology and prevention of certain side effects. Brit. J. Radiol. **25**, 625 (1952). — JOSEPHSON, B.: Examination of diodrast clearance and tubular excretory capacity in man by means of two single injections of diodrast (Umbradil). Acta med. scand. **128**, 515 (1947). — JULIANI, G., e A. GIBBA: Note di semeiotica roentgenchimografica pielo-ureterale. Radiol. med. (Torino) **43**, 209 (1957). — KÅGSTRÖM, E., P. LINDGREN and G. TÖRNELL: Changes in cerebral circulation during carotid angiography with sodium acetrizoate (Triurol) and sodium diatrizoate (Hypaque). Acta radiol. (Stockh.) **50**, 151—159 (1958). — KAUFMAN, S. A.: The acceleration of delayed excretory urograms with ingested ice water. J. Urol. (Baltimore) **74**, 243—244 (1955). — KEATES, P. G.: Improving the intravenous pyelogram: an experimental study. Brit. J. Urol. **25**, 366—370 (1954). — KENAN, P. B., G. T. TINDAL, G. MARGOLIS and R. S. WOOD: The prevention of experimental contrast medium injury to the nervous system. J. Neurosurg. **15**, 92—95 (1958). — KIIL, F.: The function of the ureter and renal pelvis. Philadelphia and London: W. B. Saunders Company 1957. — KILLMANN, S., S. GJØRUP and J. H. THAYSEN: Fatal acute renal failure following intravenous pyelography in patient with multiple myeloma. Acta med. scand. **158**, 43—46 (1957). — KITABATAKE, T.: Solidography of kidney study on rotatography, 16 report. Nagoya J. med. Sci. **18**, 159 (1955). — KNOEFEL, P. K.: The nature of the toxic action of radiopaque diagnostic agents. Radiology **71**, 13 (1958). — LAME, E. L.: Vertebral osteomyelitis following operation on the urinary tract or sigmoid. The third lesion of an un common syndrome. Amer. J. Roentgenol. **75**, 938 (1956). — LAPIDES, J., and J. M. BOBBIT: Preoperative estimation of renal function. J. Amer. med. Ass. **166**, 866 (1958). — LASIO, E., G. ARRIGONI e A. CIVINO: Indicazioni e limiti dell'aortografia addominale in urologia. Minerva chir. (Torino) **13**, 1096 (1958). — LEIGHTON, R. S.: Nephrography. Radiology **53**, 540 (1949). — LICHTENBERG, A. v.: Grundlagen und Fortschritte der

Ausscheidungsurographie. Langenbecks Arch. klin. Chir. **171**, 3 (1932). — LINDGREN, P., and G. TÖRNELL: Blood circulation during and after peripheral arteriography. Acta radiol. (Stockh.) **49**, 425—440 (1958). — MADSEN, E.: Effectiveness of urologic contrast media. Comparison between diodone and triiodyl (sodium acetriozoate). Acta radiol. (Stockh.) **47**, 192 (1957). — MALUF, N. S. R.: Role of roentgenology in the development of urology. Amer. J. Roentgenol. **75**, 847 (1956). — MANFREDI, D., R. BEGANI e L. G. FREZZA: La roentgencineangiografia renale selettiva. Minerva chir. (Torino) **13**, 1100 (1958). — MARION, G.: Traité d'urologie, T. 1—2. Paris 1928. — MARTIN, E. C., J. H. CAMPBELL and C. M. PESQUIER: Cystography in children. J. Urol. (Baltimore) **75**, 151 (1956). — MAY, F., u. M. SCHILLER: Urografin, ein neues Mittel zur Ausscheidungsurographie. Med. Klin. **49**, 1403 (1954). — McCHESNEY, E. W., and J. O. HOPPE: Studies of the tissue distribution and excretion of sodium diatrizoate in laboratory animals. Amer. J. Roentgenol. **78**, 137—144 (1957). — McDONALD, H. P., and W. E. UPCHURCH: Twenty-five years of progress in intravenous urography. Amer. Surg. **21**, 989 (1955). — MIGLIORINI, M.: Condizioni necessarie per una valutazione sommaria della funzionalità renale in corso di urografia. Radiol. med. (Torino) **43**, 462 (1957). — MIGLIORINI, M., e I. TODDEI: Sull'uso dell' E.D.T.A. di Pb come di contrasto in radiologia. Atti Accad. Fisiocr. Siena **3**, 279—284 (1956). — MÖCKEL, G.: Medikamentöse Ganglienblockade zur Verbesserung der Röntgendiagnostik der Harnwege. Dtsch. med. Wschr. **79**, 1169 (1954). — MOORE, T. D., and N. SANDERS: Reaction to urographic agents with and without antihistamines. J. Urol. (Baltimore) **70**, 538 (1953). — NALBANDIAN, R. M., W. T. RICE and W. O. NICKEL: A new category of contrast media: water-soluble radiopaque polyvalent chelates. Ann. N.Y. Acad. Sci. **78**, 779—792 (1959). — NARATH, P. A.: The hydromechanics of the calyx renalis. J. Urol. (Baltimore) **43**, 145 (1940). — Renal pelvis and ureter. New York: Grune & Stratton 1951. — The physiology of the renal pelvis and the ureter, in M. F. CAMPBELL, Urology. Philadelphia: W. B. Saunders Company 1954. — NECKER, F., u. W. v. WIESER: Die Fehldeutung der Ausscheidungssperre und andere Irrtümer bei der intravenösen Pyelographie sowie Bemerkungen zur Indikationsstellung und Untersuchungstechnik. Radiol. clin. (Basel) **9**, 105, 129 (1940). — NESBIT, R. M.: Experience with the avoidance of allergic reactions to pyelographic media by the use of antihistamine drugs. Ann. N.Y. Acad. Sci. **78**, 852—860 (1959). — The incidence of severe reactions from present day urographic contrast materials. J. Urol. (Baltimore) **81**, 486—489 (1959). — NICOLAI, C. H.: Major reactions to intravenous urographic media. Arch. Surg. (Chicago) **73**, 285—289 (1956). — Miokon, a new intravenous urographic medium. J. Urol. (Baltimore) **75**, 758 (1956). — NICOLICH, G., e G. B. CERRUTI: La nostra esperienza in angiografia renale e vescicale. Minerva chir. (Torino) **13**, 1109 (1958). — NITSCH, K., u. F. ALLIES: Kurze Hinweise zur i.v. Urographie bei Kindern. Z. Urol. **50**, 353 (1957). — OLIVERO, S., F. MORINO e F. MARGAGLIA: Comportamento delle curve glicemiche a seguito dell'arteriografia addominale selettiva. Minerva chir. (Torino) **13**, 1111 (1958). — OLSSON, OLLE: On hepatosplenography with „jodsol". Acta radiol. (Stockh.) **22**, 749—761 (1941). — Contrast media in diagnosis and the attendant risks. Acta radiol. (Stockh.) Suppl. **116**, 75—83 (1954). — PAUL, L. E., and J. H. JUHL: The essentials of roentgen interpretation. New York: Paul B. Hoeber 1959. — PAYNE, W. W., W. H. MORSE and S. L. RAINES: A fatal reaction following injection of urographic medium: a case report. J. Urol. (Baltimore) **76**, 661 (1956). — PENDERGRASS, E. P., PH. J. HODES, R. L. TONDREAU, C. C. POWELL and E. D. BURDICK: Further consideration of deaths and unfavourable sequelae following the administration of contrast media in urography in the United States. Amer. J. Roentgenol. **74**, 262—287 (1955). — PENDERGRASS, H. P., R. L. TONDREAU, E. P. PENDERGRASS, D. J. RITCHIE, E. A. HILDRETH and S. I. ASKOVITZ: Reactions associated with intravenous urography: Historical and statistical review. Radiology **71**, 1—12 (1958). — PERILLIE, P. E., and H. O. CONN: Acute renal failure after intravenous pyelography in plasma cell myeloma. J. Amer. med. Ass. **167**, 2186—2189 (1958). — PETTINARI, V., e M. SERVELLO: L'indagine arteriografica e flebografica del rene. Minerva chir. (Torino) **13**, 1117 (1958). — PIEMONTE, M., e L. MAGNO: Sulla eliminazione renale dei mezzi di contrasto iodati. Radiol. med. (Torino) **44**, 225—248 (1958). — PIERCE, W. V., and W. R. MINER: Benign tumors of the ureter. Sth. med. J. (Bgham, Ala.) **45**, 485 (1952). — PIRONTI DI CAMPAGNA, G. M., e L. SERENO: Contributo sperimentale al problema dell'eliminazione urografica. Tubulo-nefrosi da tetrationato di sodio e glomerulonefrite sperimentale da normali proteine eterogenee. Nunt. radiol. (Firenze) **22**, 1 (1956). — PIZON, P.: Les accidents de l'urographie intraveineuse. Presse méd. **64**, 1107 (1956). — POPPEL, M. H., and B. E. ZEITEL: Roentgen manifestations of milk drinker's syndrome. Radiology **67**, 195—199 (1956). — PRATHER, G. C.: Medial ptosis of the kidney. New Engl. J. Med. **238**, 253 (1948). — PUIGVERT, A.: Un caso de inhibicion renal prolongada. Cirug. Ginec. Urol. **8**, 273 (1954). — RAPOPORT, S., W. A. BRODSKY, C. D. WEST and B. MACKLER: Urinary flow and excretion of solutes during osmotic diuresis in hydropenic man. Amer. J. Physiol. **156**, 433 (1949). — RAVASINI: Studium der Nierenfunktion in der Nierenchirurgie. Z. urol. Chir. **40**, 470 (1935). — REINHARDT, K.: Ein Fall von Gallenblasendarstellung nach Perabrodilinjektion. Radiol. clin.

(Basel) **23**, 193 (1954). — REITAN, H.: Prinzipien und Erfahrungen betreffend die Urographie. Acta radiol. (Stockh.) **18**, 578 (1937). — RIBBING, S.: Über das sog. „Psoasrandsymptom" bei Pyelographie. Z. Urol. **28**, 306 (1934). — ROLLINS, M., F. J. BONTE, F. A. ROSE and D. R. KEATING: Clinical evaluation of a new compound for intravenous urography. Amer. J. Roentgenol. **73**, 771 (1955). — ROSE, D. K.: Early diagnosis of cancer of the kidney. Surg. Clin. N. Amer. **29**, 1483 (1949). — ROSSI, A.: Aortografia addominale translombare, o arteriografia renale selettiva? Minerva chir. (Torino) **13**, 1131 (1958). — SALZMAN, E., and M. R. WARDEN: Telepaque opacification of radiolucent biliary calculi. The „rim sign". Radiology **71**, 85—89 (1958). — SALZMAN, E., D. H. WATKINS and W. R. RUNDLES: Opacification of radiolucent biliary calculi. J. Amer. med. Ass. **167**, 1741—1743 (1958). — SANDERS jr., P. W.: Medial renal ptosis. J. Urol. (Baltimore) **77**, 24 (1957). — SANDSTRÖM, C.: Contrast media for the kidneys, heart and vessels, and their toxicity. Acta radiol. (Stockh.) **39**, 281—298 (1953). — SAPEIKA, N.: Lead EDTA complex; a water-soluble contrast medium. S. Afr. med. J. **28**, 759—762 (1954). — Lead EDTA complex; further radiographic studies. S. Afr. med. J. **28**, 953—956 (1954). — SAUPE, E.: Magen- und Dünndarmfüllung nach Injektion von Per-Abrodil zur Durchführung einer Ausscheidungsurographie. Fortschr. Röntgenstr. **65**, 143 (1942). — SCHERMULY, W.: Die heterotope Ausscheidung von Nierenkontrastmittel. Fortschr. Röntgenstr. **89**, 220—227 (1958). — SCHLUNGBAUM, W., u. H. BILLION: Untersuchungen der Verteilung von radioaktivem Urografin im menschlichen Organismus. Klin. Wschr. **34**, 633—635 (1956). — SCHOEN, H.: Zur Darstellung von Gallensteinen nach intravenösem Urogramm. Fortschr. Röntgenstr. **72**, 738 (1949—1950). — SCHOLTZ, A.: Kontrasterzeugende Magenfüllung im Laufe einer Ausscheidungspyelographie. Z. Urol. **35**, 209 (1941). — SECRÉTAN, M.: Les accidents au cours des urographies intraveineuses. Urol. int. (Basel) **2**, 81 (1955). — Les accidents au cours des urographies intraveineuses. J. belge Radiol. **39**, 76 (1956). — SHAPIRO, J. H., and H. G. JACOBSON: Oral 76 per cent sodium and methylglucamine diatrizoate, a new contrast medium for the gastrointestinal tract. Ann. N.Y. Acad. Sci. **78**, 966—986 (1959). — SHAPIRO, R.: Chelation in contrast roentgenography with special reference to lead disodium EDTA. Amer. J. Roentgenol. **76**, 161—167 (1956). — SINGER, P. L.: The use of antispasmodic drugs as preparation for intravenous pyelography. J. Urol. (Baltimore) **58**, 216 (1947). — SOUTHWOOD, W. F. W., and V. F. MARSHALL: A clinical evaluation of nephrotomography. Brit. J. Urol. **30**, 127—141 (1958). — SPEICHER, M. E.: A report on hypaque, a new intravenous urographic medium. Series of 800 cases. Amer. J. Roentgenol. **75**, 865 (1956). — STRANDNESS jr., D. E.: The unilateral nonfunctioning kidney. A.M.A. Arch. intern. Med. **101**, 611 (1958). — STRAUSS, M. B., R. K. DAVIS, J. D. ROSENBAUM and E. C. ROSSMEISL: „Water diuresis" produced during recumbency by the intravenous infusion of isotonic saline solution. J. clin. Invest. **30**, 862 (1951). — SUSSMAN, R. M., and J. MILLER: Iodide „Mumps" after intravenous urography. New Engl. J. Med. **255**, 433—434 (1956). — TEPLICK, J. G., and M. W. YARROW: Arterial infarction of the kidney. Ann. intern. Med. **42**, 1041 (1955). — THEANDER, G.: On the visualization of the renal pelves in cholegraphy. Acta radiol. (Stockh.) **45**, 283—288 (1956). — Precipitation of contrast medium in the gallbladder. Acta radiol. (Stockh.) **44**, 467—470 (1955). — THESTRUP ANDERSEN, P.: On tomography as an adjunct to urography. Acta radiol. (Stockh.) **30**, 225 (1948). — TONIOLO, G.: Considerazioni critiche sull'uso delle alte percentuali di jodio nell'urografia funzionale. Nunt. radiol. (Firenze) **20**, 495 (1954). — TUCKER, A. S., and G. DI BAGNO: Intravenous urography, a comparative study of neoiopax and urokon. Amer. J. Roentgenol. **75**, 855 (1956). — UTZ, D. C., and G. J. THOMPSON: Evaluation of contrast media for excretory urography. Proc. Mayo Clin. **33**, 75 (1958). — VESEY, J., C. T. DOTTER and I. STEINBERG: Nephrography: simplified technic. Radiology **55**, 827 (1950). — VESTERDAL, J., and F. TUDVAD: Studies on the kidney function in premature and full-term infants by estimating of the inulin and paraamino-hippurate clearances. Acta paediat. (Uppsala) **37**, 429 (1949). — WALL, B., and D. K. ROSE: The clinical intravenous nephrogram: preliminary report. J. Urol. (Baltimore) **66**, 305 (1951). — WALLINGFORD, V. H.: General aspects of contrast media research. Ann. N.Y. Acad. Sci. **78**, 707—719 (1959). — WARDENER, H. E. DE: The kidney. London 1958. — WECHSLER, H.: Further studies of reactions due to intravenous urography. J. Urol. (Baltimore) **78**, 496 (1957). — WEENS, H. S., and T. J. FLORENCE: Nephrography. Amer. J. Roentgenol. **57**, 338 (1947). — WEIGEN, J. F., and S. F. THOMAS: Reactions to intravenous organic iodine compounds and their immediate treatment. Radiology **71**, 21 (1958). — WINTER, C. C.: The value of chlor-trimeton in the prevention of immediate reactions to 70 per cent urokon. J. Urol. (Baltimore) **74**, 416 (1955). — A clinical study of a new renal function test: The radioactive diodrast renogram. J. Urol. (Baltimore) **76**, 182—196 (1956). — WINZER, K., H. LANGECKER u. K. JUNKMAN: Zur Frage der Verträglichkeit von Nieren- und Gallekontrastmitteln. Sonderdruck aus Ärztl. Wschr. **9**, 950—952 (1954). — WOHL, G. T.: Vertebral metastasis in renal carcinoma. An anatomic correlation. Amer. J. Roentgenol. **75**, 930 (1956). — WOODRUFF, M. W.: The five minute intravenous pyelogram as a measure of renal function. Amer. J. Roentgenol. **82**, 847—848 (1959). —

WRIGHT, F. W.: Intravenous hydrocortisone in the treatment of a severe urographic reaction. Brit. J. Radiol. **32**, 343—344 (1959). — WYATT, G. M.: Excretory urography for children. Radiology **36**, 664 (1941). — ZEITEL, B. E., W. LENTINO, H. G. JACOBSON and M. H. POPPEL: Renografin: A new intravenous urographic medium. J. Urol. (Baltimore) **76**, 461 (1956). — ZINNER, G., u. R. GOTTLOB: Die gefäßschädigende Wirkung verschiedener Röntgenkontrastmittel, vergleichende Untersuchungen. Fortschr. Röntgenstr. **91**, 507—512 (1959). — ZOLLINGER, H. U.: Thorotrast damage of kidneys with hypertension. Schweiz. med. Wschr. **87**, 1089 (1957).

Vascular changes

BOHNE, A. W., and G. L. HENDERSON: Intrarenal arteriovenous aneurysm: case report. J. Urol. (Baltimore) **77**, 818 (1957). — CEDERMARK, J., K. LINDBLOM och F. HENSCHEN: Om diagnosen av njurinfarkt, särskilt med hjälp av aortografi. Nord. Med. **10**, 1793 (1941). — CORDONNIER, J. J.: Unilateral renal artery disease with hypertension. J. Urol. (Baltimore) **82**, 1—9 (1959). — EIKNER, W. C., and C. J. BOBECK: Renal vein thrombosis. J. Urol. (Baltimore) **75**, 780 (1956). — GLAZIER, McC., and L. J. LOMBARDO: Diseases of renal artery. J. Urol. (Baltimore) **81**, 27 (1959). — HARROW, B. R., and J. A. SLOANE: Aneurysm of renal artery: report of five cases. J. Urol. (Baltimore) **81**, 35 (1959). — HUGHES, F., A. BARCIA, O. FIANDRA and J. VIOLA: Aneurysm of the renal artery. Acta radiol. (Stockh.) **49**, 117 (1958). — LEGER, L., et L. A. GEORGE: Thrombose de la veine rénale. Presse méd. **62**, 721 (1954). — LIEDHOLM, K.: Total vänstersidig njurinfarkt hos hjärtfrisk pojke. Nord. Med. **23**, 1530 (1944). — MATHÉ, C. P.: Aneurysm of renal artery causing hypertension: report of three cases. J. Urol. (Baltimore) **82**, 412—416 (1959). — MOLDENHAUER, W.: Nierenarterienverkalkungen. Fortschr. Röntgenstr. **90**, 522—523 (1959). — MUNGER, H. V.: Renal thrombosis. J. Urol. (Baltimore) **71**, 144 (1954). — POUTASSE, E. E.: Renal artery aneurysm: report of 12 cases, two treated by excision of the aneurysm and repair of renal artery. J. Urol. (Baltimore) **77**, 697 (1957). — RÍO, G. DEL: Trombosis de la vena renal. Progr. Pat. Clin. **7** (1960). — SCHÄFER, H.: Nierenvenenverkalkungen. Fortschr. Röntgenstr. **91**, 531—533 (1959). — SCHWARTZ, J. W., A. A. BORSKI and E. J. JAHNKE: Renal arteriovenous fistula. Surgery **37**, 951 (1955). — SLOMINSKI-LAWS, M. D., J. H. KIEFER and C. W. VERMEULEN: Arteriovenous aneurysm of the kidney: case report. J. Urol. (Baltimore) **75**, 586 (1956). — SMITH, G. I., and V. ERICKSON: Intrarenal aneurysm of the renal artery: case report. J. Urol. (Baltimore) **77**, 814 (1957). — SPROUL, R. D., R. G. FRASER and K. J. MACKINNON: Aneurysm of the renal artery. J. Canad. Ass. Radiol. **9**, 45 (1958). — TEPLICK, J. G., and M. W. YARROW: Arterial infarction of the kidney. Ann. intern. Med. **42**, 1041 (1955). — WESTERBORN, A.: Embolie in der Arteria renalis. Z. Urol. **21**, 687 (1937).

Supplement to references

ASK-UPMARK, K. E. F., and D. INGVAR: A follow-up examination of 138 cases of subarachnoid hemorrhage. Acta med. scand. **138**, 15—31 (1950). — DAVIDSON, C. N., J. M. DENNIS, E. R. McNINCH, J. K. V. WILLSON and W. H. BROWN: Nephrocalcinosis associated with sarcoidosis. Radiology **62**, 203—214 (1954). — HECHT, G.: Röntgenkontrastmittel. In Handbuch der experimentellen Pharmakologie, Bd. 7, S. 79—163. Berlin: Springer 1938. — HIGGINS, C. C., and N. F. HICKEN: Perinephritic Abscess. Ann. Surg. **96**, 998—1013 (1932). — IDBOHRN, H., and A. NORGREN: Personal communications. Siehe: OLLE OLSSON, Renal angiography in the pre-diagnostic phase. IX. I. C. R. München 1959. — MATTSON, O.: Practical photographic problems in radiography. Acta radiol. (Stockh.) Suppl. **120** (1955). — NOGUEIRA, A.: Spontane Gasfüllung der Harnwege. Z. Urol. **29**, 275 (1935). — OLIN, T.: Personal communications. Siehe: OLLE OLSSON, Renal angiography in the pre-diagnostic phase. IX. I. C. R. München 1959. — RISHOLM, L., and K. J. ÖBRINK: Pyelorenal backflow in man. Acta chir. scand. **115**, 144—148 (1958). — SCHMERBER, F.: Les artères de la capsule graisseuse du rein. Int. Mschr. Anat. Physiol. **13**, 269 (1896). — STAEHLER, W.: Klinik und Praxis der Urologie. Stuttgart: Georg Thieme 1959. — STEINBOCK, A.: Intravenous urography and retrograde pyelography in subcutaneous injuries of kidney. Ann. Chir. Gynaec. Fenn. **37**, Suppl. 4 (1948). — TROELL, A.: Intravenöse Pyelographie zur Prüfung der Nierenfunktion bei Prostatikern. Chirurg **7**, 513—517 (1935).

Roentgen examination of the distal urinary tract and of the male genital organs

By

K. LINDBLOM and R. ROMANUS

With 128 figures

I. General indications for roentgenologic examination of the distal urinary tract and its value in relation to that of endoscopy

At every site in the body where natural contrast media are present, or an artificial contrast medium can be introduced, roentgenologic examination is able to provide information about the shape and position of the relevant organs. Moreover, roentgenologic examination of organs in movement can—in the degree that the contours are visible—depict this event, or various phases of it, in a more physiologic way than the majority of other methods of examination. A further advantage is that the morphologic and physiologic data recorded on the roentgenograms can be filed. This implies that they can be compared—with the objectivity inherent in the photographic method—with the condition of the patient on other occasions, or with that of other patients.

Although the natural contrast media offered by the distal parts of the urinary tract and their surroundings are few, they are nevertheless important. They consist chiefly of layers of adipose tissue and of calcifications. In most individuals, the urinary bladder has a perimuscular layer of fat that is lacking only in the region of the prostate gland, but that cannot, as a rule, be identified on the roentgenogram in the posterior direction, towards the seminal vesicles and their surroundings (Fig. 1). The layer of fat also embraces the greater part of the muscles of the pelvic floor. However, only in corpulent subjects do these muscles appear so distinctly that this can be utilized for morphologic studies.

Prostatic calculi are common, and can be visualized distinctly. They do not, however, provide any topographic information about the prostate and its surroundings unless they fill a large portion of the gland. This also applies to the rare calcifications of the vas, ampullae and seminal vesicles (Fig. 2). Vesical and urethral calculi (Figs. 3—6) are naturally important indications of disease, but they may have such low absorption that they cannot be identified until the bladder and urethra are opacified. Other calcifications consist of phleboliths—generally localized to the pelvic venous plexus—but their diagnostic significance is slight or lacking (Fig. 2, 6).

Adjacent parts of the intestinal tract, particularly the rectum and sigmoid, also provide topographic data on the pelvis by means of their gas content. They are, however, seldom of diagnostic value for the lower urinary tract.

Although the pelvic skeleton is, in fact, merely the topographic framework, its reactions to pathologic processes of the pelvic organs are of great importance, and may even be decisive for the diagnosis.

Artificial contrast media can be introduced into the urethra and bladder (Fig. 7), and in pathological conditions pass into paraurethral ducts: in the anterior urethra, in the glands of Cowper and in the prostate. The prostatic utricle

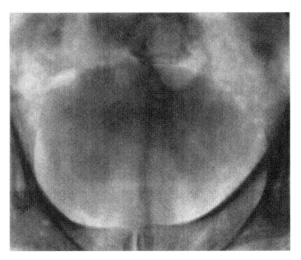

Fig. 1. Plain roentgenogram illustrating the urinary bladder with a residual urine of approximately 200 ml

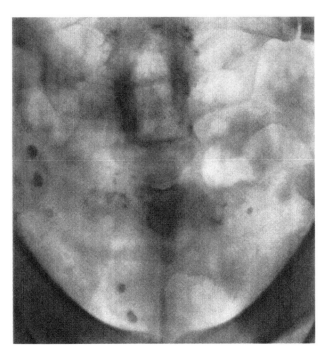

Fig. 2. Phleboliths and vesicular calcifications

the vas, the ampullae and the seminal vesicles can in various ways be contrast filled and their vascular system studied by arteriography and phlebography. The intestinal and peritoneal cavities can also be opacified. Finally, certain information can be obtained by injecting contrast medium—preferably a water-soluble iodine salt—into the pelvic tissue. The medium spreads into the existing spaces, but the data which it provides are difficult to interpret. This is because the spaces in question are not preformed, and the spreading in them is governed by the least resistance in the tissues.

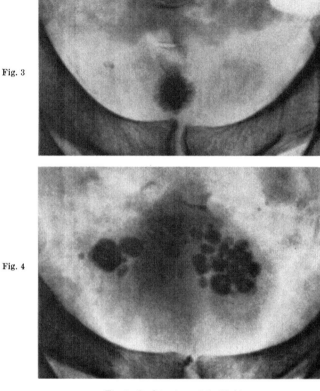

Fig. 3

Fig. 4

Fig. 3. Oxalate stone of the bladder
Fig. 4. Multiple phosphate stones in the bladder

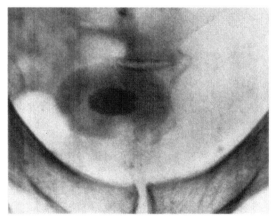

Fig. 5. Bladder stone with a center of calcium oxalate and a periphery of tripelphosphate

Evaluation of the state of the lower urinary tract is also facilitated by roentgenologic examination of the upper urinary tract. In at least half of the cases in which this examination of the lower urinary tract is indicated, urography is required as well. Micturition pictures taken at urography provide an additional basis for studies of the urethra.

A common error is to regard roentgenologic examination as a competitive method to clinical methods of examination, such as palpation and endoscopy. As a rule, it is not a matter of "either/or", but of "both/and". The methods complement each other and only making use of both gives a complete picture of the

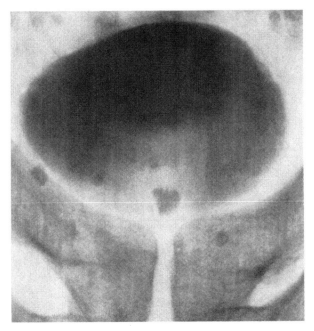

Fig. 6. Oxalate stone in the supracollicular portion of the urethra

conditions, facilitating the selection between various methods of treatment. Endoscopy gives, for example, information about the appearance of the surface of a pathologic process presented towards a lumen and gives opportunity to biopsy; palpation about its consistence, mobility and possible tenderness. Roentgenologic examination is informative chiefly with respect to such factors as the position of the pathologic process and its influence on the surroundings, the presence of communicating cavities, and sphincter function. Endoscopy or other forms of instrumentation are, as a rule, obligatory preliminaries to opacification of the seminal vesicles and ejaculatory ducts. On the other hand, in the presence of a narrow urethra, roentgenologic examination may necessarily be a complete substitution for endoscopy.

II. Complications of roentgenologic examination and its contraindications

Like most other instrumental forms of examination, the roentgenologic methods which include injection of contrast medium are associated with certain sources of danger. In urethrocystography—which is the most important means of studying the lower urinary tract—there is a possibility of complications by the

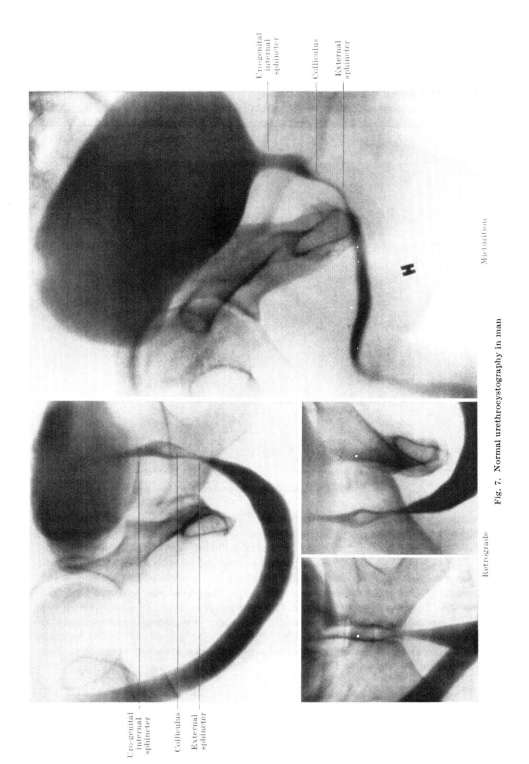

Fig. 7. Normal urethrocystography in man

introduction and spreading of infectious substances, and of trauma to the wall by instruments and pressure of injection (Fig. 8).

As far as the risk of infection is concerned, the contraindications are the same as those to other instrumental examinations of the urethra, such as urethroscopy. The examination should therefore be avoided in acute inflammatory changes especially acute urethritis. When balanitis is present, it should be treated first. After examination, the patient should be kept under observation, so that suitable therapy can be instituted if infection supervenes. Many prefer prophylactic treatment with sulpha drugs during 5 days, before and after the examination.

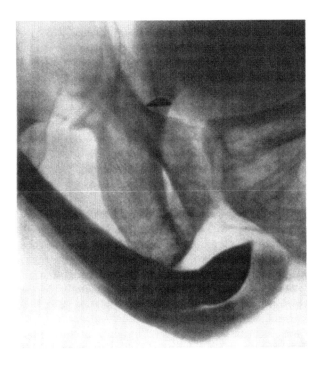

Fig. 8. Urethrocavernous reflux from a rupture at the external orifice

To prevent damage to the mucosa by the pressure of injection, urethrocystography preferably should be performed before endoscopy, in any case not on the days immediately after cystoscopy or probing, particularly if they can be suspected to have injured the mucosa. Furthermore—as on introduction of the cystoscope—the patient should be instructed to try to micturate during the injection of contrast medium. This is because the decrease in tonus of the external sphincter of the urethra produced by the attempt to micturate facilitates the inflow of contrast medium. Should an urethrocavernous reflux arise as a result of mucosal rupture, antibiotics should always be given and the patient kept under careful observation.

The risk of mucosal rupture seems to be less with more viscous contrast solution. Since urethro-cavernous reflux, however, may occur a water-insoluble or unabsorbable contrast medium should not, in any circumstances, be used for retrograde injection. Emulgated oil preparations are not suitable, as embolies may appear and periurethrally deposited contrast material may cause chronic inflammation (thorotrast even secondary sarcoma). Only if the contrast medium is introduced directly into the bladder through a catheter, is it permissible to use such contrast media as barium sulphate or gaseous substances.

The roentgen irradiation to which the gonads of a fertile patient are exposed also belongs to the contraindications. Only in men can this risk be practically eliminated by means of a lead shield around the scrotum. Otherwise, the size of the dose to the gonads amounts to about 0.5 r per exposure.

III. Urethrocystographic technique: instruments, contrast medium, procedure

The instrument most commonly used for injection of contrast medium into the urethra consists of a cannula with a cone-shaped mouthpiece of rubber. After introduction into the external urethral orifice, the cannula is secured by a penis clamp. The cannula can be replaced by a small-bore catheter introduced into the anterior urethra, and kept in position by tying around the glans penis; this is particularly useful in hypospadias. If the urethra has a perineal orifice, the cannula with a rubber cone is used, the cone being kept pressed into the orifice by hand.

The contrast medium generally used is a water-soluble iodine salt of the same type as in urography, e.g. a 35 per cent solution of diiodide (Perabrodil, Perjodal). It is suitable to add a viscosity-raising medium such as dextran (Perjodal H), to get better distension of the posterior urethra. Contrast medium with wetting properties miscible with urine and the secretions of the paraurethral ducts are preferable, especially for relief studies of the mucous membrane.

High concentrations should be avoided, on the grounds of unduly strong chemical and osmotic irritation. As far as irritation is concerned, the length of time for which the contrast medium is in contact with the mucosa is of paramount importance. Consequently, injection should be performed as rapidly as possible. Moreover, the retrograde fase of filling of the concentrated contrast medium should be followed by injection of a less concentrated solution, appropriately 40 ml of the contrast medium diluted with 60 ml of water.

In view of the irritant properties of the contrast medium, it is advisable —before it is injected—to inject a mucosal anaesthetic, e.g. 12 ml of 0.5 per cent Xylocaine.

The use of a viscous contrast medium facilitates a study of the posterior urethra, since its transient opacification is prolonged and fortified with increasing viscosity of the medium. This allows, for example, the voluntary muscle function of the urethra to be studied. If a highly fluid contrast medium is used, the injection must be made much more rapidly to obtain sufficient distension of the posterior urethra. It must be emphasized that the viscosity-raising medium should not be of such a nature that it can produce foreign-body irritation if the mucosa is injured. At the present time, dextran is the viscosity-raising substance that can be recommended for this purpose.

The examination takes place as follows. The patient tries to empty his bladder completely, after which a survey picture is taken. This discloses whether or not residual urine is present. If the vesical shadow is still large and the bladder should be examined it is emptied with a catheter.

Before injecting the contrast medium, the urethral orifice and its immediate surroundings are swabbed with an antiseptic. The injection instrument is then introduced, and the mucosal anaesthetic is injected.

During the initial part of the examination, the patient is in the supine position, and the exposures are taken with the rays directed sagittally. First, 20 ml of the concentrated contrast medium are injected, of which the greater portion is required to fill the anterior urethra. This is followed by rapid injection of an additional 10 ml, during which the patient tries to micturate, simultaneously holding his breath. The exposures are made during this second injection. The patient is then rotated to the semi-lateral position, and exposure takes place in the oblique view, during rapid injection of a further 10 ml, also with an attempt to micturate and apnoea. This is repeated a third time in the semi-lateral position in the opposite direction (Fig. 7).

For special topographic studies, a true lateral projection may also be desirable. In this case, the procedure is repeated for the fourth time. Exposures during voluntary contraction of the pelvic floor may sometimes be of value.

This retrograde examination of the urethra is followed directly by injection of the dilute contrast solution, after which the instrument is removed.

If the bladder capacity is small, the patient may experience such intense urgency that the quantity of contrast medium injected must be decreased. If, on the contrary, the bladder capacity is abnormally large, a greater quantity of the dilute contrast medium may be required to permit the subsequent micturition study.

The micturition study is preferably made with the patient in the erect position, using oblique projections with the rays directed horizontally. The exposures are not made until urination has started properly. If the cause of dribbling is to be studied, pictures are also taken after the end of micturition. With a little patience, exposures can be obtained during micturition in most cases. Even if the patient is unable to micturate, his attempts to do so should be depicted.

For a study of the extent of vesico-ureteric reflux, and for possible simultaneous filling of the renal pelvis, it is better to make the micturition examination with the patient supine, instead of erect.

In adults, a micturition examination in the lateral view, with injection of the water-soluble contrast medium in question, provides such indistinct details that they suffice only for a topographic study. The bladder must instead be filled with a sterile 25 per cent suspension of barium sulphate. This contrast medium may also be used for cinematographic studies of the course of micturition. Air has also been used as a contrast medium in cystography *i.e.* mixed with high viscous contrast solution as in "double contrast enema" of the colon. However, in view of the constant risk of intravenous reflux, even during micturition, such contrast media as barium sulphate and air should be avoided as far as possible.

Another means of obtaining better depiction of the prostate by artificial reflux into the prostatic ducts is based on injection under positive pressure, after blocking the bladder neck with a balloon (Figs. 113 and 114). Because of the risk of infection, caution should be observed.

IV. The urinary bladder

1. Normal and pathologic roentgenologic features

At rest and when moderately distended, the frontal cross-section of the normal urinary bladder has the shape of a recumbent oval. In the resting bladder, the roof assumes the shape of its surroundings, and a slight impression may be produced in it by a distended loop of the sigmoid or the uterus. The bladder floor is a mould of the underlying tissue. The lower margin of the retroureteric fossa is marked by a downwardly convex line, which is completely symmetric. It appears in the supine position, and is most distinct in the beginning of the examination,

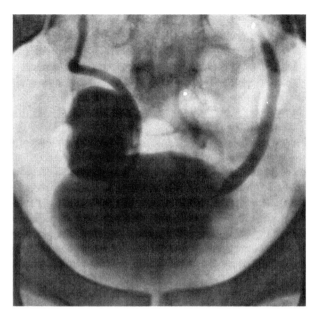

Fig. 9. Paraurethral diverticulum of the bladder (see also Fig. 33)

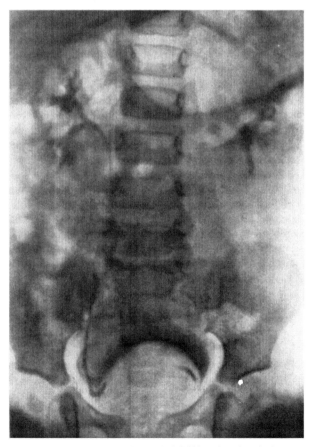

Fig. 10. Ureterocele from the ureter of an upper pelvis of the left kidney (non-functioning upper pole). The ureter
ends in the posterior urethra (ectopic ureter with ureterocele)

when the posterior wall is covered by a relatively thin layer of contrast medium. Its visualization is facilitated if the direction of the rays is not truly ventrodorsal, but concurrently somewhat caudocranial. The transition of the trigone into the urethra often has the appearance of a shallow funnel. In the prone position, or in the lateral view, the upper contour of the bladder is often conical, following the anterior abdominal wall in the direction of the remnants of the urachus.

Greater filling of the bladder takes place essentially by raising of its roof. Its cross-section then changes from a recumbent to an erect oval, with its upper pole directed towards the umbilicus. The bladder tends to assume the raised shape characterizing it during detrusor contraction. During micturition, the characteristic shape of the bladder is that of an erect oval, with an often pointed

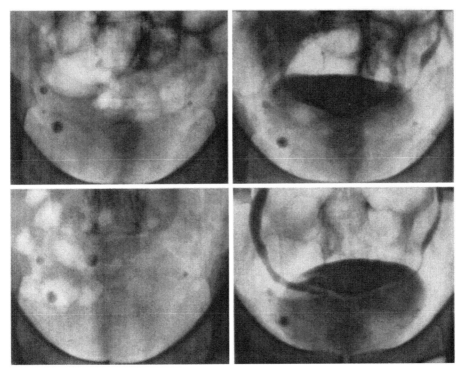

Fig. 11. Case with ureterocele examined before (upper figures) and after blockage caused by a stone (lower figures)

upper pole. Under normal conditions, the contour of the bladder remains even. Its floor—which, at rest, is on the level of the upper margin of the symphysis— descends during micturition or straining to the level of the middle of the symphysis or its lower margin and is during voluntary contraction of the pelvic floor lifted about one cm.

The mucosa is folded only when the bladder is empty or practically empty. In the normal bladder, the thin folds are then represented by an irregular pattern of small defects.

Normal variants in the appearance of the bladder occur. Among them is a waist-like constriction between the postero-inferior and supero-anterior part of the bladder; it may be so marked that the anterior part resembles a large diverticulum. With a flaccid abdominal wall, the bladder may seem to hang over the symphysis, owing to the symphysis region making an impression in the bladder floor. Faint trabeculation of the bladder during micturition is not necessarily pathologic.

In the female, the uterus produces a broad impression in the bladder roof. In view of this impression, and of the usually large bladder capacity, a greater degree of filling is, as a rule, required for the female bladder to assume the shape of an erect oval instead of a recumbent one. The retroureteric fossa is shallower in the female than in the male. Consequently, its lower contour—produced by the interureteric ridge—is more often lacking in the former.

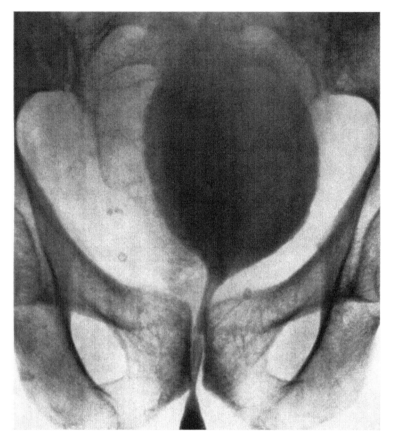

Fig. 12. Dislocation of the bladder from an extraperitoneal hematoma (after operation of a hernia)

2. Developmental anomalies

Developmental anomalies of the bladder are determined by embryologic factors. Incomplete closure gives rise to exstrophy of the bladder, and a persistent urachal duct to a fistula from the vertex to the umbilicus. Supernumerary ureteric buds are the cause of ectopic ureters, and possibly also of the para-ureteric diverticula that may be present in the posterior bladder wall, without any demonstrable signs of an impediment to emptying (Fig. 9).

The bladder may also be affected by developmental anomalies of the ureteric primordia. Thus, saccular bulgings of the ureters, of congenital origin, may appear in the bladder (Figs. 10 and 11).

If a supernumerary ureter is combined with ureterocele, it is generally the ureter of the upper renal pelvis that is involved. Such a ureter not infrequently has an ectopic orifice in the upper part of the posterior urethra.

3. Positional changes

The urinary bladder is an extraperitoneal organ, which has intimate relations only with the pelvic floor and its organs, and with the anterior abdominal wall.

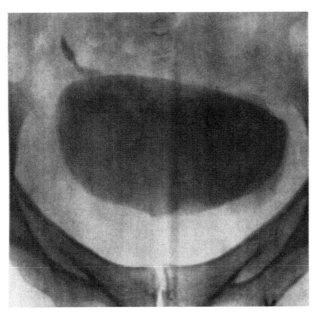

Fig. 13. Increased distance between the bladder and the symphysis caused by a postoperative edema

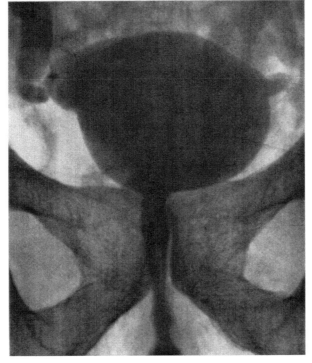

Fig. 14. Dislocation of the bladder wall and the urethra because of an abscess from a vesiculitis

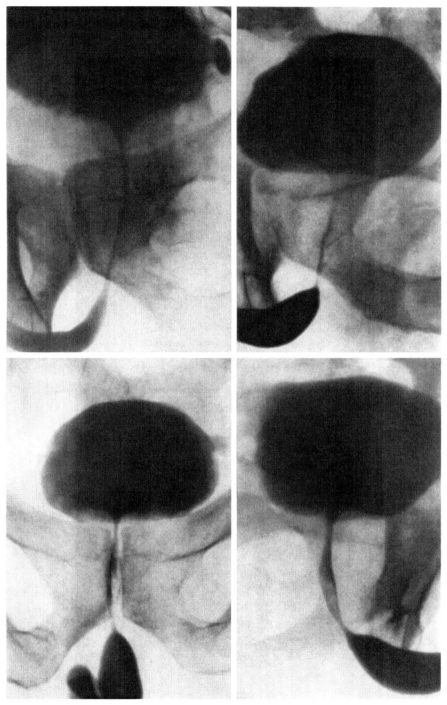

Fig. 15. Elevated bottom of the bladder because of prostatitis with marked swelling: to the left, during acute
fase with bullous edema in the bladder; to the right, six weeks later during healing

Consequently, processes in these regions can affect the position of the bladder as a whole. Widespread oedema and large tumours of the pelvic floor may lift not only the bladder floor, but the entire bladder (Figs. 12—16). Pressure from the peritoneal cavity, on the contrary, merely compresses the bladder. Only on relaxation of the muscles of the pelvic floor does the bladder descend with it, and if a defect is present in the pelvic floor, the bladder may protrude concurrently, forming a cystocele. A cystocele may also arise in the anterior abdominal wall if a suprapubic separation of the rectus muscles of the abdomen has taken place. A rare occurrence is for part of the bladder wall to protrude through the mouth of an inguinal hernia.

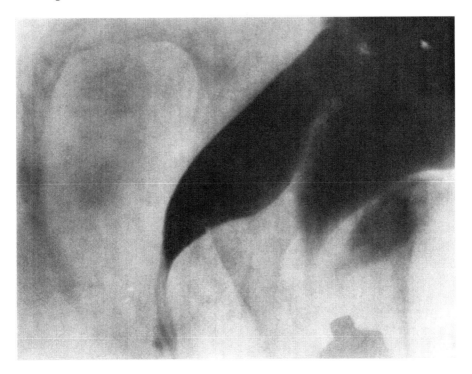

Fig. 16. Bladder and rectum elevated by a pelvic edema originating from the presacral region. In this case the edema was caused by a lymphogranuloma inguinale

A cystocele in the pelvic floor may occur in women who have undergone pregnancy. It appears on bearing down, when the bladder floor behind the urethral orifice protrudes through a gap in the levator muscles. The size of the herniating part of the bladder varies from case to case. The lower part of the ureters may even be included. The fact that the cystocele is a hernia is shown by the presence of a constriction corresponding to the mouth of the hernia. This feature distinguishes a cystocele from generalized relaxation of the pelvic floor, which is essentially comparable to a pendulous abdomen. For further details regarding cystocele, reference is made to page 40.

4. Traumatic changes

An indirect injury can lead to total or partial rupture of the bladder, which may be extra- or intraperitoneal. An extraperitoneal rupture produces a haematoma or infiltrate, which displaces the bladder lumen upwards and to one side.

The roentgenologic features of an intraperitoneal rupture are the same as those of free fluid. To visualize the rupture, cystography must be performed, when leakage of contrast medium can be demonstrated.

5. Inflammatory changes

In most cases of so-called trigonal cystitis, the roentgenogram is normal, with the possible exception of a more rounded bladder than usual, as a sign of increased tonus. As a rule, there is reason to interpret such conditions as urethritis rather than as cystitis.

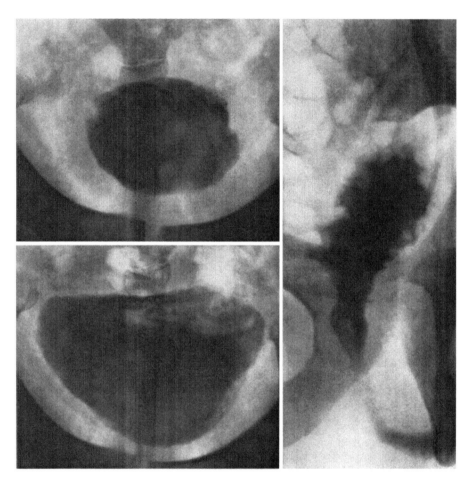

Fig. 17. Case of acute urogenital infection and Reiters syndrome, appearing as a severe cystitis with haematuria. Upper figures, during acute fase; lower left figure, two months later when healed

True cystitis, on the contrary, also produces roentgenologic signs. In order to interpret these signs and their implications, the features that can be reproduced on the roentgenogram must be understood. They are primarily the thickness of the bladder wall and the breadth of the mucosal folds. Secondary to them are such indirect signs as the bladder capacity and tonus, and the state of the ureteric and urethral orifices.

The more oedematous and deep-reaching is the process, the greater is the thickening of the bladder wall (Figs. 17—21). Whereas under normal conditions, the distance from the lumen to the subperitoneal layer of fat in the bladder roof —measured in the moderately distended bladder—is a few millimetres, it is increased to $^1/_2$ cm or more in most cases of cystitis. In acute cystitis associated with bleeding, a wall thickness of 1 cm is common (Fig. 17). Such marked thickening of the wall is also characteristic of the contracted bladder, *e.g.* in tuberculosis (Fig. 21) or after lengthy catheter treatment.

The oedema leading to generalized thickening of the wall is not infrequently in the form of a bullous oedema of the mucosa, which then has an undulating outline instead of a smooth one. When oedema is present in a trabeculated bladder, the trabeculae are seen to have a thickness of $^1/_2$ cm or more. If the

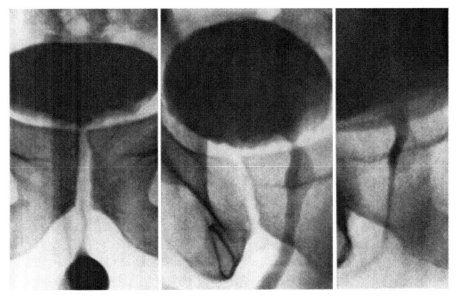

Fig. 18. Bullous edema in the bottom of the bladder, caused by acute prostato-vesiculitis

oedematous bladder is studied after the end of micturition, the extremely slender folds normally present are found to be replaced by coarse ones.

Cystitis may be local, *e.g.* superimposed on acute seminal vesiculitis or prostatitis (See V/2 and VIII), around the orifice of an inflamed diverticulum (Fig. 19) or an occluded, inflamed ureter, or in the roof of the bladder, as a result of irritation of the wall by a catheter tip, or caused by radiation injury. Roentgenologically, localized cystitis is seen as a local thickening of the wall, and a coarse mucosal relief, bulging into the lumen. Both roentgenologically and at cystoscopy, it may be difficult to make a differential diagnosis between localized cystitis and a tumour. In many cases this can, in fact, be done only by means of deep biopsy or exploratory operation.

In this connexion, it is necessary to recall the incidence of inflammatory changes often found when a tumour is present. They will also be stressed in connexion with the roentgenologic features of tumours of the bladder.

The indirect roentgenologic signs of cystitis are more difficult to evaluate. All degrees of increased tonus and reduced capacity occur. They are most conspicuous in the constricted bladder, and in interstitial cystitis in general. When tonus is increased, the bladder neck has a tendency to remain open like a funnel during retrograde injection of contrast medium. The ureteric orifices—which, normally, do not allow any passage from the bladder—are often open in cystitis, with consequent vesico-ureteric reflux.

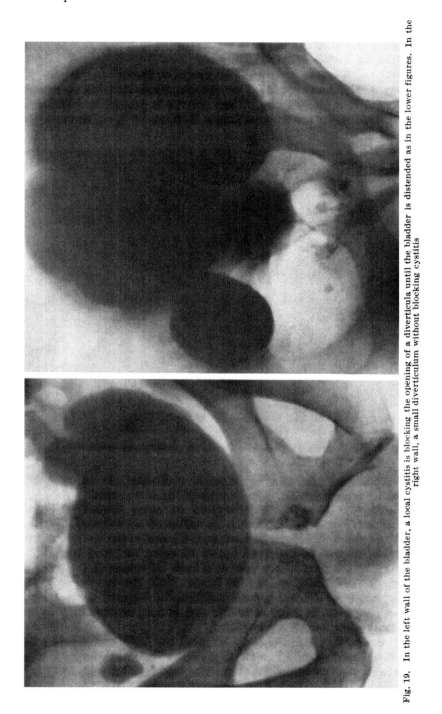

Fig. 19. In the left wall of the bladder, a local cystitis is blocking the opening of a diverticula until the bladder is distended as in the lower figures. In the right wall, a small diverticulum without blocking cystitis

A variant of acute, deep-penetrating cystitis is emphysematous cystitis, in which a discontinuous layer of gas can be observed in the bladder wall.

In interstitial cystitis (Hunner's ulcer), the capacity of the bladder is reduced, but its general shape is ordinary. When the bladder is emptied, the normal

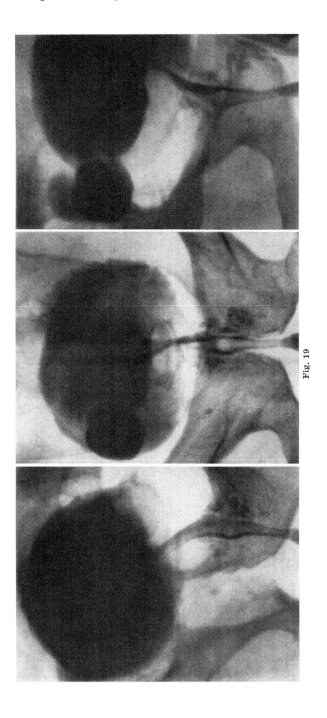

Fig. 19

slender folds in the mucosa are lacking to a varying degree. When it is distended, an indentation in the bladder contour will appear corresponding to the site of an ulcer. On the other hand, the generally shallow ulcerations cannot, as a rule, be identified on the roentgenogram. The roentgenologic features are understandable,

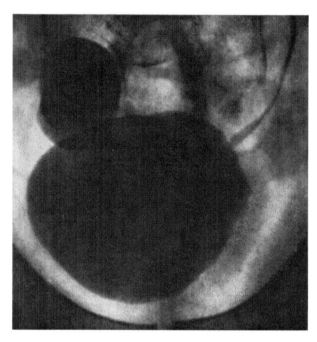

Fig. 20. Thickening of the left wall of the bladder corresponding to a local cystitis with leukoplakia

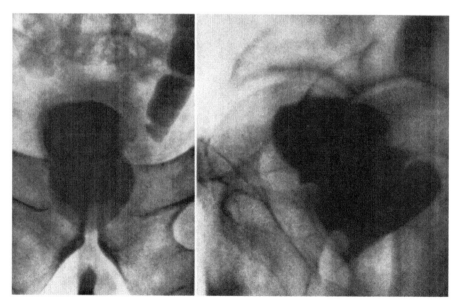

Fig. 21. Chronic cystitis in a stage of fibrosis

against the background of the atrophic and fibrosing lesions of the bladder wall in this disease (Fig. 22).

6. Calculi and foreign bodies

Vesical calculi may originate in the bladder, or be passed down from the kidney into the bladder, where they may enlarge. Their chief components are uric acid and urates, but since calcium salts are generally present as well, they are visible

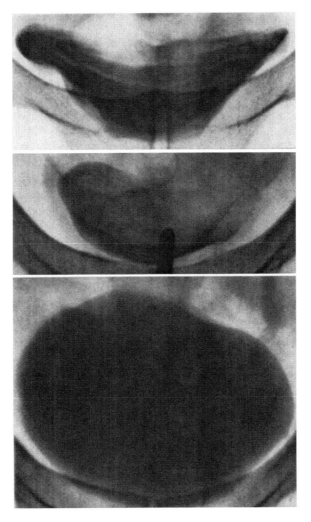

Fig. 22. Atrophic cystitis (Ulcus simplex): at sparse filling appearing as decreased folding of the mucous membrane; at complete filling seen as indentations of the contours. Compare with normal folding in upper figure representing a normal case

roentgenologically. In view of their low calcium content, they most often appear as thin shadows on plain roentgenograms, and as filling defects when contrast medium is injected.

Vesical calculi almost invariably arise with concurrent urinary retention and infection of the bladder. Consequently, when a stone is demonstrated in the bladder, a search should be made for an urethral impediment. Conversely, when signs of an impediment to emptying of the bladder are present, particular attention should be focused on the possible existence of vesical calculi.

Bladder stones may lie in a diverticulum, and in the rare cases in which the mouth of a concretion-bearing diverticulum is closed, it may be difficult to make a differential diagnosis between vesical calculus and extravesical calcifications, particularly sloghed appendices epiploicae. The latter are visible as a calcium shell, and are a not altogether uncommon finding in the pouch of Douglas in elderly patients who are—or who have been—corpulent. Concretions lying freely in the bladder lumen can be distinguished from extravesical calcifications by examination in the lateral view with the rays directed horizontally, when a vesical calculus falls towards the lateral wall.

Foreign bodies, such as a broken-off catheter tip, pieces of a ruptured Foley bag or nonresorbable sutures may be present in the bladder and constitute the nucleus of calculi. When a catheter is allowed to remain in the bladder for some time, salts are apt to be precipitated in and around it.

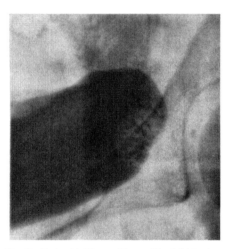

Fig. 23. Benign bladder papilloma without thickening of the wall at the base of the tumour

7. Tumours

The chief tumours of the urinary bladder are papilloma and carcinoma. Although the trigone and its immediate surroundings are the sites of predilection, a tumour may be present in any part of the bladder. In addition, there are urachal tumours of the vertex and, in rare cases, other tumours, such as pedunculated polyps.

On the cystogram, a tumour of the urinary bladder is seen as a filling defect, its shape and size corresponding to the part of the tumour bulging into the lumen. If the tumour is only slightly raised above its surroundings, or consists of an extremely small papilloma, it cannot always be identified on the cystogram, but is more easily detected at cystoscopy. On the other hand, cystography can, in most cases, provide information about the thickness of the bladder wall in the vicinity of the tumour; it thus gives an indication of the infiltration of the wall in a way that essentially complements the cystoscopic picture. If urography is performed as well, it can be ascertained whether dilatation of the ureter or cessation of renal function is present on the side of the tumour, as an expression of its manner of growth. Roentgenologic examination and cystoscopy are thus intended, to a high degree, to complement each other as methods of examination.

A comparison between the roentgenologic and palpatory signs of infiltration of the bladder wall also show that these forms of examination are complementary. It is, for example, especially difficult to evaluate the degree of infiltration by means of palpation when the tumour is situated retropubically. Perivesical fixation may be revealed by comparing routine radiograms with pictures exposed during micturition or voluntary contraction of the pelvic floor.

The roentgenologic estimation of the thickness of the bladder wall is based not only on the distance from the lumen, outlined by the contrast medium, to the extravesical layer of fat. It is also based on a local disappearance of the layer of fat in the tumour region, and a displacement of the bladder lumen. Evaluation of the exact site of the outer wall of the bladder is sometimes facilitated by opacification of adjacent cavities, such as the rectum, sigmoid and peritoneal cavity. Contrast medium can also be injected into the retropubic space.

At the base of a benign papilloma, the bladder wall is generally of normal thickness, *i.e.*, the distance from the lumen to the extravesical adipose tissue amounts to a few millimetres (Fig. 23). However, despite the absence of malig-

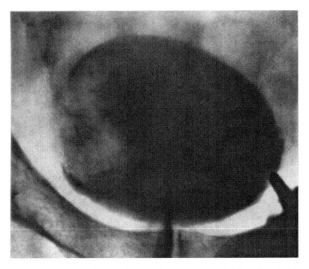

Fig. 24. Broad-based tumour of the bladder with a nodular surface and thickened wall at the base of the tumour as sign of malignancy

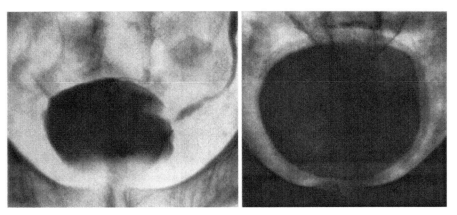

Fig. 25. Malignant tumour with nodular surface and wide-spread thickening of the bladder wall (right figure). The absence of ureteral blocking (left figure) speaks against a perivesical growth

nancy, there may occasionally be thickening of the bladder wall. It is in the form either of perifocal oedema, or of a generalized cystitic change, and in such cases roentgenologic examination may appear misleading. In most cases, however, thickening of the wall in the tumour region is a sign of infiltrative growth (Figs. 24 to 25). This sign is often associated with a closely-related feature, namely, that the tumour is not sharply delimited, but has gently outlines merging with the surroundings. In the presence of marked infiltration, the bladder lumen is distinctly displaced towards the healthy side.

The urographic sign of blocking of the ureteric lumen often appears when the tumour infiltrates the posterior wall of the bladder (Fig. 26). Only in rare cases can a benign papilloma of the ureteric orifice cause blocking of the ureter. On careful examination, the villous papilloma can be seen to project into the ureteric lumen as a filling defect.

Calcifications on the tumour surface generally represent a precipitation of salts in the necrotic tissue, and are a sign of malignancy (Fig. 27).

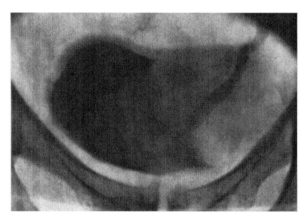

Fig. 26. Malignant tumour with marked thickening of the bladder wall and ureteral blocking indicating perivesical growth

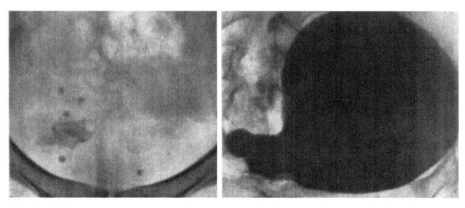

Fig. 27. Calcifications in a necrotic tumour tissue as a sign of malignancy. The tumour is situated close to a diverticulum

A tumour of the bladder, especially when it is of low malignancy, is not infrequently associated with growth in the adjacent parts of the pelvic bone (Fig. 28).

The major portion of an urachal tumour often extends perivesically into the bladder roof. Since part of the sigmoid usually lies against the bladder roof, there is reason—particularly in these cases—to opacify the sigmoid, and study its position in relation to the bladder.

From the differential-diagnostic point of view, it should be borne in mind that an inflammatory infiltrate may resemble a tumour, both cystoscopically and cystographically. Thus, vesiculitis may cause a localized bullous oedema bulging into the bladder with a change in its mucosal relief and, in rare cases, may even produce stenosis of the adjacent ureter (Fig. 110, see further VIII). Also important from the practical standpoint is a tumour-like diverticulitis originating in the sigmoid, as well as local cystitis of a tuberculous nature around an ureteric orifice with a dilated ureter, and such greatly impaired function of the corresponding kidney that the tuberculous pyelonephritis is not manifest at urography. Such features can be misinterpreted as a tumour of the bladder with malignant in-filtration into the ureter (Fig. 29).

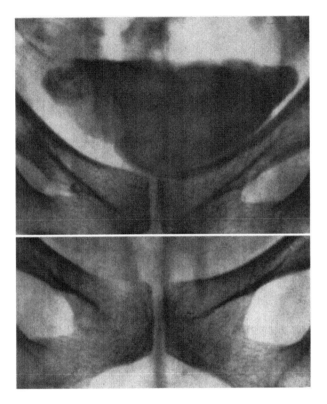

Fig. 28. Malignant bladder tumour. Five months after resection of the bladder (lower figure) a tumour destruction is seen in the adjacent part of the pubic bone

Irradiation reactions of the bladder in the acute stage behave like acute cystitis, and in the chronic stage—if the irradiation damage is severe—like a contracted bladder. Local irradiation damage, *e.g.* after implantation of radium in the uterus and vagina, may give rise to a vesico-vaginal fistula.

8. Influence of extravesical processes

The influence of extravesical processes on the bladder has been partly described in connexion with changes in position of the bladder, cystitis and tumours of the bladder, but processes at other sites may also give rise to vesical changes.

Enlargement of the prostate due to prostatitis or hypertrophy pushes the bladder floor upwards at the urethral orifice. Generalized oedema of the pelvic tissues not only displaces the whole bladder floor upwards, but compresses the walls of the bladder so that its lower part assumes the shape of a funnel, narrowing towards the urethra, with concurrent elongation of the latter. Tumours of the uterus and its adnexa compress the bladder from behind and above. Other large tumours or abscesses in the vicinity may also produce changes in shape and position of the bladder.

9. Endometriosis of the bladder

Since the distance from the uterine cervix to the trigone of the bladder is short, endometriosis of the uterus may result in direct involvement of this part of the bladder. This may occur when endometriosis arises as a result of evacuation of the uterine cavity by vaginal section.

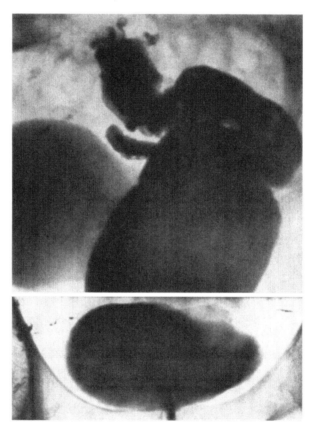

Fig. 29. Bullous edema in the roof of the bladder (lower figure) caused by perisigmoiditis with abscess in a case of diverticulitis of the sigmoid (upper figure)

If, in this condition, a change is present in the trigonal region of the bladder, there is reason to suspect that it is a question of endometriosis. On the cystogram, endometriosis has the appearance of a round tumour, only slightly elevated above its surroundings (Fig. 30). The roentgenologic features are not pathognomonic, but require a differential-diagnostic investigation with biopsy, in view of the possibility that it may actually be a malignant tumour of the bladder.

10. Bladder fistulas

The bladder fistulas for which roentgenologic diagnosis plays an important role are the spontaneous fistulas between the intestine and the bladder roof, between the posterior part of the bladder and the vaginal fornix, and possibly the rectum as well, as a result of obstetric or gynaecologic interventions (Fig. 31). Paraurethral false passages to the bladder, as a result of prostatectomy or probing, will be described later in connexion with urethral injuries.

A vesico-intestinal fistula may be difficult to opacify from the bladder, in which case only signs of local cystitis are visible in the bladder roof. Nor can the

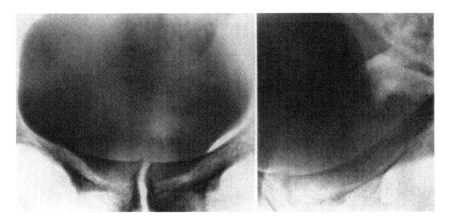

Fig. 30. Endometriosis bulging into the bladder adjacent to the cervix of the uterus

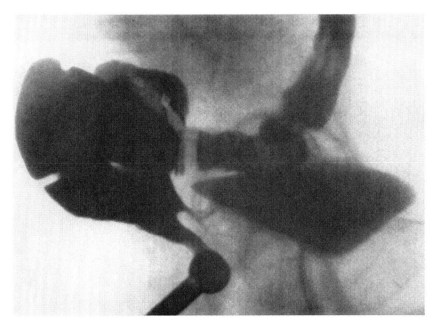

Fig. 31. Fistula between the bladder and the rectum caused by utero-vaginal application of radium followed by exstirpation of the uterus

fistula invariably be filled from the intestine; however, in this case as well, indirect signs of a fistula may appear on opacification. If, for example, there is a communication with the sigmoid, a perforated diverticulum is generally present at the roof of the bladder. A raised mucosal relief around the opacified diverticulum, as well as an increased tendency of the sigmoid to contract, may then appear as an expression of sigmoiditis and perisigmoiditis.

A fistula between the bladder and the vaginal fornix is usually short and wide. The contrast medium then passes rapidly from the bladder into the vagina. To visualize the communication, the examination must be made in the lateral view during injection of contrast medium into the bladder, preferably with concurrent blocking of the vagina with a distended rubber balloon.

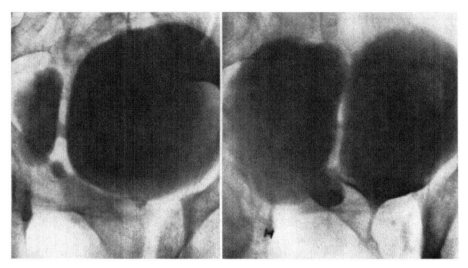

Fig. 32. Bladder diverticula of acquired type, distended during voiding (right figure), so called internal micturition

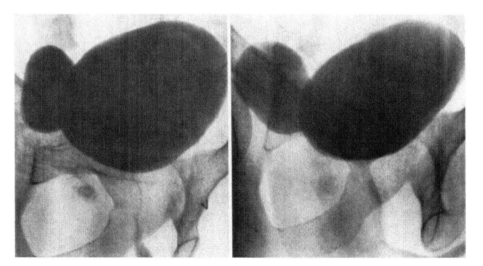

Fig. 33. Paraureteral diverticulum of congenital type, not distended during voiding (right figure)

11. Changes due to urinary obstruction

A chronic impediment to emptying of the bladder generally results in muscular hypertrophy, which is seen as trabeculation and moderate thickening of the wall. The trabeculae appear on the cystogram as folds in the bladder wall even when it is distended; as a rule, the folds become more conspicuous during micturition. Obviously, trabeculation is increased by chronic irritation.

If there is coincident cystitis, the folds become coarser, and the wall is still more thickened. The lumen may bulge between the folds, giving an impression of small diverticula, although they do not exist. True diverticula are present only when the bulges protrude beyond the rest of the bladder wall. These true diverticula—which are herniations of the mucosa through gaps in the muscles— have a deficient ability to contract, and increase in width during micturition, i.e., an often considerable portion of the bladder content is emptied into the diverticulum, with residual urine as a result (Figs. 32 and 33). This phenomenon can be denoted as internal micturition. Internal micturition can also take place to the ureters and renal pelves, by means of vesico-ureteric reflux (see the following).

Acute retention of urine leads to an over-distended bladder. On plain roentgenograms, it is seen as a large soft-tissue formation filling the lower part of the abdomen.

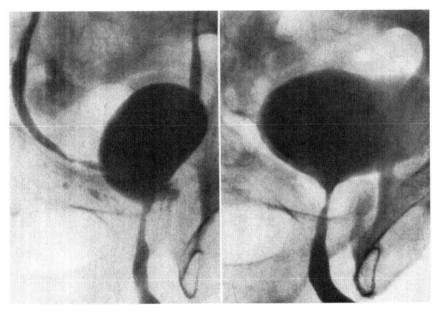

Fig. 34. Ureteral reflux during acute cystitis. In the right figure same case four months later in a free interval without reflux

12. Vesico-ureteric reflux

Vesico-ureteric reflux is a result of deficient closure of the ureter and its orifice, usually due to inflammatory changes in the bladder wall with partial stricture and rigidity of the orifice (Fig. 34). Thus, reflux is a common occurrence in chronic cystitis. It takes place more often during micturition than at rest. The ureter and renal pelvis may be distended by the high pressure in the bladder, so that a considerable part of what appears to be the bladder capacity is, in fact, the volume of the upper urinary tract. Consequently, in cases of vesico-ureteric reflux, roentgenologic examination should include the kidney.

Although vesico-ureteric reflux not infrequently occurs in acute cystitis as well, its true incidence cannot be determined by ordinary cystography. This is because in such cases, the reflux has a tendency to be transient, and cannot be induced on repeated examination of the same patient. It may even be so transient that reflux is visible on only one of several micturition pictures taken on the same occasion (Fig. 35). The occurrence of reflux seems to be favoured by marked distension of the bladder.

The existence of reflux to the ureters has contributed to focusing attention on ascending urinary infection, and transmission of the vesical pressure to the upper urinary tract, with rupture of the renal pelvis as a possible consequence. No final solution of these questions has been reached. An incontrovertible fact is that vesico-ureteric reflux is a prerequisite for the retrograde tumour implantation which may take place from the bladder to the renal pelvis.

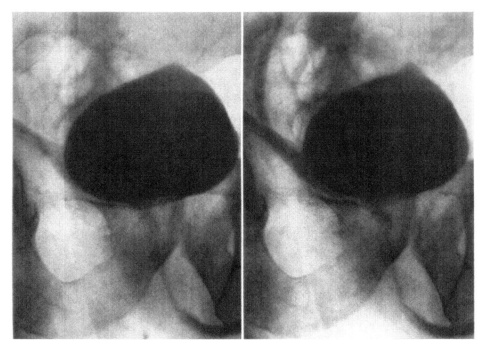

Fig. 35. Ureteral reflux appearing temporarily during micturition. The right figure represents a later fase of the same micturition as in the left figure

13. The neurogenic bladder. — Nocturnal enuresis

From the urethrocystographic point of view, neurogenic disturbances of the bladder are of three basic types. Two of them appear in lesions of the central nervous system, and the third in the absence of such lesions.

With a lesion of the central nervous system above the spinal bladder centre in the conus terminalis (at the level of Th_{12}), the urethrocystogram has a normal appearance on retrograde filling, apart from the bladder having a more rounded shape than usual when moderately filled, as a sign of hypertension. The patient's ability to micturate spontaneously is lost. When micturition occurs—either involuntarily or by peripheral stimulation, e.g. by filling the bladder to overflow, or by scratching the inside of the thighs—it is accompanied by marked dilatation of the posterior urethra. Micturition is, however, often interrupted before the bladder is completely emptied; the posterior urethra once more closes, and residual urine of moderate degree is present. This type is denoted as *supranuclear* (Figs. 36 and 37).

With chronic lesions of the spinal cord and cauda equina below the spinal bladder centre, the urethrocystogram is characteristic. During both retrograde

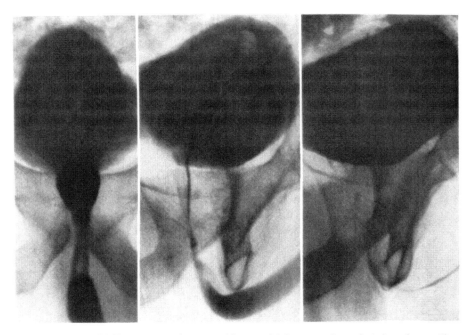

Fig. 36. Neurogenic bladder of supranuclear type without cystitis in a case of paraplegia from the mamillary level due to an injury level with Th 6. Left and mid figures during injection; right figure during an attempt to void. During one injection a temporary voiding occurred. No external sphincter spasm and no openstanding bladder neck

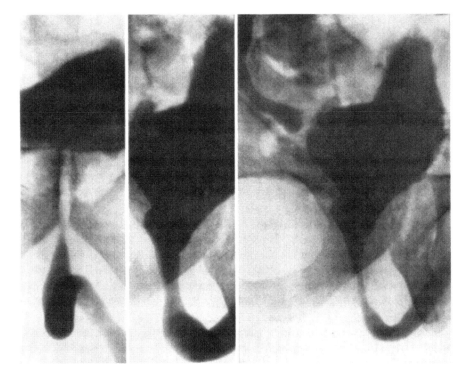

Fig. 37. Neurogenic bladder of supranuclear type with cystitis in a case of paraplegia following fracture of C 5. Left and mid figure during injection; right figure during voiding. Note no external sphincter spasm

filling and micturition, the posterior urethra—except for the region of the external sphincter—remains wide open like a funnel. This corresponds to the Schramm phenomenon seen at cystoscopy. The bladder is permanently raised in the micturating position, and—if the lesion is long-standing—is greatly trabeculated, with numerous small diverticula. Retrograde filling takes place without any signs of impediment in the region of the external sphincter, which then dilates normally. However, when the patient tries to micturate, the lumen does not relax at the external sphincter; the latter remains contracted, and only

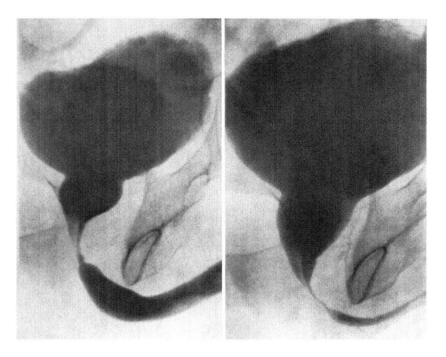

Fig. 38. Neurogenic bladder of infranuclear type in a case of paraplegia after fracture of L 1. Left figure during injection; right figure during voiding. External sphincter spasm and constantly open bladder neck as well as raised bladder are the typical features

allows passage of small portions of urine through the narrow lumen. The spasm of the external sphincter can be temporarily relieved by parasympatholytic drugs, and by blocking the superior lumbar ganglia. This type is denoted as *infranuclear* (Fig. 38).

The third basic type of neurogenic bladder is the so-called *atonic bladder*. Its pathogenesis is more uncertain. It may be a result of a peripheral injury leading to impaired sensitivity of the bladder and urethra, but it cannot be distinguished roentgenologically from an over-distended bladder. Cystographically, the atonic bladder has a large capacity, without the presence of trabeculation or diverticula. Attempts to micturate fail, or result in only inappreciable dilatation of the whole posterior urethra.

In *nocturnal enuresis* in adults, the urethrocystographic features have some resemblance to those in the supranuclear type of nerve lesion, although the patient can micturate voluntarily. As in the supranuclear type, the dilatation of the posterior urethra may be more marked than usual. Regarding Enuresis in children see VII, p. 443.

V. The male urethra and its adnexa

1. Normal anatomy

In retrograde filling, the normal anterior urethra of the adult male is distended to a width of 1—1$^1/_2$ cm (Fig. 7), provided that erection is not present, when the width decreases to $^1/_2$ cm. This distension is due to the high pressure of injection required to force the sphincters of the posterior urethra. At the border-line of the posterior urethra, the lumen narrows conically. A moderate constriction may be present at the sides of the cone, due to contraction of the bulbocavernous muscles. A special portion of this muscle (M. compressor hemisphericum bulbi, M. compressor nudae or sphincter nudae) may be found at the boundary between the posterior part of the pars anterior—the pars nuda (lacking cavernous tissue in its wall)—and the remainder of the anterior urethra (being surrounded by corpus spongiosum). Contraction of this muscle causes indentation of the anterior and lateral walls, which can be mistaken for a stricture. Otherwise, the wall of the anterior urethra is even.

The apex of the conical termination of the anterior urethra marks the transition into the posterior urethra which, during retrograde injection, is distended to a width of a few millimetres, and has a slight curvature, concave forwards. The function and the boundaries of the diaphragmatic portion (pars membranacea) can be more thouroughly studied using high viscous solution and active contraction of the pelvic floor. In the posterior wall of the prostatic part the colliculus forms a spindle-shaped bulge. The upper and lower poles of the colliculus continues into the crista urethralis, a millimetre-wide ridge which becomes flattened caudad and proximally. The sides of this ridge supracollicularly are marked by two shallow grooves, which can be followed as far as the bladder neck. Another groove, which normally is also shallow, is present in the anterior wall, running from the bladder to the leved of the colliculus. These grooves are obliterated on the greater distension of the lumen occurring during micturition.

Measured on the urethrogram, the posterior urethra is 3—4 cm in length. The site of the colliculus varies in the individual case, from the middle to the lower part of the posterior urethra. When the collicle is situated very low, it is reason to suspect a big prostatic utricle (see V, 13).

The prostatic and other paraurethral ducts or cavities are not opacified from the normal urethra, unless the pressure of injection is greatly raised by artificial blocking of the bladder neck.

During micturition, the appearance of the urethra changes from that during retrograde injection. The bladder neck dilates into a funnel, resulting in obliteration of the folds in the supracollicular part of the posterior urethra. As far as the external sphincter, the posterior urethra is more widened than earlier, with an average diameter of $> ^1/_2$ cm, in the lateral view slightly wider at the colliculus. The lumen is usually narrower from the external sphincter onwards. With the patient in the erect position, the anterior urethra behind the penile root may, however, show a slight spindle-shaped bulge, due to tension of the ligamentum suspensorium penis (cf. V, 6).

The position of the posterior urethra also changes during micturition, due to the descent of the pelvic floor . Since this descent is most marked in the upper and posterior part of the pelvic floor, it produces displacement of the bladder neck and upper portion of the prostatic part downwards and backwards, whereas the region of the external sphincter is only slightly depressed—thus the prostatic part is lowered and at the same time "tipped backwards". The posterior urethra is therefore less vertical. The degree of deformity varies with the intensity of intra-abdominal pressure during micturition.

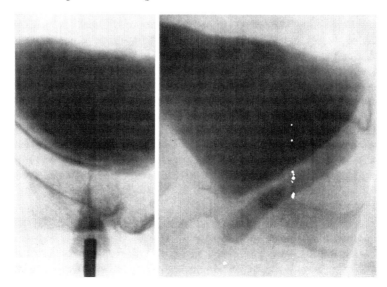

Fig. 39. Female with the vagina opening into the posterior urethra. The vagina became filled during micturition (right figure)

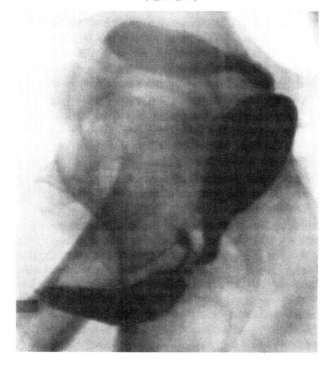

Fig. 40. Intersex-malformation with short anterior urethra of male type and a vagina with uterus opening into the posterior urethra

2. Developmental anomalies of the urethra

In epispadias, the posterior urethra forms the floor of the fissure. In hypospadias, the lower aspect of the anterior urethra is split to a varying degree, and difficulties may be encountered in introducing the instrument for injection.

The developmental anomalies of intersex nature which involve the urethra appear as an abnormal vaginal formation from the Müllerian ducts and their caudal continuation. Normally, a remnant of the Müllerian ducts is present in the male, in the form of the masculine utricle, a small blind sac behind the upper part of the colliculus, ending on the top of it. Unless urethritis is or has been present, the utricle is not filled at urethrography. In female hermaphrodites, the vagina and urethra may merge below the external sphincter region into the anterior urethra (Figs. 39 and 40). In the male, a medially situated diverticulum is sometimes

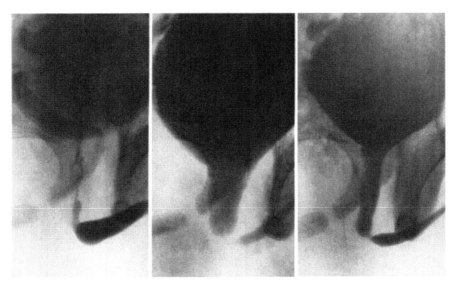

Fig. 41. Infracollicular valve in the posterior urethra appearing during micturition (mid figure). After resection of the valve the micturition is normal (right figure)

present on the underside of the posterior part of the anterior urethra; it is considered likely to be a distal vaginal primordium. On the other hand, bilateral diverticula-like formations in this region, or a single diverticulum on one side of the midline, are regarded as belonging to the excretory ducts of Cowper's glands.

In foetuses and children, sail-shaped congenital impediments may be present at the level of the colliculus. They are discovered only during micturition, when they unfold like a valve, and cause a varying degree of urinary obstruction (Fig. 41).

An ectopic ureter may open into the posterior urethra, and is often not opacified until micturition (Fig. 42; cf. Ureterocele).

3. Positional changes of the urethra

A change in position of the posterior urethra may be brought about by pathologic conditions in its surroundings. As a rule, it is a question of expansion, inflammatory processes or a tumour of the prostate. Acute Cowperitis may produce inappreciable displacement in the region of the external sphincter. Generalized oedema of the small pelvis stretches and elongates the posterior urethra. Scarring after acute inflammatory processes or operations (e.g. for rectal carcinoma) may also cause deviations of the urethral lumen.

4. Traumatic lesions of the urethra

The portion of the urethra with the strongest fixation to the pelvis is the region of the external sphincter. Its outer voluntary fibres—which chiefly sweep

backwards in a horseshoe-shape around the lower end of the posterior urethra—are
to some extent interlaced with other striated muscles in the pelvic floor, with
smooth muscles surrounding the urethra and with the connective tissue delimiting
the urogenital diaphragm and the fascial coverings of the obturator muscles.

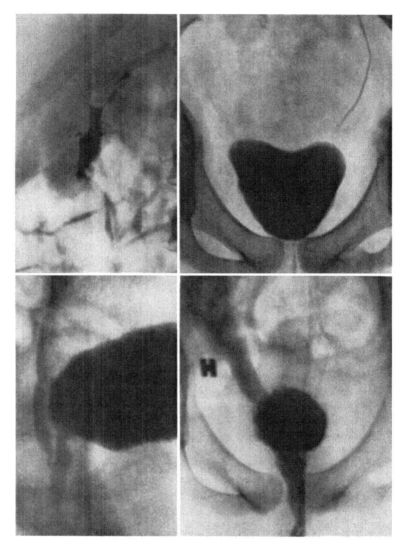

Fig. 42. Ectopic ureter opening into the posterior urethra appearing during micturition (lower figures). The
upper pole of right kidney was previously resected because of an infected hydronephrosis of an upper kidney pelvis

Consequently, a fracture of the anterior part of the pelvis is apt to lead to a lesion
of the urethra in this segment, often in the form of total rupture. In the acute
stage, the urethrogram shows a leakage of contrast medium into the pelvic tissue
below the prostate which is lifted upwards (Figs. 43 and 44). At a later stage, the
change is in the form of a short, irregular stricture, this segment of the urethra
often having a Z-shaped course. A false passage is a not infrequent outcome (Figs. 45
and 46).

Traumatic changes due to external violence also occur, *e.g.* in the form of a perineal contusion or pole injury, which may lead to rupture and subsequent stricture of the posterior portion of the anterior urethra (Fig. 47).

Instrumental damage is described under the heading of urethral stricture.

5. Inflammatory changes in the urethra

Urethrography should not be performed in acute urethritis, but gives often important informations in more chronic stages. Inflammation of the urethra — like that of other mucous membranes — leads in the first place to swelling of the mucosa, visible roentgenologically as a coarsening of its folds (Figs. 48 and 49). In posterior urethritis, the folds in the supracollicular region are broader than usual. In the collicular region—around the orifices of the prostatic and ejaculatory ducts—swelling of the mucosa often causes the grooves at the sides of the colliculus to be narrowed, or even obliterated. The surface of the mucous membrane, especially on the colliculus, may be finely or more coarsely granulated—even inflammatory pseudopolyps may be seen.

Scarring and shrinking causes the orifices of the prostatic ducts to be insufficient to the reflux of contrast medium, whereas the ejaculatory ducts and the utricle, which are surrounded by pseudocavernous tissue, are more able to withstand it. Reflux into the Cowperian ducts is considerably less common than reflux into the prostatic ducts. Filling of small, paraurethral

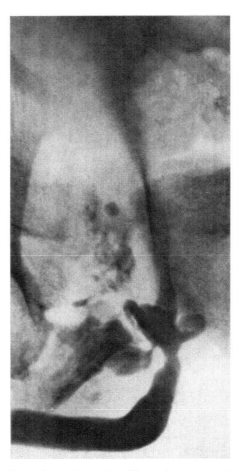

Fig. 43. Incomplete rupture of the urethra in a case of pelvic fracture. Beside leakage into the pelvic tissue dye has passed into the posterior urethra and the bladder

glandular ducts in the anterior urethra may occur, on the same grounds as reflux into the prostatic ducts. All demonstrable contrast filling of paraurethral ducts and cavities is thus a sign of chronic inflammation.

Irritation of the posterior urethra produced by urethritis leads to an increased urge to micturate, while dysuria with burning or pain is caused by anterior urethritis. This explains why—despite the fact that the bladder is often hypertonic, and is in constant readiness for micturition—this is frequently interrupted before the bladder is emptied. The result is often residual urine, demonstrable roentgenologically even before injection of contrast medium. This also explains why the external sphincter region often presents greater resistance than normally to both retrograde injection and micturition, although no stricture exist. In cinematography, this urethritic spasm of the external sphincter is visible as jerky contractions interrupting micturition, whereas the posterior urethra above the stricture is more dilated than usual (Figs. 48 and 98). The smooth muscle does not, on the contrary, seem to partake in this spasm.

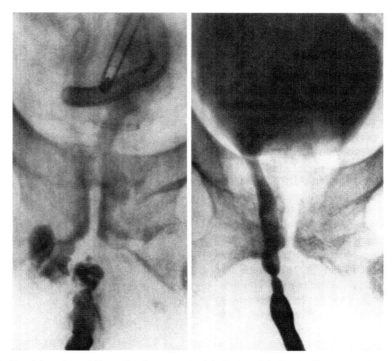

Fig. 44. Complete rupture of the urethra in a case of pelvic fracture (left figure). Non-successful suture, and healing with a false passage outside the external sphincter, consequently with incontinence (right figure)

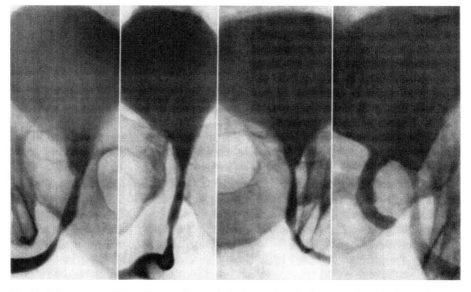

Fig. 45. False passage with incontinence after pelvic fracture and urethral rupture. In right figure, the true posterior urethra is visualized during micturition

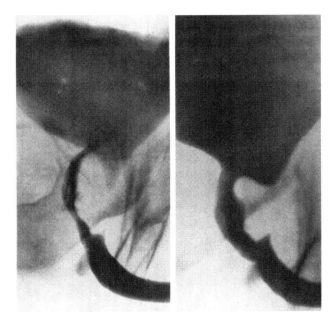

Fig. 46. Same case as in Fig. 45 after reconstruction of the urethra in the region of the external sphincter. Healed with continence

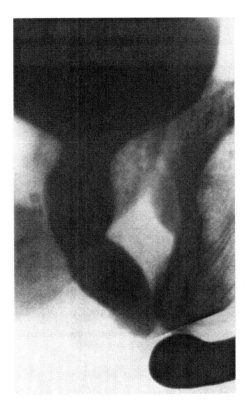

Fig. 47. Complete urethral stricture from a pole injury of the perineum. Anterior urethra is filled by retrograde injection, posterior urethra by urography and attempt to micturate

26*

In the anterior urethra, chronic urethritis and its sequels produce decreased distensibility, *i.e.*, some degree of stricturition which initially can be identified only on retrograde filling, but which in more advanced cases is a cause of urinary impediment.

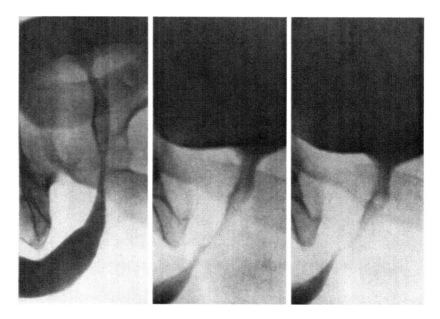

Fig. 48. Acute posterior urethritis. External sphincter spasm during micturition (right figures)

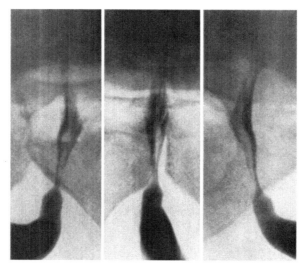

Fig. 49. Thick folds in supracollicular part of posterior urethra as sign of urethritis in case with prostatitis and utriculitis with hemospermia

6. Urethral stricture

Congenital valves in the posterior urethra have already been described in connexion with developmental anomalies, and the strictures resulting from pelvic injuries under the heading of traumatic changes. It remains to account for the two common forms of stricture, *i.e.*, that appearing after urethritis, and that due to instrumental damage. For so-called sclerosis of the bladder neck, reference

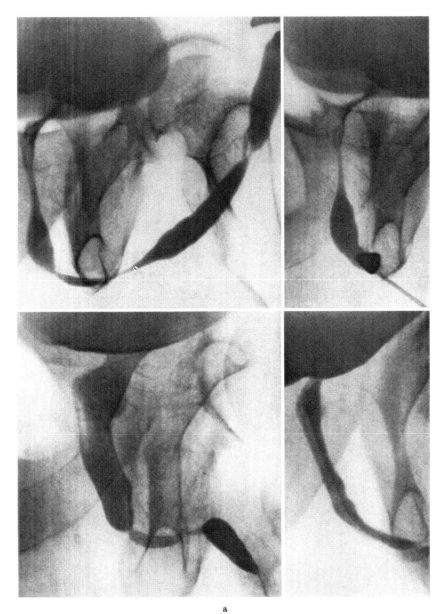

a

Fig. 50 a and b. Strictures of the anterior urethra, both at the base of the penis and at the opening of the Cowper ducts, visualized by reflux. Upper figures, during retrograde injection; lower figures, during micturition. a To the left, before operation, to the right, after perineal urethrostomy, b (following page) after reconstruction and recurrence of stricture proximal to the earlier ones

is made to the section on the prostate gland. This also applies to strictures developing after interventions on the prostate.

Posturethritic and instrumental post-traumatic strictures involve the anterior urethra. The posturethritic are of two kinds, *i.e.*, a short stricture of valvular nature, and the elongated processes that generally extend more deeply, as an indication that cavernitis has also been present (Fig. 50). The strictures produced by instrumental injury are, as a rule, of the latter type. The valvular strictures

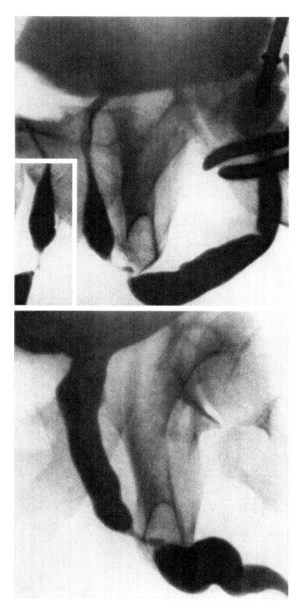

Fig. 50 b

are essentially confined to the bulbous part, whereas the elongated processes are further forward, and sometimes involve the whole anterior urethra.

The retrograde phase of the urethrocystogram provides information about the nature and extent of the stricture, and the micturition studies allow visualization of the degree to which the stricture produces urinary obstruction. During micturition, prestenotic dilatation of the whole urethra takes place. This is often accompanied by filling of the duct system of the prostate. The appearance of the

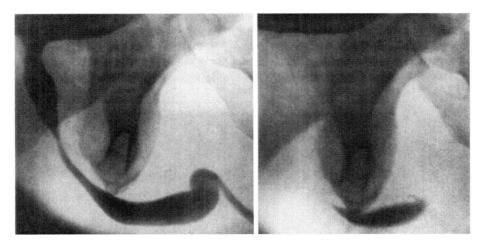

Fig. 51. Strangulating effect of the suspensory ligament of the penis during micturition (left figure) causing residual urine in the urethra after micturition (right figure). After learning to empty his urethra by manual pressing the patient was free from after-drip

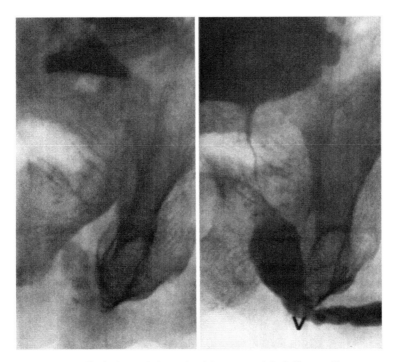

Fig. 52. Urethral stone in front of serial strictures of the bulbous portion

bladder is also helpful for conclusions regarding the degree and duration of a stricture. This is because a considerable urinary impediment of long duration results in the formation of trabeculae and diverticulae of the bladder.

Even if a stricture does not produce any definite impediment to urinary outflow, it can unquestionably hinder erection and even ejaculation. The data provided by the micturition pictures are confined to the conditions on micturition.

If a highly irritant contrast medium in strong concentration is used at urethrography, it may lead to such damage that a secondary stricture arises. With the contrast media in use nowadays for urography, this risk does not exist, provided that moderate concentrations are used, and the medium is not in contact with the mucosa for longer than is necessary (cf. Urethrocystographic technique).

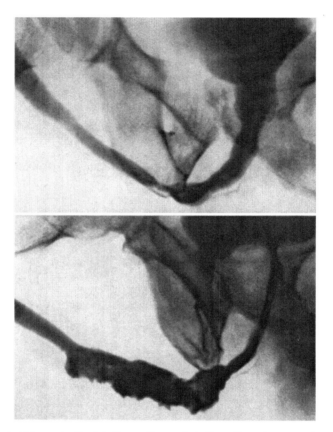

Fig. 53. Urethral stricture and reflux into the one Cowper duct. Lower figure, two years after reconstruction, an irregular lumen from hair and epithelial desquamation

During micturition, tension of the ligamentum suspensorium penis may cause a functional stricture, which can give rise to dribbling, when the small amount of residual urine stagnating behind it in the bulbar part is emptied after the end of micturition (Fig. 51).

7. Stones and foreign bodies in the urethra

An ejected ureteric calculus may become arrested in the urethra, either above the external sphincter or at the site of a stricture (Fig. 52). After partial prostatectomy, a prostatic stone may pass into the urethra. Reconstruction of the anterior urethra is not infrequently followed by the formation of a foreign body —composed of desquamated epithelium and hair—in the urethra, usually at the level of the neck of the scrotum (Fig. 53). In rare cases, such a body may become partly calcified; otherwise, it is visible only as a filling defect in the urethra.

8. Tumours of the urethra

Primary tumours of the urethra are rare. As a rule, they consist of a papilloma or a benign polyp (Figs. 54 and 55). Small polyp-like formations of inflammatory

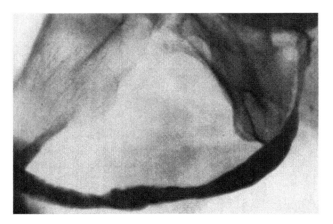

Fig. 54. Papilloma of the anterior urethra

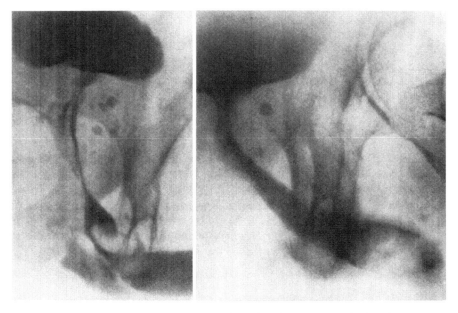

Fig. 55. Tumour of the bulbus portion of the urethra; the tumour was a benign polyp

origin are occasionally observed in chronic urethritis, especially around the colliculus.

A vesical papilloma not uncommonly extends into the posterior urethra, and a large part of the urethra may occasionally be involved. The extent of spreading is easily established at urethrography. Malignant papilloma or squamous cell carcinoma of the urethra is rare but the latter may occur in a chronic stricture.

It is not unusual for carcinoma of the prostate to grow in the form of a small-nodulated mass into the posterior urethra, usually at the colliculus and its immediate surroundings and even small nodules of benign hypertrophy may cause rounded defects in the contrast contour in the same region.

9. Urethral fistulas

A fistula extending towards the perineum may develop in inflamed prostatic tissue with cavity formation, particularly in tuberculosis of the prostate. A fistula from the anterior urethra, on the other hand, is associated with severe urethritis, usually of gonorrhoeal nature. Such fistular systems are opacified at urethro-

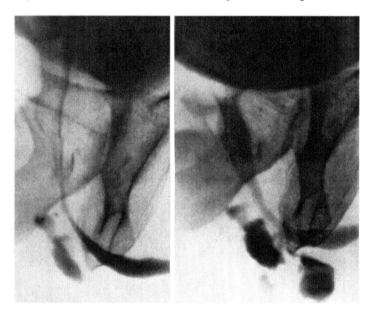

Fig. 56. Perineal fistula following gonorrhoic urethritis and cowperitis with abscess

cystography, when their topography can be determined. In the latter type of fistula, this can be done by retrograde filling, whereas the former can sometimes be identified only in micturition studies (Fig. 56).

A fistula can also develop between the urethra and rectum, most commonly after total prostatectomy. Injection of contrast medium into the rectum, in addition to micturition urethrography, may be required for visualization of such fistulas.

10. The prostate and prostatic utricle: normal anatomy

Although the prostate gland is not directly visible on the roentgenogram, much indirect information can be obtained about changes in this organ. This information consists both of the presence of prostatic concretions, and of the passage of contrast medium from the urethra into the prostatic ducts and other cavities. In addition, particularly valuable information is provided by the way in which the urethra and the bladder floor are deformed by pathologic processes of the prostate.

In order to understand the urethrocystographic features of such processes, it is necessary to be acquainted with the structure of the prostate (Fig. 57). The major portion of its glandular tissue lies behind the urethra, extending from the bladder floor to the external sphincter. Only the lower part of the gland surrounds the urethra like a horseshoe from behind, but its anterior mass is relatively slight, and sometimes does not reach the midline in front of the urethra. All the associated

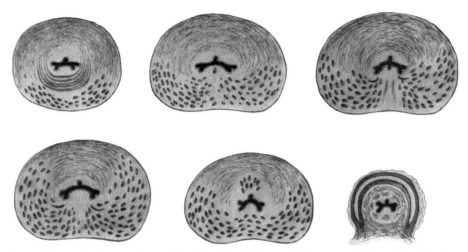

Fig. 57. Topographic diagrams from serial sections through the prostate transverse to the urethra, from the bladder neck to the external sphincter. Anterior direction upwards in the figures

glandular orifices in the urethra lie in the paracollicular grooves and their continuations caudad along the crista urethralis. The openings of a few short ducts belonging to an exceedingly small anterior primordium of the prostate are,

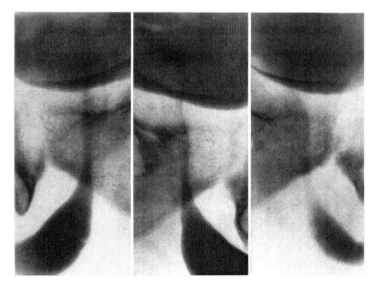

Fig. 58. Acute prostatitis causing obliteration of mucosal folds and collicular sulci

however, present furthest down in the prostatic part of the urethra. The upper part of the posterior urethra is surrounded on the ventral side by smooth muscle and connective tissue devoid of prostatic glands. On the dorsal side, the uppermost portion of the urethra is separated from the prostatic glands by powerful smooth musculature.   A considerable part thereof form a transverse sphincter, which surrounds the lumen from behind, and in the anterior direction merges

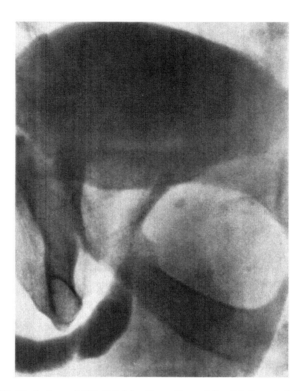

Fig. 59. Acute prostatitis dislodging the urethra and the utriculus anteriorly

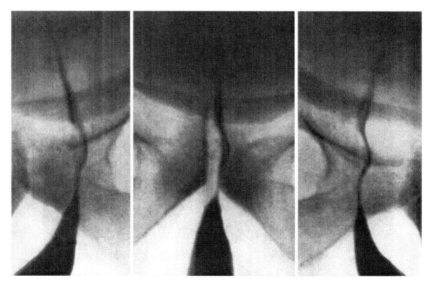

Fig. 60. Obliteration of the right paracollicular sulcus from acute prostatitis in the right lobe

with the fibromuscular tissue present at this site. This sphincter (M. sphincter internus) has an important sexual function, shutting of the urethra from the bladder at erection and ejaculation. The submucosa contains small paraurethral glands, and an often highly developed vascular network, resembling a thin layer of cavernous tissue.

The normal prostatic utricle is a slit-shaped cavity behind the superior portion of the colliculus. The ejaculatory ducts run forwards and downwards through the prostatic tissue into the colliculus, like slender tubes (Fig. 115).

In view of the position of the prostatic glands proper, the essential result of an expansile process in this region is a ventral displacement of the urethral lumen (and a constriction from behind). A unilateral expansile process is able,

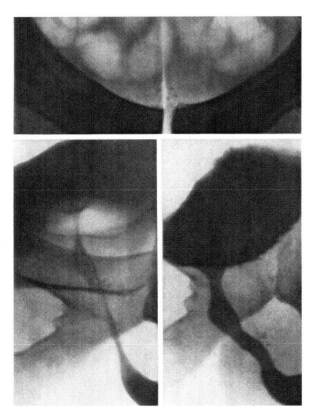

Fig. 61. Urethra dislodged anteriorly by acute prostatitis in the main portion of the gland. Concretions and openstanding ducts in the anterior lobe as sign of chronic prostatitis

in addition, to displace the lumen to one side, particularly in the apical part of the prostate. In fibromuscular hypertrophy, on the contrary, the main bulk usually lies anterior to (and beside) the upper half of the posterior urethra and at its sides, but may also be localized dorsally, directly beneath the floor of the bladder.

Anatomical details and pathological features regarding the seminal vesicles are described in VIII.

11. Prostatic calculi

Prostatic calculi may provide both diagnostic and topographic information. The latter applies particularly when calculi are present in large parts of the glandular tissue, and this is displaced by an expansive process. In hypertrophy of the prostate, the stones frame the lower pole of the fibroadenomatous masses. When there is an expansile process in the region of the prostate, carcinoma, an abscess or a large cyst, it is, on the contrary, more or less surrounded by the calculi.

Which pathologic conditions of the prostate are reflected by the presence of calculi is a difficult question to answer. Large stones are an indication of dilated ducts and cavities which are always an expression of inflammatory processes. Large

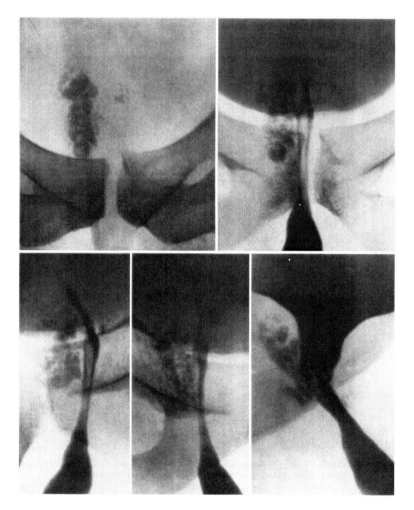

Fig. 62. Chronic prostatitis with concretions in widened ducts in the lateral lobes and in the anterior one

stonefilled cavities in the prostate are seen particularly in tuberculosis. Retention of secretion and inflammatory changes are often present behind small stones in the prostatic ducts, and thus a sign of chronic prostatitis. Whether or not this prostatitis is of clinical importance cannot, however, be determined by the mere presence of calculi but as the treatment and prognosis of prostato-vesiculitis is influenced thereof such findings on roentgenograms should always be pointed out.

12. Prostatitis

Prostatitis and seminal vesiculitis are usually combined and from a clinical point of view they should always be discussed together. However, as contrast studies of the seminal vesicles are described in VIII both anatomical and pathological data are gathered there.

Prostatitis leads to a varying degree of swelling of the glandular parts of the prostate, which affects the shape, length and position of the posterior urethra (Figs. 58—67). Generalized swelling elongates and stretches the posterior urethra.

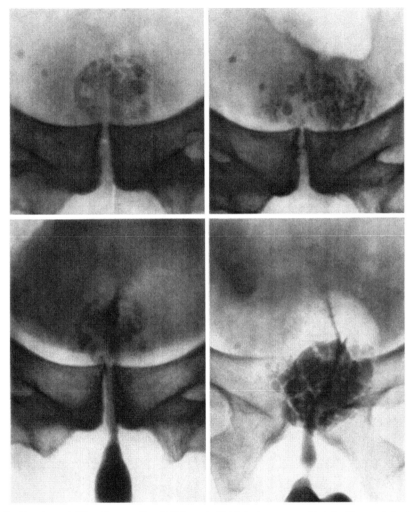

Fig. 63. Chronic prostatitis with concretions (left figures) which later became complicated with a prostatic abscess dislodging the concretions and the urethra (right figures)

With moderate swelling, its course is straight instead of having a curvature, concave forwards, and in the most pronounced cases it has a backward concavity, particularly conspicuous in exposures during micturition (Fig. 59). Unilateral swelling produces displacement of the lumen in the lateral direction, or more often ventrolaterally towards the healthy side or the side with more chronic, not acute exudative changes. Lateral displacement occurs chiefly in the collicular and infracollicular part, due to the fact that appreciable amount of glandular tissue on the lateral aspect of the urethra is present mostly in this region. Extremely marked lateral displacement can be observed when a prostatic abscess is present (Fig. 63).

The swollen prostatic tissue obliterates the grooves around the colliculus and below it, so that they, especially the contours of the colliculus, are less conspicuous than usual, blurred or completely lacking. A contributory factor is

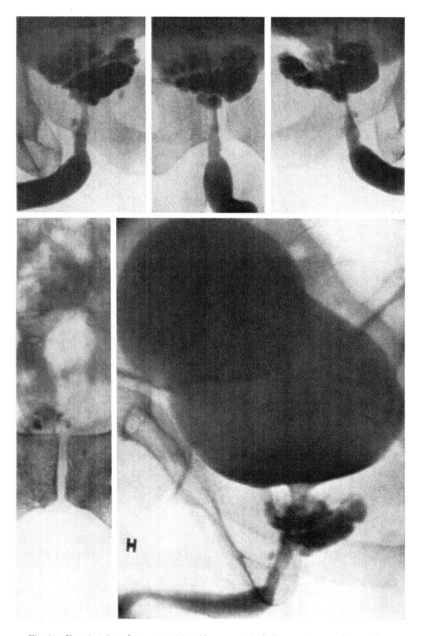

Fig. 64. Chronic tuberculous prostatitis with comparatively large cavities and concretions

local swelling of the urethral mucosa at the orifices of the glands, the ejaculatory ducts and the utriculus as an expression of local posterior urethritis (Fig. 58).

Since posterior urethritis and prostatitis (and seminal vesiculitis) usually are associated conditions, the signs of urethritis described earlier are found in a large number of cases of prostatitis. The tendency of the urethritic process to cause the orifices of the prostatic glands to remain open produces reflux of the urethral contents into the prostatic ducts. Although such spontaneous filling of the ducts

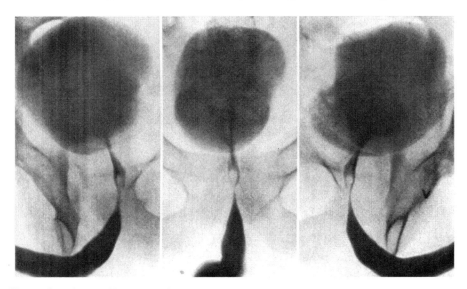

Fig. 65. Case of reumatoid arthritis and acute prostato-vesiculitis elevating the bladder with broad impressions level with the ureters

at urethrography is, strictly speaking, a feature of urethritis, it can in actual fact also be regarded as an expression of prostatitis. In many cases, contrast medium does not pass from the urethra into large cavities in the prostate, since they are in the nature of retention cysts. The contrast filling of prostatic ducts and cavities is, however, often facilitated by stripping of stagnating prostatic secretion just before the roentgen examination.

13. Dilatation of the prostatic utricle. — Utriculitis and haemospermia

When the prostatic utricle is large and dilated—more than $1^1/_2$ cm in length—its active drainage is impaired and its secretions is therefore not completely emtied. Acute posterior urethritis and prostato-vesiculitis usually engage the utricle. The risk of relapse of these diseases is therefore increased in patients with a large utricle. Thus a large utricle is relatively often found in patients with chronic prostato-vesiculitis. Symptoms indicating this state are recurring discharge

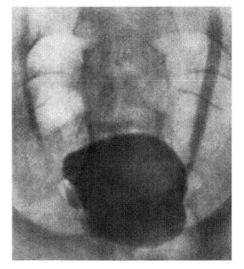

Fig. 66. Same case as in Fig. 65. Urography reveals in addition to the bladder deformity a mild stasis in the ureters

(especially discharge and/or a burning urethral sensation at defecation), prostatorrhea, haemospermia or terminal haematuria, slow micturition alternating with normal (depending on whether the utricle is distended or empty).

A dilated prostatic utricle causes expansion also of the posterior urethral wall in front of it, above the colliculus (Fig. 68). Instead of having a narrow crista between two parallel grooves, the posterior wall has a broad elevation with the grooves displaced laterally. The margin of the elevation towards the colliculus may be indistinct, so that one has the impression of a broad upper continuation of the colliculus. An utricle that has undergone a change of this kind and is causing urogenital symptoms is relatively seldom in such open communication with the urethra that it is filled with contrast at urethrography. When this does occur, it is more

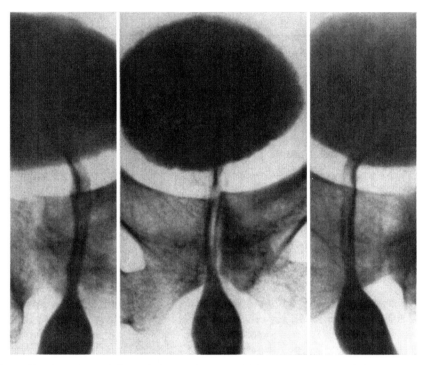

Fig. 67. Chronic prostato-vesiculitis on the left side elevating the bladder and dislocating the bladder neck anteriorly and to the right

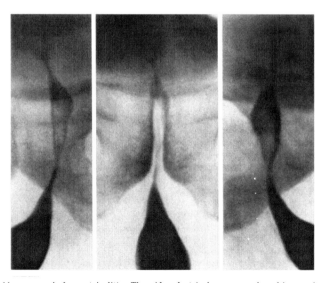

Fig. 68. Case of hemospermia from utriculitis. The widened utriculus causes a broad impression appearing as a cranial continuation of the colliculus. A left-sided acute cowperitis causes a lateral impression of the membranous portion, while on the right side the Cowper duct becomes filled as sign of chronic Cowperitis

common during micturition than during retrograde filling and the contrast fluid is then usually retained after the micturition, indicating incomplete emptying capacity.

The suspicion as to a large utricle ought to be aroused by such findings as a low seminal collicle (usually situated apically in the prostate), which often is large and broad, while the supracollicular portion of the urethra is long and the bladder neck often narrow. Further signs are that the urethral lumen immediately supracollicularly is very wide, especially when the contour is bulging dorsolaterally. This is not atrophy, but increased dilating capacity, caused by a primary defect of the prostatic parenchyma. Such a picture is combined with typical changes found at rectal palpation; pressure produces emptying of a large volume of thin secretion and reveals a sharply-defined dimple in the centre of the prostate, which can in marked cases reach right up to the base of the prostate, the central part of which is un-developed. Chronic inflammation both in the prostate and the seminal vesicles may, however, blur the edges of the dimple and make the judgement difficult.

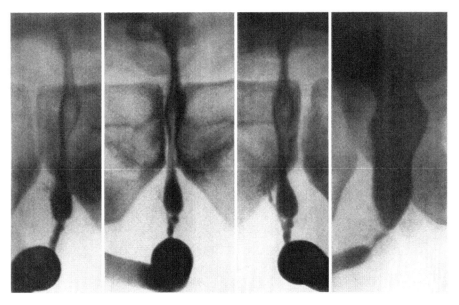

Fig. 69. Chronic cowperitis with reflux into the ducts and stricture of the urethra adjacent to the openings of the Cowper ducts

The utricle can be contrast-filled with a catheter using a urethroscope—see VIII. The ejaculatory ducts seldom open into the utricle—primarily or even secondarily due to inflam-matory destruction of the thin wall between them. (Fig. 119 and 120.) With normal sepa-ration of the ejaculatory ducts and the utricle infection from stagnating secretions may, however, spread through the walls, causing vesiculitis and epididymitis (Fig. 120).

A large utricle is found in developmental anomalies of intersex nature, sometimes also in hypospadia and nocturnal enuresis but most often without such anomalies. A totally blocked utricle may appear as a very large cyst between the bladder floor and the rectum.

A dilated big prostatic utricle is generally the site of inflammation, *i.e.*, utriculitis. This is not unusual in association with posterior urethritis and prostato-vesiculitis (Figs. 59 and 72), but may occur as an isolated phenomenon, especially in chronic essential haemospermia. Haemospermia is a frequent symptom of utriculitis; consequently, when it is present, particular attention should be focused on the region of the prostatic utricle.

14. Cowperitis

In acute Cowperitis, the swelling may cause a shallow impression in the urethra, at the level of the membranous part (Fig. 68). It may, however, be difficult to determine whether a displacement is to be ascribed to unilateral expansion in the apex of the prostate, or to Cowperitis. In occasional cases of chronic Cowperitis, calcifications may be present in the gland.

The changes in Cowper's glands most often seen on the urethrocystogram are of a chronic nature, in the form of reflux of contrast medium into one or both excretory ducts, sometimes as far as the region of the gland itself (Fig. 69). The excretory duct not infrequently has a slightly irregular outline, and is often dilated in the immediate vicinity of the urethra. If, on the contrary, the duct ends anteriorly in a true sac or pouch on the underside of the urethra, there is reason to interpret it as a malformation.

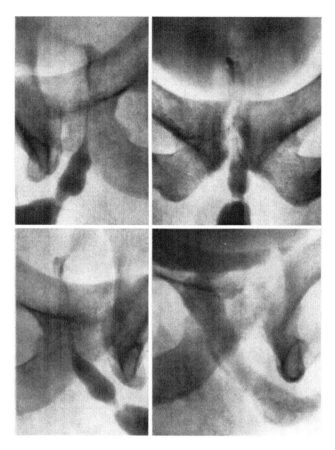

Fig. 70. Chronic inflammatory complex: urethritis, prostato-vesiculitis, bladder neck sclerosis, urethral stricture and destructions in the symphysis

In cases of chronic Cowperitis, a stricture of the urethra is generally present at the level of the opening of the Cowperian ducts. For this reason, strictures at this site are presumably a result of the chronic irritation produced by the underlying Cowperitis.

15. The inflammatory complex of the urethra and its adnexa. — Pelvospondylitis and symphysitis

In reality, the inflammatory changes in the posterior urethra and its surroundings are not limited to one segment or to a single gland, but appear concurrently in various combinations, merely with greater severity in one or the other region (see also VIII). Moreover, an inflammatory reaction in the bones or joints is present in many cases, manifested as a rheumatoid disease. Consequently, there is reason to speak of an inflammatory complex.

As a rule, such an inflammatory complex has the following components: slight residual urine in the bladder, a coarse or granulated mucosal relief in the posterior urethra, and groups of small prostatic calculi. In addition, there is often reflux from the urethra to prostatic ducts, a raised bladder floor owing to vesiculitis, urethral stricture—particularly at the openings of the Cowperian

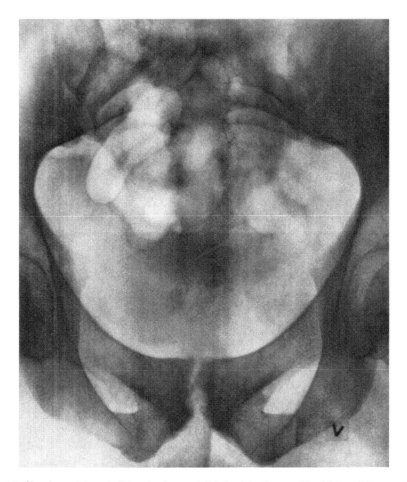

Fig. 71. Chronic prostato-vesiculitis and pelvospondylitis involving the sacroiliac joints and the symphysis

ducts, possibly with filling of these ducts—and some degree of sclerosis of the bone around the symphysis pubis (Fig. 70). More sporadic findings are *e.g.* bladder-neck obstruction and a trabeculated bladder with a thickened wall, with or without diverticula, and the signs of utriculitis described earlier. In the acute stage, the most conspicuous features are swelling of the prostate and seminal-vesicle regions, with its effect on the urethra and bladder, and often a tendency to spasm of the external sphincter, appearing on micturition.

Of importance in this connexion are the rheumatoid complications, particularly pelvospondylitis ossificans (= Ankylosing spondylitis) (Figs. 71 and 72). The roentgenologic changes appear only in the subacute or chronic stage. They then consist initially of erosion of the sacroiliac joints and anterior margins of the vertebrae, in the latter case giving the spine an appearance of having been planed off anteriorly. Erosions also appear at other sites, especially in the symphysis pubis, the manubrio-sternal synchondrosis, the sternoclavicular and acromio-clavicular joints, and in the insertions of various tendons and muscles.

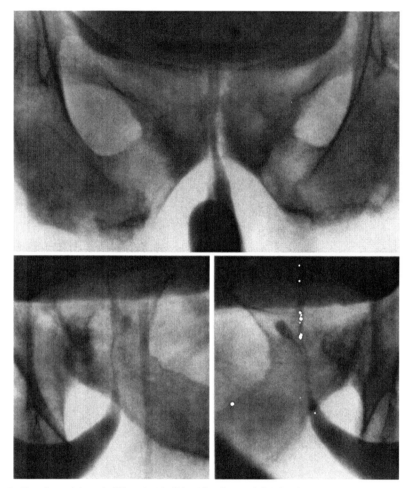

Fig. 72. Chronic prostato-vesiculitis and utriculitis with pelvospondylitis involving also the symphysis and the tubera ischii

Destructive arthritis is sometimes present in one or both hip joints. Sclerosis gradually takes place around the erosions, as well as ossification of granulation tissue, adjactheent to ligaments—so-called syndesmophytes. In the spine, the appearance of these syndesmophytes on the surfaces of the intervertebral discs is a relatively early manifestation. The end result is usually synostosis in the sacroiliac joints and in large segments of the spine, which—due to overgrowth of the syndesmophytes—resembles a bamboo stem.

Relatively more common than this fully developed pelvospondylitis are local changes in the symphysis pubis, in the form of sclerosis, with or without sub-chondral erosions (Fig. 73). In the individual case, this may be impossible to distinguish from the normal state; in this event, the changes can, in fact, be disclosed only by means of serial pictures showing the development. Sclerosis of the symphysis seems to be essentially associated with chronic urethritis and prostatitis. The osteitis of the symphysis which may be a sequel of prostatectomy (Fig. 74) is well-known; it usually regresses spontaneously, and is relatively asymptomatic. Urethritis in the female may also be accompanied by local changes in the symphysis pubis of the same nature as in the male (Fig. 75).

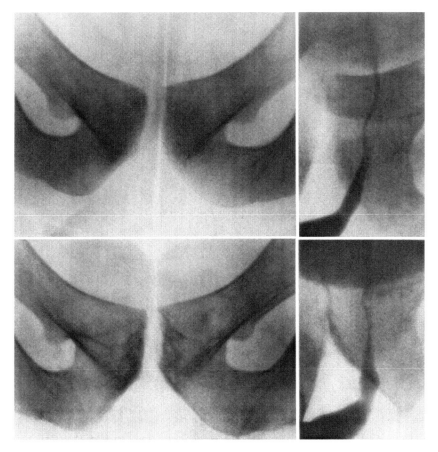

Fig. 73. Destructions appearing in the symphysis in a case of prostatitis. Six years between the upper and the lower figures

16. Tumours of the prostate

Like other tumours, it lies in the nature of a prostatic tumour to expand, and in carcinoma of the prostate, this expansion takes place primarily in the regions where glandular tissue is present (Fig. 76). On principle, this expansion should produce the same displacement of the urethral lumen on the urethrocystogram as prostatitis. In actual fact, it is more difficult to identify in carcinoma of the prostate, possibly because in prostatitis the urethrographic changes are accentuated by coincident urethritis. Thus, experience shows that deformity of the urethra is a relatively late sign in carcinoma of the prostate, as compared to the palpatory findings. An exception is a carcinoma of such extent that it spreads towards the urethra at an early stage, producing small-nodular tumour masses bulging into the urethral lumen, usually at the colliculus and directly above it (Figs. 77 and 78).

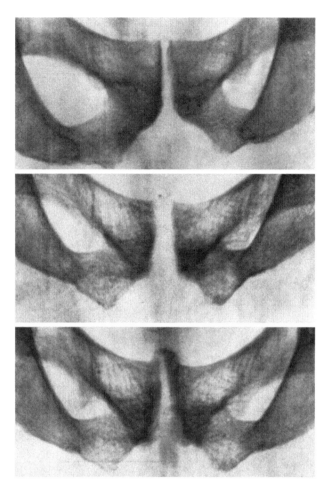

Fig. 74. Destruction in the symphysis after suprapubic prostatectomy. Upper figure before operation: normal. Mid figure two months after operation: destruction. Lower figure four months after operation: healing

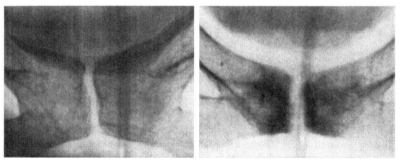

Fig. 75. Destruction in the symphysis in a case of urethritis with rheumatoid arthritis in a virgin female. Four years between the figures

The possibilities of roentgenologic diagnosis are enhanced by vasography, since the expansile process may displace and block the ejaculatory ducts (see VIII. Figs. 124—127).

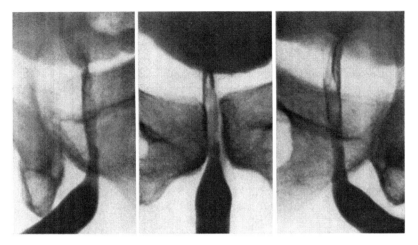

Fig. 76. Prostatic carcinoma expanding the one lobe in the region of the glands

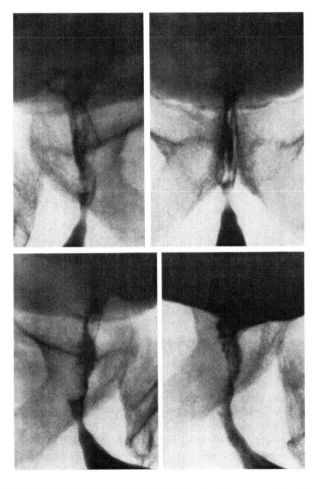

Fig. 77. Prostatic carcinoma growing into the urethral lumen as small nodules

When a carcinoma breaks through the prostatic capsule and extends into the pelvic tissue, it is apt to lift the bladder floor on the affected side. The adjacent ureter may also be involved, with urinary stasis as a result. The rectal wall may also be invaded with eventual intestinal obstruction, but ulceration of the rectal mucosa is very rare.

The combination of carcinoma and hypertrophy of the prostate is a common one. In typical cases, a postero-inferior impression is seen as an expression of

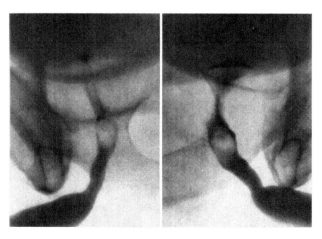

Fig. 78. Prostatic carcinoma growing into the region of the colliculus

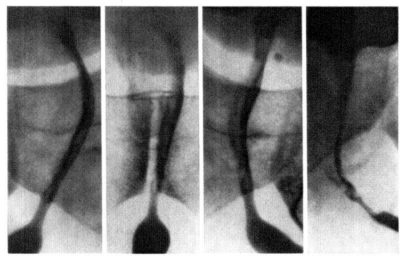

Fig. 79. Prostatic hypertrophy and carcinoma. Supracollicular expansion anteriorly on the right side from an asymmetric hypertrophy. Infracollicular expansion of the right lobe with carcinomatous growth into the urethra

carcinoma, together with bilateral anterosuperior compression due to hypertrophy (Fig. 79). As a rule, the predominant features are those of hypertrophy.

Myosarcoma of the prostate (Fig. 80) is rare, and it is impossible to recapitulate its urethrocystographic features.

The presence of skeletal metastases is of great practical importance in the diagnosis of carcinoma of the prostate. The metastases occur both in the usual osteosclerotic form, and in an osteolytic form. They are often amenable to hormone therapy (Fig. 81).

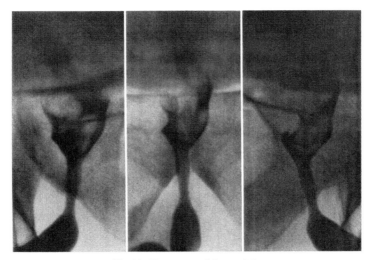

Fig. 80. Myosarcoma of the prostate

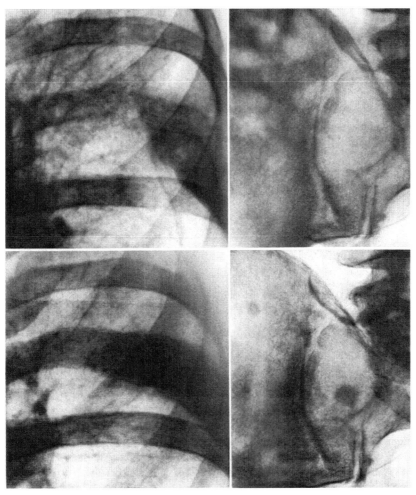

Fig. 81. Metastases of prostatic carcinoma. The original osteolysis (upper figures) was replaced by an osteosclerosis after hormonal treatment (lower figures)

17. Hypertrophy of the prostate

Since the fibroadenomatous proliferation takes place chiefly above the glands of the prostate, it results in an increase in the distance between them and the bladder floor. On the urethrocystogram, this is seen as an elongation of the supracollicular portion of the posterior urethra. The elongation is not, however,

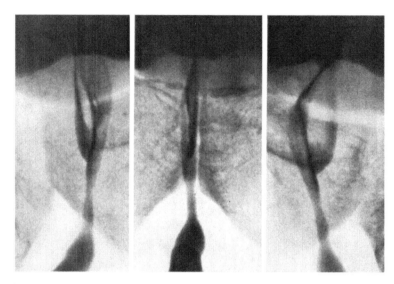

Fig. 82. Prostatic hypertrophy. The ventro-lateral expansion in the supracollicular region makes the urethra lumen Y-shaped in cross sections

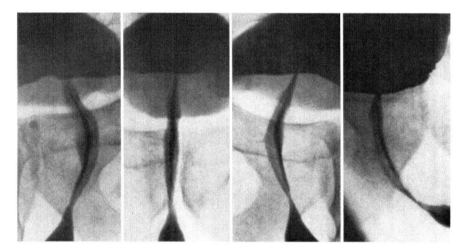

Fig. 83. Prostatic hypertrophy appearing as a diffuse hyperplasia along the entire posterior urethra

confined to the longitudinal axis of the urethra, but takes place sagitally as well, in view of the proliferation on both sides of the urethral lumen. The normally shallow anterior groove in the supracollicular portion is then converted into a sagittally-directed slit, often more than a centimetre deep. There is concurrent backward displacement of the lateral grooves of the urethra. The normal T-shape of the cross-section of the lumen in this region is replaced by a Y-shape, the elongated lower limb of the Y representing the ventral groove. It is this feature in particular which makes the urethrocystogram characteristic in hypertrophy of the prostate (Figs. 82—84). If the hypertrophy is not completely symmetric,

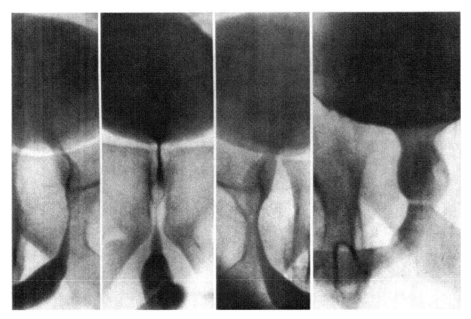

Fig. 84. Prostatic hypertrophy with typical deformity of the supracollicular portion of the urethra. The micturition reveals that the hindrance is a stricture of the anterior urethra

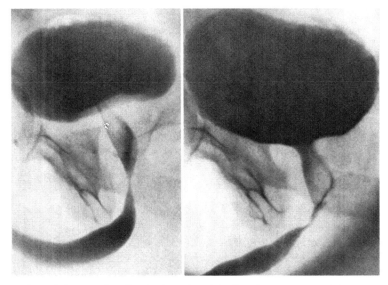

Fig. 85. Prostatic hypertrophy. The plugging effect of the fibroadenomas appears during micturition

lateral displacement is superadded, but the difference between the two sides is usually inappreciable.

If dorsal hyperplasia is present, it lies in the midline at the urethral orifice in the bladder, resulting in the development of a so-called third lobe. This condition also has a characteristic appearance on the urethrocystogram, *i.e.*, in the form of a half-spherical protrusion dorsally into the urethral orifice and bladder floor (Fig. 86). Lateral and dorsal proliferation are not infrequently combined. In marked cases, the bladder floor with the ureteric orifices is displaced so far upwards that the lumen of the urethra and bladder have the shape of an umbrella.

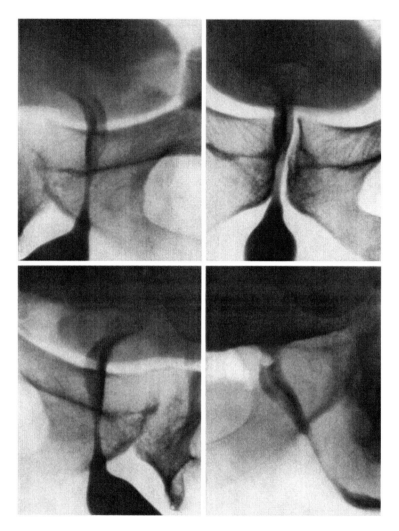

Fig. 86. Prostatic hypertrophy with a posterior lobe prolabating during micturition

The classical features of hypertrophy of the prostate generally include trabeculation of the bladder, and not infrequently vesical diverticula as well, as a sign of long-standing urinary obstruction. The way in which this impediment to emptying arises can be illustrated in early cases by exposures during micturition. They show that the inward bulging fibroadenoma is to some extent forced downwards in the urethra, with an evident blocking effect, due to its acting as a ball-valve (Figs. 85 and 86). It has not been possible to establish to what extent this also applies in advanced cases. Even after operation, the adenomas—or their remnants—may play a role as an impediment to urinary outflow (Figs. 87 and 88).

Hypertrophy of the prostate is not seldom combined with other complaints. Retention of urine in the bladder favours the development of cystitis. Vesical calculi are another frequent complication. Prostatitis and hypertrophy of the

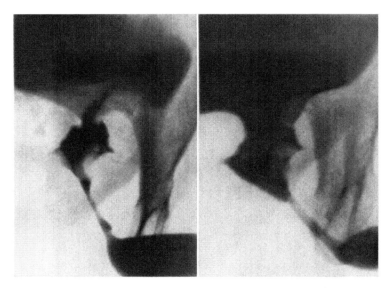

Fig. 87. Status after prostatectomy with naked adenomas bulging into the irregular operation cavity

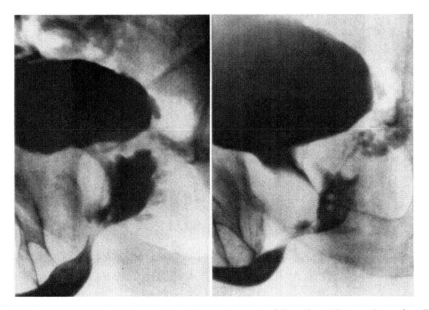

Fig. 88. Prostatic hypertrophy treated ad modum Deisting with forced distension of the posterior urethra. The micturition demonstrates the blocking effect of fibroadenoma (right figure). Remnants of a posterior rupture of the prostate opening the seminal ducts

prostate may coexist, and the latter is stated to be present in about half of all cases of carcinoma of the prostate. The combination of hypertrophy of the prostate and prostatitis leads not only to the posterior urethra being elongated and deformed by the hypertrophy as already described, but also to its course being straightened, due to expansion in the lower glandular region of the prostate. The depressed glandular tissue encircles the lower part of the proliferation like a bowl (Fig. 89).

Regarding vasographic studies in hypertrophy of the prostate see VIII (Figs. 122 and 123).

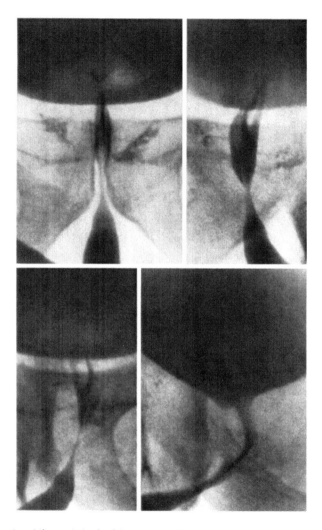

Fig. 89. Compression of the prostatic gland from prostatic hypertrophy; the prostatic gland is represented by concretions

The value of urethrocystography for the diagnosis of hypertrophy of the prostate is twofold. Although the diagnosis can, as a rule, be established by rectal palpation, there is not seldom a considerable difference between the size of the part deforming the urethra and bladder, respectively (Fig. 90). The urethrocystogram therefore complements rectal palpation, and provides better topographic information than urethrocystoscopy. Still more important are the urethrographic data regarding the combination of prostatic hypertrophy and inflammatory changes in the prostate and urethra. Micturition studies may disclose the real impediment (Fig. 84). If prostatic hypertrophy of a blocking nature is absent, it should—in many cases—point to the inadvisability of attempts

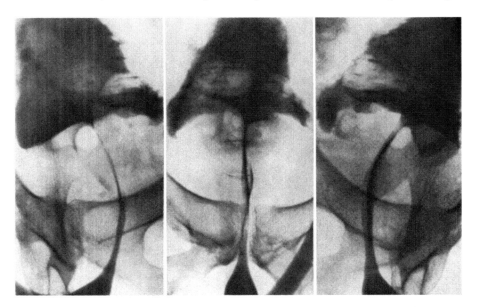

Fig. 90. Prostatic hypertrophy which appears as large in the urethrocystogram though the rectal palpation gave the impression of a moderate enlargement

to enucleate the fibrodenoma from a chronically fibrosed prostatic tissue, which may lead to sphincter disturbances and a rectal fistula.

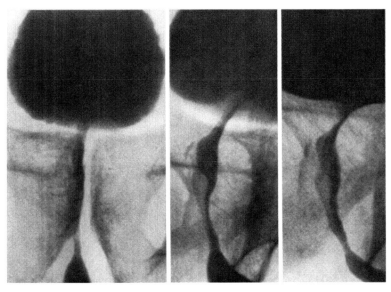

Fig. 91. Chronic prostato-vesiculitis with bladder neck sclerosis

18. Vesical-neck contraction

By vesical-neck contraction—also known as vesical-neck sclerosis—is meant a contraction of the smooth muscle which, at the internal urethral orifice, extends forwards in a half-circle around the urethra. Although a number of conditions have been suggested as its cause, prostatitis and seminal vesiculitis seems to

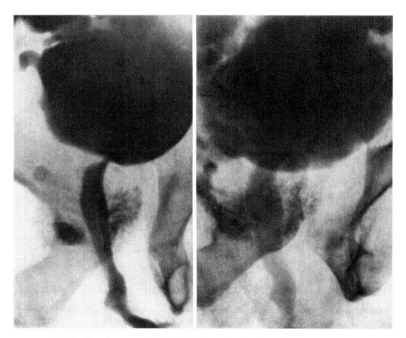

Fig. 92. Chronic prostatitis with bladder neck sclerosis and urethral stricture

be the prime aetiologic factor, since it is present in the overwhelming number of cases of vesical-neck contraction (Figs. 91 and 92). It can be presumed that

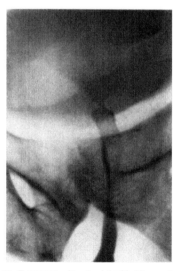

Fig. 93. Recurrent sclerosis of the bladder neck after transurethral resection

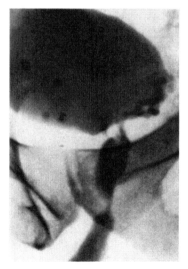

Fig. 94. Secondary bladder neck sclerosis after prostatectomy. The seminal ducts open into the operation cavity

the muscle in question has an essential genital task, which in the male is to occlude the posterior urethra from the bladder during ejaculation.

On the urethrocystogram, vesical-neck contraction is seen—both in retrograde injection and during micturition—in the form of a barrier protruding from behind, to which the alternative name posterior bar refers. The barrier is only a few millimetres wide, and its contours are even. If it is combined with hyper-

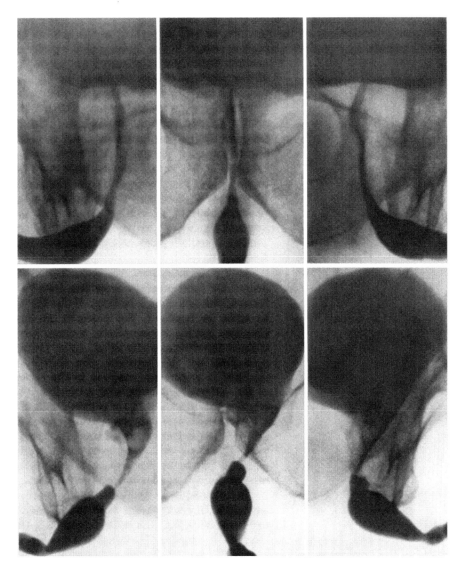

Fig. 95. Prostatic hypertrophy and prostatitis (upper figures). Postoperative incontinence because of a false passage outside the external sphincter (lower figures)

trophy of the prostate in the same region, the barrier is wider. It should not be confused with pure hypertrophy of the prostate of the third lobe type. On the whole, vesical-neck contraction is found in considerably younger age groups than is hypertrophy of the prostate.

In severe cases, vesical-neck contraction produces an impediment to emptying of the bladder, with trabeculation as a result. The contraction has a marked tendency to recur after surgical resection (Fig. 93). Secondary constriction of the vesical neck may occur after prostatectomy, and is denoted as secondary vesical-neck sclerosis (Fig. 94).

19. Postoperative changes in the posterior urethra. — False passages in the prostatic region

Surgical interventions on the prostate, as well as probing of the urethra for prostatic disease, may produce a complete change in the features of the posterior urethra. Partial prostatectomy for hypertrophy of the prostate is apt to cause the bladder neck and the part down to the collicular region to remain constantly wide open, without the ability to close, so called Vorblase. Small, irregular tissue fragments or small rounded adenomas may protrude into an operative cavity (Fig. 87) where concrements may be formed. It is fairly exceptional for the lumen to resume a more normal appearance after prostatectomy. The closing function of the internal sphincter region is often lacking, causing ejaculation to occur backwards into the bladder.

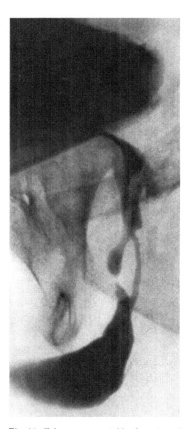

If the transurethral resection has been deeper, or total prostatectomy has been performed, the colliculus is lacking. If the ability to close is regained, the posterior urethra therefore has the appearance of a short tube, without the characteristic relief. After radical operations on the prostate, the ability to contract is sometimes confined to the region of the external sphincter with a tendency to urinary incontinence. This occurs strikingly often in cases where preoperative urethrocystography showed features more compatible with prostatitis than with hypertrophy of the prostate. A fistula to the rectum may develop after such deep resection or total prostatectomy.

Fig. 96. False passage outside the external sphincter after pelvic fracture with rupture of the urethra

False passages in the prostatic region are of two types. One is a passage which runs upwards and backwards from the collicular region in the prostatic tissue and, in rare cases, reaches the bladder. The other is a passage at the side of the prostate or in front of it; it starts below the external sphincter, passes outside the anterolateral portion of the prostate, and opens in the bladder floor or at some site in the posterior urethra (Figs. 95 and 96).

VI. The female urethra

1. Urethrocystographic technique and normal anatomy

From the technical point of view, urethrocystography in the female involves some difficulty in attaching the instrument to the urethral orifice. If a cannula with a rubber cone is used, it must be pressed against the orifice, which results in deformation of the external part of the urethra. A Kjellman suction cup is not invariably leakproof. The most practicable instrument seems to be a cannula ending in an oblique metal plate, $^1/_2$ to 1 cm in diameter. It is coaxed beyond the meatus by gentle twisting, after which slight traction makes it straighten the urethra, at the same time as it stops leakage.

The female urethra is 3—4 cm long; about $^2/_3$ of it consists of a sphincter portion, and about $^1/_3$ of an intercavernous part. The former corresponds to the posterior urethra in the male, except that the prostate is lacking as a glandular organ. Numerous paraurethral glands are present instead, the majority lying

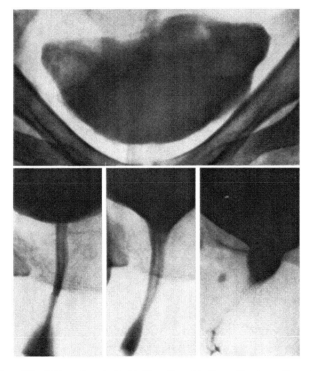

Fig. 97. Urethritis-cystitis. Bullous edema in the bladder adjacent to the urethra (upper figures); thickened folds in the urethra (lower left figures); external sphincter spasm during micturition (lower right figures)

posterolaterally. The glands are most plentiful in the middle third. The sphincter muscles have essentially the same appearance and structure as in the male. Like the prostatic glands, the female paraurethral glands are partly embedded in smooth muscle. The external sphincter runs backwards around the urethra in the shape of a horseshoe, its posterior limbs merging with the retrourethral tissue; it also surrounds part of the vagina. As in the male, the urethral mucosa has longitudinal folds, which appear on moderate distension.

2. Urethritis, urethral diverticula, diverticulitis

In the female as well, inflammatory changes of the urethral mucosa lead to swelling of its folds, sometimes with granulation of the mucosa and small polyps (Figs. 97—100). Inflammation may also produce insufficiency of the glandular orifices, so that retrograde filling occurs at urethrography. With concurrent dilatation of the ducts, they get the appearance of diverticula. As in the male, urethritic processes are associated with a tendency to spasm of the external sphincter. It is particularly evident during micturition, when it produces prestenotic

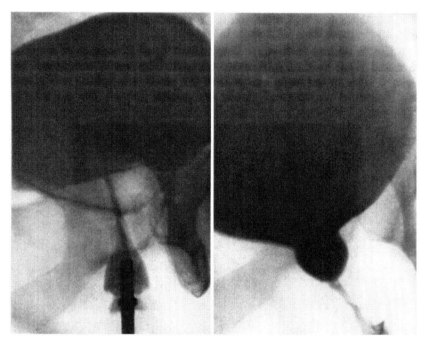

Fig. 98. Urethritis with obliterated folds at retrograde injection (left figure), and external sphincter spasm during micturition (right figure)

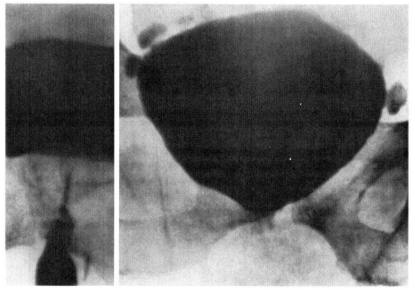

Fig. 99. Chronic urethritis with nodular mucosal pattern, urethral stricture, and bladder diverticula

dilatation of the superior part of the urethra (Figs. 97 and 98). A posterior barrier at the vesical neck may appear in connexion with chronic urethritis, although it is a much rarer occurrence than in the male.

Diverticula of the urethra may be congenital, or they may be acquired on various grounds. The congenital type may be due to anomalous primordia with retention of secretion, and retention probably plays the essential role in the acquired type as well. A definite relation also exists between urethritis and urethral

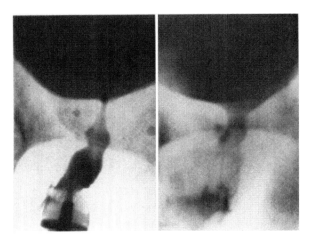

Fig. 100. Chronic urethritis with polypous mucous membrane

diverticula. As a rule, the large diverticula open above the external sphincter, and in these cases spasm of the external sphincter with a resultant rise in pressure in the posterior urethra is strikingly common. Such diverticula have, in addition,

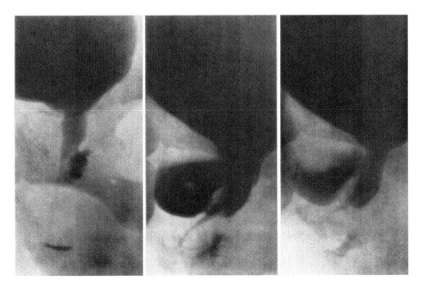

Fig. 101. Urethritis with external sphincter spasm and urethral diverticulum (left figures). Postoperative recurrence of the diverticulum (right figure)

a marked tendency to recur after excision, which can also be ascribed to the pressure of micturition (Fig. 101).

Filling defects can occasionally be observed in large urethral diverticula, representing the presence of solid secretion or possibly of tissue fragments. The diverticula may also contain calculi.

A paraurethral abscess displaces the urethral lumen forwards and laterally. The position of such abscesses is well compatible with that of the paraurethral glands, in which they are believed to originate (Fig. 102).

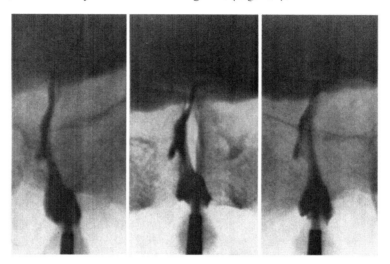

Fig. 102. Paraurethral abscess dislocating the urethra. In the opposite wall of the urethra the opening of a diverticulum is filled

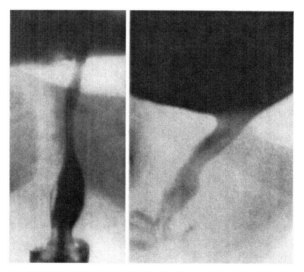

Fig. 103. Urethritis with obliterated folds. On the one side a Skene's duct is filled

Paraurethral ducts belonging to the external part of the urethra are not affected by the aforementioned hypertension caused by spasm of the external sphincter (Fig. 103).

In the meatal syndrome, constriction of the external urethral orifice may be present, causing prestenotic dilatation.

3. Cystocele and stress incontinence

Since the pelvic floor is part of the abdominal wall, its position is dependent on the intraabdominal pressure and on the muscle tonus, particularly that of the

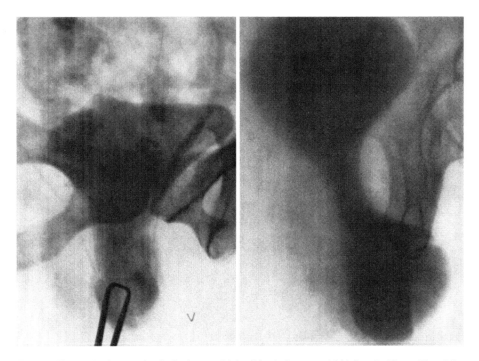

Fig. 104. True cystocele appearing during increased intraabdominal pressure (right figure). The position of the ureters in relation to the cystocele is illustrated (left figure)

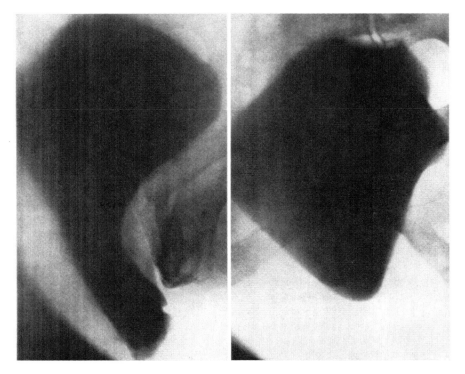

Fig. 105. Case with cystocele: normal appearance during resting; herniating bladder during pressing (left figure). After closure of the deficiency of the levator muscle no herniation remains (right figure)

levator muscles. Bearing down is accompanied by sinking of the pelvic floor, which takes place to a varying degree in the individual case, so that no borderlines can be drawn for the normal range. The bladder descends concurrently and, since this is strongest in the middle of the pelvic canal, the retroureteric fossa sinks most. Consequently, during micturition, the course of the urethra—whose membranous part is relatively immobile—is more or less dorsoventral above this part.

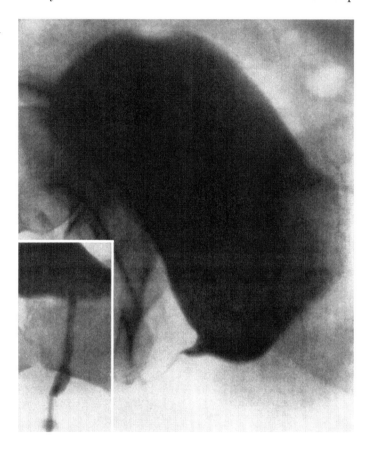

Fig. 106. Case of stress incontinence. Irregularity of the mucosal pattern in the urethra, and external sphincter spasm as signs of urethritis, but no cystocele. Operated with "reconstruction" of the pelvic muscles though without influence on the symptoms

A definitely pathologic feature is, on the contrary, for the bladder floor to protrude through the mouth of a hernia in the pelvic floor, producing a circular constriction of the bladder which makes it more or less resemble a dumb-bell. In contrast to the generalized descent of the pelvic floor, this herniation of the bladder is to be regarded as a true cystocele (Figs. 104 and 105), of which the lowest point is the retroureteric fossa. In pronounced cases, adjacent parts of the bladder are involved in the herniation, as are the ureters, which then open into the anterior wall of the cystocele (Fig. 104).

A true cystocele of this kind is not necessarily associated with any difficulty in urination. This may, however, apply in some cases, whereas stress incontinence is present in others.

Urethrocystographically, stress incontinence is of two distinct types. One is the herniation of the bladder just described; the other occurs without such herniation. In the latter type, the bladder neck is often seen to be open even at rest, forming a funnel which is a few millimetres long (Fig. 106). A roentgenologic feature common to both types is the usual presence of signs of urethritis, in the form of spasm of the external sphincter, as well as coarsening and irregularity of the urethral folds, or their obliteration by swelling (Fig. 107).

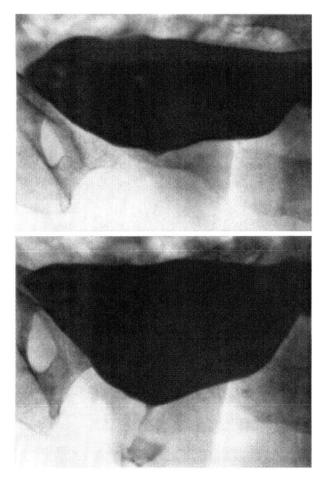

Fig. 107. Case of stress incontinence with openstanding bladder neck during resting (upper figure), and polypous mucosal relief of the urethra as signs of urethritis (lower figure)

VII. Urethrocystography in children

The task of urethrocystography in children differs to some extent from that in adults. Thus, in the former, anomalies producing urinary obstruction (ureterocele and urethral valves), as well as those consisting of cavities opening into the posterior urethra (ectopic ureter and certain types of intersexuality), are relatively common indications for urethrocystography. Since their visualization is dependent chiefly on the micturition studies, one can refrain from retrograde injection, and fill the bladder through a catheter instead. A sterile suspension of barium sulphate has been recommended as contrast medium in these cases. A prerequisite for the use of such contrast medium is that there has been no trauma to the urethra or bladder.

Urinary obstruction is frequently associated with hydronephrosis and infection. The presence of infection is of particular importance for interpretation of the urethrocystographic features. Thus, when an urethral valve is present, it is not unusual to find—in addition to a trabeculated bladder with a swollen mucosa— a posterior barrier and opacification of the seminal vesicles and prostatic utricle.

Urethrocystography is of special interest in children for investigating the cause of enuresis. Apart from urethral valves, which are a relatively uncommon cause, urethrocystography has been able in many of the cases to demonstrate changes indicative of infection. Examples are an irritated bladder with a greatly contracted region in the trigone, vesico-ureteric reflux, vesical-neck contraction, and urethral spasm, the latter to be ascribed to increased irriability of the external sphincter. It has not, on the other hand, been possible in paediatric series to demonstrate any changes on the urethrocystogram specific to enuresis.

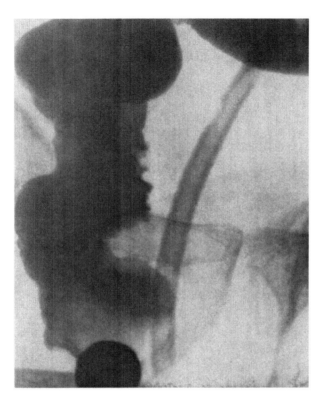

Fig. 108. Barium enema roentgenogram of a case with acute seminal vesiculitis with involvement of the rectal mucosa (catheter in the urethra and bladder)

VIII. Vaso-vesiculo-epididymography

Unfortunately the seminal vesicles are organs which are often ignored, particularly in connection with nonspecific inflammation (which is common). It is of importance that they be considered, since they not only can cause local symptoms but also may act as foci of infection, causing remote signs and symptoms(see V: 15, e.g. Pelvospondylitis ossificans or relapsing iritis), especially when local symptoms are lacking. As has already been mentioned (V: 12, V: 15), infections spread readily throughout the male urogenital system so that the term *male adnexitis* is suitable, comprising changes in the prostate, seminal vesicles, ampullae, vas deferens, epididymis, posterior urethra, COWPER's glands, prostatic utricle and sometimes even in portions of the urinary bladder and the ureters. In many ways chronic seminal vesiculitis is the most important factor in such a complex of symptoms but it may easily escape detection in the course of routine clinical examination.

When only mildly affected the vesicles remain mobile and may be difficult to discern at rectal palpation. Not infrequently the main pathology is perivesiculitis with induration of the tissues around the vesicles. They are then concealed beneath the thickened but smooth recto-genital septum (fascia Denonvilliers). The upper concave border of this septum can often be palpated as a slight shelf but the contours of the vesicles, ampullae and the prostatic base are blurred or even totally obscured. Of great importance in the diagnosis of seminal vesiculitis are rectal palpation, which sometimes may be difficult to interpret, and microscopic examination of expressed content, which in conjunction with complete occlusion of the vesicle (empyema) may prove to be misleading. Thus vesiculography may provide valuable information in difficult cases and ought to be utilized much more than it has been up to the present. Moreover suitable techniques for rectal palpation and for stripping of the contents of the vesicles (for diagnostic microscopy as well as therapy) must be based on the knowledge of their topography gained by vesiculography (see below).

The seminal vesicles are situated above the prostatic base, between the bladder floor and the rectal wall (Fig. 116). Seminal vesiculitis may thus cause dislocation of the bladder wall and the urethra (Fig. 14) or bullous oedema of the bladder floor (as may also prostatitis, see Fig. 15, 17, 18 and page 381) and of the rectal wall (Fig. 108). The distal portion of the ureter may because of its intimate contact with the vesicle (Fig. 109) in perivesiculitis be constricted, resulting in hydroureter and hydronephrosis (Fig. 110).

Such changes may regress completely after successful treatment of the vesiculitis (possibly first after vesiculectomy, as in the case shown in Fig. 110).

Contrast examination of the spermatic tract has originated from methods for treatment of inflammatory conditions in the vesicles by local injections and instillations of antiseptics. Roentgen examination may suitably be combined with irrigation

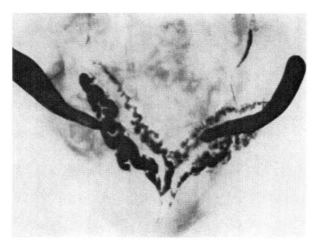

Fig. 109. Simultaneous contrast filling of the ureters, ampullae and seminal vesicles in an autopsy specimen to show the juxtaposition of the distal portion of the ureter and the vesicle—just that portion of the ureter, where the stricture in Fig. 110 is located

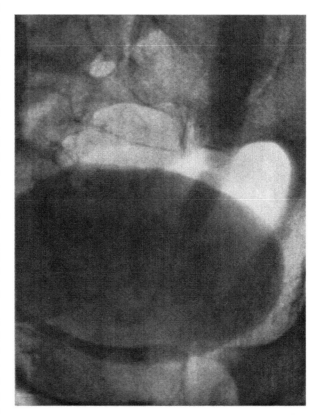

Fig. 110. Chronic prostatitis, seminal vesiculitis and perivesiculitis with inflammatory stricture of the distal 2—3 cm of the left ureter with secondary hydroureter (and hydronephrosis)

of the vas deferens, ampulla and vesicle, from which the stagnant contents are thus removed. This procedure has therapeutic value in inflammatory conditions, and increases to some extent the indication for vesiculography in conjunction with nonspecific adnexitis. In most instances the investigation is confined to the ampulla, vesicle, and ejaculatory duct, but under special circumstances may include the was deferens and even the epididymis.

Contrast filling can be accomplished in two ways,

1. the deferential route by means of vasopuncture or vasotomy and

2. the transurethral route with retrograde catheterization of the ejaculatory duct through a urethroscope.

Moreover epididymography may be carried out by means of vasopuncture.

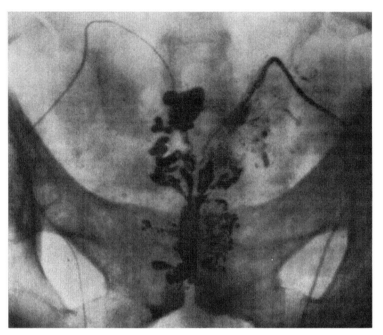

Fig. 111. Vaso-seminal vesiculography with iodized oil in a case of leftsided perivesicular, inflammatory process. Rupture of the left ampulla permitted the oil to penetrate into the vesicorectal tissue, showing that nonsoluble contrast matter is unsuitable. An abundance of dilated prostatic ducts and cavities are seen, particularly on the left side

1. Vaso-vesiculography or *vesiculography via the deferential route*, introduced by BELFIELD in 1905—1913, is the oldest and most used method, because the technique is easy and complications are few.

A scrotal incision is better than percutaneous puncture. If vasectomy is performed, for example, prophylactically in hypertrophy or carcinoma of the prostate, or in tuberculous epididymitis, a fine plastic catheter is inserted on each side and secured with a ligature. Thereafter roentgen exposures are made during simultaneous injection into both catheters (see VESTBY). If, on the other hand, the passage through the vas is to remain functional, puncture with a fine needle is preferred. Since the ampulla and the ejaculatory duct are comparatively rapidly emptied after cessation of injection, exposure of the roentgenograms should commence during the injection or immediately thereafter. Adequate fixation of the needle to avoid its slipping out is essential. If this is made with a ligature, a rupture within a pathologically changed area, usually in the ampulla (Fig. 111) may occur (in about 2—4%). Using a very fine needle held by hand during the injection the contrast fluid will leak back along the needle if there is complete stenosis of the spermatic tract.

The vesicle is filled from the opening of its excretory duct in the ejaculatorysinus.

When water soluble contrast is employed and the vesicular content is markedly fluid a ready mixing is obtained and the vesicle is completely filled with contrast.

If the vesicular content is highly viscous, however, it may be forced back during the injection into the apical coils and diverticula which thereby may be only partially or not at all filled with contrast medium. Employment of a water insoluble agent (such as iodized oil) may result in incomplete mixing with the vesicular content and consequent defective filling of the vesicle. A frequently disregarded source of error is thus high viscosity of the vesicular content, which, however, may be avoided by irrigating the vesicle prior to roentgen examination. 3—4 thorough washings with 2—3 ml physiological saline, interspersed by short intervals is sufficient. In this way pictures with a wealth of detail and demonstrating good contrast filling even of narrow passages and small diverticula may be obtained. (Moreover the mechanical irrigation has a therapeutic value in cases of chronic vesiculitis.)

2. *The transurethral route* is based on catherization of the ejaculatory duct (introduced by KLOTZ and LUYS before 1900) and later development of the irrigating urethroscope by, among others, McCARTHY, VON LICHTENBERG, LOWSLEY & PETERSEN. The examination requires a special instrumentarium, considerable experience, and has had noteworthy use by only few clinicians (Fig. 119, 120). It is accompanied by a greater incidence of complications than the deferential route, and should not be employed in cases of acute inflammatory conditions.

The catheter usually passes from the ejaculatory duct into the vesicle due to the anatomical relationships (see below). Thus at injection the vesicle is filled first, and in order to obtain a picture of the ampulla and possibly a part of the vas repeated injections of small quantities of contrast are required.

Spontaneous filling of the ejaculatory duct, ampulla and vesicle at urethrography because of a rigid and persistently open ostium of the ejaculatory duct or perforation of an abscess and open fistula between the urethra and some part of the spermatic tract (most often the vesicle) is very rare, but can occur with tuberculosis, after a perforated pyogenic abscess in the prostate (or in the vesicle), after prostatectomy or in conjunction with chronic non-specific prostato-vesiculitis. Such a retrograde contrast filling of the prostatic ducts but also of the prostatic utricle and the ejaculatory ducts, can be facilitated by producing increased pressure in the posterior urethra using a special technique (according to GULLMO): The bag of a Foley catheter placed in the urinary bladder is pressed against and occludes the internal orifice of the urethra, while the posterior part of the penile urethra is compressed from without around the catheter by a rubber tourniquet and the contrast agent via many small holes in the catheter is forced into the prostatic part of the urethra (Fig. 112, 113).

3. *Epididymography.* Since the epididymis is readily available for palpation and epididymitis hardly occurs without vesiculitis on the same side the necessity of roentgen examination is not great—the possibility of irradiation damage to the testis also diminishes its utilization. The injection of contrast medium, however, can give information as to whether the passage through the duct system is open or some obstruction is present. By means of epididymography anatomical details have been clarified within the cauda and its transition into the vas deferens. Indications for epididymography are, therefore, pathologic lesions of the lower vas and epididymis, and the study of male infertility (naturally combined with vesiculography in the latter case).

The deferential route is employed (see page 446). The vas is punctured with a fine needle and 0.2—0.3 ml (70% contrast) is injected. Thereafter gentle massage of the epididymis during injection of an additional 0.2 ml as "un véritable barbotage" (BOIREAU) in order to facilitate the passage of the contrast medium to the very small calibre duct system in the epididymis. Such a technique permits the contrast to pass into the corpus and even into the caput but separated coils of the duct system can no longer be distinguished. If a very fine needle is employed it is possible for the contrast to leak back along the needle and the risk of rupture of the duct wall is thereby eliminated.

Roentgenological technique. Water soluble, highly fluid triiodated contrast mediums are most suitable: for vesiculography a 30—40% solution and for epididymography about 70%. As a rule 1.5—2.0 ml of contrast is sufficient for filling the vas deferens, ampulla, vesicle and ejaculatory duct. An excess of injected contrast passes via the urethra into the urinary bladder whereby the contour of the bottom of the bladder is outlined and its position in relation to the ampulla and vesicle can be determined. This provides an indication of the thickness of the walls of the organs. On the other hand a large amount of contrast in the urinary bladder easily masks the ampullae and vesicles, making it difficult to interpret the pictures. As a rule the contrast material is resorbed within 3 hours and does not cause any permanent injury to the mucosa of the spermatic tract. In certain cases—especially with acute inflammatory conditions in the vesicles and ampullae—it is advisable immediately to wash away the contrast solution with physiological saline or a nonirritating antiseptic. Routine use of prophylactic antibiotics is not necessary.

As standard projections (as mentioned before preferably during injection) a frontal exposure is taken, usually with the central ray directed 15⁰ to 30⁰

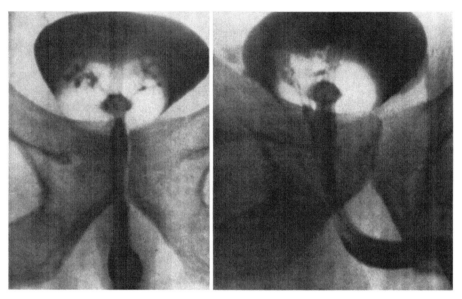

Fig. 112   Fig. 113

Fig. 112 and 113. Urethrography according to Gullmo with occlusion of the internal urethral orifice with a Foley catheter and compression of the posterior part of the penile urethra. The opening of the enlarged prostatic utricle (depth 2 cm) had earlier been widened by coagulation. The rigid orifices of the ejaculatory ducts are situated in the utricle (which is unusual) and the contrast therefore fills not only the utricle but also the ejaculatory ducts, ampullae and seminal vesicles

caudally, semi-lateral pictures as in urethrography and sometimes also a true lateral picture (Fig. 117) (in order to improve the contrast effect for topographical studies the lumen of the rectum can then be filled with air).

Contrast filling of the spermatic tract provides much valuable information regarding the anatomy and topography of the male adnexal glands under normal and pathological conditions and have in certain circumstances diagnostic importance; particularly in tuberculosis and nonspecific prostato-vesiculitis, in prostatic abscess and for differential diagnosis between prostatic carcinoma and chronic prostato-vesiculitis (both nonspecific and tuberculous), especially with co-incidental hypertrophy.

Anatomy and normal roentgenograms. The *vas deferens* courses from the inner orifice of the inguinal canal straight distally, medially and far dorsally, thereafter it takes a sharp bend medially forward (Fig. 111, 116). The ducts from both sides converge toward the prostatic hilus in the center of the base of the prostate.

The last centimeters of the duct are widened to the *ampulla ductus deferentis* (Fig. 114). This is as rule a little longer than the corresponding vesicle and runs parallel with and close up to it. Its main duct is slightly convoluted with closely placed small diverticula, which show individual variations. The angle between the two ampullae in the frontal view is 45⁰ to 90⁰ but may approach 180⁰ and varies somewhat with the filling of the urinary bladder and rectum.

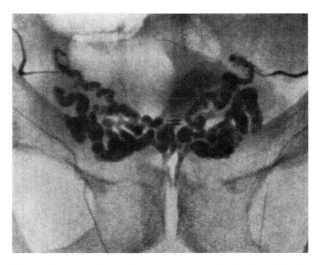

Fig. 114. Vaso-seminal vesiculography of a normal individual. Note the looping of the vesicular canal, the small diverticula on the ampulla and the broad vesiculo-ampullar junction

The seminal vesicle is composed of a more or less convoluted main duct with large or small branches, into which gracile diverticula, variable in size and number open (Fig. 115). The whole is enveloped and joined together by connective tissue to form a lengthy pears-shaped coarsely-knobbed entity. The apical portion of the main duct is as a rule bent back like a hook (Fig. 109). The shape, size and volume are individually variable: length 25—55 mm, width 15—20 and thickness 10 mm. The capacity in cadavers is stated to be from 1.5 to 7 ml but in vivo it is seldom over 2.5 ml. A prototype of a "normal vesicle" cannot be given but the arrangement is usually principally the same on both sides with regular convolutions and gracile ramifications or a more unitarily coarsely knobbed duct system. The structure may, however, show many variations in details. Thus various morphological subdivisions proposed by different authors have not been useful for practical clinical work.

During puberty a very rapid development of the vesicles occurs with enlargement of the lumen and appearance of many

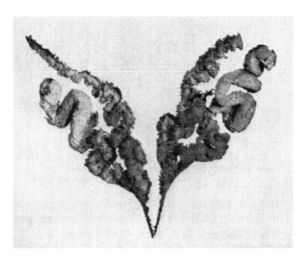

Fig. 115. Plastic corrosion model of the normal seminal vesicles of a 47 year old man. (From S. NILSSON 1962)

small plicae and crypts. During the active sexual period the lumen is widened a little more but later it gradually shrinks somewhat and the mucosa is smoothered.

The vesicular main duct is funnel-shaped, narrows down to the excretory duct and is in confluence with the distal part of the tapering ampulla forming the ejaculatory duct. Its direction usually coincides with that of the vesicle, while the ampulla opens into it at a more or less acute angle (Fig. 109, 111, 114). This explains why a catheter introduced through the ejaculatory duct usually proceeds into the vesicle.

The ejaculatory duct is the terminal part of the spermatic tract (length about 15 mm). The ducts on both sides run parallel and almost totally within the prostate (Fig. 109). The lumen tapers from the wider part—sinus ejaculatorius— which sometimes is found immediately distal to the confluens, towards the opening on the seminal collicle, which is situated distal to the middle of the pars

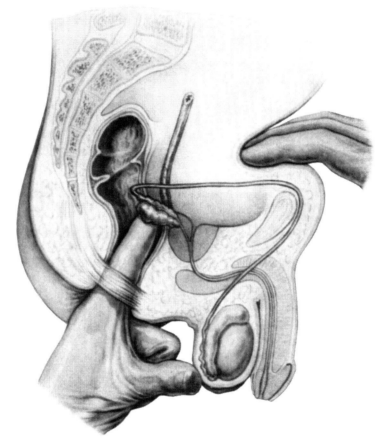

Fig. 116. Schematic drawing showing bimanual palpation of the prostate and the seminal vesicles with the patient in standing position

prostatica urethrae. Small gracile diverticula occasionally open into the ejaculatory ducts (Fig. 109, 114). The duct orifices are seldom situated in a normal prostatic utricle, but when this is large and chronically inflamed the orifices may be so placed that contrast fluid can pass from the utricle into the ducts (Fig. 112, 113, 119, 120). Thus there are possibilities for infection to spread in the same way. When the utricle is large, the ejaculatory ducts pass quite near the wall for a long distance and then infectious processes can encroach directly and also cause a pathological communication.

The topography of the seminal vesicles. Inability to palpate the seminal vesicles is often said to be due to inadequate length of the doctor's index finger. Sufficient knowledge of the topographical anatomy of the vesicles reveals, however, that the length of the finger usually is quite enough—the position of the finger is the determining factor. When the patient is standing and the bladder empty or half filled but not contracted, the bladder base is almost horizontal (Fig. 116). The vesicles are then not vertical (as they are usually said to be) but horizontal, pointing towards the sacro-coccygeal junction (Fig. 117). They embrace the rectum in front and laterally and also a palpating finger in the rectal lumen which advances along the prostatic posterior surface. When the finger in the rectum is moved laterally it meets the vesicle more or less at its middle part and tends to push it upward and laterally, because the normal vesicles are quite mobile. To get around the apical part of vesicle—which is important not only to judge its consistency and fixation but also to express its contents—the palpating finger must therefore first be circumducted: posteriorly so that it is free in the

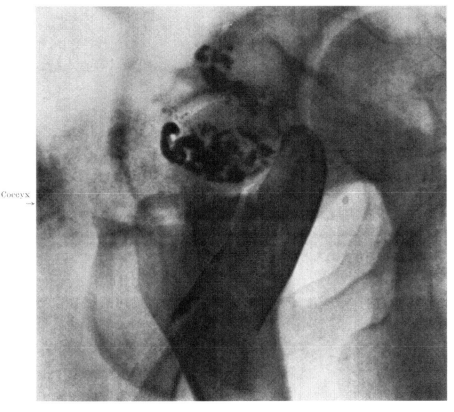

Coccyx

Fig. 117. Roentgenogram showing the same as Fig. 116: The index finger is shown in the rectum because of contrast matter around it in the glove. The seminal vesicles are filled with contrast injected at vasotomy, they are horizontally located and pointing toward the coccyx

rectal lumen, then laterally and finally forward pressing against the other hand which is depressing the abdominal wall dorsally and medially just above the inguinal ligament (Fig. 116).

Diagnostic vesiculography

Nonspecific inflammation—male adnexitis—preferably prostato-vesiculitis, cannot be excluded by normal roentgen examinations (neither by urethrocysto-graphy nor vaso-vesiculography), but especially if vesiculitis is dominating, vesiculography may offer very important information (see *e.g.* STAEHLER).

Acute seminal vesiculitis may be unilateral or, in certain cases, particularly when a chronic prostato-vesiculitis exacerbates, is often dominant on one side. In acute nonspecific epididymitis usually changes occur first and are best revealed

29*

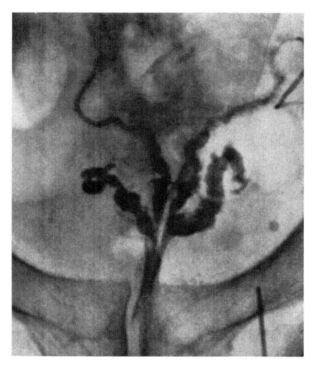

Fig. 118. Vaso-seminal vesiculography in a case of chronic prostatitis and vesiculitis with diffuse irregular contours of the vesicles and distal ampullae. Note the increased distance between the vesicle and ampulla, especially on the right side

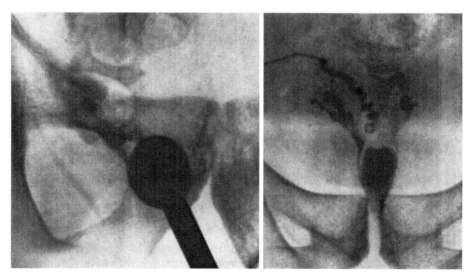

Fig. 119   Fig. 120

Fig. 119 and 120. Chronic non-specific uro-genital infection in a 36 year old male with prostatitis, seminal vesiculitis, right epididymitis and hemospermia. Fig. 119. Very large prostatic utricle (capacity more than 10 ml) injected with contrast matter through a urethroscope. From the utricle diffuse contrast filling of the right ampulla and seminal vesicle. Fig. 120. 1¹/₂ years after treatment the dilated utricle had shrunk as shown: At vasography contrast filling of right ampulla and seminal vesicle and of the utricle. From the utricle via the left ejaculatory duct also faint filling of the left vesicle (which is quite unusual). Signs of bilateral vesiculitis in the vesicle and the confluens region (on the same side as the epididymitis) where the lumen because of swelling of the mucosa is a good deal more narrow than normal with blurred contrast contours. The ramifications and diverticula of the ampulla may be less visible and the convolutions diminished but broadly speaking it looks normal—quite the contrary to the appearence of the ampulla in tuberculous epididymitis (see below 454). Often in acute inflammation—as also in some cases of chronic process—an increased distance can be noted between the contrast in the ampulla and the vesicle. Their normally parallel course is then more acutely angulated because of inflammatory oedema in the walls and the tissues separating them (Fig. 118).

In *chronic* (prostato-) *vesiculitis* (which often has a chronic onset without urethral symptoms) three main types may be distinguished clinically, particularly by palpation.

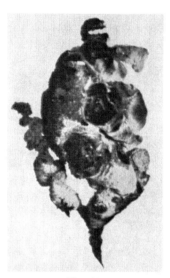 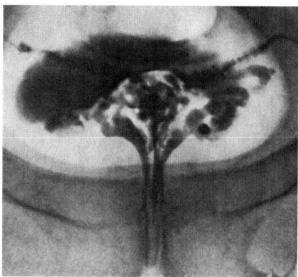

Fig. 121   Fig. 122

Fig. 121. Plastic corrosion model of the seminal vesicle of a 65 year old man with total occlusion of the ejaculatory duct due to posterior urethritis. Marked dilation of the vesicle and ampulla. (From S. NILSSON 1962)

Fig. 122. Vaso-seminal vesiculography in a case of benign hypertrophy with simultaneous chronic prostatitis and seminal vesiculitis. The increased distance between the vesicle and the corresponding ampulla may be considered as an indication of inflammatory thickening of the walls

1. Interstitial vesiculitis mainly showing thickening of the walls.

2. Catarrhal vesiculitis with greater or lesser distension of the lumen—most pronounced apically—caused by catarrhal (seldom pyogenic) inflammation of the mucosa, stagnating secretions and some hypotonicity of the wall. Totally occluded empyema (pyovesiculosis) is rare.

3. Perivesiculitis with more or less organized oedema around the vesicles and thickening of the whole rectogenital septum (Fig. 111).

From roentgenograms it is often difficult to differentiate such types, partly because the initial anatomic structure, as mentioned before, can vary so much.

In chronic conditions the ampulla may take a more gross wave-like course with good contrast filling but the roentgenogram may show somewhat blurred contours and less wealth of details. After a period of time the width of the lumen is diminished due to scarification in and around the wall accompanied by shrinkage of the diverticula and convolutions, resulting in a more irregular lumen size than in acute conditions (Fig. 118, 120). The vesicle changes more slowly with chronic nonspecific processes and not to such a high degree, showing a smoothing of the contours of the wall. The lumen is sometimes broadened especially apically (see above type 2). A very marked dilatation—with hydrops or empyema—is rare, but occurs with obstruction of the ejaculatory duct (Fig. 121). Under such circumstances vesiculography is of great diagnostic value. Defects in the contour of the vesicle or inadequate contrast filling to a greater or lesser degree, particularly of the apical portion or of diverticula, can be due to high viscosity of residual vesicular content (see page 447) or to a tuberculous process. The ampullae are normal or show insignificant changes with nonspecific inflammations, however, with tuberculosis the ampullae show marked typical changes (see below). More or less local constriction of the lumen of the vesicle (or ampulla) can depend on swelling of the mucous membrane or granuloma formation while actual constriction alternating with dilitation of the lumen, particularly in the vas, is typical of tuberculosis. Rupture of the ampullar or vesicular wall resulting in contrast leakage occasionally occurs (Fig. 111), but contrast filling of pathological cavities connected with the lumen is seldom accomplished (as in tuberculosis).

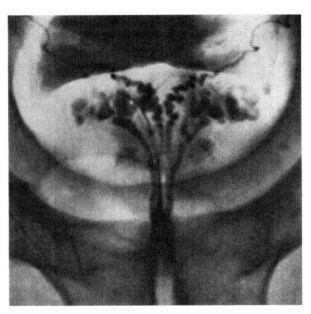

Fig. 123. Vaso-seminal vesiculography in a case of benign hypertrophy of the prostate showing typical curved dislocation and elevation of the vesicles by the adenomas. There was no enlargement of the vesicles indicating no compression of the ejaculatory ducts

Chronic prostato-vesiculitis can be *combined with benign hypertrophy* of the prostate (or even carcinoma), and accurate diagnosis may in some cases be important both for the treatment and prognosis (Fig. 122). The occurrence of seminal vesiculitis in hypertrophy increases the indications for vasectomy and vas-irrigation and it may influence the choice of treatment of the hypertrophy. Finally, totally occluded or badly drained inflamed vesicles may explain why complaints of "prostatism" sometimes persist after prostatectomy.

Since *urogenital tuberculosis* often occurs without symptoms vaso-vesiculography has diagnostic significance (see E. Ljunggren, part IX, 2). Spread of the tuberculous changes within the male adnexa may be determined more accurately with vesiculography than by palpation or endoscopy. When a tuberculous epididymitis is diagnosed, the tuberculous process has usually became widely disseminated so that in addition to the changes in the vas deferens, ampulla and vesicle on the same side, in approximately half of the cases, the so-called healthy side has become involved (first in the ampulla by direct encroachment from the diseased ampulla).

In recent cases shrinkage and constriction of the lumen have not developed but the contrast filling is patchy, the apical portion of the vesicle often dilated and the contours of the confluens and adjacent portion of the ampulla blurred.

In typical cases of long duration the most marked changes are within the vesicles and as a rule even the vas and ampulla are clearly pathological. The lumina are narrowed through shrinkage so that the convolutions of the ampulla and vesicle look like fine chased spirals (such as arabesques). Occasionally ill-defined out-lines and irregular lumina dominate, sometimes lens-shaped defects in the con-trast contour, or eroded contours or larger filling defects are seen. Particularly the lateral loops of the vesicles may show incomplete filling and sometimes gracile patterns with bowshaped convolutions and very small lumina—similar to the changes found around the confluens and ejaculatory duct in prostatic cancer (Fig. 124, 126). Shrinkage and occlusion with alterating narrowed and dilated portions, resulting in a beaded pattern of the ampulla, vesicle, and even the vas are most usual; within the vas—ampulla the changes are sometimes likened to an old fashioned lamp brush. Such constriction can comple-tely occlude, for example, the transition of the vas and the ampulla with match-like dis-tension of the vas and occasio-nal contrast leakage into the surrounding tissues. (In such cases disseminated tuberculous changes of the same vesicle and ampulla can usually be palpa-ted). Occasionally such an ob-stacle is situated at the con-fluens so that the vesicle is not filled at all, or in the middle of the vesicle with poor or no fill-ing of the apical portion. Such stoppages, as the aforementio-ned local contour defects of the

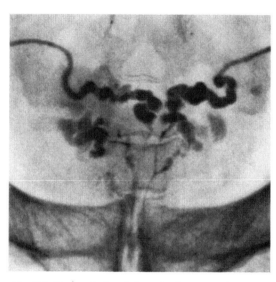

Fig. 124. Vaso-seminal vesiculography in a case of prostatic carcinoma with involvement of the junction of the vesicles and ampullae. The narrowed, rigid contours of the central duct system indicates the encroachment of invading tumour tissue, but the lateral portions of the vesicles and ampullae are unaffected

vesicle, usually are caused by caseous masses. Often smallnecked cavities or dilated ducts are filled with contrast from the urethra or by a fistula from the vesicle or the ampulla (see also page 447), while the contours of the urethra itself are remarkably unchanged.

In chronic cases the changes especially of the vesicles are as a rule more asymmetrical than with nonspecific inflammation.

Primary carcinoma of the seminal vesicles is extremely rare and in published cases the diagnosis has been made too late. Uni- or bilateral defective contrast filling at vesiculography has been described. Differential diagnosis is mainly concerned with secondary tumours (metastases in DOUGLAS' pouch from some abdominal organ, projecting into the rectal lumen as a shelf, see also page 457), with rectal cancer, endometriosis or prostatic sarcoma.

Even *pathological conditions of the male adnexa but outside the spermatic tract proper* can influence the vaso-vesiculogram, *i.e.,* prostatic hypertrophy, prostatic cancer, prostatic abscess, and enlargement of the prostatic utricle or so-called MÜLLER's cyst.

Hypertrophy of the prostate causes according to the size of the adenomas a more or less symmetrical elevation of the vesicles and ampullae with curved dis-location of the ejaculatory ducts (Fig. 122, 123). Even if the enlargement at rectal palpation seems mostly unilateral usually the changes noted by roentgen examination are symmetrical. The interampullary angle—usually below 90° (see page 449)—can increase because of such displacement but this is not pathognomonic for adenomatous hypertrophy. It has been considered that the emptying of the vesicles might be impaired by local pressure on the ejaculatory and excretory ducts, followed by stagnation of secretions and distension of the vesicle and the ejaculatory duct. In cases with such distension, however, pure hypertrophy is not likely but instead chronic inflammation of the vesicles has probably occurred, i.e. hypertrophy combined with prostato-vesiculitis (Fig. 122). The volume of the vesicles does not seem to be increased with prostatic adenomas—provided that this comparison is made within corresponding age groups. A large prostatic hypertrophy causes lengthening of the ejaculatory duct and a length over 2 cm thus supports such a diagnosis.

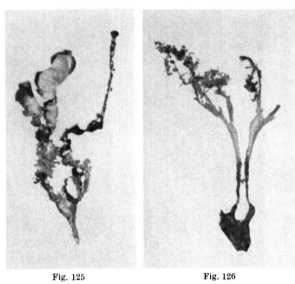

Fig. 125   Fig. 126

Fig. 125. Plastic corrosion model of the seminal vesicle of an 82 year old man with prostatic carcinoma with involvement of the vesicles and ampullae except for the distal portions. Compare Fig. 124. (From S. Nilsson 1962)

Fig. 126. Plastic corrosion model of the seminal vesicles of an 82 year old man with prostatic carcinoma with involvement of the entire vesicular and ampullar system. Compare Fig. 127

Carcinoma of the prostate usually spreads to the spermatic tract first in the confluens region. Thus vesiculography shows the earliest changes in the ejaculatory ducts and the terminal portions of the ampullae and vesicles. The lumina become constricted to narrow, rigid threads without normal circular folds (Fig. 124, 125, 126). The contrast filling of the vesicles may be incomplete (Fig. 127), presumably due to the stagnating content in a very narrow portion, which prevents contrast filling of the apical part. However, this totally or partially occluded portion is usually not distended. These changes are more often bilateral with varying degrees of asymmetry but may be purely unilateral.

When benign adenoma and carcinoma occur at the same time their effect on the vesicles, ampullae and ejaculatory ducts are additive. But an adenoma as such does not complicate the vesiculographic diagnosis of prostatic carcinoma. As carcinoma may arise anywhere in the prostatic parenchyma proper, influence on some part of the spermatic tract is not, however, necessarily an early sign but can appear comparatively late.

Acute prostatic abscess often shows typical vesiculograms with dislocation of a distended vesicle and an often incompletely filled ejaculatory duct. "The genital median line" is thus displaced to the healthy side by an expansive process in one of the prostatic lobes. Unilateral prostatic hypertrophy causes a similar curved dislocation of the vesicle neck around the confluens but the genital median line is then not displaced and the confluens and ejaculatory duct are usually normally contrast filled (see Fig. 123). This latter fact is important for the differential diagnosis of very rare bilateral abscesses (or grave diffuse parenchymatous prostatitis).

Enlarged prostatic utricle or cyst (from the MÜLLER's ducts) without communication with the urethra is situated in the median line between the ejaculatory ducts, which are thus curved laterally (Fig. 120). A large cyst, reaching far over the prostatic base, may, however, be displaced over to one side but is still located between the ampullae.

Processes outside the male adnexa can also influence the vaso-vesiculogram. Vesiculography may thus give valuable information regarding possible encroachment of a *rectal carcinoma* into the ampullar-vesicular region. The whole vesicular lumen is then compressed and the contours possibly blurred. This picture is quite different from the earlier described gracile ramifications caused by prostatic carcinoma (see Fig. 124, 127) where the pathological changes are always found at the prostatic hilus but often not in the apical portion of the vesicle.

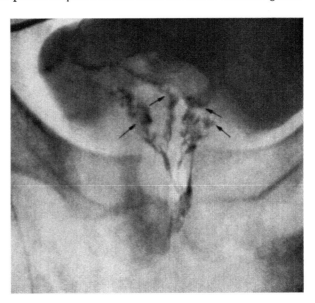

If pain occurs in the small pelvis some time after rectal extirpation for carcinoma with suspicion of local relapse, vaso-vesiculography may be of value.

This also holds true in analyses of the cause of so-called *shelf tumour of the rectum*, i.e. infiltration of the anterior rectal wall by an extra-rectal process at the bottom of the DOUGLAS' pouch (see page 455).

Simultaneous contrast filling of both the urinary bladder and the ampullae-vesicles may better elucidate the extension of a *tumour of the urinary bladder* and thus help in planning the treatment.

Fig. 127. Vaso-seminal vesiculography in a case of prostatic carcinoma with malignant infiltration to the line indicated by the arrows. On the left side there may be complete occlusion of the vesicular lumen at this site

Calcifications and calculi in the spermatic tract are uncommon (prostatic calculi see V: 11). True calculi are very rare and their content of calcium is often not sufficient for their clear visualization. Stagnating secretions and low grade chronic inflammation in older persons may have etiologic importance. Localized calcifications are most often seen in the vesicles or ampullae and are caused by chronic inflammation, especially tuberculosis, in younger individuals. Such findings therefore are an indication for more thorough investigation. More extensive calcifications, particularly of the Tunica muscularis circularis of the vas but also of the ampullae and vesicles (Fig. 2), are usually due to degenerative processes—old age, diabetes, scar tissue—and do not have any diagnostic importance.

In *analysis of male sterility* vaso-vesiculo-epididymography can give valuable information, especially by showing a mechanical obstacle in the spermatic tract or inflammatory adnexitis.

The cause of total stenosis may be: a) congenital defect or stricture, e.g. at the transition vas-epididymis or at the opening of the ejaculatory duct; b) posttraumatic stenosis after a closed or open lesion, most often after an operation for inguinal hernia; c) postinflammatory stricture within the cauda epididymidis (rarely within the ejaculatory duct) after nonspecific process.

Both tuberculous and nonspecific adnexitis can depress the fertility in spite of free passage from the testis to the urethra. Recovery is possible after conservative or operative treatment of the adnexitis (e.g. uni-or bilateral vesiculectomy with retaining vas-ampulla-ejaculatory duct at least on one side). However, there are many examples of intact fertility in grave inflammatory changes with pyospermia.

Megavesicles and megaampullae have been considered to exist with disturbed hormonal stimulation and microvesicles with secretory sterility, but the limits for normal and pathological variations are still too ill-defined to permit such classifications.

Wider use of vaso-vesiculo-epididymography would at present offer valuable information in many cases and by more extensive use a more complete and systematized knowledge of the spermatic tract could thus be accumulated.

IX. Angiography of the bladder, urethra and male genital organs

Hitherto, the angiographic methods of examination that play an important role for so many organs have not—with one exception—proved to be of any practical significance as far as the genitourinary tract is concerned. It is true that

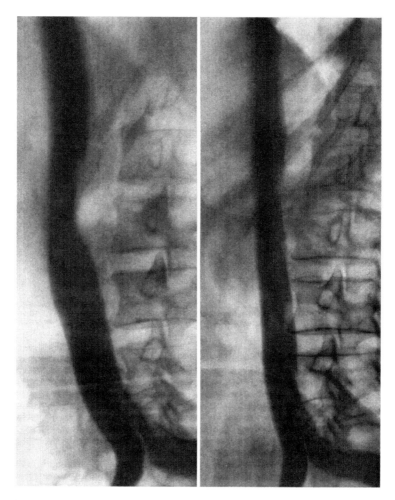

Fig. 128. Cavograms in a case of testicular tumour with metastases in lymph nodes level with L 2. To the left: a marked bulge into the posterior wall of the caval vein; to the right: the bulge almost disappeared after radiation treatment

the vesical and pudendal arteries, and sometimes the corpora cavernosa as well, can be depicted arteriographically, but this has up to now been of little diagnostic value. Although a displacement of vessels and sparse hypervascularization can be observed in the presence of expansile processes such as carcinoma of the prostate, and bladder tumours, they are by no means typical, as they may be due to an inflammatory process. Even if at least part of the pelvic venous plexus can be visualized at phlebography, this cannot be denoted as a diagnostic improvement. This also applies to direct puncture of the corpora cavernosa by injection of contrast medium. Nor have encouraging results been obtained in attempts to study tumour metastases by mean of lymphography, combined with exposure of the vas deferens.

The only angiographic method that has been able to justify its existence is cavography for visualization of retroperitoneal metastases of tumours of the testis. This also holds good, to a certain extent, for that part of the same examination intended to depict the iliac veins, for a study of metastases in the true pelvis.

Cavography is best performed by introducing a catheter into the iliac vein on one or both sides, according to Seldinger's technique. The rapid passage into the inferior vena cava requires a quantity of 30—40 ml of an iodine solution to be injected within a few seconds.

The expansion of the lymph-node region intended to be depicted by cavography in tumours of the testis lies retrocavally, at the level of the renal arteries. The best information is provided by an oblique projection, anteriorly to the left and posteriorly to the right. The deformity that can then be identified consists of displacement of the posterior wall of the vena cava, usually on a broad front. This is illustrated in Fig. 128. The possibility of giving information about tumour metastases by means of phlebography are, however, limited to the definitely positive findings. The absence of an impression in the venous wall merely implies that the metastases—if they exist—are not voluminous.

References

ABESHOUSE, B. S., E. HELLER and J. O. SALIK: Vaso-epididymography and vaso-seminal vesiculography. J. Urol. (Baltimore) 72, 983—991 (1954). — ABESHOUSE, B. S., and M. E. RUHEN: Prostatic and periprostatic phlebography. J. Urol. (Baltimore) 68, 640—646 (1952). — ADLER, U., u. J. NICK: Die Bedeutung der Tonometrie und Urethro-Cystographie bei der funktionellen Urininkontinenz. Gynaecologia (Basel) 146, 283—289 (1958). — ÅLKEN, C. E.: Leitfaden der Urologie für Studium und Praxis. Stuttgart: Georg Thieme 1955. — ALONSO, A.: Un nuevo modelo de uretrógrafo. Rev. argent. Urol. 10, 348—350 (1941). — ALVAREZ IERENA, J. J.: La uretro-cistografia. Pren. méd. mex. 11, 72, 79 (1946). — AMSELEM, A., y L. PALOMEQUE: Accidentes vasculares de la uretrocistografia. Clin. y Lab. 49, 426—430 (1950). — ANDERSEN, P. E.: Calcification of the Vasa deferentia. Acta radiol. (Stockh.) 34, 89—95 (1950). — ANDERSON, H. E.: Diagnosis of placenta praevia by use of cystogram. Urol. cutan. Rev. 42, 577—581 (1938). — ARANALDE BLANNO, J.: Estudio radiologico de la vena cava como medio diagnostico en urologia. Tesis México 1953. — ARENAS, N., y A. FOIX: Importancia de la cistouretrografia en el tratamiento de la incontinencia de orina de esfuerzo. Sem. méd. (B. Aires) 106, 160—166 (1955). — ARRIGONI, G., e G. LOVATI: Studio uretrocistografico del collo vescicale dopo prostatectomia ipogastrica e perineale. Arch. ital. Urol. 22, 190—206 (1947). — ASTRALDI, A., and E. L. LANARI: Radiographic diagnosis of malignancy of bladder tumors—personal method. Urol. cutan. Rev. 37, 222—226 (1933). — ASTRALDI, J.: Sur une radiographie de la vésicule séminale. Bull. Soc. franç. Urol. 1952, 6—8. — ATTWATER, H. L.: Inflammation of the seminal vesicles, epididymes, vasa deferentia and testes. In H. P. WHINSBURY-WHITE, Textbook of genito-urinary surgery. Baltimore: Williams & Wilkins 1948.

BACH, H.: Ventil-polyp udgået fra prostata. Ugeskr. Laeg. 120, 495—496 (1958). — BAENSCH, W.: Zur Technik der Harnröhrenfüllung. Warnung vor öligen Kontrastmitteln. Röntgenpraxis 8, 316—317 (1936). — BALL, H., u. H. PELZ: Tödlicher Zwischenfall bei der Urethrographie mit Bariumsulfat. Z. Urol. 46, 539—545 (1953). — BALL, T. L., and R. G. DOUGLAS: Topographic urethrography in "continent" and "incontinent" women. Trans. New Engl. obstet. gynec. Soc. 4, 65—80 (1950). — BALLENGER, E. G., O. F. ELDER and H. P. McDONALD: Collapsed bladder skiodan cystograms. Sth. med. J. (Bgham, Ala.) 27, 938—939 (1934). — BARRINGTON, F. J. F.: The diagnosis of stone in the urinary tract. II. Bladder and urethra. Med. Wld (Lond.) 74, 515—518 (1951). — BÁRSONY, T., and E. KOPPENSTEIN:

New method for roentgenoscopy. Orv. Hetil. 76, 989—991 (1932). — Bársony, T., u. E. Pollák: Intravenöse Urozystographie. Röntgenpraxis 4, 956—957 (1932). — Bauer, K. M.: Seltene Erkrankungen der Samenblasen. Z. Urol. 49, 287—295 (1956). — Das Rücklaufzystogramm. Medizinische 1957, 47—48. — Die Klinik der Samenblasenerkrankungen. Med. Klin. 55, 529—531 (1960). — Baumgart, R.: Diagnosestellung eines Blasenkarzinoms durch intravenöses Pyelogramm bei Unmöglichkeit der Cystoskopie wegen starker Hämaturie. Z. Urol. 47, 382—384 (1954). — Beard, D. E., W. E. Goodyear and H. S. Weens: Radiologic diagnosis of the lower urinary tract. Springfield, Ill.: Thomas 1952; Oxford: Blackwell 1952; Toronto: Ryerson 1952. — Beck, A. C., and F. P. Light: Use of x-ray (cystogram) in diagnosis of placenta praevia. N.Y. St. J. Med. 39, 1678—1684 (1939). — Begg, R. C.: The verumontanum in urinary and sexual disorders. Brit. J. Urol. 1, 237—253 (1929). — Belfield, W. T.: Vasotomy-radiography of the seminal duct. J. Amer. med. Ass. 61, 1867—1869 (1913). — Belfield, W. T., and H. Rolnick: Roentgenography and therapy with iodized oils. J. Amer. med. Ass. 86, 1831—1833 (1926). — Bell, J. C., G. W. Heublein and H. J. Hammer: Roentgen examination with special reference to methods and findings. Amer. J. Roentgenol. 53, 527—566 (1945). — Benedini, E.: L'uso dei raggi x nelle cistiti tubercolari a scopo preparatorio all'esame endoscopico (contributo, clinico). Ann. ital. Chir. 24, 128—136 (1947). — Beneventi, F. A., and V. F. Marshall: Some studies of urinary incontinence in men. J. Urol. (Baltimore) 75, 273—284 (1956). — Bengmark, S., and S. Nilsson: Human seminal vesicle, their embryonic development, studies with morphologic methods. Acta radiol. (Stockh.) (1961, to be published). — Benjamin, J. A., F. T. Joint, G. H. Ramsay, J. S. Watson, S. Weinberg and W. W. Scott: Cinefluorographic studies of bladder and urethral function. Trans. Amer. Ass. gen.-urin. Surg. 46, 43—53 (1954). — J. Urol. (Baltimore) 73, 525—535 (1955). — Bentzen, N.: Urethrographic studies of prostatic tuberculosis. Thesis Copenhagen 1960. — Bernardi, R., y J. C. Chiozzi: Anestesia retroprostático-vesical; su visualización, radiográfica. Rev. argent. Urol. 17, 431—436 (1948). — Berri, H. D.: La importancia de la radiologia en las fistulas uretrales. Sem. méd. (B. Aires) 1, 480—487 (1933). — Bertelsen, A., and H. H. Wandall: Vaso-seminal vesiculography and its clinical application. Acta radiol. (Stockh.) 26, 36—45 (1945). — Berti-Riboli, E. P., G. B. Cerruti, C. Malchiodi e G. Reggiani: Studio angiografico dei tumori vesicali. Minerva pediat. (Torino) 9, 11—18 (1957). — Bezzi, E., L. Rossi, G. Macaluso e A. Rabaiotti: Aspetti arteriografici della patologia prostatica. Minerva chir. (Torino) 12, 867—875 (1957). — Bianchini, A.: Su di un caso di calcificazione quasi totale della vie deferenziali. Arch. Radiol. (Napoli) 6, 228—233 (1930). — Birkun, A. A.: Smertel naia gazovaia emboliia pri tsistografii. (Fatal gas embolism in cystography.) Urologija 22, 65—66 (1957). — Bladdertumors. A symposium. Philadelphia: J. B. Lippincott Company 1957. — Blanc, H., et M. Negro: La cystographie; étude radiologique de la vessie normale et pathologique. Paris: Masson & Cie. 1926. — Blum, E.: Renseignements fournis par l'urographie et la prostatographie dans les maladies de la prostate. Strasbourg méd. 10, 423—425 (1959). — Blum, E., et D. Sichel: La radiographie de la prostate; technique, résultats, indications. Acta urol. belg. 25, 381—390 (1957). — Blum, E., D. Sichel, R. Wolff et J. P. Wagner: L'exploration radiologique du prostatique; valeur comparée de l'urographie intraveineuse et de la prostatographie. J. Urol. méd. chir. 63, 308—317 (1957). — Bobbio, A., E. Bezzi and L. Rossi: Pelvic angiography in diseases of the prostatic gland. Amer. J. Roentgenol. 82, 784—792 (1959). — Boeminghaus, H. W.: Urologische Diagnostik und Therapie für Ärzte und Studierende, 2. erw. Aufl. Jena: Gustav Fischer 1931. — Urologie. Operative Therapie, Klinik, Indikation, 2. Aufl. München: Werk-Verlag 1954. — Boeminghaus, H. W., u. U. Baldus: Zur Physiologie der Samenblasen und der Spermien. Z. Urol. 28, 433—462 (1934). — Boeminghaus, H., u. L. Zeiss: Erkrankungen der Harnwege im Röntgenbild. Leipzig: Johann Ambrosius Barth 1933. — Boevé, H. J.: Pyelography and cystography in children. Ned. T. Geneesk. 16, 690—694 (1929—1930). — Boone, A. W.: Cystourethrograms before prostatectomy. J. Urol. (Baltimore) 67, 358—363 (1952). — Boreau, J.: L'étude radiologique des voies séminales normales et pathologiques. Paris: Masson & Cie. 1953. — Boreau, J., A. Ellim, P. Hermann, B. Vassel et R. Fua: L'épididymographie. Presse méd. 59, 1406—1407 (1951). — Boreau, J., P. Hermann, B. Vasselle et R. Fua: L'étude radiologique et radiomanométrique des voies génitales de l'homme appliquée à la clinique et à la physiologie. Sem. Hôp. Paris 28, 1549—1556 (1952). — Boreau, J., S. Jagailloux, B. Vasselle and P. Hermann: Epididymography. Med. Radiogr. Photogr. 29, 63—66 (1953). — Boreau, J., B. Vasselle et S. Jagailloux: Étude radiologique des voies génitales normales et pathologiques de l'homme. Presse méd. 61, 1—4 (1953). — Bortolin, F.: Studio anatomo-radiologico delle vie spermatiche. Quad. Radiol. 7, 165—168 (1942). — Bosch Sola, P.: Diverticulosis y diverticulitis vesical. Exploración roentgenólogica. Clin. y Lab. 20, 217—222 (1932). — Boulland, G.: Rétention vésicale chez les prostatiques par la cysto-radiographie de profil. Paris: Le Grand 1928. — Bowen, D. R., and L. Heiman: Combined roentgenoscopic and roentgenographic cystoscopic table. Amer. J. Roentgenol. 23, 85—88 (1930). — Boyce, W.

H., J. A.Harris and S. A. Vest: The dorsal cystogram or "squat shot": a technique for roentgenography of posterior bladder and pelvic ureters. J. Urol. (Baltimore) **70**, 969—974 (1953). — Boyd, M. L., and W. A. Smith: Are cystometrograms indispensable for explanation of bladder function disturbances? J. Urol. (Baltimore) **42**, 410—419 (1939). — Boyd, R. W.: Pneumocystogram. Canad. med. Ass. J. **43**, 221—224 (1940). — Braasch, W. F., and J. L. Emmett: Clinical urography. Philadelphia: Lea & Febiger 1951. — Brailsford, J. F., H. Donovan and E. H. Mucklow: A simple estimation of residual urine in cases of prostatic disease following the ingestion of hippuran by mouth. Brit. J. Radiol. **27**, 183—186 (1954). — Brandstetter, F.: Prüfungsverfahren zur Objektivierung der funktionellen Harninkontinenz unter besonderer Berücksichtigung der Urethrozystographie. Zbl. Gynäk. **77**, 1269—1272 (1955). — Brelland, P. M.: Relationship of bladder shadow to bladder volume on excretion urography. J. Fac. Radiol. (Lond.) **9**, 152—153 (1958). — Briney, A. K., and P. J. Hodes: Urinary incontinence in women; roentgen manifestations. Radiology **58**, 109—112 (1952). — Brodny, M. L.: New instrument for urethrography in male. J. Urol. (Baltimore) **46**, 350—354 (1941). — Urethrography: its value in the study of male fertility and sterility. Fertil. and Steril. **4**, 386—411 (1953). — Brodny, M. L., and S. A. Robins: Enuresis; use of cystography in diagnosis. J. Amer. med. Ass. **126**, 1000—1006 (1944). — Use of new viscous water-miscible contrast medium rayopake (iodine preparation) for cystourethrography. J. Urol. (Baltimore) **58**, 182—184 (1947). — Value of roentgenography of male urethra following infection. Amer. J. Syph. **32**, 272—285 (1948). — Urethrocystography in male child. J. Amer. med. Ass. **137**, 1511—1517 (1948). — Morbidity after prostatectomy: an urethrocystographic study. J. int. Coll. Surg. **14**, 143—158 (1950). — Urethrocystographic study; a guide for selective prostatectomy. J. int. Coll. Surg. **21**, 351—361 (1954). — Urethrocystographic classification of prostatism. Schweiz. med. Wschr. **86**, Suppl., 541—543 (1956).— Brodny, M. L., S. A. Robins, H. A. Hershman and A. Denuccio: Epididymography, varicocelography, and testicular angiography; their uses in the study of the infertile male. Fertil. and Steril. **6**, 158—168 (1955). — Browning, W. H., D. C. Reed and H. O'Donnell: Delayed cystography; a valuable diagnostic tool. J. Kans. med. Soc. **60**, 22—24 (1959). — Bruni, P.: Angioma dell'uretra e reflusso uretro-venoso. G. ital. Chir. **4**, 515—523 (1948). — Buchmann, E.: Röntgenologisch diagnostizierte Blasenruptur. Fortschr. Röntgenstr. **82**, 823—824 (1955). — Bugyi, B.: Urethrography with umbradil viscous U preparation. Mag. Sebész. **10**, 375—378 (1957). — Bunge, R. G.: Further observations with delayed cystograms. J. Urol. (Baltimore) **71**, 427—434 (1954). — Burstein, H. J.: Cystography as aid in urologic diagnoses. Illinois med. J. **64**, 344—346 (1933). — Butler jr., W. W. S., and C. H. Peterson: Roentgen ray study of prostatic urethra with special reference to resection. Sth. med. J. (Bgham, Ala.) **27**, 690—693 (1934); also Virginia med. Monthly **61**, 276—282 (1934). — Butten, F., J. R. Sullivan and W. D. Birnbaum: Radiographic evidence indispensable aid in diagnosis of intraperitoneal rupture. West. J. Surg. **43**, 410—413 (1935).

Camerini, R., V. Zaffagnini and G. Lolli: Tomography as a research means of bladder walls. Radiol. clin. (Basel) **22**, 421—424 (1953). — Campbell, M. F.: Cystography in infancy and in childhood. Amer. J. Dis. Child. **39**, 386—402 (1930). — Cancrini, A., e A. Napolitano: Il pneumoperitoneo pelvico associato alla cistografia gassosa nello studio delle neoplasie vescicali. Ann. ital. Chir. **36**, 364—375 (1959). — Caporale, L.: Manuale di urologia. Torino: Minerva medica 1952. — Capua, A.: Possibilità della radiologia nell'accertamento delle cause di sterilità. Recenti Progr. Med. **4**, 389—409 (1948). — Carneiro Monteiro, J.: Da uretrografia no homem e suas vantagens no diagnostico das afecções uretrais. Rev. Radiol. clin. **2**, 580—588 (1933). — Carrai, P. E.: L'uretrografia negli ipospadici operati associando i procedimenti di plastica dell'Ombrédanne e del Leveuf. Arch. ital. Chir. **79**, 505—510 (1955). — Cartelli, N.: Es suficiente la radiografia simple para asegurar una litiasis vesical. Sem. méd. (B. Aires) **1**, 1460—1463 (1940). — Cartelli, N., C. Comotto y H. D. Berri: Gran reflujo uretro venoso por uretrografía. Rev. argent. Urol. **15**, 59—62 (1946). — Carvalho, M. A.: Study of 111 cystograms for diagnosis of placenta previa. Amer. J. Obstet. Gynec. **39**, 306—312 (1940). — Castellanos, A., y R. Pereiras: La cistografía en el niño. Arch. Med. infant. **9**, 160—175 (1940). — Cella, C.: Ricerche anatomoradiografiche sull'ampolla deferenziale dell'uomo nelle varie età. Ann. Radiol. diagn. (Bologna) **24**, 3—26 (1952). — Chandrachud, S.: Carcinoma in a urinary bladder diverticulum. Amer. J. Roentgenol. **75**, 925—929 (1956). — Charbonneau, J.: Du diagnostic des tumeurs de la vessie par la cystographie. J. Hôtel-Dieu Montréal **14**, 357—361 (1945). — Chauvin, E.: Maladies des vésicules séminales, anatomie, pathologie et chirurgie. Paris: Maloine 1929. — Chauvin, H. F., et A. Orsoni: Rétrécissement du col vésical après prostatectomie. Présentation de radiographie. J. Urol. méd. chir. **57**, 739—740 (1951). — Chavigny, C. L.: Beaded chain and catheter for cystograms. Obstet. and Gynec. **10**, 296—302 (1957). — Chevassu, M.: L'uréthrographie dans la tuberculose génitale mâle. Bull. Soc. franç. Urol. **1936**, 274—279. — Etude uréthrographique des cavités de prostatectomie sus-pubienne. Bull. Soc. franç. Urol. **1937**, 109—119. — L'uréthrographie à la diodone visqueuse. J. Urol. méd. chir. **58**, 149—150

(1952). — CHEVASSU, M., et E. MOREL: L'exploration radiographique de l'urètre et de la prostate. Strasbourg méd. **95**, 101—104 (1935). — CHRISTIAN, E., u. N. N. CONSTANTINESCU: Urethrography. Rev. rom. Urol. **2**, 112 (1935). — CHWALLA, R.: Die endokrine Situation beim Prostatiker. Klin. Med. (Wien) **13**, 469—477 (1958). — CIBERT, J., et H. CAVAILHER: L'exploration radiographique chez les prostatiques. J. Urol. méd. chir. **52**, 35—38 (1944). — CIVINO, A., e G. LOVATI: Controllo clinico-radiologico di un gruppo di prostatectomizzati secondo il metodo di Hryntschak. Osped. maggiore **44**, 558—562 (1956). — COE, F. O., and P. S. ARTHUR: New medium (visco-rayopake, iodine preparation) for cystourethrography. Amer. J. Roentgenol. **56**, 361—365 (1946). — COLBY, F. H.: Early carcinoma of the prostate; diagnosis and treatment. J. Mich. med. Soc. **54**, 463—465 (1953). — COLBY, F. H., and H. I. SUBY: Cysto-urethrograms; roentgen visualization of urethra, bladder and prostate. New Engl. J. Med. **223**, 85—92 (1940). — COLOMÉ BOUZA, A.: La cistografía en la práctica urológica. Vida nueva **53**, 17—24 (1944). — COMARR, A. E.: Position of the patient for roentgenologic interpretation of prostatogram. Amer. J. Roentgenol. **75**, 893—895 (1956). — COMARR, A. E., and E. BORS: Spermatocystography in patients with spinal cord injuries. J. Urol. (Baltimore) **73**, 172—178 (1955). — COMARR, A. E., and L. DODENHOFF: A safe, simple method of performing urethrograms. J. Urol. (Baltimore) **70**, 980—981 (1953). — CONRADT, J.: Les suites opératoires locales de la prostatectomie suspubienne étudiées par l'urétrographie. J. belge Urol. **11**, 31—35 (1938). — COOK, E. N.: Diverticulum of the female urethra: problems in diagnosis and treatment. Surg. Gynec. Obstet. **99**, 273—276 (1954). — COTTALORDA, J., H. RUFF et J. SAVELLI: Résultats uréthrographiques de l'opération de Millin. Marseille chir. **8**, 5—31 (1956). — COTTENOT, P., et BINET DU JASSONEIX: Un cas d'opacité totale des vésicules séminales. Bull. Soc. Radiol. méd. France **17**, 109 (1929). — COUTES, W. E., et F. A. CANTIN: Contribution à la vésiculographie séminale. J. Urol. méd. chir. **41**, 553—555 (1936). — COUVELAIRE, R.: Pathologie de l'appareil urinaire et de l'appareil génital masculin. Nouveau précis de pathologie chirurgicale, tome VI/I. Paris: Masson & Cie. 1949. — COUVELAIRE, R., et J. FORET: Sur la signification de l'asymétrie urographique des images urétéro-pyélo-calicielles du prostatique. J. Urol. méd. chir. **59**, 17—27 (1953). — COUVELAIRE, R., et C. LEVEY: Sur la deferentovésiculographie en exploration génito-urinaire. J. Urol. méd. chir. **59**, 447—469 (1953). — CRABTREE, E. G.: Venous invasion due to urethrograms made with lipiodol (iodized oil). Trans. Amer. Ass. gen.-urin. Surg. **38**, 19—30 (1947) also J. Urol. (Baltimore) **57**, 380—389 (1947). — CRABTREE, E. G., and M. L. BRODNEY: Estimate of value of urethrogram and cystogram in diagnosis of prostatic obstruction. J. Urol. (Baltimore) **29**, 235—276 (1933). — CRABTREE, E. G., M. L. BRODNEY, H. A. KONTOFF and S. R. MUELLNER: Roentgenologic diagnosis of urologic and gynecologic diseases of female bladder. J. Urol. (Baltimore) **35**, 52—69 (1936). — CROOKS, M. L.: Roentgen examination of the urinary tract in children. X-Ray Techn. **23**, 24—26 (1951). — CRUZ, M.: Über dynamische Störungen der Urethra posterior und ihre Untersuchung mit Hilfe der Urethrographie. Z. Urol. **28**, 675—681 (1934).

DAMANSKI, M., and A. S. KERR: The value of cysto-urethrography in paraplegia. Brit. J. Surg. **44**, 398—407 (1957). — DAMM, E.: Die funktionelle Cysturethrographie. Z. Urol. **42**, 68—70 (1949). — DA MOTTA PACHECO, A. A.: Diagnóstico radiológico do adenoma da próstata. S. Paulo méd. **2**, 360—370 (1944). — DA MOTTA PACHECO, A. A., J. M. DE CASTRO, J. JANY y H. TUFF: Cineuretrocistografia indireta. Arch. bras. Urol. **4**, 7—17 (1946). — DA MOTTA PACHECO, A. A., y O. L. DO ROSARIO: A imagem do veru-montanum na uretrografia. An. paul. Med. Cir. **42**, 293—305 (1941). — DANNENBERG, M., J. S. BEILLY, M. B. RODNEY and C. STORCH: Cystographic studies in placenta praevia. Amer. J. Roentgenol. **64**, 53—60 (1950). — DARGET, R.: L'exploration par l'air du rein et de la vessie. Bull. Soc. Chir. Bordeaux et Sud-Ouest **1932**, 69—74. — Nuove ricerche radiografiche in urologia. Minerva chir. (Torino) **10**, 367 (1955). — DEAN, A. L.: Carcinoma of the male and female urethra; pathology and diagnosis. J. Urol. (Baltimore) **75**, 505—513 (1956). — DEAN jr., A. L., J. K. LATTIMER and C. B. MCCOY: The standardized Columbia University cystogram. J. Urol. (Baltimore) **78**, 662—668 (1957). — DE AZEVEDO, G. V., y J. M. CABELO CAMPOS: Da uretrografia na mulher e seu valor pratico. Rev. Ass. paul. Med. **1**, 400—405 (1932). — DE FIGUEIREDO, A.: Uretroscopia e uretrografia. Med. Cirurg. Farm. **1942**, 789—829. — DE LAMBERT, B. M., and N. F. GREENSLADE: Cystourethrography in the male. Med. J. Aust. **41**, 159—162 (1954). — DE LA PEÑA, A., y E. DE LA PEÑA: Diverticular or cavitary chronic prostatitis. J. Urol. (Baltimore) **55**, 273—277 (1946). — DEL NEGRO, O.: Epididimografia; técnica y ventajas. Sem. méd. (B. Aires) **113**, 701—706 (1958). — DELPORTE, T. V.: La uretrografia. Su importancia en urología. Rev. méd. Rosario **33**, 165—181 (1943). — DE MORAES BARROS, C., y A. A. DA MOTTA PACHECO: O refluxo uretro-vesiculodeferencial na uretrografia. An. paul. Med. Cir. **42**, 47—50 (1941). — O cistograma nas pericistites. Arch. bras. Urol. **1**, 87—97 (1942). — Ensaio de sistematisação dos sináis radiológicos das afecções da prostata. Arch. bras. Urol. **1**, 17—85 (1942). — DE MOURA, C., y P. DE CARVALHO: Neumo-testiculo. Arch. esp. Urol. **10**, 39—49 (1954). — DENCK, H., u. R. HOHENFELLNER: Über die chronische, unspezifische

Prostatitis. Klin. Med. (Wien) 13, 245—250 (1958). — DESY, J.: L'uréthro-cystographie et ses déductions cliniques. Rev. méd. Liège 4, 491—493 (1949). — DEUTICKE, P.: Klinik der Erkrankungen von Hoden und Samenblase. Wien. klin. Wschr. 56, 356—358 (1943). — DEVOS, R.: Tumeur testiculaire; intérêt des radiographies systématiques du médiastin. Acta urol. belg. 23, 274—275 (1955). — DIAZ CASTRO, H. B., y C. ROVIRA BURZACO: Consideraciones sobre uretrografía. Arch. urug. Med. 1, 380—391 (1932). — DI GRAETA, S., e F. ORRENTINO: La policistografía: metodologia ed indicazioni. Rif. med. 73, 1224—1227 (1959). — DILLON, J. R.: Excretory cystograms after voiding. Calif. Med. 67, 17—22 (1947). — DIONISI, H., y A. FERNIOT: La cistografia en el prolapso genital. Bol. Soc. Cir. Córdoba 8, 275—287 (1947). — DOSSOT, R., et M. PALAZZOLI: Les urétrites chroniques; diagnostic et traitement. Paris: Masson & Cie. 1932. — DOTTA, J. S., y T. V. DELPORTE: El reflujo venoso en la uretrografia. Rev. argent. Urol. 13, 133—137 (1944). — DRAPER, J. W., and J. G. SICELUFF: Excretory cysto-urethrograms. J. Urol. (Baltimore) 53, 539—544 (1945). — DRESSLER, L.: Neuere Untersuchungen zur röntgenologischen Darstellung der männlichen Harnröhre, Prostata und Samenblase. Fortschr. Röntgenstr. 39, 872—882 (1929). — DUCLUZAUX, J. Q.: A propos des remainements radiographiques du bassin chez les cancéren prostatiques. Thèse Paris 1952. — DUFOUR, A.: Réflexions sur l'exploration radiologique de la vessie. Sem. Hôp. Paris 33, 4324 SP (1957). — DUVERGEY, H., u. PUJO: Was wird aus der Wundhöhle nach Prostatektomie? Z. Urol. 36, 343—351 (1942).

EBERHART, C.: The etiology and treatment of urethritis in the female patients. J. Urol. (Baltimore) 79, 293—299 (1958). — EDLING, N. P. G.: Urethrocystography in male with special regard to micturition. Acta radiol. (Stockh.) Suppl. 58, 1—144 (1945). — On roentgen aspect of prostatic cancer by urethrocystography. Acta radiol. (Stockh.) 29, 461—474 (1948). — On the roentgen aspect of prostatic atrophy. Acta radiol. (Stockh.) 31, 145—151 (1949). — Radiologic aspect of utriculus prostaticus during urethrocystography. Acta radiol. (Stockh.) 32, 28—32 (1949). — Die Darstellung der Harnröhre und der Harnblase mittels wasserlöslicher Kontrastmittel. Fortschr. Röntgenstr. 72, 18—29 (1950). — Roentgendiagnostik der Harnorgane. In SCHINZ, BAENSCH, FRIEDL u. UEHLINGER, Lehrbuch der Roentgendiagnostik, 5. Aufl., Bd. 7/8. Stuttgart: Georg Thieme 1952. — The roentgen diagnosis of the diseases of the prostate. J. Urol. (Baltimore) 67, 197—207 (1952). — The radiologic appearances of diverticula of the male cavernous urethra. Acta radiol. (Stockh.) 40, 1—8 (1953). — EDSMAN, G.: Roentgenologic changes in the urinary bladder and the distal portion of the ureters in spermatocystitis. Acta radiol. (Stockh.) 29, 371—382 (1948). — EDWARDS, D.: Cineradiography of the congenital neurogenic bladder. Proc. roy. Soc. Med. 49, 898—899 (1956). — Cineradiology of congenital bladder-neck obstruction and the megaureter. Brit. J. Urol. 29, 410—415 (1957). — EISLER, F.: Röntgenuntersuchung der Harnblase. Röntgenpraxis 6, 204—210 (1934). — EKMAN, H.: Views on the value of urethrocystography in determining indications for surgery in prostatic hypertrophy. Acta chir. scand. 115, 18—24 (1958). — Late results of prostatectomy for benign prostatic hyperplasia. A clinical study based on 370 cases. Acta chir. scand. Suppl. 250, 1—140 (1959). — ENGEL, W. J.: Uretral ectopia opening into the seminal vesicle. J. Urol. (Baltimore) 60, 46—49 (1948). — Intravenous urography in study of vesical neck obstructions. Amer. J. Roentgenol. 62, 661—669 (1949). — ENGELS, E. P.: Sigmoid colon and urinary bladder in high fixation; roentgen changes simulating pelvic ulcer. Radiology 72, 419—422 (1959).

FAZEKAS, I. G.: Plötzlicher Tod infolge des durch die Harnröhrenperforationen in den Blutkreislauf gelangten Röntgenbreies (Bariumsulfatschock). Z. Urol. 47, 673—679 (1954), also Orv. Hetil. 95, 669—672 (1954). — FERDINAND, L.: Technic of urethrography. Rozhl. Chir. 35, 24—26 (1956). — FERNICOLA, A. R.: Extra-urethral confines of urethrographic contrast medium. J. Urol. (Baltimore) 66, 132—144 (1951). — FERULANO, O. e D. NAPOLI: La proiezione assiale dorso-perineale nella indagine cistografica. Arch. Radiol. (Napoli) 30, 225—241 (1955). — FETTER, T. R.: Prostatitis and seminal vesiculitis: acute and chronic. Penn. med. J. 50, 812—822 (1947). — FEY, B., F. STOBBAERTS, P. TRUCHOT et G. WOLFROMM: Exploration radiologique de l'appareil urinaire inférieur (vessie, urètre, prostate). Avec la collaboration de L. SABADINI et al. Paris: Masson & Cie. 1949. — FICHARDT, T.: Screening urethrocystography of adult Bantu males under manometric control; normal and pathological findings. Brit. J. Radiol. 32, 120—131 (1959). — FILHO MATTOSO, S.: El empleo del doble contraste en uretrografia. Arch. esp. Urol. 5, 330—332 (1949). — FINKELSHTEIN, S. I.: Axial roentgen projections in urology. Urologija 24, 50—53 (1959). — FIRSTATER, M.: Cistografia de eliminación y uretroprostatografia. Rev. argent. Urol. 22, 151—156 (1953). — FITZPATRICK, R. J., and L. M. ORR: Pelvio-prostatic venography; preliminary report. J. Urol. (Baltimore) 68, 647—651 (1952). — FLECKER, H.: Position of urinary bladder. Med. J. Aust. 2, 823 (1934). — FLOCKS, R. H.: The roentgen visualization of the posterior urethra. J. Urol. (Baltimore) 30, 711—736 (1933). — FOCHEM, K.: Die Bedeutung der Röntgendiagnostik im Rahmen der Sterilitätsuntersuchungen. Wien. klin. Wschr. 71, 388—390 (1959). — FOCHEM, K., u. A. H. PALMRICH: Zur zystographischen Symptomatik der relativen

Harninkontinenz. Zbl. Gynäk. **76**, 1741—1746 (1954). — FORBES, K. A., and J. J. CORDON-NIER: Circulatory collapse following combined use of rayopake and air for urethrocystography. J. Urol. (Baltimore) **70**, 975—979 (1953). — FORSYTHE, W. E.: Prostatic abscess with particular reference to use of urethrogram in diagnosis. Urol. cutan. Rev. **46**, 613—617 (1942). — FORSYTHE jr., W. E.: Cystourethrographic diagnosis of prostatic disease. Urol. cutan. Rev. **47**, 669—673 (1943). — FRAIN-BELL, L., and J. GRIEVE: The micturating cystourethrogram in relation to function after prostatectomy. Brit. J. Urol. **29**, 15—19 (1937). — FRANCKE jr., P., and J. W. LANE: Cystitis emphysematosa, case report. Amer. J. Roentgenol. **75**, 921—924 (1956). — FRANKSSON, C., and K. LINDBLOM: Roentgenographic signs of tumor infiltration of the wall of the urinary bladder. Acta radiol. (Stockh.) **37**, 1—7 (1952). — FRANKSSON, C., K. LINDBLOM and W. WHITEHOUSE: The reliability of roentgen signs of varying degrees of malignancy of bladder tumors. Acta radiol. (Stockh.) **45**, 266—272 (1956). — FRANZ, R.: Die Bedeutung der Cystographie für die Wahl der Therapie bei Harninkontinenz. Wien. klin. Wschr. **68**, 2170 (1956). — FREIRE, J. G. DE CAMPOS: Valôr diagnóstico das radiografías contrastadas das vias espermáticas. Tése de concurso São Paulo 1943. — FRIEDHOFF, E.: Die intravenöse Urographie bei der Blasenhalsgeschwulst. Langenbecks Arch. klin. Chir. **274**, 132—138 (1953). — FRIEDMAN, P. S., L. SOLIS-COHEN and S. M. JOFFE: Urethral calculus; its roentgen evaluation. Radiology **62**, 248—250 (1954). — FRÜHWALD, R.: Urethrographie bei Gonorrhoe des Mannes und bei der Frau. Derm. Wschr. **90**, 133—143 (1930). — Die röntgenologische Darstellung der männlichen Harnröhre. Bemerkungen zu der Arbeit von OSWALD GRIMM. Dtsch. med. Wschr. **62**, 2102—2103 (1936). — Ein Urethrogramm bei Balanitis xerotica obliterans. Z. Haut- u. Geschl.-Kr. **24**, 157—161 (1958). — FRUMKIN, A. P.: Röntgenographie von Hyperthrophien der Vorsteherdrüse. Röntgenpraxis **1**, 498—504 (1929). — FULTON, H.: Delayed cystography in children. Amer. J. Roentgenol. **78**, 486—491 (1957).

GAIGNEROT, J.: La radiographie dans les tumeurs de la vessie. Arch. Mal. Reins **10**, 461—515 (1936). — GAMBETTA, G., et L. BORINI: La vésiculographie dans la tuberculose génitale; notre expérience personelle et présentation de dix radiogrammes. Acta urol. belg. **23**, 285—301 (1955). — La stratigraphie des vésicules séminales normales et pathologiques. Acta urol. belg. **25**, 11—34 (1957). — L'investigation radiologique des vésicules séminales dans le carcinome vésical. Acta urol. belg. **25**, 391—399 (1957). — GANDINI, D., e A. GIBBA: Modoficazione alla tecnica della cistografia combinata. Ann. Radiol. diagn. (Bologna) **26**, 64—78 (1953). — GARCIA, A. E., y J. CASAL: El diagnóstico uretrográfico de la enfermedad del cuello vesical. Rev. méd. Hosp. esp. (B. Aires) **23**, 83—87 (1953). — El diagnóstico uretrográfico de la enfermedad del cuello vesical. Rev. argent. Urol. **23**, 49—54 (1954). — GARCIA, A. E., J. CASAL y A. ROCCHI: El reflujo uretro-venoso como accidente de la uretrografia. Rev. argent. Urol. **15**, 423—430 (1946). — GAUDIN, H.: Roentgen examination of male urethra. N.Z. med. J. **45**, 376—383 (1946). — Fatal embolism following urethrography. J. Urol. (Baltimore) **62**, 375—377 (1949). — GAUSA, P.: Una nueva técnica urográfica. Visualizacion radiográfica de las neoformaciones vesicales. Rev. méd. Barcelona **25**, 223—240 (1936). — GAUTIER, E. L.: Urologie, 4. edit. Rev. corr. et mise à jour par J. L. Gaillard. Paris: Malonie 1954. — GÉRARD, P. L., A. DUFOUR et C. HELENON: Intérét de l'exopneumopéritoine dans l'étude des tumeurs de la vesic. J. Radiol. Électrol. **40**, 341—343 (1959). — GERNER-SMIDT, M.: Vesiculography as a diagnostic aid in cancer and hypertrophy of the prostate. Acta chir. scand. **114**, 387—397 (1958). — GIBBA, A., e D. GANDINI: Su di una recente modalita di tecnica cistografia combinata. Arch. ital. Urol. **25**, 245—254 (1951/52). — GIBSON, T. E.: Tumors of the seminal vesicle. Urology **2**, 1170—1176 (1954). — GIERTZ, G., and K. LINDBLOM: Urethro-cystographic studies of nervous disturbances of the urinary bladder and the urethra; a preliminary report. Acta radiol. (Stockh.) **36**, 205—216 (1951). — GILLIES, C. L., and H. D. KERR: Diagnosis of lesions of lower urinary tract. Radiology **26**, 286—294 (1936). — GINESTIE, J.: L'urétrographie en position debout en particulier dans l'hypertrophie de la prostate. J. Urol. méd. chir. **50**, 171—174 (1942). — GIORDAMENGO, G.: Sulle reazione della vesica ai vari mezzi di contrasto radiografico. Boll. Soc. piemont. Chir. **4**, 1330—1341 (1934). — GIROTTO, A.: Pneumourethrography in diagnosis of foreign bodies of male urethra. Ann. ital. Chir. **21**, 651—657 (1942). — GISCARD, J. B., et DE BERTRAND-PIBRAC: L'utilité de la radiographie dans les formations diverticulaires de la prostate. Presentation de clichés. Bull. Soc. Radiol. méd. France **22**, 438—442 (1934). — GIULIANI, L., e E. PISANI: L'intestino nella chirurgia plastica e sostitutiva della vesceca: Valutazione cistomanometrica e cestografica dei risultati. Arch. ital. Urol. **32**, 165—217 (1959). — GÖTZEN, F. J.: Über eine cystographische Besonderheit bei nerval gestörter Harnblase. Z. Urol. **49**, 340—343 (1956). — GOLDBERG, V. V.: X-ray diagnosis of cancer of the prostate. Urologija **3**, 24—37 (1955). — GOLJI, H.: Clinical value of epididymo-vesiculography. J. Urol. (Baltimore) **78**, 445—455 (1957). — GONZALES, J. V.: Urétro-cystographie dans un cas de diaphragme intervésicoprostatique. J. Urol. méd. chir. **26**, 236—237 (1928). — GONZALES-IMAN, F.: Retrograd seminal vesiculography. J. Urol. (Baltimore) **49**, 618—627 (1943). —

GOODWIN, P. B.: Roentgen study of lesions of urinary bladder. Illinois med. J. **69**, 58—62 (1936). — GOODYEAR, W. E., D. E. BEARD and H. S. WEENS: Urethrography: diagnostic aid in diseases of lower urinary tract. Sth. med. J. (Bgham, Ala.) **41**, 487—495 (1948). — GORRO, A.: Vesikulographie. J. Urol. méd. chir. **28**, 781—791 (1934). — GOUVÊA, G. S.: Iconografia urológica; bexiga. Rev. bras. Cir. **31**, 526—531 (1956). — GRAAS, G., u. H. MIL-LER: Eine neue Methode zur Darstellung der Blase und ihrer pathologischen Inhalte. Fortschr. Röntgenstr. **87**, 218—221 (1957). — GRAJEWSKI, L. E., and R. F. HOFFMAN: Conditions of male and female urethra as demonstrated by cystourethrography. Alex. Blain Hosp. Bull. **5**, 87—97 (1946). — GRANBERG, P. O., and F. SVARTHOLM: Urethral diverticula in the female; with special reference to the roentgenographic diagnosis and the result of surgery. Acta chir. scand. **115**, 78—88 (1958). — GRASHEY, R.: Atlas des chirurgisch-pathologischen Röntgen-bildes. Lehmanns medizinische Atlanten, 3. Aufl., Bd. VI. München: J. F. Lehmann 1931. — GRAUHAN, M.: Zur Klinik und Anatomie des venösen Refluxes bei der Urethrographie. Zbl. Chir. **66**, 1692—1701 (1939). — GREENBERG, G.: Treatment of gonorrheal arthritis by vaso-tomy with special reference to the study of vesiculograms. Med. J. Rec. **124**, 76—79 (1926). — GRENADINNIK, J. S.: Cystography in nocturnal incontinence. Vestn. Rentgenol. Radiol. **31**, 54—56 (1956). — GRIESBACH, W. A., R. K. WATERHOUSE and H. Z. MELLINS: Voiding cysto-urethrography in the diagnosis of congenital posterior urethral valves. Amer. J. Roentgenol. **82**, 521—529 (1959). — GRIMALDI, A., y A. R. ERASO: Impregnación persistente del medio de contraste urografico; pielografia retrograda y eretrografia. Rev. argent. Urol. **24**, 680—683 (1955). — GRIMM, O.: Die röntgenologische Darstellung der männlichen Harnröhre. Dtsch. med. Wschr. **62**, 1671—1673 (1936). — GUDBJERG, C. E., L. K. HANSEN and E. HASNER: Mic-turition cysto-urethrography; automatic serial technique. Acta radiol. (Stockh.) **50**, 310—315 (1958). — GÜNTHER, G. W.: Röntgenuroskopie: Nierenbecken und -kelche, Harnleiter, Blase, Harnröhre. Stuttgart: Georg Thieme 1952, New York: Grune & Stratton 1952. — GUICHARD, R., et H. DUVERGEY: L'urethrographie. Paris: Masson & Cie. 1948. — GULLMO, Å.: A simple instrument for urethrocystography and fistulography in adults and children. Acta radiol. (Stockh.) **45**, 473—478 (1956). — GULLMO, Å., and J. SUNDBERG: A method for roentgen examination of the posterior urethra, prostatic ducts and utricle (utriculogra-phy). Acta radiol. (Stockh.) **45**, 241—247 (1957).

HAAS, L., et K. FILLENZ: Contribution au radiodiagnostic de la prostate. J. Radiol. Électrol. **22**, 103—108 (1938). — HACKWORTH, L. E.: Urethrography in infants and children. J. Urol. (Baltimore) **60**, 947—951 (1948). — HAENISCH, F.: Die Röntgenuntersuchung des Uropoëtischen Systems. In H. LOSSEN, Röntgendiagnostik, 7/1, S. 902, Lehmanns medi-zinische Atlanten, 5. Liefg. München: J. F. Lehmann 1938. — HAGEMANN, E.: Eine rationelle Methode zur Röntgenuntersuchung der Harnblase. Dtsch. Gesundh.-Wes. **12**, 846—847 (1957). — HAGNER, R.: The operative treatment of sterility in the male. J. Amer. med. Ass. **107**, 1851—1855 (1936). — HAJOS, E.: Methodik des Röntgenschichtverfahrens in der Uro-logie. Fortschr. Röntgenstr. **91**, 366—382 (1959). — HALLGREN, B.: Enuresis. Köpenhamn: Munksgaard 1957. — HANAFEE, W. N., and R. D. TURNER: Some uses of cinefluorography in urologic diagnostic problems. Radiology **73**, 733—739 (1959). — HARDER, E.: The micturi-tion cystourethrography in children. Radiography **21**, 255—258 (1955). — HARLIN, H.: Seminal vesiculitis. J. Amer. med. Ass. **143**, 880—884 (1950). — HARTL, H.: Die Ergebnisse der Urethrographie bei der Frau. Fortschr. Röntgenstr. **82**, 680—686 (1955). — HARTUNG, W., and R. H. FLOCKS: Diverticulum of bladder, method of roentgen examination and roentgen and clinical findings in 200 cases. Radiology **41**, 363—370 (1943). — HECKEN-BACH, W.: Physiologie und Pathologie der Harnleiterdynamik bei der Ausscheidungsuro-graphie unter besonderer Berücksichtigung der Adnexerkrankungen. Z. urol. Chir. **35**, 34—77 (1932). — HEDERRA, R.: Cistografia con doble medio de contraste. Arch. Soc. Ciruj. hosp. **13**, 210—211 (1943). — HEIKEL, P. E., and K. V. PARKKULAINEN: A comparison between the results obtained by urography and mictiocystography in pediatric urological disease. Acta paediat. (Uppsala) **48**, Suppl. 118, 149—150 (1959). — The value of mictio-cystourethrography in pediatric urological diagnosis. Ann. Med. intern. Fenn. **48**, Suppl. 128, 25—34 (1959). — HEISE, G. W., u. A. KULESSA: Mitteilung über eine verbesserte Röntgendiagnostik der Samenblasenerkrankungen. Z. Urol. **48**, 295—315 (1955). — HEITZ-BOYER, M.: L'urétrographie dans la polypose urétrale. Bull. Soc. franç. Urol. **1934**,88—92. — Formations diverticulaires prostatiques et orchites à répétition (dites sans cause); intérêt de l'urétrographie en pareil cas. Bull. Soc. franç. Urol. **1934**, 119—128. — Urétrographie et formations diverticulaires prostatiques; son utilité pour la technique de l'évidement. Bull. Soc. franç. Urol. **1935**, 46—49. — Maladie diverticulaire de la prostata et septicémie. Bull. Soc. franç. Urol. **1935**, 49—67. — Maladie diverticulaire de la prostata et calculs pro-statique. Bull. Soc. franç. Urol. **1935**, 108—130. — Maladie diverticulaire prostatique et cancer de la prostate. Bull. Soc. franç. Urol. **1935**, 131—139. — Urétrographie avec "rem-plissage variable". Bull. Soc. franç. Urol. **1935**, 316—323. — HELLER, M.: L'étude radio-logique de la vésicule séminale. J. Radiol. Électrol. **29**, 151—152 (1948). — HENDRIOCK,

A.: Beobachtungen von urethrovenösem Übertritt des Kontrastmittels bei der Urethrographie. Zbl. Chir. **59**, 1415—1423 (1932). — Hendriock, A.: Gefahren bei der Harnröhrenanästhesie und Urethrographie und ihre Vermeidung. Dtsch. med. Wschr. **59**, 171—172 (1933). — Henline, R. B.: Prostatitis and seminal vesiculitis: acute and chronic. J. Amer. med. Ass. **123**, 608—615 (1943). — Hennig, O.: Die röntgenologische Darstellung der Prostatikerblase mit Bariumaufschwemmung und Luft am liegenden und stehenden Kranken; ein wirtschaftliches Verfahren. Langenbecks Arch. klin. Chir. **275**, 418—439 (1953). — Herbst, R. H., and J. W. Merricks: Visualization and treatment of seminal vesiculitis by catheterization and dilatation of the ejaculatory ducts. J. Urol. (Baltimore) **41**, 733—750 (1939). — Herbut, P. A.: Urological pathology. Philadelphia: Lea & Febiger 1952. — Herman, L.: The practice of urology. Philadelphia and London: W. B. Saunders Company 1943. — Herzog, A.: Die röntgenologische Darstellung der Harnblase ohne Kontrastmittel. Z. Urol. **28**, 200—203 (1934). — Hickel, R.: Technique et résultats de l'exploration radiologique de la vessie. Sem. Hôp. Paris **33**, 4311—4323 SP (1957). — Hindse-Nielsen, S.: Cystoradiographie mit Bromnatriumlösung — Cystitis gravis — Exitus letalis. Zbl. Chir. **56**, 1681—1683 (1929). — Hinman jr., F., G. M. Miller, E. Mickel and E. R. Miller: Vesical physiology demonstrated by cineradiography and serial roentgenography; preliminary report. Radiology **62**, 713—719 (1954). — Hinman jr., F., G. M. Miller, E. Mickel, H. L. Steinbach and E. R. Miller: Normal micturition; certain details as shown by serial cystograms. Calif. Med. **82**, 6—7 (1955). — Hock, E.: Diverticula of the prostate. J. Urol. (Baltimore) **56**, 353—367 (1946). — Hodgkinson, C. P., and H. P. Doub: Roentgen study of urethrovesical relationships in female urinary stress incontinence. Radiology **61**, 335—345 (1953). — Hodgkinson, C. P., H. P. Doub and W. T. Kelly: Urethrocystograms: metallic bead chain technique. Clin. Abst. (N.Y.) **1**, 668—677 (1958). — Hofer, R., u. H. Lossen: Teilweise verkalkte Ductus deferentes. Z. Urol. **26**, 153—156 (1932). — Holder, E.: Die Harnröhrenstriktur im Röntgenbild. Langenbecks Arch. klin. Chir. **272**, 224—240(1952). — Horne, G. O.: Examination of prostatic secretion for leukocytes. Brit. J. Urol. **27**, 61—62 (1955). — Hortolomei, N., et T. Katz-Galatzi: Contribution à l'étude de l'urétrographie. J. Urol. méd. chir. **36**, 321, 437 (1933). — Roentgenologic study of urethral strictures. Rev. Ştiinţ. med. **22**, 1125—1143 (1933). — Urethrographic study of rupture of urethra. Român. med. **11**, 311—313 (1933). — Value and indications for roentgenography of urethra and its accessory organs. Român. med. **11**, 289—291 (1933). — Howard, F. S.: Hypospadias with enlargement of the prostatic utricle. Surg. Gynec. Obstet. **86**, 307—316 (1948). — Hudson, E.: Urethro-cystography. Radiography **23**, 316—224 (1957). — Huggins, C.: The prostatic secretion. Harvey Lect. **92**, 148—193 (1946). — Huggins, C., and R. S. Bear: Course of prostatic ducts and anatomy, chemical and X-ray diffraction analysis of calculi. J. Urol. (Baltimore) **51**, 37—47 (1944). — Huggins, C., and W. Webster: Duality of human prostate in response to estrogen. J. Urol. (Baltimore) **59**, 258—266 (1948). — Hulse, C. A.: Radiographic procedures in urology. X-Ray Techn. **21**, 348—353 (1950). — Hultborn, K. A., O. Morales and R. Romanus: The so-called shelf tumour of the rectum. Acta radiol. (Stockh.) Suppl. **124**, 1—46 (1955). — Hyams, J. A., H. R. Kenyon and S. E. Kramer: Urethrocystography in male. J. Amer. med. Ass. **101**, 2030—2035 (1933).

Iacapraro, G., y R. Iacapraro: La cistografía en los tumores de vejiga; su importancia. Bol. Inst. Med. exp. Cáncer (B. Aires) **15**, 173—182 (1938). — Ichikawa, T.: Über unsere Methode der Prostatographie. Z. Urol. **48**, 114—115 (1955). — Inclán Bolado, J. L.: Algunas consideraciones sobre la vesiculografia. Arch. esp. Urol. **12**, 26—36 (1956). — Isnardi, U.: La uretrografía en el adenoma de próstata. Sem. méd. (B. Aires) **1**, 1661—1663 935). — Ivanizky, M.: Beiträge zur Anatomie des Ductus ejaculatorius. Z. Anat. Entwickl.-Gesch. **87**, 11—21 (1928).

Jablonski, K., u. E. Meisels: Der diagnostische Wert der Cystographie bei Placenta praevia. Zbl. Gynäk. **62**, 532—538 (1938), also Ginek. pol. **17**, 22—28 (1938). — Jagailloux, S.: Contribution apportée à l'étude clinique des affections de l'appareil génito-urinaire par la radiographie des voies séminales de l'homme. Thèse Paris 1952. — Jakhnich, I. M.: Metodicheskie ukaraniia k provedeniiu rentgenologiche skogo issledovaniia nochevykh organov. Moskva: Medgiz 1957. — Jakoleff, A. A.: Value of roentgen diagnosis in hernia of bladder. Vestn. Rentgenol. Radiol. **6**, 331—335 (1928). — Janker, R.: Ein Beitrag zur Verkalkung der Samenblasen und Samenleiter. Fortschr. Roentgenstr. **52**, 36—43 (1935). — Jensen, V.: A simple device for urethrocystography. Acta radiol. (Stockh.) **45**, 403—404 (1956). — Jianu, S., and Z. Borza: Clinical use of urethrography. Rev. chir. (Bucureşti) **21**, 483—492 (1929). — Jomain, J.: L'uréthrographie: Technique et résultats. Paris: Le François 1936. — Prévention des embolies huileuses au cours de l'urethrographie par l'emploi d'un moyen de contraste hydrosoluble en solution visqueuse. J. Urol. méd. chir. **58**, 134—136 (1952). — Diagnostic radiographique des tumeur vésicales par une technique de cystographies tandard; pseudo-tomographies par la méthode de la flaque améliorée. J. Urol. méd. Chir. **63**, 536—539 Jones, R. F.: Symposium on prostatic cancer. V. Conclusion. J. nat. med. Ass. (N.Y.) **47**,

157 (1955). — JOSEPH, E., u. S. PERLMANN: Archiv und Atlas der normalen und pathologischen Anatomie in typischen Röntgenbildern. Die Harnorgane im Röntgenbild. Fortschr. Röntgenstr., Erg.bd. 37, herausgeg. von Prof. GRASHEY, 2. Aufl. Stuttgart: Georg Thieme 1931. — JOUBERT, J. D.: Kistografie en uretragrafie. S. Afr. med. J. 32, 748—752 (1958). — JULES, R.: L'information déférento-vésiculographique dans le diagnostic de la tuberculose génitale profonde et dans celui du cancer de la prostate. Thèse Lille 1958. — JULIANI, G., e A. GIBBA: Quadri deferento-vesiculografici negzi adenomi e nei carcinomi della prostata. Nunt. radiol. (Firenze) 21, 165—187 (1955). — JUNGHANNS, H.: Darstellung der Samenblasen im Röntgenbild durch Füllung mit Jodipin. Röntgenpraxis 8, 21—24 (1936).

KADRNKA, S., et J. PONCET: Vessie géante par cancer papillaire. Contribution à la cysto-radiographie de l'épithélioma. Rev. méd. Suisse rom. 54, 789—796 (1934). — KAISER, R.: Selten lange Verweildauer des Kontrastmittels nach urethro-venösem Übertritt bei der Urethrographie. Chirurg 11, 61—63 (1939). — KANAUKA, V.: Roentgen diagnosis of male urethra. Medicina (Kaunas) 16, 487—492 (1935). — KATZ-GALATZI, T.: Le reflux uréthroveineux et les dangers de l'emploi des huiles dans l'urèthre. J. Urol. med. chir. 44, 300—310 (1937). — KAUFMANN, J. J., and M. RUSSEL: Cystourethrography, clinical experience with the newer contrast media. Amer. J. Roentgenol. 75, 884—892 (1956). — KAUFMAN, P., u. A. IKLÉ: Beitrag zur Beurteilung der relativen Urininkontinenz mit der lateralen Zystourethrographie. Geburtsh. u. Frauenheilk. 16, 29—43 (1956). — KELLER, J.: Urologie. Ein Leitfaden für den Urologen und den urologisch interessierten Praktiker, 2. neubearb. Aufl. Dresden u. Leipzig: Theodor Steinkopff 1958. — KELLER, O.: Value of urethrography from practical and clinical viewpoint. Hospitalstidende 73, 583—596 (1930). — Om urethro-venös reflux. Ugeskr. Laeg. 96, 750—751 (1934). — KEMBLE, J.: Urethrography, technique, interpretation and utility. Brit. med. J. 2, 683—686 (1939). — KENNEDY, W. T.: Incontinence of urine in female; functional observations of urethra illustrated by roentgenograms. Amer. J. Obstet. Gynec. 33, 19—29 (1937). — Incontinence of urine in female. Study of urethral sphincter under hydrostatic pressure with roentgenograms—sphincter mechanism, loss of control, restoration. N.Y. St. J. Med. 38, 256—261 (1938).—KERR, H. D., and C. L. GILLIES: The urinary tract. A handbook of roentgen diagnosis. Chicago: Year Book Publ. 1944. — KIDD, F.: Cystogram of hernia of bladder. Brit. J. Urol. 2, 166—169 (1930). — Catheterisation of the ejaculatory ducts and seminal vesiculogram. Lancet 1931, 864. — KIMBROUGH, J. C.: Symposium on prostatic cancer. II. Importance of early detection. J. nat. med. Ass. (N.Y.) 47, 149—152 (1955). — KINGREEN, O.: Röntgendiagnostik des Chirurgen, 4. überarb. Aufl. Leipzig: Johann Ambrosius Barth 1958. — KJELLBERG, S. R., N. O. ERICSSON and U. RUDHE: The lower urinary tract in childhood; some correlated clinical and roentgenologic observations. Chicago: Year Book Publ. 1957. — KLIKA, M.: Die neueren Ansichten über die Anatomie und das Adenom der Prostata und ihre praktische Ausnützung. Urol. int. (Basel) 6, 232—242 (1958). — KNEISE, O., u. K. L. SCHOBER: Die Röntgenuntersuchung der Harnorgane, 4. Aufl. Leipzig: Georg Thieme 1952. — KNUTSSON, F.: On the technique of urethrography. Acta radiol. (Stockh.) 10, 437—441 (1929). — Urethrography. Examination of male urethra and prostate after injection of contrast material into urethra; experience gained from examination of 154 patients in Maria Hospital, Stockholm. Acta radiol. (Stockh.) Suppl. 28, 1—150 (1935). — KOHNSTAM, G. L. S., and E. H. P. CAVE: The radiological examination of the male urethra. London: Baillière, Tindall & Cox 1925. — KORABEL'NIKOV, I. D.: Contrast cystography in diagnosis of retroperitoneal hematomas. Vestn. Rentgenol. Radiol. 2, 91—93 (1955). — KORIN, D. L.: Cystography method in diagnosis of injuries of the bladder. Chirurgica 1952, 64—68. — KORKUD, G.: L'épididymographie. Sem. Hôp. Paris 28, 2427—2433 (1952). — KOTAY, P., et L. SZERÉMY: Nos expériencens sur l'examen combiné röntgen de la vessie. Acta urol. belg. 3, 46—53 (1949). — KRAAS, E.: Die röntgenologisch gleichzeitige Darstellung der männlichen Harnröhre und Blase. Langenbecks Arch. klin. Chir. 178, 361—375 (1933). — KRAATZ, H.: Der Einfluß der vaginalen Radikaloperation auf die Harnblase. Ein Versuch, die postoperativen urologischen Komplikationen nach funktionellen Gesichtspunkten unter Zuhilfenahme der Zystoradiographie zu klären. Z. Geburtsh. Gynäk. 123, 1—65 (1941). — Die Bedeutung der Cystoradiographie für die gynäkologische Urologie. Zbl. Gynäk. 65, 793—812 (1941). — KÜSS, R., et NOIX: Étude radiocinématographique de la miction des vessies iléales. J. Urol. méd. chir. 62, 519—520 (1956). — KURITA, T.: Über die intravenöse Pyelographie und Cystographie. Nagoya J. med. Sci. 6, 8—15 (1932).

LACCETTI, C.: Importanza di alcune ricerche nella diagnostica radiologica della vescica e del rene. Arch. ital. Chir. 39, 967—973 (1933). — LAMIAUD, H.: Le lipiodol en urologie. Paris: Maloine 1931. — LANGE, J.: La tomographie dans les tumeurs de la vessie. J. Urol. méd. chir. 60, 158—163 (1954). — LANGER, E.: Roentgenography of male urethra. Vestn. Vener. Derm. 6, 36—40 (1929). — Zur Diagnose der Harnröhren- und Blasenmißbildungen. Z. Urol. 23, 324—327 (1929). — Die Röntgendiagnostik der männlichen Harnröhre. Leipzig: Voss 1931. — Zu der Arbeit von PAUL EICHLER, zur Frage bei Embolie-Gefahr bei der Verwendung von Jodölen in der Röntgendiagnostik der unteren Harnwege. Röntgenpraxis **4**, 405—406 (1932). — Langer, E., u. C. Engel: Fortschritte in der Röntgendiagnostik der männlichen Harnröhre und ihrer Anhängegebilde. Z. Urol. **26**, 30—35 (1932). — Die Deutung des Röntgenbildes der sogenannten Nebenharnröhre. Z. urol. Chir. **36**, 428—432 (1933). — Die Deutung des Röntgenbildes der sogenannten Nebenharnröhre. Z. Urol. **27**, 566—567 (1933). — Langreder, W., u. F. Brandstetter: Grundlagen zur röntgenologischen Inkontinenzdiagnostik. Arch. Gynäk. **188**, 344—363 (1957). — Lasio, E.: I tumori maligna della vesica. Milano: Delfino 1950. — Lasio, E., G. Arrigoni e A. Gvino: L'aortografia addominale in chirurgia urologica. Minerva urol. (Torino) **7**, 8—10 (1955). — Laurent, G., et G. Conradt: Étude radiographique de l'urètre masculin. Ann. Soc. méd.-chir. Liège **2**, 198—204 (1933). — Étude radiographique de l'urètre masculin. Liège méd. **27**, 200—215 (1934). — Leal, H.: Das vesiculografias. Rev. Urol. S. Paulo **3**, 32—41 (1935). — Ledoux-Lebard, R., J. Garcia-Calderon et J. Petetin: L'urétrographie. Paris méd. **1**, 105—111 (1932). — La uretrografia. Rev. méd. cubana **45**, 674—686 (1934). — Le Fur, R.: De la vésiculographie. Bull. Soc. Chirurgiens Paris **22**, 21 (1930). — Legueu, F., B. Fey et P. Truchot: Cystographie au collothor. Bull. Soc. franç. Urol. **1933**, 156—161. — Lemaitre, G., G. Defrance et C. Dupuis: Radiologie des valvules urétrales du nourrisson et de l'enfant. J. Radiol. Électrol. **39**, 436—438 (1958). — Lemaitre, G., et R. Jules: La déférento-vésiculographie. Application au diagnostic de la tuberculose séminale. J. Radiol. Électrol. **40**, 535—544 (1959). — Lemaitre, L.: La cystographie. Gaz. méd. Fr. (Suppl. Radiol.) **1933**, 101—103. — Lepontre, C.: Urétrographie postérieure et indications opératoires. Bull. Soc. franç. Urol. **1938**, 164—167. — Décalage de l'urètre prostatique. Bull. Soc. franç. Urol. **1940**, 103—105. — Lerique, J.: Vesicule seminale fistulisée à la fesse à l'age de 6 mois; diagnostic établi à l'age de 11 ans. J. Radiol. Électrol. **38**, 375 (1957). — Lespinasse, V. D.: Urethrograms of male urethra. Quart. Bull. Northw. Univ. med. Sch. **19**, 298—302 (1945). — Levey, C.: La déférento-vésiculographie en exploration génito-urinaire. Étude critique. Thèse Paris 1953. — Levi, I.: Sull'uretrografia nelle affezioni blenorragiche. G. ital. Derm. Sif. **71**, 1353—1360 (1930). — Sopra due casi di "falsa strada", accertati mediante l'uretrografia. Arch. ital. Derm. **7**, 501—505 (1931). — Levine, M. H., and S. Crosbie: The value of a routine abdominal film. J. Amer. med. Ass. **156**, 220—222 (1954). — Levy, C. S.: Value of cystogram in cases of very large prostatic hypertrophies. Urol. cutan. Rev. **44**, 644—646 (1940). — Lewis, L. G.: Symposium on prostatic cancer. III. Surgical approach for diagnosis and treatment. J. nat. med. Ass. (N.Y.) **47**, 152—155 (1955). — Liang, D. S.: Hemangioma of the bladder. J. Urol. (Baltimore) **79**, 956—960 (1958). — Lichtenberg, A. v., u. W. Heinemann: Über die technischen Bedingungen der Sondierung der Ductus ejaculatorii. Z. urol. Chir. **25**, 286—291 (1928). — Liess, G., u. K. Berwing: Fehlermöglichkeiten bei der röntgenologischen Darstellung der Prostatahypertrophie mit Hilfe der Abrodilpfütze nach Kneise-Schober. Z. Urol. **48**, 240—250 (1955). — Lievre, J. A.: Le diagnostic des métastases osseuses du cancer de la prostate et de l'osteite fibreuse. Presse méd. **60**, 85—89 (1952). — Lloyd, F. A., and T. L. Cottrell: Diatrizoale sodium. Ann. N.Y. Acad. Sci. **78**, 987—992 (1959). — Loizzi, A.: La deferento — epididimografia. Arch. ital. Urol. **26**, 63—73 (1953). — Loughnane, F. McG.: Examination of the male urethra. In: H. P. Whinsbury-White, Textbook of genito-urinary surgery, p. 374. Baltimore: Williams & Wilkins Company 1948. — Lower, W. E., and B. H. Nichols: Roentgenographic studies of the urinary system. St. Louis: Mosby Comp. 1933. — Lowsley, O. S., and T. J. Kirwin: Clinical urology, 2. edit., I—II. Baltimore: Williams & Wilkins Company 1944. — Lowsley, O. S., and A. P. Peterson: The Lowsley—Peterson universal endoscope. A new instrument and its uses. Amer. J. Surg. **79**, 168—170 (1938). — Lund, C. J., J. A. Benjamin, T. A. Tristan, R. E. Fullerton, G. H. Ramsey and J. S. Watson: Cinefluorographic studies of the bladder and urethra in women. I. Urethrovesical relationships in voluntary and involuntary urination. Amer. J. Obstet. Gynec. **74**, 896—908 (1957). — Lund, C. J., R. E. Fullerton and T. A. Tristan: Cinefluorographic studies of the bladder and urethra in women. II. Stress incontinence. Amer. J. Obstet. Gynec. **78**, 706—711 (1959). — Lurá, A.: Valore diagnostico del pneumovaginale e dell'insufflazione della spazio scrotale. Ann. Radiol. diagn. (Bologna) **18**, 379—387 (1946). — Luys, G.: Le cathétérisme des canaux éjaculateurs. Clinique (Paris) **23**, 73—76 (1928). — Traité des maladies des vésicules séminales. Paris: Maloine 1929.

Mac Laren, J. W.: Modern trends in diagnostic radiology. New York: Hoeber 1948. — Macnish, J. M.: Cysto-urethrography in male. Urol. cutan. Rev. **40**, 77—81 (1936). — Macquet, P., et G. Lemaitre: La cystographie à la flaque dans les tumeurs vésicales. J. Radiol. Électrol. **34**, 418—420 (1953). — Mainzer, F., u. E. Yaloussis: Über latente Lungenerkrankung bei manifester Blasenbilharziose. Nach Röntgenuntersuchungen. Fortschr. Röntgenstr. **54**, 373—381 (1936). — Mándi, J., u. G. Tompa: Pelvic venography in prostate surgery. Orv. Hetil. **97**, 1169—1171 (1956). — Marchand, J. H., N. Barag, G. Clement, L. Le Vizon et M. Grimberg: Contribution à l'étude radiologique de la prostate. J. Radiol.

Électrol. **38**, 838—839 (1957). — MARCHAND, J., LE VIZON, CLEMENT, GRIMBERG, BARAG et PINSKY-MOORE: Étude d'un rétrécissement urétral par le double procédé de l'urographie veineuse et de l'urétro-cystographie rétrograde. J. Radiol. Électrol. **38**, 1146—1147 (1957). — MARION, G.: Des erreurs dans l'interprétation des uréthrographies. Bull. Soc. franç. Urol. **1936**, 40—47. — De la nécessité de pratiquer une exploration complète de la vessie avant toute prostatectomie. J. Urol. méd. chir. **46**, 139—143 (1938). — Traité d'urologie. Paris: Masson & Cie. 1940. — MARKMAN, B. J.: Two mechanical devices for reducing risk of radiation exposure during certain types of roentgen examinations. Acta radiol. (Stockh.) **27**, 388—391 (1946). — MARKS, J. H., and D. P. HAM: Calcification of vas deferens. Amer. J. Roentgenol. **47**, 859—863 (1942). — MARSHALL, V. F.: Diagnosis of genito-urinary neoplasms. New York: Amer. Cancer. Soc. 1949. — Textbook of urology. London: Harper 1956. — MARTINELLI, V., G. MICIELI e L. SARACCA: Quadri deferentovesiculografici nella ipertrophia prostatica. Ann. ital. Chir. **37**, 34—49 (1960). — MARTINET, R.: La uretrografía retrograda. Arch. esp. Urol. **4**, 318—323 (1948). — MARTINI, M.: Röntgendarstellung der Samenblasen am Lebenden. Z. urol. Chir. **44**, 326—339 (1938). — MARTIN-LUQUE, T.: La radiographie de la miction dans les affections prostato-urétrales. J. Urol. méd. chir. **28**, 237—249 (1929). — MARTINS COSTA, J., e B. NEGRINI: Cateterismo dos canais ejaculadores e vesiculografia com o aparelho de McCarthy. Arch. bras. Urol. **1**, 209—220 (1942). — MASON, J. T., and W. B. CRENSHAW: Rectal obstruction by carcinoma of the prostate. Amer. J. Surg. **96**, 319—323 (1958). — MATHEY-CORNAT, R., et H. DUVERGEY: Sur l'exploration urétrographique des cancer de la prostate. J. Radiol. Électrol. **25**, 199—201 (1942/43). — MAYNE, G. O.: Urethrography in urethral stricture. Brit. J. vener. Dis. **32**, 119—126 (1956). — MAZUREK, L. J.: Radiodiagnostyka kliniczna chorob narzada moczowego. Warszawa: Panstwowy Zaktad Wydawn. Lekarskich 1957. — McCARTHY, J. F., and J. S. RITTER: The seminal vesicles. J. Amer. med. Ass. **98**, 687—691 (1932). — McCREA, L. E.: Primary carcinoma of the seminal vesicles—report of two cases—review of the literature. Urol. cutan. Rev. **46**, 700—703 (1942). — Clinical urology. Essentials of diagnosis and treatment. Philadelphia: F. A. Davis & Co. Publ. 1948. — Primary carcinoma of the seminal vesicles. J. Amer. med. Ass. **136**, 679—682 (1948). — McDONALD, H. P., W. E. UPCHURCH and M. F. ARTIME: Visualization of vesical masses by excretory urography. Amer. Practit. **10**, 2140—2142 (1959). — McDOWELL, J. F.: Cystographic diagnosis of placenta praevia. Amer. J. Obstet. Gynec. **33**, 436—443 (1937). — McIVER, J.: Use of cystogram in diagnosing placenta praevia. Tex. St. J. Med. **32**, 471—474 (1936). — McKENNA, C. M., and J. H. KIEFER: Congenital enlargement of the prostatic utricle with inclusion of the ejaculatory ducts and seminal vesicles. Trans. Amer. Ass. gen.-urin. Surg. **32**, 305—320 (1939). — McMAHON, S.: An anatomical study by injection technique of the ejaculatory ducts and their relations. J. Anat. (Lond.) **72**, 556—574 (1937) also in J. Urol. (Baltimore) **39**, 422 (1938). — Contrast cystogram. Brit. J. Urol. **11**, 133—141 (1939). — MÉAN, L.: La cystographie dans le diagnostic des diverticules vésicaux. Liège méd. **29**, 577—581 (1936) also Ann. Soc. méd.-chir. Liège **1936**, 92—96. — MELLINGER, G. T., and P. B. KLATTE: Neocystoscopy and neocystography. Proc. N. cent. Sect. Amer. urol. Ass. **1957**, 144—146 also J. Urol. (Baltimore) **79**, 459—462 (1958). — MENTHA, C.: L'examen radiologique de la vessie (stéréo-pneumo-iodocystographie). J. Urol. méd. chir. **53**, 89—97 (1946/47). — MERRICKS, J. W.: The modern conception of the diagnosis and treatment of infections of the seminal vesides; with roentgenologic visualization of these organs by catherization of the ejaculatory ducts. Int. Clin. **2**, 193—199 (1940). — MIDDLEMISS, J. H.: Radiology in diseases of the prostate. J. Fac. Radiol. (Lond.) **4**, 115—124 (1952). — MIGLIARDI, L.: La cistouretrografia discendente. Radiol. med. (Torino) **21**, 136—150 (1934). — L'indagine radiologica del collo vesicale e delli uretra posteriore maschili. Boll. Soc. piemont. Chir. **5**, 345—354 (1935). — La cysto-urétrographie descendante; sa technique et ses indications. J. Urol. méd. chir. **40**, 499—511 (1935). — MIKALOVICI, I.: L'urétrographie chez les nourrissons avec un cas de strictures congénitales. J. Urol. méd. chir. **37**, 516—519 (1934). — MILLER, A.: Radiology in diseases of the prostate. J. Fac. Radiol. (Lond.) **4**, 125—129 (1952). — MILLER, J. D.: Studies on cystocele and urinary incontinence in female by use of cystograms and urethrograms. J. Urol. (Baltimore) **40**, 612—623 (1938). — MOCK, J., et R. GAMBIER: Urétrographie dans un cas de rétrécissement serré de l'urètre avec fistule périnéale. Bull. Soc. Chirurgiens Paris **24**, 5—9 (1932). — *Modern trends in urology*, edit. by E. W. RICHES. London: Butterworth & Co. 1953. — MONTENEGRO, N.: Cálculos vesicales invisibles a la radiografía. Rev. argent. Urol. **9**, 531—539 (1940). — MORALES, O., and R. ROMANUS: Urethrography in the male with a highly viscous, water soluble contrast medium, umbradilviscous U. Acta radiol. (Stockh.) Suppl. **95** (1952). — Urethrography in the male; delimitation of the anterior and posterior urethra, the pars diaphragmatica, the pars nuda and the presence of a musculus compressor nudae. Acta radiol. (Stockh.) **39**, 453—476 (1953). — Urethrography in the male: the boundaries of the different urethral parts and detail studies of the urethral mucous membrane and its motility. J. Urol. (Baltimore) **73**, 162—171 (1955). — MOREAU, M. H., y J. E. MOREAU: Contribución a la técnica de la uretrografía; pinza para uretrografía. Radiologia (B. Aires) 8, 174—176 (1945), also Rev. Asoc. méd. argent. 60, 818—819 (1946) and Pren. méd. argent. 33, 2041—2044 (1946). — MORTENSEN, H.: Use of cystourethrogram in diagnosis of various conditions in lower portion of urinary tract. Med. J. Aust. 1, 157—160 (1942). — MUELLNER, S. R., and F. G. FLEISCHNER: Normal and abnormal micturition; study of bladder behavior by means of fluoroscope. J. Urol. (Baltimore) 61, 233—243 (1949). — MUND, E.: Zur Kontrastdarstellung der männlichen Harnröhre. Dtsch. med. J. 7, 126—129 (1956). — MUÑOZ, H. D.: Uretrografia. Tesis. Universidad Buenos Aires. Buenos Aires: S. A. Casa Jacobo Penser 1942. — MURAYAMA, M.: Recherches sur des calculs de la vessie au point de vue chimique et radiographique. J. orient. Med. (Abstr. sect.) 20, 76 (1934). — MUSIANI, A.: Aspects cystoscopiques et cystographiques de la rétraction inflammatoire de l'urétère. J. Urol. méd. chir. 57, 11—20 (1951). — MYGIND, H. B.: Urogenital tuberkulose hos manden; undersøgelse med vesikulografi og urethrografi; foreløbig meddelelse. Ugeskr. Laeg. 121, 449—454 (1959). — Urogenital tuberculosis in the human male. Vesiculographic and urethrographic studies. Dan. med. Bull. 7, 13—18 (1960).

NAMIKI, J., and T. HANAOKA: On lateral urethrography. Jap. J. Derm. (Abstr. sect.) 38, 44—47 (1935). — NAMIKI, J., J. KAGAYA u. J. YOSHIHIRO: Zwei Fälle von Barrierebildung. Jap. J. Derm. 45, 105—109 (1939). — NAVARRETE, E.: A propósito de un signo radiológico que presenta la cistografia en la mujer. Rev. méd. peru. 19, 459—465 (1946). — NÉDELEC, M.: Vérification des résultats anatomiques des prostatectomies sus-pubiennes par l'urétrographie. Arch. Mal. Reins 8, 147—175 (1934). — NEGRO, M.: La cistografia combinata idrobarina, olio gomenolato, aria. Minerva urol. (Torino) 5, 179—182 (1953). — NESBIT, R. M.: Problems in urological diagnosis; series 1. Ann Arbor, Mich.: Edwards bros. 1948. — NEY, C., and J. DUFF: Cysto-urethrography: its role in diagnosis of neurogenic bladder. J. Urol. (Baltimore) 63, 640—652 (1950). — NIIZAWA, S., and H. MAEHARA: Calcification of lymph nodes in true pelvis; roentgenography in differential diagnosis between shadows of vesical calculi and similar extravesical shadows. J. orient. Med. (Abstr. sect.) 30, 270 (1939). — NILSEN, P. A.: Cystourethrography in stress incontinence. Acta obstet. gynec. scand. 37, 269—285 (1958). — NILSSON, A. E.: The palpability of infiltrative bladder tumours; a diagnostic comparison with roentgenographic findings. Acta chir. scand. 115, 132—137 (1958). — NILSSON, S.: Human seminal vesicle, studied with plastic corrosion method under normal and pathological conditions. Acta radiol. (Stockh.) 1962, to be published. — NÖLTING, D. E., R. CASO y J. R. STRATICO: Contribución al diagnóstico radiológico de la placenta previa por medio de la cistografía. Bol. Inst. Matern. (B. Aires) 11, 261—268 (1942). — Contribución al diagnóstico radiológico de la placenta previa por medio de la cistografía; a propósito de su utilización en el diagnóstico diferencial de 40 observaciones de hemorragias genitales del último trimestre del embarazo. Pren. méd. argent. 30, 368—371 (1944). — NORDENSTRÖM, B. E. W.: A method of topographic urethrocystography in women. Acta radiol. (Stockh.) 37, 503—509 (1952). — Some observations on the shape and course of the female urethra during miction. Acta radiol. (Stockh.) 38, 125—132 (1952). — Roentgenologic demonstration during micturition of pathologic changes in the female urethra. Acta radiol. (Stockh.) 38, 254—272 (1952). — NOTTER, G., u. C. G. HELANDER: Über den Wert der Cavographie bei Diagnose und Behandlung retroperitonealer Testistumormetastasen. Fortschr. Röntgenstr. 89, 409—417 (1958).

O'CONOR, V. J., and E. CROWLEY: Bilateral calcification of the vasa deferentia. Quart. Bull. Northw. Univ. med. Sch. 21, 28—30 (1947). — ODISCHARIA, S.: Zur Kontrast-Röntgenuntersuchung der männlichen Harnröhre. Fortschr. Röntgenstr. 40, 1108—1110 (1929). — OLIVIER, C., et P. FELLUS: Diagnostic cystographique d'un hématome pelvien sous-peritonéal. Presse méd. 61, 1243—1244 (1953). — OLSSON, O.: Cystography with graduated compression. Acta radiol. (Stockh.) 29, 429—434 (1948). — OLTRAMARE, J. H., et R. MARTINET: De l'uréthrographie. Schweiz. med. Wschr. 68, 12—25 (1938). — ORANTES SUAREZ, A.: Radiografía clínica de la uretra. Rev. Urol. (Méx.) 2, 322—331 (1944) also Rev. méd. Hosp. gen. (Mex.) 6, 111—117 (1944). — ORAVISTO, K. J., and S. SCHAUMAN: Urethrocystography in the differential diagnosis of cancer of the prostate. Duodecim (Helsinki) 71, 395—408 (1955). — Urethrocystography in the differential diagnosis of prostatic cancer. J. Urol. (Baltimore) 75, 995—999 (1956). — ORSOLA MARTI, J.: La cistografía en el diagnóstico de los tumores de vejiga. Rev. méd. Barcelona 24, 21—28 (1935) also Medicina (Méx.) 15, 241—243 (1935). — ORTMANN, K. K., and H. CHRISTIANSEN: Roentgenologic studies of male urethra, closing mechanism of bladder, and micturition under normal and pathologic conditions. Acta radiol. (Stockh.) 15, 258—283 (1934). — Roentgenologic studies of male urethra and vesical sphincter and mechanism of micturition under normal and pathologic conditions. Hospitalstidende 77, 921—940 (1934). — OSADCHUK, V. I.: Experiences in the roentgenological investigation of seminal vesicles. Urologija 25, 35—40 (1960).

PAALANEN, H.: Malignant prostate. Ann. Chir. Gynaec. Fenn. 45, Suppl. 10 (1956). — PALMER, B. M.: Study of air cystograms in prostatic hypertrophy. Urol. cutan. Rev. 44, 795—797 (1940). — PANZIRONI, P. E., e G. IANNACCONE: La vesica urinaria nel lattante;

studio anatomo-radiologico. Radiol. med. (Torino) 40, 1109—1126 (1954). — PARKER, G.: Uses and interpretation of urethrogram. Brit. J. Urol. 4, 1—10 (1932). — PARONYAN, R. L.: Air embolism during cystography. Nov. hir. Arh. 44, 321—322 (1939). — PARTSCH, F., u. BREITLÄNDER: Die Darstellung der Harnröhre bei Strikturen und Rupturen im Röntgenbild. Z. urol. Chir. 25, 108—123 (1928). — PEREIRA, A.: Fundamentos para a interpretacāo das radiografia contrastadas das vesiculas seminaes e das vias espermaticas. Rev. Urol. (S. Paulo) 2 (1935). — Vesiculographias. Rev. Urol. (S. Paulo) 3, 42—52 (1935). — Vesiculas seminaes patologicas. Rev. Urol. (S. Paulo) 3 (1935). — Diagnóstico radiológico das disetasias do colo vesical. S. Paulo méd. 2, 437—452 (1943). — Importance of roentgen examination in diagnosis of adenoma of prostate. Amer. J. Roentgenol. 51, 600—613 (1944). — Roentgen diagnosis of diseases of neck of bladder. Amer. J. Roentgenol. 56, 489—499 (1946). — Information derived from examination of neck of bladder and of prostatic urethra. J. Urol. (Baltimore) 57, 1054—1068 (1947). — Roentgen interpretation of vesiculograms. Amer. J. Roentgenol. 69, 361—379 (1953). — PEREZ CASTRO, E.: Diagnostic value of lacunar cystography. J. Urol. (Baltimore) 64, 484—498 (1950). — PERUZZO, L., e R. ANTONINI: L'epididimografia; ricerche cliniche e sperimentali. Arch. ital. Urol. 26, 540—544 (1934). — PERVES, J., et H. DUVERGEY: Du reflux urétro-vésiculo-deferential. J. Urol. méd. chir. 48, 97—113 (1939). — PETCHERSKY, B. L., F. Y. STROKOFF and I. F. SHISHOFF: Urethrography and cysto-urethrography. Vener. Derm. 7, 54—60 (1930). — Röntgen diagnosis of paraurethral sinuses and urethral anomalies. Urol. cutan. Rev. 34, 673—679 (1930). — Roentgenography in urethral stenosis. Sovet. Vestn. Vener. i Derm. 1, H. 8, 47—54 (1932). — PETERSON, A. P.: Retrograde catheterization in diagnosis and treatment of seminal vesiculitis. J. Urol. (Baltimore) 39, 662—677 (1938). — On the digital examination of the seminal vesicles with reference to the significance of findings. Surg. Clin. N. Amer. 19, 317—323 (1939). — Comparative studies on the active and passive drainage of the seminal vesicles. Urol. cutan. Rev. 43, 241—246 (1939). — PETKOVIĆ, S.: Die Bedeutung der Malignität von Blasentumoren. Z. Urol. 46, 511—523 (1953). — PÉTRIGNANI, R.: Indications et technique de l'urétrographie. Arch. Élect. méd. 41, 243—254 (1933) also Bull. Soc. Radiol. méd. France 21, 315—319 (1933). — PEZZI, G.: L'urethrografia. Ann. Med. nav. colon. 41, 475—490 (1935). — PFAHLER, G. E.: Die Röntgendiagnostik und -therapie der Blasenkrebse. Kontrolle des Behandlungserfolges durch Serien von Pneumozystogrammen. Strahlentherapie 54, 538—548 (1935). — Diagnosis and treatment of cancer of the bladder by means of roentgen rays. Penn. med. J. 39, 572—575 (1936). — Roentgen rays in diagnosis and treatment of tumors of bladder. Amer. J. Roentgenol. 41, 962—969 (1939). — Los rayos Roentgen en el diagnóstico y en el tratamiento de los tumores de la vejiga. Sem. méd. (B. Aires) 1, 1525—1532 (1940). — PFEIFER, K.: Eine rationelle Methode zur Röntgenuntersuchung der Harnblase. Dtsch. Gesundh.-Wes. 12, 809—812 (1957). — PFEIFER, W.: Grundlagen der funktionellen urologischen Röntgendiagnostik. Stuttgart: Georg Thieme 1949. — PIGANIOL, G., A. HERVÉ et A. BRUNEAU: La vésiculodéférentographie chez les bilharziens. J. Urol. méd. chir. 63, 773—785 (1957). — PINCELLI, C., e F. PROSPERI: L'indagine pneumocistostratigrafica associata a retropneumoperitoneo nello studio delle neoplasie vescicali. Minerva urol. (Torino) 11, 215—220 (1959). — POHJOLA, R., and P. I. TUOVINEN: Vesiculography in vesiculoprostatitis. Ann. Chir. Gynaec. Fenn. 38, 221—237 (1949). — POMEROY, E. S.: Diagnostic value of cystograms. Urol. cutan. Rev. 40, 35—37 (1936). — PONS, H., Y. DENARD et Y. MOREAU: Un signe radiologique du diabète: la calcification des canaux déférents. J. Radiol. Électrol. 38, 237 (1957). — POTSAID, M. S., and L. L. ROBBINS: Diprotrizoate sodium. Ann. N.Y. Acad. Sci. 78, 993—1008 (1959). — PRAETORIUS, G.: Zur Röntgendarstellung chronischer Prostata-Abszesse. Z. Urol. 26, 689—698 (1932). — PRATHER, G. C., and B. PETROFF: Spinal cord injuries; urethrographic study of bladder neck. J. Urol. (Baltimore) 57, 274—284 (1947). — PRENTISS, R. J., and W. W. TUCKER: Cystography in diagnosis of placenta praevia. Amer. J. Obstet. Gynec. 37, 777—787 (1939). — Cystographic diagnosis of placenta praevia. J. Iowa St. med. Soc. 29, 252—256 (1939). — PUGH, W. S.: Seminal vesiculitis. A cause of ureteral obstruction. J. Amer. med. Ass. 91, 1443—1446 (1928). — Seminal vesiculitis or appendicitis. J. Urol. (Baltimore) 22, 313—320 (1929). — PUHL, H.: Die Röntgenuntersuchung der männlichen Harnröhre. Dtsch. Z. Chir. 220, 372—417 (1929). — Fortschritte der Röntgenologie und Endoskopie der Harnröhre und des männlichen Genitale. Zbl. Chir. 57, 2552—2573 (1930). — PUIGVERT GORRO, A.: Technique et résultats de la vésiculographie. J. Urol. méd. chir. 37, 193—205 (1934). — Diverticulos vesicales: aportación a su diagnóstico y tratamiento. Arch. esp. Urol. 2, 263—284 (1946), also Ann. med. Barcelona 33, 341—348 (1946). — Cistovesiculografía simultánea. Arch. esp. Urol. 4, 135—141 (1947). — PUIGVERT, A., y C. ROMERO-AGUIRRE: La vesiculografia para el diagnostico de las afecciones de la prostata y vejiga. Acta ibér. radiol.-cancer. 3, No 9, 1—31 (1954).

QUACKELS, R.: Propos sur la spermato-cystographie. Acta urol. belg. 25, 413—419 (1957). — QUENU, L., et B. TRUCHOT: La pariétographie vésicale dans l'étude des tumeurs de vessie. J. Radiol. Électrol. **40**, 596—598 (1959). — Quinn, W. P.: Radiologic methods in diagnosis and treatment of carcinoma of the prostate and urinary bladder. J. nat. Cancer Inst. **20**, 109—113 (1958).

Raffaelli, M.: Studio radiologico del fondo vescicale nella diagnosi differenziale tra ipertrofia prostatica semplice e tumore maligno della prostata. Quad. Radiol. **1**, 41—60 (1937). — Raffo, V., et A. Vallebona: Quelques remarques à propos de la cystoradiographie. J. Urol. méd. chir. **27**, 216—219 (1929). — Rating, B.: Zur Darstellung von Urethravarizen. Fortschr. Röntgenstr. **63**, 214—221 (1941). — Rebaudi, L., y M. Moreau: Radiografia de próstata. Rev. argent. Urol. **27**, 40—41 (1958). — Renander, A.: Roentgenologic differentiation of vesical uroliths. Acta radiol. (Stockh.) **26**, 329—333 (1945). — Reygaerts, J.: Aspects de la cystographie après opération de Michon et leur signification. Brux.-méd. **37**, 1483—1490 (1957). — Riba, L. W.: Carcinoma of the female urethra. Quart. Bull. Northw. Univ. med. Sch. **28**, 347—351 (1954). — Riba, L. W., C. J. Schmidlapp and N. L. Bosworth: Ectopic ureter draining into the seminal vesicle. J. Urol. (Baltimore) **56**, 332—338 (1946). — Richards, C. E.: Visco-rayopake (iodine preparation) in cystography. J. Urol. (Baltimore) **58**, 185—191 (1947). — Ringleb, O.: Die Grundlagen für die richtige Beurteilung der Tiefenerstreckung in der Blase. Z. Urol. **30**, 673—685 (1936). — Zur radiologischen Klinik der Blasengeschwülste. Strahlentherapie **105**, 530—550 (1958). — Ritter, J. S., and I. N. Rattner: Umbrathor (thorium dioxide preparation) in urography. Amer. J. Roentgenol. **28**, 629—633 (1932). Roberts, H.: Cystourethrography in women. Brit. J. Radiol. **25**, 253—259 (1952). — Roberts, M. S., and J. K. Lattimer: Advantages of floating lipiodol as further test for voiding efficiency. J. Pediat. **54**, 68—75 (1959). — Robertson, J. P., and J. W. Headstream: The use of the cystogram and urethrogram in the diagnosis and management of rupture of the urethra and bladder. Sth. med. J. (Bgham, Ala.) **44**, 895—901 (1951). — Robles Fontan, W.: Diagnostico de las neoplasmas genito-urinarias. Thesis Mexico 1955. — Rollestone, G. L.: Lower urinary tract disorders in children. J. coll. radiol. Aust. **4**, 15—20 (1960). — Rolnick, D., R. R. Cross jr. and F. A. Lloyd: Urethrograms in the diagnosis and management of benign prostatic hypertrophy. J. int. Coll. Surg. **31**, 683—691 (1959). — Rolnick, H. C.: Catherization of the ejaculatory ducts. Surg. Gynec. Obstet. **42**, 667 (1926). — Romanus, R.: Pelvo-spondylitis ossificans in the male (Ankylosing spondylitis, Morbus Bechterew-Marie-Strümpell) and genito-urinary infection. Acta med. scand. Suppl. **280**, 1—368 (1953). — Romanus, R., and S. Ydén: Pelvo-spondylitis ossificans. Rheumatoid or ankylosing spondylitis. Copenhagen: Munksgaard 1955. — Romero-Aguirr, C.: Estudo radiologico algunas afecciones extrinsecas de las vias espermáticas. Deferento-vesiculografia. Thesis Madrid. 1953. — Roper, R. S.: Gonococcal infections of the seminal vesicles. Lancet **1931**, 793—800. — Rose, D. K.: Various cystourethrograms and their interpretation; study of preoperative and postoperative incontinence in male. J. Urol. (Baltimore) **27**, 207—227 (1932). — Ross, N.: Radiographic diagnosis of prostatic enlargement. Lancet **1933**, 14—16. — Value of aerocystography. Lancet **1934**, 124—128. — Rothfeld, S. H., and B. S. Epstein: The size of the bladder in intravenous urography and retrograde cystography; a potential source of diagnostic error in children. J. Urol. (Baltimore) **78**, 817—820 (1957). — Rotstein, T.: Zur Methodik der Röntgenuntersuchung der männlichen Harnröhre. Fortschr. Röntgenstr. **44**, 785—787 (1931). — Rotstein, Z. J., u. Z. V. Chaskina: Zur Frage der Röntgenuntersuchung der männlichen Urethra bei der Gonorrhoe. Röntgenpraxis **2**, 885—890 (1930). — Rubi, R. A., y J. A. Goldarecena: Uretrografias con un nuevo medio de contraste: umbradil U. Rev. argent. Urol. **21**, 205—209 (1953). — Rubin, A., and O. Snobl: Cystoradiography in infants and in elder children. Pediat. Listy **8**, 244—246 (1953). — Ruckensteiner, E.: Die Urethro-zystographie. Wien. med. Wschr. **109**, 168—171 (1959). — Ruggero, A.: Pathologie delle vesiculo seminale. Milano 1933.

Sabadini, L.: L'importance des renseignements fournis par l'urétrographie préopératoire, et résultats de l'urétrectomie et de la réfection immédiate de l'urétre au cours des phlegmons diffus du périne. Mém. Acad. Chir. **74**, 515—528 (1948). — Utilité des uréthro-cystographies immédiates post traumatique pour le diagnostic des ruptures de la vessie. Presse méd. **56**, 231—232 (1948). — Sack, H.: Pneumo-Zystographie bei Blasentumor. Röntgenpraxis **8**, 826 (1936). — Sáenz, M.: La cistorradiografia en el diagnóstico de los tumores vesicales. Rev. méd. Rosario **27**, 1086—1097 (1937). — Saigrajeff, M. A.: Pathogenesis of gonorrheal inflammation of the seminal vesicles as revealed by anatomical, histological and roentgenological examinations. Urol. cutan. Rev. **37**, 485—493 (1933). — Sala, S. L., y E. G. Bergdolt: El diagnóstico radiólogico de la placenta previa por medico de la cistografía. Bol. Soc. Obstet. Ginec. B. Aires **19**, 131—141 (1940). — Nuevas experiencias sobre el diagnóstico de la placenta previa por medio de la cistografia. An. bras. Ginec. **12**, 123—129 (1941). — Nuevas experiencias sobre el diagnóstico de la placenta previa por medico de la cistografia. Arch. Clín. obstet. ginec. "Canton" (B. Aires) **1**, 164—172 (1942). — Salgado, C., y A. H. Rocha: A cistografia no diagnóstico da placenta prévia. Rev. paul. Med. **24**, 319—322 (1944). Salleras, J.: La cistorradiografía de los tumores de la vejiga. Sem. méd. (B. Aires) **1**,

1284—1287 (1934). — Cystoradiography of tumors of bladder. Urol. cutan. Rev. **39**, 25—27 (1935). — SALLERAS, J., y J. GRIMBERG: Consideraciones sobre la uretrografía en las afecciones de la uretra anterior y posterior. Rev. Asoc. méd. argent. **46**, 794—799 (1932), also Sem. méd. (B. Aires) **1**, 13—21 (1933). — SANCHEZ SALVADOR, A.: La cistografia lacunar en el prostatismo; su valor en el diagnóstico del carcinoma de prostata. Arch. esp. Urol. **12**, 49—59 (1956). — SANTA MARIA, M.: Cateterismo dos canaese ejaculadores para lavagem das vesiculas seminaes sob controle radioscopico e radiografico. II. Congr. Amer. e I Argent. Urol. 1937. — Lavagem das vesiculas seminais por cateterismo endoscópico dos canais ejaculadores; espermatocistografía; tecnica do autor. An. paul. Med. Cir. **65**, 253—265 (1953). — SANTE, L. R.: Manual of roentgenological technique, 14 ed. Ann Arbor: Edwards 1947. — SARGENT, J. C.: Interpretation of seminal vesiculogram. Radiology **12**, 472—483 (1929). — SAVONA, B.: Cistoradioscopia e cistografia nelle vescicle normali e nei prolassi vaginali. Folia gynaec. (Genova) **30**, 477—491 (1933). — SCHAEFER, O.: Die Bedeutung der urologischen Röntgenuntersuchung für die Frauenheilkunde. Thesis Würzburg 1956. — SCHAPIRA, A.: Neoplasia secundaria de las vesículas seminales. Contribución al diagnóstico por medio de la vesiculografía seminal. Sem. méd. (B. Aires) **2**, 612—614 (1936). — SCHEELE, K.: Gefahren der Urethrographie. Z. Urol. **48**, 141—147 (1955). — SCHELLENBURG, W.: Über einen Fall von Verkalkung der Samenleiter und Ampullen. Frankfurt. Z. Path. **40**, 298—301 (1930). — SCHIAPPAPIETRA, T.: Ventajas e inconvenientes de las preparaciones de contraste para uso uretrografico. Rev. argent. Urol. **12**, 15—19 (1943). — SCHIFFER, E.: Urologiai röntgendiagnostica. Budapest: Tudományos Könyvkiadó 1950. — SCHINZ, H. R., W. E. BAENSCH, E. FRIEDL and E. UEHLINGER: Roentgen-diagnostics. Vol. 4: Gastro-intestinal tract, gynecology, urology. Cumulative index. English transl. arr. and edit. by JAMES T. CASE. 1. Am. ed. (based on 5. German ed.). New York: Grune & Stratton 1954. — SCHOBER, K. L.: Die Abrodilpfütze nach Kneise-Schober und ihre Bedeutung für die Diagnose der Prostatahypertrophie. Z. Urol. **34**, 139—148 (1940). — SCHREUS, H. T.: Röntgenologische Darstellung der hinteren Harnröhre mittels der Rektumkassette. Münch. med. Wschr. **80**, 1177—1198 (1933). — SCHULTHEIS, T.: Zur Deutung des Kontrastbildes der Harnblase bei Ausscheidungsurographie. Langenbecks Arch. klin. Chir. **264**, 586—588 (1950). — SCHULZE-MANITIUS, H.: Wie entwickelte sich die Photographie und Kinematographie des Blaseninneren? Z. Urol. **52**, 376—381 (1959). — SCHUMANN, E.: Klärung eines jahrzehntelangen Harnröhrenleidens durch Urethrocystographie. Z. Urol. **46**, 703—706 (1953). — SCHÖNFELD, A., u. F. KRAFT: Die Erkrankungen der Harnblase im Röntgenbilde. Leipzig u. München: Mennich 1925. — SÉDAL, P., et M. COTTALORDA: Les complication urinaires de l'hysterotomie: étude radio-clinique. Marseille chir. **9**, 17—20 (1957). — SERANTES, A., y A. E. GARCIA: Visualización de la mucosa vesical. Diagnóstico radiológico de los tumores. Hosp. argent. **3**, 566—580 (1932). — SGALITZER, M.: Technic of roentgen diagnosis of tumors of bladder. Türk Tip Cem. Mec. **5**, 308—319 (1939). — SHEA, J. D., and J. W. SCHWARTZ: Calcification of the seminal vesicles; case report. J. Urol. (Baltimore) **58**, 132—133 (1947). — SHIGA, H.: Roentgendiagnosis of the kidney and urethra. Tokyo: Kanekara 1933. — SICHEL, D., et E. BLUM: Radiographie et tomographie de la prostate. J. Radiol. Électrol. **39**, 487—493 (1958). — SICHEL, D., E. BLUM, J. P. WALTER et R. WOLFF: Étude radiographique et tomographique de l'hypertrophie et du cancer de la prostate. J. Radiol. Électrol. **39**, 321—322 (1958). — SILVA DE ASSIS, J.: Klinische Beobachtungen der Samenblase und Samenwege durch Katheterismus der Ducti ejaculatorii. Z. urol. Chir. Gynäk. **43**, 427—451 (1937). — Vesiculografia e cateterismo dos canais ejaculadores. Hospital (Rio de J.) **16**, 993—1005 (1939). — SINGER, P. L.: Seminal vesiculitis in the young. Urol. cutan. Rev. **50**, 328—330 (1946). — SITKOWSKI, W.: Roentgen diagnosis of bladder tumors. Pol. Przegl. radiol. **13**, 153—154 (1938). — SMITH, W. H.: The reliability of excretion urography in the diagnosis of bladder tumours. J. Fac. Radiol. (Lond.) **6**, 48—54 (1954). — SMYRNIOTIS, P. C.: Vessie bilharzienne calcifiée, dilatation des uretères et tumeur greffée sur la vessie, diagnostic radiologique. J. Radiol. Électrol. **21**, 489—493 (1937). — Vingt-quatre années de radiodiagnostic de la bilharziose en Egypte. J. Radiol. Électrol. **30**, 514—517 (1949). — SOIFER, S.: Prostatography; preliminary report. J. Urol. (Baltimore) **39**, 410—413 (1938). — SPÉDER et FOURNIER: Une infestation bilharzienne décelée par la radiographie. Arch. Élect. méd. **40**, 23—26 (1932). — SQUIRE, F. H., and H. L. KRETSCHMER: Limitations of roentgen rays in diagnosis of bladder stone. J. Amer. med. Ass. **145**, 81—82 (1951). — SRIVASTAVA, S. P.: Prostatic calculi. J. Indiana med. Ass. **25**, 404—408 (1955). — STAEHLER, W.: Die Behandlung der männlichen Adnexitis. Z. Urol. **38**, 72—93 (1944). — Die Samenblase im Röntgenbild. Z. Urol. **38**, 93—126 (1944). — Die Diagnose des Prostataabszesses im Röntgenbild. Z. Urol. **40**, 161—164 (1947). — Die Diagnose der inneren männiichen Genitaltuberkulose im Röntgenbild. Helv. chir. Acta **15**, 476—486 (1948). — Röntgendiagnostik der eitrigen unspezifischen Samenblasenentzündungen. Z. Urol. (Sonderh.) **1949**, 230—234. — Über die Röntgendiagnostik der entzündlichen Erkrankungen der inneren männlichen Genitalorgane. Fortschr. Röntgenstr. **72**, 202—207 (1949/50). — Klinik und Praxis der Urologie. Stuttgart: Georg Thieme 1959. — STÄHLI, G.: Anwendung und Leistungsfähigkeit des Röntgenbildes bei der

Untersuchung der Harnorgane. Med. Welt **20**, 927—930 (1951). — Eine einfache Urethrographiemethode beim Manne mit gutem Strahlenschutz. Helv. chir. Acta **22**, 96—98 (1953). — STEGEMAN, W.: Cystourethrograms; use, technic and advantages, especially before prostatectomy. J. Urol. (Baltimore) **46**, 549—564 (1941). — STEINHARTER, E. C., and S. BROWN: Urethrocystography. Amer. J. Obstet. Gynec. **18**, 259—260 (1929). — STENSTRÖM, B.: Das Röntgenbild der Prostatatuberkulose. Acta radiol. (Stockh.) **20**, 303—313 (1939). — STEPHENS, F. D.: Urethral obstruction in childhood; the use of urethrography in diagnosis. Aust. N. Z. J. Surg. **25**, 89—109 (1955). — STEVENS, W. E., and S. P. SMITH: Examination of female urethra. J. Urol. (Baltimore) **37**, 194—201 (1937). — STEWART, C. M.: Delayed cystograms. J. Urol. (Baltimore) **70**, 588—593 (1953), also Trans. west. Sect. Amer. urol. Ass. **20**, 18—23 (1953). — Delayed cystography. Bull. Moore-White med. Fdn. **5**, 49—52 (1954). — STILSON, W. L., and P. H. DEEB: Unusual problems in urologic radiology. Urol. cutan. Rev. **54**, 325—330 (1950). — ST. MARTIN, E. C., J. H. CAMPBELL and C. M. PESQUIER: Cystography in children. Trans. s.-east. Sect. Amer. urol. Ass. **19**, 86—95 (1955), also J. Urol. (Baltimore) **75**, 151—159 (1956). — STOBBAERTS, F.: L'urétrocystographie mictionnelle à double contraste. Procès-verb. Congr. franç. Urol. **40**, 264—267 (1946). — STOETER, E.: Röntgenuntersuchungen mit Kontrastmitteln bei alten Harnröhrenzerreißungen. Beitr. klin. Chir. **160**, 369—398 (1934). — STRAUSS, B.: Roentgen demonstration of the perivesical spaces. J. Urol. (Baltimore) **46**, 520—527 (1941). — STRÉJA, M.: Considérations sur l'image urétrographique de la portion susmontanale de l'urètre. J. Urol. méd. chir. **48**, 193—199 (1939). — STROM, G. W., and E. N. COOK: Excretory cystogram as aid in diagnosis. Proc. Mayo Clin. **17**, 170—176 (1942). — STÜMPKE, G., u. H. STRAUSS: Erfahrungen mit Urethrographien. Derm. Wschr. **95**, 1367—1374 (1932). — SWEETSER, T. H.: Cystography, especially pneumocystography as guide in treatment of vesical neck lesions. J. Urol. (Baltimore) **40**, 285—293 (1938). — Cystography in study of difficulties following prostatic surgery. Trans. west. surg. Ass. **48**, 59—67 (1939). — Cystography in study of postoperative difficulties. Minn. Med. **23**, 40—43 (1940).

TAGER, I., u. M. SANTOCKIJ: Die Darstellung der Harnblasentumoren mit Hilfe der Kontrastpneumographie. Fortschr. Röntgenstr. **53**, 882—888 (1936). — TALANCÓN, G., y R. ENGELKING LOPEZ: Estenosis en longitud total de la uretra. Reflujo uretro-venoso durante uretrografia. Rev. Urol. (Méx.) **6**, 374—378 (1948). — TAUBER, A.: A new catheter for urethrography. J. Urol. (Baltimore) **81**, 700—701 (1959). — TAVOLARO, M.: Espermatocistografia por via retrógrada. Med. Cirurg. Pharm. **1943**, 115—122. — TELTSCHER, E.: Große Cyste am Blasenhals. Z. Urol. **44**, 172—173 (1951). — TEMELIESCO, J.: La cystopolygraphie. J. Urol. méd. chir. **62**, 482—486 (1956). — TEMPORAL, A.: A uretra normal e patologica aos raiosx. Arch. bras. Cir. Ortop. **3**, 101—168 (1935). — TESCHENDORF, W.: Lehrbuch der röntgenologischen Differentialdiagnostik, 2. Aufl., S. 533. Stuttgart: Georg Thieme 1950. — THOMSEN, E.: Roentgen examination of female urethra, especially in cases of prolaps and incontinence. Acta radiol. (Stockh.) **11**, 527—535 (1930). — Röntgenundersögelse af kvindens urethra, specielt ved prolaps og incontinens. Ugeskr. Laeg. **92**, 533—548 (1930). — Studies of female urethra, especially closing mechanism of bladder. Acta radiol. (Stockh.) 433—457 (1932). — TRABUCCO, A., y E. B. BOTTINI jr.: Persuflacion quimografica del deferente. Rev. argent. Urol. **17**, 241—248 (1948) also Obstet. Ginec. lat.-amer. **6**, 499—504 (1948). — La radiografia del epididimo. Obstet. Ginec. lat.-amer. **12**, 52—54 (1954). — TRABUCCO, A., E. B. BOTTINI jr. y F. MARQUEZ: Epididimigrafias. Rev. argent. Urol. **23**, 205—216 (1954). — TRABUCCO, A., B. OTAMENDI y J. C. LURASCHI: Persuflacion y vesiculografia en la obstruccion de los conductas deferentes. Obstet. Ginec. lat.-amer. **16**, 279—281 (1958). — TRABUCCO, A., y R. E. SANDRO: Técnica de la exploración radiológica de las vesículas seminales. Sem. méd. (B. Aires) **1**, 355—356 (1940). — TRATTNER, H. R.: Introduction of solution into tubulo—alveolar system (by catheterization); new method useful in diagnosis and therapie. J. Urol. (Baltimore) **48**, 710—734 (1942). — TREUTLER, H.: Beitrag zur Röntgendiagnostik des männlichen Chorionepithelioms. Fortschr. Röntgenstr. **82**, 338—341 (1955). — TRUC, E.: Le radiodiagnostic des tumeurs du rein et de la vessic. Montpellier méd. **5**, 387—395 (1934). — Diagnostic urgent du cancer du testicule. Montpellier méd. **19—20**, 377—383 (1941). — TRUC, E., P. GUILLAUME, J. CANDON, M. PÉLISSIER et P. LEENHARDT: Les tumeurs de la vessie; leur exploration par le double contraste et la péripneumocystographie. J. Radiol. Électrol. **35**, 278—289 (1954). — TRUC, E., MARCHAL et R. PALEIRAC: Le pneumo-exopéritoine pas voie sus-pubienne; nouvelle technique d'insufflation. Semeilogie, radiologique de l'espace sous péritoneal abdomino-pelvien. J. Urol. méd. chir. **57**, 125—140 (1951). — TRUC, E., R. PALEIRAC, P. GUILLAUME, Y. BONNET e J. CANDON: L'impiego della parietografia vesicale nell esplorazione della vesica. Minerva urol. (Torino) **7**, 26—27 (1955). — TRUCCHI, O.: L'associazione del pneumo-peritoneo pelvico e della pneumocistografia nell'esame radiologico della parete della vesica urinaria con particolare riguardo alla ricerca delle neoplasie. Radiol. med. (Torino) **44**, 421—429 (1958). — TRUCHOT, P.: Cystographie au collothor. Bull. Soc. radiol. méd. France **21**, 423—426 (1933). — A propos de la technique de l'urétrographie. Bull. Soc. radiol. méd. France **23**, 339—343 (1935). — TUCKER, A. S., H. YANAGIHARA and A. W. PRYDE: A method roentgenography of the male genital tract. Amer. J. Roentgenol. **71**, 490—500 (1954). — TUKHSHNID, D. I., and F. T. EPSHTEGN: Practical value of urethrography in diagnosis of diseases of urethra in male. Vrač. Delo **17**, 269—274 (1934). — TURANO, L.: Diagnostica radiologica dell'apparato uropoietico, edit. 2. Roma: Soc. ed. Universo (Tip. S. Guiseppe) 1948. — TZSCHIRNTSCH, K.: Die anamnestisch verheimlichte Lues im urologischen Röntgenbild. Z. Urol. **44**, 479—481 (1951).

ÜBELHÖR, R.: Urologie. Therapie und Praxis H. 11. Wien u. Innsbruck: Urban & Schwarzenberg 1958. — UHLÍR, K.: Tuberculosis of seminal vesicles: vesiculography. Acta urol. belg. **25**, 53—60 (1957). — ULTZMANN, H.: Die Deferentographie bei Obstruktions-azoospermie. Wien. med. Wschr. **106**, 52—53 (1956). — *Use of sodium acetrizoate for urethro-graphy.* J. Amer. med. Ass. **164**, 282 (1957). — USON, A. C., D. W. JOHNSON, J. K. LATTIMER and M. M. MELICOW: A classification of the urographic patterns in children with congenital bladder neck obstruction. Amer. J. Roentgenol. **80**, 590—602 (1958).

VACCARI, F.: La calcolosi endogena della prostata e il contributo della uretrografia alla sua diagnosi. Arch. ital. Urol. **17**, 241—276 (1940). — VALLIER, G. R. M.: Possibilité de mettre en évidence par l'urographie intra-veineuse le contour intra-vésical des lobes prostatiques sans manoeuvre instrumentale. Thèse. Paris: Clermont-Ferraud 1950. — VALVERDE, B.: Le lavage des vésicules dans le traitment des spermatocystites chroniques. J. Urol. méd. chir. **36**, 262—277 (1933). — Concerning vesiculography and lavage of the seminal vesicles through the ejaculatory ducts. Urol. cutan. Rev. **37**, 595—600 (1933). — Sobre a vesiculo-grafia e a lavagem des vesiculas seminaes pelos canaes ejacula dores. Arch. Serv. Vias Urin. Policlin. Rio de Jan. 1936. — Lavage of the seminal vesicles. Urol. cutan. Rev. **55**,159—165 (1951). — VAQUIER, P. M.: La technique actuelle du radio diagnostic des affections urinaires Thèse Paris 1949. — VASSELLE, B.: Étude radiologique des voies séminales de l'homme. Thèse Paris 1953. — VERNET, S. GIL: La tuberculose génitale masculine. Acta urol. bélg. **27**, 264—329 (1959). — VERRIERE, P., H. NOOEL, R. NOVEL et P. BURLET: Présentation d'un nouvel uréthrographe. J. Urol. méd. chir. **62**, 700—702 (1956). — VESTBY, G. W.: Vaso-seminal vesiculography in hypertrophy and carcinoma of the prostate with special reference to the ejaculatory ducts. Oslo: Oslo University Press 1960. — Vasoseminal vesiculography in hypertrophy and carcinoma of the prostate. Acta radiol. (Stockh.) **50**, 273—284 (1958). — VIEHWEGER, G.: Zur Kontrastdarstellung der Harnröhre. Ärztl. Wschr. **7**, 318—321 (1952). — VILLELA ITIBERE, D., E. W. DE SOUZA ARANHA y O. MELLONE: Refluxo uretrovenose na uretrografia. Rev. méd. bras. **12**, 187—193 (1942). — VINCENT, P.: L'uréthrographie par voie mictionelle. Thèse Paris 1935. — L'uréthrographie dans les rétrécissements. Arch. méd.-chir. Province **26**, 2—8 (1936). — VITALI-MAZZA, L.: Le modificazioni strutturali delle veschi-chette seminali nelle varie età. Riv. Anat. pat. **11**, 739—761 (1956).

WALDRON, E. A.: Urethrocystography. J. Fac. Radiol. (Lond.) **4**, 54—63 (1952). — WANGERMEZ, C., et P. BONJEAN: Appareil destiné à l'urétrographie rétrograde ches la femme. J. Radiol. Électrol. **49**, 206 (1959). — WEBER, B., u. A. WEBER: Urethrographie mit blut-verträglichen viskösen Kontrastmitteln. Z. Urol. **49**, 79 (1956). — WELFLING, J., et P. POY-AUD: Utilisation d'un appareil à hystérographie pour l'uréthrographie rétrograde chez l'homme. J. Urol. méd. Chir. **65**, 492—493 (1959). —WELKENHUYZEN, P. VAN: Les modifications radiolo-giques des voies séminales par les lésions de la prostate. Acta urol. belg. **25**, 34—52 (1957). — Re-marques sur l'interprétation des vésiculographies en cas de lésions de la prostate. Acta urol. belg. **26**, 38—47 (1958). — WELKENHUYZEN, P. VAN, et R. ZALCMAN: Radiocinématographie des vesicules séminales; premiers resultats. Acta urol. belg. **27**, 121—125 (1959). — WELLS, W. W.: Placenta praevia with discussion of x-ray aid. J. Okla. St. med. Ass. **30**, 285—289 (1937). — WENIG, H.: Eine vereinfachte Methode der funktionellen röntgenologischen Sphinkterometrie. Zbl. Gynäk. **80**, 1906—1910 (1958). — WESSON, M. B., and H. E. RUGG-LES: Urological roentgenology: A manual for students and practitioners, 3. edit. Phila-delphia: Lea and Febiger 1950. — WHINSBURY-WHITE, H. P.: Textbook of genito-urinary surgery. Baltimore: Williams & Wilkins 1948. — WILHELM, S. F.: Observations on the emplying of vasa deferentia and seminal vesicles. J. Urol. (Baltimore) **34**, 284—287 (1935). — Vasoseminal vesiculography; clinical and experimental application. J. Urol. (Baltimore) **41**, 751—757 (1939). — WILLICH, E.: Röntgendiagnostik der Harntraktanomalien im frühen Kindesalter. Mschr. Kinderheilk. **107**, 474—482 (1959). — WINTER, C. C.: The problem of rectal involvement by prostatic cancer. Surg. Gynec. Obstet. **105**, 136—140 (1957). — WOL-FROMM, G., G. DULAC et M. GILSON: Sur trois méthodes de cystographie: la "flaque", la "flocculation", la "réplétion". J. Urol. méd. chir. **52**, 175—184 (1944/45). — WOLFROMM, G., et M. GILSON: De quelques perfectionnements dans la cystographie par la méthodede la "flaque" (Kneise et Schobert). J. Urol. méd. chir. **53**, 332—337 (1946/47). — WOLFROMM, G., et M. ROUFLÉ-NADAUD: Diverticule de la vessie étudié grâce au perfectionnement apporté par M. J. Jomain à la méthode de la flaque (Abrodilpfütze) de Kneise et Schober. J. Urol. méd. chir. **63**, 801—803 (1957). — WOLFROMM, G., et A. SORIN: La cystographie par la méthode de précipitation de Stobbaerts. J. Urol. méd. chir. **53**, 33—34 (1946/47). — Wug-meister, I.: Die röntgenographische Darstellung divertikulärer Gebilde der hinteren Harn-röhre. Röntgenpraxis **8**, 313—316 (1936).

Yanagihara, H., and T. Miyata: Radiography of vas deferens (ampulla) and seminal vesicles. J. orient. Med. (Abstr. sect.) **23**, 85—94 (1935). — Young, B. W., W. L. Anderson and G. G. King: Radiographic estimation of residual urine in children. J. Urol. (Baltimore) **75**, 263—272 (1956). — Young, H. H., and C. A. Waters: Urological roentgenology. Annals of roentgenology, 2. edit., vol. 7. A series of monographic atlases, edit. by James T. Case. New York: Hoeber 1931. — Youssef, A. F., and M. M. Mahfouz: Sphincteromethrography, a new technique for studying the physiology and pathology of urinary continence in the female. J. Obstet. Gynaec. Brit. Emp. **63**, 19—25 (1956).

Zaigraeff, M. A., and N. S. Liakhovitsky: Roentgenography of seminal vesicles of cadavers. Vener. Derm. **8**, 43—53 (1931). — Zak, K.: Cystographic evaluation of surgical results in urinary incontinence in women. Čsl. Gynaek. **19**, 178—180 (1955). — Zeman, E.: Pelveovenographie; ein neues diagnostisches Hilfsmittel bei den Blasentumoren. Z. Urol. **48**, 129—141 (1955). — Zimmer, W.: Innendrüsenkarzinome der Prostata. Wien. med. Wschr. **108**, 1039—1041 (1958). — Zoedler, D.: Beitrag zur Endometriose der Harnblase. Z. Urol. **50**, 243—250 (1957).

Diagnostic radioactive isotopes in urology

By

RUBIN H. FLOCKS and CHESTER C. WINTER

With 16 figures

Introduction

The use of radioactive isotopes for diagnostic Urology has had limited clinical application to date. Most of the published work has dealt with experimental studies pointing the way to possible clinical usefulness.

There appear to be four divisions in diagnostic nuclear Urology: 1. tests of organ function, 2. cancer detection, 3. fluid and electrolyte exchange, and 4. diagnostic radiography. The first category would include renal function tests utilizing contrast media tagged with I-131. The second classification would include attempts to follow the course of metabolites through the use of tagged elements (P-32, Na-24, and Zn-65) in an effort to determine whether health or disease exists. Thirdly, various isotopes (Na-24, K, albumin-I-131, rose bengal-I-131) have been used in studying exchanges of electrolytes and fluids in the urinary and intestinal tracts as related to urological conditions and procedures. Finally, isotopes, notably thulium-170, have been used to make radioautographs of the kidney. All of these applications have been experimental, except the kidney function test and the vesical-ureteral reflux test which are being used clinically in an increasing number of medical centers. Nevertheless, the experimental work is worthy of mention since it precedes clinical application and may suggest new areas of usefulness.

A. Diagnostic tests of organ function
I. The radioisotope renogram

In 1955, TAPLIN, MEREDITH, and KADE working with rabbits, and WINTER and TAPLIN working with humans, developed a new method of determining several aspects of individual kidney function through use of isotopes. Using intravenously injected diodrast-I-131, they were able to detect changing levels of γ-radiation over each kidney area with scintillation probes connected through rate meters to recorders (Fig. 1)[1]. A characteristic tracing for the normal kidney as compared with the lung is shown in fig. 2. The height of the initial leg of the renogram (a) reflects the vascular capacity of the kidney plus that of the immediately adjacent tissue. The rapidity and height of the secondary rise (b) in the tracing indicates the degree of tubular cell function. The tracing also shows a third segment, the terminal fall (c). The rapidity of the descent indicates the ability of the kidney to evacuate urine or the presence of stasis. The procedure has been shown to be rapid, safe and nontraumatic in over 1500 tests. While results are qualitative

---

[1] Unknown to the authors was the experimental work of OESER and BILLIN (1952) who used diodrast-I-131 in a similar manner but plotted tracings from collected urine samples.

only and not diagnostic, they do yield information regarding renal vascularity, secretory function, and excretory ability. Thus, distinctive tracings are obtained for such medical and urological renal disorders as absent or non-functioning kidney (Fig. 3), ureteral obstruction (Fig. 4), and various degrees of dysfunction (Fig. 5). It is possible, for example, to differentiate anuria due to acute renal failure from bilateral ureteral obstruction (Fig. 6). The test is particularly applicable in children and seriously ill patients where standard urological procedures would

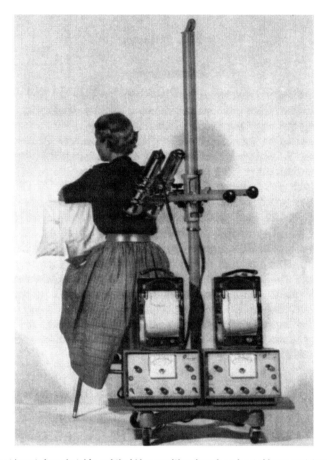

Fig. 1. The patient is seated comfortably and the kidney positions have been located by an upright roentgenogram. Two scintillation probes are connected through two rate meters to two recorders. Following the intravenous injection of Hypaque I-131, continuous tracings are made of the gamma ray level in each kidney region and the tracings may be interpreted immediately

be dangerous or extremely difficult. Another valuable use is in following patients' renal status after surgery (Figs. 7 and 8).

The renogram's main usefulness, however, has been found to be for screening hypertensive individuals in order to find those few with curable unilateral renal disease or renal arterial disease as the cause of their high blood pressure (WINTER 1957 and 1959). Most of those with abnormal renograms would require extensive urological investigation (Fig. 9). However, those with normal renograms bilaterally could be spared extensive urological investigation and aortography. In a series of 214 patients, 56 were found to have one abnormal renogram. Further investigation with conventional individual renal function tests plus aortography

proved 85% of the renograms to be correct. "This compared favorably with
the consistency of the individual renal clearance test results (creatinine, 83%;

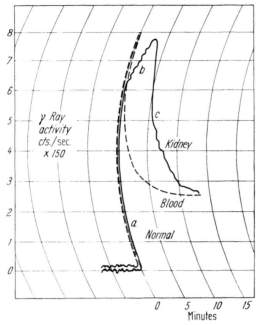

Fig. 2. The normal radioactive hypaque renogram tracing (solid line) has three segments: a vascular spike,
b functional segment and c excretory leg. While the level of radioactivity in the blood (dotted line) is rapidly
falling, the renal tubular cells are actively picking up the hypague-I-131 (b)

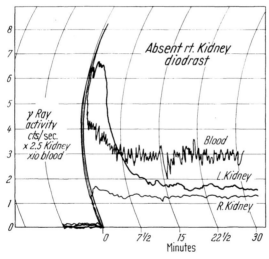

Fig. 3. The right renogram representative of an absent or non-functioning kidney shows a short initial vascular
spike since no renal blood is present. Only the blood level of radioactive tissue under the scintillation probe is
detected. There is no secondary rise since tubular cell secretion is present

inulin, 88%; para-aminohippuric acid, 80%) and dye excretion tests (PSP,
90% and indigo carmine, 83%). All tests including the renogram showed greater
value when used merely to bring out differences between two kidneys (90 to
95%)." Twentytwo of these individuals underwent urological or renal arterial

surgery with resulting cure in nine and marked improvement in an additional eight (80% total).

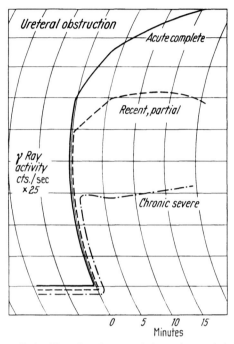

Fig. 4. Tracings taken from patients with various degrees and stages of ureteral obstruction are shown. In the acute and complete obstruction, the function is intact and produces a sharp secondary rise. As obstruction becomes chronic both the initial vascular spike and secondary functional segment decrease

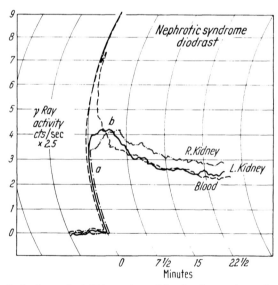

Fig. 5. In the Nephrotic Syndrome, the initial vascular and functional segments are decreased proportional to the severity of the disease

In addition to Diodrast-I-131, other contrast media have been tried as test agents (Winter and Taplin 1957). Hypaque, Miokon, and Renografin were found to have qualities similar to Diodrast, since they are actively secreted by the renal tubules (Fig. 10). Urokon and Sodium Iodide were found to give nondistinctive renogram patterns, since they are passively filtered by the renal glomeruli. Since Diodrast is picked up by the liver, false right renograms are

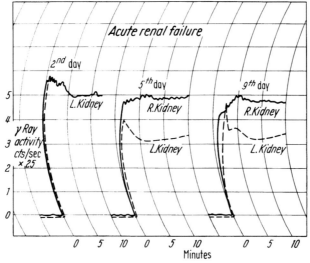

Fig. 6. At the onset of acute renal failure the vascular spike is intact but function is almost absent. Note the gradual increase in function of the right kidney compared to the failure of the left renal function to return by the ninth day. If anuria were due to acute bilateral ureteral obstruction, the secondary segments would rise sharply

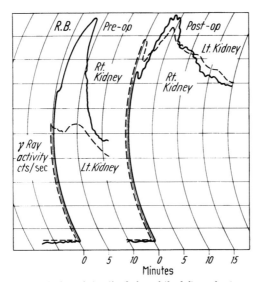

Fig. 7. Preoperatively the patient had an obstructive lesion of the left renal artery represented by diminished vascular and functional segments. Following left renal endarterectomy, both the vascular and functional aspects returned to normal

obtained occassionally. Hippuran has been found to have all the good characteristics of Diodrast without the liver effect. The authors now prefer Hippuran or Hypaque-I-131 as the test agents of choice.

In order to test the hypothesis that the renogram would detect renal arterial lesions, experiments were carried out in dogs (WINTER 1958). The results of varying degrees of renal arterial ligation are shown in Fig. 11. Other dogs were made hypertensive by applying a silver clamp to one renal artery after the technique of Goldblatt. Differences between the affected kidney and the normal contralateral kidney were easily discernible (Fig. 12). Thus, it seemed likely that renal arterial lesions would be detectable in humans by the renogram. This has been borne out in a high percentage of clinical cases.

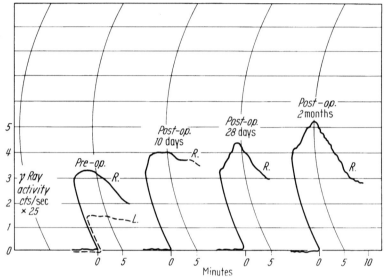

Fig. 8. A young girl had malignant hypertension, uremia and a solitary right kidney. The preoperative renogram shows a left tracing indicative of an absent kidney and decreased vascularity and function of the right kidney. Following removal of a sarcoma of the aorta which had extended into the right renal artery, the uremia disappeared and the vascular and functional segments of the right renogram returned to normal

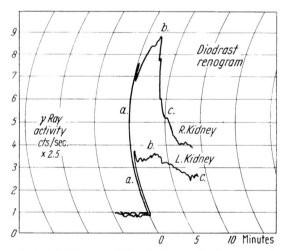

Fig. 9. An eighteen-month-old boy had hypertension of six months duration. At age six months he developed acute gastroenteritis and pyuria. An atrophic, poorly functioning left kidney was discovered. An aortogram revealed a marked decrease in vascularity of the left kidney. The right renogram was found to be normal, while the left tracing showed unilateral renal disease, as depicted by decreased vascularity (A) and function (B). Left nephrectomy has resulted in a cure for over three years

Large carrier doses of Diodrast, Miokon, and Hypaque have been given prior to and with tracer amounts of I-131 tagged contrast media. They cause the functional segment (b) to rise more slowly to a lesser height. These findings suggest the possibility of determining the extent of renal damage in certain diseases.

BLOCK, HINES and BURROWS in 1959 described the intravenous injection of 1 gram of carrier Diodrast just prior to starting the Diodrast I-131 renogram

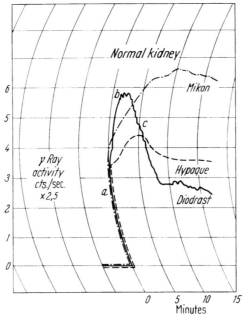

Fig. 10. A comparison of three common contrast media show that they are all actively secreted by the renal tubular cells. Diodrast is secreted most rapidly, while Hypaque is handled slightly slower, and Miokon, more slowly yet. Hypaque and Miokon have the advantages of not being selected by the liver, as is 10—15% of Diodrast

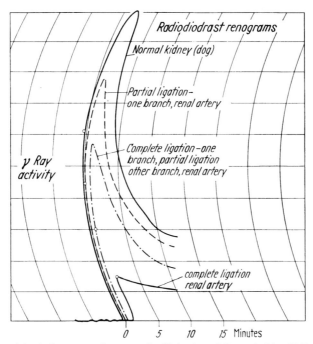

Fig. 11. The normal (control) renogram is compared with tracings of the contralateral kidney in the course of varying degrees of ligation of the renal artery. Note step-like diminution of initial vascular spike and secondary functional rise in tracings

in order to effectively block out the liver pickup of I-131. Their patients were given approximately a liter of water by mouth in the hour prior to the reno-

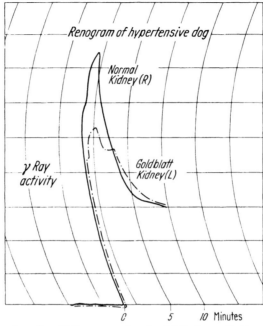

Fig. 12. The initial vascular spike of left renogram is reduced following application of GOLDBLATT clamp to renal artery producing hypertension

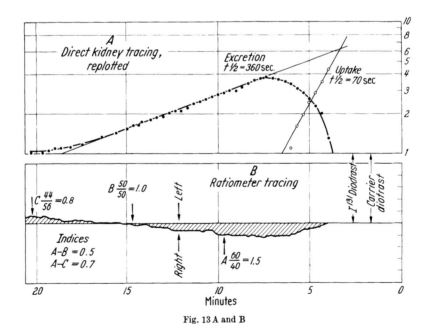

Fig. 13 A and B

gram. After being placed in the upright position with the kidney monitors directed horizontally toward the kidney, an intravenous infusion of 300 ml. of 5% dextrose in water containing an additional 1 gram of carrier Diodrast was administered slowly throughout the study. In addition to a direct recording of radioactivity, they also utilized a ratiometer, which compared the counting rates of the renal areas.

From their direct kidney tracing, replotted on semilogarithmic paper, a rate of uptake of I-131 Diodrast by one kidney was derived (Fig. 13a). The slope of the excretory phase was extended back to its intercept with the ordinant. At 20 second intervals following injection of the dose, the recorded uptake was subtracted from the extended excretory slope and the difference plotted. The half time value in seconds of the straight line so obtained was termed "$T^1/_2$ uptake". "$T^1/_2$ excretion" was derived from the excretory slope and the time required to reach peak uptake was noted. From the ratiometer tracing the ratio of the counting rates of the separate kidney could be derived at selected times after the dose (Fig. 13b). With equal counting rates from the two kidneys the plotted ratio of one count rate to the combined count rates was 0,5 (midline on the graph). Differences in the counting rates of the separate kidneys were shown by shift in the ratiometer tracing away from the midline. The direction of this shift (right or left) was determined in relation to a unilaterally diseased kidney. The percentage of the total count rate from each kidney could be determined from the graph at selected intervals and the ratio of the two count rates expressed as a ratio of these percentages. An index of the change in one count rate relative to the other, shown by a change in this ratio, was derived as follows. Near the peak uptake, ratio "A" was determined placing the higher percentage in the numerator. A straight line was drawn from this point along the ratiometer tracing over a 5 minute interval, and the ratio was also determined ("C"). Changes in the ratio (A—B and A—C) were calculated as indices of secondary shift. The tracings were continued for 30 minutes, at which time a urine sample was collected to determine the per cent of the dose excreted.

An initial shift of the ratiometer indicated a diminished uptake of I-131 diodrast by one kidney as compared to the other. If there was no significant difference in the subsequent rates of excretion by the two kidneys, a relatively constant ratiometer recording was obtained after the peak uptake (Type I). Such differences in uptake usually were not observed with proved unilateral renal ischemia and could also be seen with differences between the kidneys and counting geometry. An obvious secondary shift occurring soon after peak uptake, with or without an initial shift of the ratiometer, indicated delayed excretion of I-131 diodrast by one kidney compared to the other (Type II). All patients in these authors' series with proved unilateral renal ischemia had this type of tracing. The authors felt that normal I-131 diodrast renogram results may rule out unilateral renal ischemia, but that an abnormal result is not in itself an indication for nephrectomy.

II. Estimation of renal blood flow with radioisotopes

PERSKEY, BONTE, and KROHMER (1957) studied the estimation of renal blood flow in animals by using intravenously injected albumin-I-131. Scintillation counters were placed in direct contact with lead-shielded dog kidneys. Following intravenous injection of albumin-I-131, counts were made of the normal blood flow and after vascular ligation. Similar studies were made with the counters outside of the body but directed towards the kidneys. The authors suggested that this method could be made into a quantitive measure of renal blood flow by comparing renal blood counts with non-renal vascular areas. (The counts in this method are comparable to the initial vascular leg of the radioisotope renogram, Fig. 2.)

Rose Parker and William Beierwaltes of the University of Michigan compared effective renal plasma flow as determined by I-131 labeled Diodrast

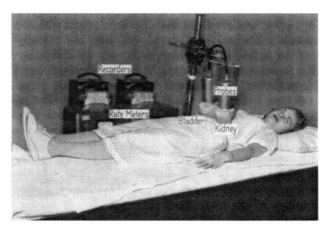

Fig. 14. The patient lies in a comfortable supine position. A catheter is placed in the bladder and a non-absorbable I-131 solution introduced. The test equipment consists of two scintillation probes directed vertically toward each anterior kidney surface and connected through rate meters to recorders. Continuous tracings are made while the test agent is in the bladder, so that immediate or delayed vesicoureteral reflux can be recorded. When the bladder is emptied the tracing returns to normal, if the kidneys empty promptly. If there is a delay in drainage this will also be revealed by a slowly descending tracing

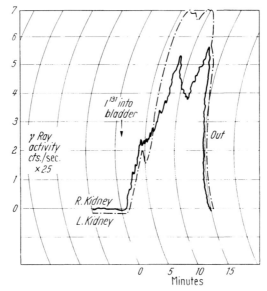

Fig. 15. Following instillation of I-131 into the bladder, reflux into kidneys is demonstrated by rise in tracings. Absence of ureteral obstruction is shown by rapid terminal fall in tracings

and by the chemical assay for inactive Diodrast[1]. The standard clearance formula

$$CD = \frac{UV}{P}$$

[1] Report to the Sixth Annual Meeting of the Society of Nuclear Medicine, Chicago, Illinois, June 17—20, 1959.

was applicable to the isotopic studies, simply substituting the counts per second per ml of plasma or urine. Seven of eight clearances fell within one standard deviation of the more laborious chemical method. Tubular mass measurements could also be made, requiring only the additional data supplied by chemically determined inulin clearance.

III. Vesical-ureteral reflux

Another use of the radiation equipment (with slight modification) as shown in fig. 14 was demonstrated by WINTER in 1958. With the patient supine and the two scintillation counters directed towards the anterior surface of the kidneys, I-131 was introduced into the urinary bladder, tagged to an agent which was not absorbable through bladder mucosa. If vesical-ureteral reflux was present, a rise occured in the tracings (Fig. 15). Thus, the degree and dynamics of reflux can be studied. The chief disadvantages of the conventional roentgenological methods are overcome; e.g. radiation hazard and absorption of contrast medium in the bladder producing excretory pyelograms.

B. Cancer detection

I. Radioactive zinc in the prostate and prostatic fluid

MASSON and FISCHER (1951) found a higher concentration of zinc in the prostate than any other soft tissue. It was of the same level of concentration in the normal as benign hypertrophied glands. However, in carcinoma and infection, the levels were lower. GUNN and GOULD (1956) studied the level of radioactive zinc in the rat prostate. Zinc was demonstrated to be present in the epithelial cells of prostatic acini by DANIEL, et al. (1956), as had previously been demonstrated by MAGER, et al. (1953). The former demonstrated the presence of zinc-65 by radioautographs. They also found higher concentrations in prostatic cancer than previous workers. Low levels were found in benign prostatic hypertrophy and chronic prostatitis. PROUT, DANIEL, and WHITMORE (1957) injected zinc-65 intravenously into dogs prepared with prostatic fistulae. They found peaks of zinc-65 in the prostatic fluid in four to twelve days. Thereafter, levels decreased steadily, but were always detectable up to three to five months. Both prostatic fluid and zinc-65 content were decreased by administration of estradial given intramuscularly. The implications of these studies are that one might be able to diagnose cancer of the prostate or other pathological conditions of that gland plus metastatic lesions through the use of zinc-65.

II. Attempts to localize metastatic lesions of the prostate with P-32

HUMMEL, HARRISON, MARBERGER, and FLOCKS (1956) attempted to localize in the prostate, the radioactive products of parenterally administered phosphate esters. Since, in the human, normal and neoplastic prostatic tissue have higher levels of phosphatase than other tissues, the test would be of great value in determining the stage of malignancy as well as the extent and location of metastases. Also, it would offer a means of determining the location of metastases that have bound the isotopes given for irradiation treatments. However, there was no conclusive evidence that the administration of radioactive esters of phosphoric acid resulted in more than a transient sojourn in prostatic tissue.

C. Fluid and electrolyte exchange

I. Electrolytes

Pyrah, Care, Reed and Parsons (1955) studied the transport of Na-24 and Cl-38 across the epithelium of an excluded intact bladder. They showed the migration of these ions in both directions in approximately equivalent amounts. When the bladder was enlarged with ileum, there was a small net absorption of chlorides and sodium ions in almost equivalent amounts. They concluded, therefore, that hyperchloremic acidosis would not occur after ileocystoplasty.

Winter (1957) studied the absorption of Diodrast-I-131 from the isolated normal bladder and confirmed the findings of Maluf (1953, 1955) that contrast media are easily absorbed through the urinary bladder and excreted by the kidneys. It was possible to produce excretory urograms in this manner.

Pyrah, Care, and Reed (1957) studied the extent of reabsorption of Cl-38 and Na-24 from the isolated rectosigmoid in two cases, eight and twenty-two months respectively after the first test. While chloride ions were absorbed in excess of sodium in the initial study, the two ions were absorbed less differentiatedly the greater the interval of time. This suggested an adjustment or adaptation of the colonic mucous membrane.

Marucci, et al. (1954) performed 37 absorption studies with 5 to $50 \mu c$ of I-131, Na-22, and P-32 in three types of dogs' bladders: reversed seromuscular ileal grafts, mucous membrane lined ileal bladder, and normal canine bladder. In each instance the test dose was diluted with 20 milliliters of isotonic saline and instilled in the bladder. Serial blood samples were collected and assayed. Only from the mucous membrane lined ileal bladder were appreciable amounts of any of the isotopes absorbed.

De Haven (1957) studied the effect of tracer amounts of P-32 and I-131 in an isotonic solution in an isolated ileal bladder in the human. He found no appreciable absorption from the bladder in a single experiment.

II. Renal lymphatics studied with isotopes

Goodwin and Kaufman in 1956 showed that renal urine could escape via the renal lymphatics and thereby into the blood stream by instilling I-131 directly into the renal pelvis. These findings added to the evidence that the renal lymphatics act as a safety valve for the obstructed kidney.

III. Effect of hormones on renal clearance of radioiodine in the rat

Perris, Ford, Lorenz, Keating and Elvert (1955) assessed renal clearance of I-131 in intact, thyroidectomized, hypophysectomized, adrenalectomized and adrenohypophysectomized rats before and after treatment with a variety of hormones. Adrenalectomy reduced the clearance by 50%, but full cortisone therapy brought this back to normal. Hypophysectomized and adrenalectomized rats or just hypophysectomized rats reduced the clearance to one-fourth. Full doses of cortisone brought the clearance back to two-thirds of normal. However, a combination of cortisone and pituitary extracts or growth hormones brought the clearance back to 100%. Intact rats treated by acute or chronic cortisone therapy showed slight depression of renal clearance, and the administration of DOCA produced no change whatsoever.

IV. The transfer of irrigating fluid during transurethral prostectomy

GRIFFIN, DOBSON and WEAVER (1955) placed Na-I-131 in irrigating fluid used for transurethral prostatectomies. Both the irrigant and interval blood samples were counted for I-131 content. These patients were given KI to block out the thyroid. The method was of value in measuring the volume of fluid transferred into the vascular system.

A similar procedure was carried out by TAYLOR, MAXSON, CARTER, BETHARD and PRENTISS (1957). They used albumin-I-131 in the irrigating solution but recorded continuously the levels of radioactivity over the chest with an apparatus similar to the one used by WINTER (Fig. 1) for the radioisotope renogram. They were able to show transfer of the irrigant in this manner.

V. Aortography timing

PORPOROUS, ZINK, WILSON, BARRY, ROYCE and ROSE (1953) added di-iodo-fluorescein-I-131 to 70% urokon to tell the optimal time for aortography, by placing a scintillation counter over the femoral artery.

VI. I-131 labelled sodium acetriozoate in excretory urography

CAVE, RANKIN and MABBS (1957) used tracer amounts of Urokon-I-131 with large carrier doses of Urokon for intravenous urography. They placed geiger counters over the kidney, liver, spleen, and urinary bladder in order to find maximum conditions for excretory urography in relation to hydration.

D. Diagnostic radioautography
I. Renal autography

In 1950, west suggested the feasibility of using Thulium as a source of γ-radiation in industry, and MAYNEORD (1952) thought it applicable to human diagnostic use. So, UNTERMYER and HASTERLIK (1954) developed a portable unit for making radiographs of extremities using Thulium-170 as a source of energy. This unit was designed for field work in the United States Armed Forces. BURKE (1956), a urologist, also prepared a portable unit for use in the operating theater in order to make radiographs of the kidneys for location of elusive calculi. He showed its feasibility by studies in the cadaver, dog, and human. His unit, called the Thul-X, consisted of a seven pound, lead shield, 9 by 7 by 6 cm., with a chrome-plated aluminium cover (Fig. 16). The thulium capsule was shielded by one inch of lead at all times, except when making exposures through an aperature. At those times, the γ-rays, in the diagnostic roentgenologic range, were used to expose x-ray film held in special 4 by 5 inch cassettes with super-speed, double intensifying screens. The leaded cassette was covered with a sterile rubber glove and placed behind the mobilized kidney, while the Thul-X was covered with a sterile plastic bag and brought to within seven inches of the kidney. This unit had the advantages of low initial cost, did not require electricity, had no explosive hazard, and was completely portable. Disadvantages were: small amounts of radiation were received by the personnel involved, necessity of complete mobilization of the kidney, and thulium source must be replaced every eight to ten months, due to a half life of 129 days. Unfortunately, the unit has never been made available commercially, and therefore sufficient experience with this method is lacking.

II. The localization of sodium in the rat kidney

Krakusin and Jennings (1955) used a direct means of studying renal mechanisms in the metabolism of electrolytes. They exposed frozen dried slices of rat kidney to x-ray film following the injection of Na-22. It was possible to visualize sodium ions in various regions of the rat kidney and to correlate these findings with theories of renal function.

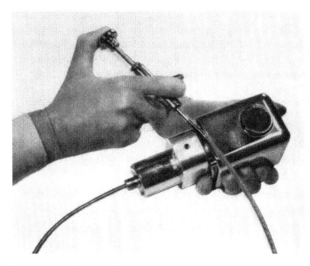

Fig. 16. The Thul-X unit is a small lead shield containing an isotope source that exposes the x-ray film when the plunger is pushed to open the aperature

III. Use of I-131 and colloidal Au-198 to study the route of urine in acute hydronephrosis in dogs

Persky et al. (1956) used I-131 and colloidal Au-198 to study the route of urine in acute hydronephrosis in dogs. They injected the isotope into the renal pelvis after ligation of the ureter. Following constant pelvic pressure for one hour, the kidneys were removed, bled, and frozen for 24 hours. Then, slices of kidney were exposed to photographic plates. After five to seven days, the radioautographs were interpreted as showing pyelotubular and pyelointerstitial backflow. These data could not be translated to the human, however.

References

Block, J. B., G. J. Hines and B. A. Burrows: The effects of carrier diodrast in excretion of I[131] Diodrast. J. Lab. clin. Med. (in Press). — Burke, D.: Isotope radiographs for localization of renal calculi during surgery: A new truly portable radiographic unit using a radioisotope (thulium-170) as an energy source. J. Urol. (Baltimore) **76**, 508—519 (1956). — Care, A. D.: Ionic migration across the mucosa of the small intestine and its significance in urology. Proc. roy. Soc. B **48**, 27 (1955). — Care, A. D., G. W. Reed and L. N. Pyrah: Changes in the reabsorption of sodium and chloride ions after uretero-colic anastomosis. Clin. Sci. **16**, 95—101 (1957). — Cave, P., J. A. Rankin and D. V. Mabes: Experiences with I-131-labelled sodium acetriozoate in excretion urography. J. Fac. Radiol. (Lond.) **8**, 252—257 (1957). — Daniel, O., F. Haddad, G. Prout and W. F. Whitmore jr.: Observations on the distribution of radioactive zinc in prostatic and other human tissues. Brit. J. Urol. **28**, 271—278 (1956). — Goodwin, W. E., and J. J. Kaufman: Renal lymphatics, II. Preliminary experiments. J. Urol. (Baltimore) **76**, 702—707 (1956). — Griffin, M., L. Dobson and J. C. Weaver: Volume of irrigating fluid transfer during transurethral prostatectomy, studied with radioisotopes. J. Urol. (Baltimore) **74**, 646—651 (1955). — GUNN, S. A., and T. C. GOULD: Difference between dorsal and lateral components of dorsolateral prostate of the rat in Zn-65 uptake. Proc. Soc..exp. Biol. (N.Y.) **92**, 70—120 (1956). — HAVEN, H. DE: Chemical interchanges in the ileal bladder. Unpublished data (Personal communication), 1957. — HUMMEL, J. P., S. A. HARRIS, H. MARBERGER and R. H. FLOCKS: Possible localization of compounds in the prostate: Distribution of diphenylphosphoramido-phenylphosphoric acid. J. Urol. (Baltimore) **76**, 637—644 (1956). — KRAKUSIN, J. S., and R. B. JENNINGS: Radio-autographic localization of Na-22 in the rat kidney. Arch. Path. (Chicago) **59**, 471—486 (1955). — MAGER, M., W. F. McNARY jr., and F. LEONETTI: The histochemical detection of zinc. J. Histochem. Cytochem. **1**, 493 (1953). — MALUF, N. S. R.: Absorption of water, urea, glucose and electrolytes through the human bladder. J. Urol. (Baltimore) **69**, 369—404 (1953). — Absorption through the human bladder. J. Urol. (Baltimore) **73**, 830—835 (1955).— MARUCCI, H. D., W. D. SHOEMAKER, A. W. WARE, H. D. STRAUSS and S. W. GEYER: Permeability of normal and artificially constructed canine urinary bladder to I-131, Na-22, and P-32. Proc. Soc. exp. Biol. (N.Y.) **87**, 569—572 (1954). — MAWSON, C. A., and M. I. FISCHER: Carbonic anhydrase and zinc in the prostate glands of the rabbit and the rat. Arch. Biochem. Biophys. **36**, 485 (1952). — The occurrence of zinc in the human prostate gland. Canad. J. med. Sci. **29/30**, 336 (1951/52). — MAYNEORD, W. V.: Radiography of the human body with radioactive isotopes. Brit. J. Radiol. **25**, 517—526 (1952). — Radiography of the human body with radioactive isotopes. Lancet **1952 I**, 276. — OESER, H., and H. BILLION: Funktionelle Strahelndiagnostik durch etikettierte Röntgenkontrastmittel. Fortschr. Röntgenstr. **76**, 431—442 (1952). — PARIS, J., E. FORD, N. LORENZ, F. R. KEATING jr. and A. ALBERT: Effect of hormones on renal clearance of radioiodine in the rat. Amer. J. Physiol. **183**, 163—166 (1955). — PERSKY, L., F. J. BONTE and G. AUSTEN jr.: Mechanisms of hydro-nephrosis: Radioautographic backflow patterns. J. Urol. (Baltimore) **75**, 190—193 (1956). — PERSKY, L., F. J. BONTE and M. A. KROHMER: Experimental external estimation of renal blood flow with radioactive iodinated albumin. J. Urol. (Baltimore) **77**, 568—570 (1957). — PORPORIS, A. A., O. C. ZINK, H. M. WILSON, C. N. BARRY, R. ROYCE and D. K. ROSE: Routine clinical experiences using urokon sodium 70% in intravenous urography. Radiology **60**, 675 (1953). — PROUT, G. R., O. DANIEL and W. F. WHITMORE jr.: The occurrence of intravenously injected radioactive zinc in the prostate and prostatic fluid of dogs. J. Urol. (Baltimore) **78**, 471—482 (1957). — PYRAH, L. N., A. D. CARE, G. W. REED and F. M. PARSONS: The migration of sodium, chloride, and potassium ions across the mucous membrane of the ileum. Brit. J. Surg. **42**, 357 (1955). — TAPLIN, G. V., O. M. MEREDITH, H. KADE and C. C. WINTER: The radioisotope renogram. J. Lab. clin. Med. **48**, 886—901 (1956). — TAYLOR, R. O., E. S. MAXSON, F. H. CARTER, W. F. BETHARD and R. J. PRENTISS: Volumetric, gravimetric and radioisotopic determination of fluid transfer in transurethral prostatectomy. J. Urol. (Baltimore) **79**, 490—499 (1958). — UNTERMYER, S., F. H. SPEDDING, A. H. DAANE, J. E. POWELL and R. HASTERLIK: Portable thulium-x-ray unit. Nucleonics **12**, 35—37 (1954). — WEST, R.: A low energy gamma ray source for radiography and thickness measurements. Nucleonics **9**, 76 (1951). — WINTER, C. C.: A clinical study of a new renal function test: the radioactive diodrast renogram. J. Urol. (Baltimore) **76**, 182—196 (1956). — Unilateral renal disease and hypertension: Use of the radioactive diodrast renogram as a screening test. J. Urol. (Baltimore) **78**, 107—116 (1957). — The absorption of diodrast-I-131 from the normal isolated human bladder. Unpublished data, 1957. — A new isotope test for vesicoureteral reflux: An external technique using radioisotopes. J. Urol. (Baltimore) **81**. 105—111 (1959). — Further experiences with the radioisotope renogram. Amer. J. Roentgenol. **82**, 862—866 (1959). — WINTER, C. C., M. MAXWELL, C. KLEEMAN and R. ROCKNEY: The radioisotope renogram as a screening test of kidney function among hypertensive individuals and comparison of the results with standard individual renal function tests and aortography. J. Urol. (Baltimore) (in press). — WINTER, C. C., and G. V. TAPLIN: A clinical comparison and analysis of radioactive diodrast, hypaque, miokon, and urokon renograms as tests of kidney function. J. Urol. (Baltimore) **79**, 573—579 (1958).

Author Index

Page numbers in *italics* refer to the references

Subject Index

Numbers in *italics* indicate the page where the subject is treated at length

REPRINT FROM

HANDBUCH DER UROLOGIE
ENCYCLOPEDIA OF UROLOGY
ENCYCLOPÉDIE D'UROLOGIE

EDITED BY

C. E. ALKEN · V. W. DIX · H. M. WEYRAUCH · E. WILDBOLZ

VOLUME V/I

SPRINGER-VERLAG / BERLIN · GÖTTINGEN · HEIDELBERG 1962
(PRINTED IN GERMANY)

ROENTGEN EXAMINATION OF THE KIDNEY
AND THE URETER

BY

OLLE OLSSON

IN COLLABORATION WITH GÖSTA JÖNSSON

WITH 258 FIGURES

REPRINT FROM

HANDBUCH DER UROLOGIE
ENCYCLOPEDIA OF UROLOGY
ENCYCLOPÉDIE D'UROLOGIE

EDITED BY

C. E. ALKEN · V. W. DIX · H. M. WEYRAUCH · E. WILDBOLZ

VOLUME V/I

SPRINGER-VERLAG / BERLIN · GÖTTINGEN · HEIDELBERG 1962
(PRINTED IN GERMANY)

ROENTGEN EXAMINATION OF THE DISTAL URINARY TRACT AND OF THE MALE GENITAL ORGANS

BY

K. LINDBLOM AND R. ROMANUS

WITH 128 FIGURES

REPRINT FROM

HANDBUCH DER UROLOGIE
ENCYCLOPEDIA OF UROLOGY
ENCYCLOPÉDIE D'UROLOGIE

EDITED BY

C. E. ALKEN · V. W. DIX · H. M. WEYRAUCH · E. WILDBOLZ

VOLUME V/I

SPRINGER-VERLAG / BERLIN · GÖTTINGEN · HEIDELBERG 1962
(PRINTED IN GERMANY)

DIAGNOSTIC RADIOACTIVE ISOTOPES IN UROLOGY

BY

RUBIN H. FLOCKS AND CHESTER C. WINTER

WITH 16 FIGURES

Handbuch der Urologie
Encyclopedia of Urology · Encyclopédie d'Urologie

Gesamtdisposition · Outline · Disposition générale

	Allgemeine Urologie	General Urology	Urologie générale
I	Geschichte der Urologie Anatomie und Embryologie	History of urology Anatomy and embryology	Histoire d'urologie Anatomie et embryologie
II	Physiologie und pathologische Physiologie	Physiology and pathological physiology	Physiologie normale et pathologique
III	Symptomatologie und Untersuchung von Blut, Harn und Genitalsekreten	Symptomatology and examination of the blood, urine and genital secretions	Symptomatologie et examens du sang, de l'urine et des sécrétions annexielles
IV	Niereninsuffizienz	Renal insufficiency	L'insuffisance rénale
V/1	Radiologische Diagnostik	Diagnostic radiology	Radiologie diagnostique
V/2	Radiotherapie	Radiotherapy	Radiothérapie
VI	Endoskopie	Endoscopy	Endoscopie

	Spezielle Urologie	Special Urology	Urologie spéciale
VII/1	Mißbildungen	Malformations	Malformations
VII/2	Verletzungen. Urologische Begutachtung	Injuries. The urologist's expert opinion	Traumatismes. L'expertise en urologie
VIII	Entleerungsstörungen	Urinary stasis	La stase
IX/1	Unspezifische Entzündungen	Non-specific inflammations	Inflammations non-spécifiques
IX/2	Spezifische Entzündungen	Specific inflammations	Inflammations spécifiques
X	Die Steinerkrankungen	Calculous disease	La lithiase urinaire
XI	Tumoren	Tumours	Les tumeurs
XII	Funktionelle Störungen	Functional disturbances	Troubles fonctionnels
XIII/1	Operative Urologie I	Operative urology I	Urologie opératoire I
XIII/2	Operative Urologie II	Operative urology II	Urologie opératoire II
XIV	Gynäkologische Urologie	Gynaecological urology	Urologie de la femme
XV	Die Urologie des Kindes	Urology in childhood	Urologie de l'enfant
XVI	Schlußbetrachtungen General-Register	Retrospect and outlook General index	Conclusions Table des matières

CPSIA information can be obtained at www.ICGtesting.com
Printed in the USA
LVOW09s1130040514

384360LV00006B/333/P